Biomedical Diagnostics and Clinical Technologies:
Applying High-Performance Cluster and Grid Computing

Manuela Pereira
University of Beira Interior, Portugal

Mário Freire
University of Beira Interior, Portugal

Medical Information Science REFERENCE

MEDICAL INFORMATION SCIENCE REFERENCE

Hershey · New York

Director of Editorial Content:	Kristin Klinger
Director of Book Publications:	Julia Mosemann
Acquisitions Editor:	Lindsay Johnston
Development Editor:	Julia Mosemann
Publishing Assistant:	Milan Vracarich, Jr.
Typesetter:	Natalie Pronio
Production Editor:	Jamie Snavely
Cover Design:	Lisa Tosheff

Published in the United States of America by
Medical Information Science Reference (an imprint of IGI Global)
701 E. Chocolate Avenue
Hershey PA 17033
Tel: 717-533-8845
Fax: 717-533-8661
E-mail: cust@igi-global.com
Web site: http://www.igi-global.com

Library of Congress Cataloging-in-Publication Data

Biomedical diagnostics and clinical technologies : applying high-performance cluster and grid computing / Manuela Pereira and Mario Freire, editors.
p. ; cm.
Includes bibliographical references and index.
Summary: "This book disseminates knowledge regarding high performance computing for medical applications and bioinformatics"--Provided by publisher.
ISBN 978-1-60566-280-0 (h/c) -- ISBN 978-1-60566-281-7 (eISBN) 1. Diagnostic imaging--Digital techniques. 2. Medical informatics. 3. Electronic data processing--Distributed processing. I. Pereira, Manuela, 1972- II. Freire, Mario Marques, 1969-
[DNLM: 1. Image Interpretation, Computer-Assisted--methods. 2. Medical Informatics Computing. W 26.5 B6151 2011]
RC78.7.D53B555 2011
616.07'54--dc22
2010016517

British Cataloguing in Publication Data
A Cataloguing in Publication record for this book is available from the British Library.

All work contributed to this book is new, previously-unpublished material. The views expressed in this book are those of the authors, but not necessarily of the publisher.

Table of Contents

Selected Readings

Detailed Table of Contents

features are then considered as random variables whose distribution may be either parametric, and then belongs to the exponential family, or non parametric and is then estimated through a Parzen window. In the proposed framework, the authors consider the optimization of divergences between such pdfs as a general tool for segmentation or tracking in medical images. The optimization is performed using a shape gradient descent through the evolution of an active region. Using shape derivative tools, the authors' effort focuses on constructing a general expression for the derivative of the energy (with respect to a domain), and on deriving the corresponding evolution speed for both parametric and non parametric pdfs. Experimental results on medical images (brain MRI, contrast echocardiography, perfusion MRI) confirm the availability of this general setting for medical structures segmentation or tracking in 2D or 3D.

Chapter 3
Modeling and Simulation of Deep Brain Stimulation in Parkinson's Disease 62
T. Heida, University of Twente, The Netherlands
R. Moroney, University of Twente, The Netherlands
E. Marani, University of Twente, The Netherlands

Deep Brain Stimulation (DBS) is effective in the Parkinsonian state, while it seems to produce rather non-selective stimulation over an unknown volume of tissue. Despite a huge amount of anatomical and physiological data regarding the structure of the basal ganglia (BG) and their connections, the computational processes performed by the basal ganglia in health and disease still remain unclear. Its hypothesized roles are discussed in this chapter as well as the changes that are observed under pathophysiological conditions. Several hypotheses exist in explaining the mechanism by which DBS provides its beneficial effects. Computational models of the BG span a range of structural levels, from low-level membrane conductance-based models of single neurons to high level system models of the complete BG circuit. A selection of models is presented in this chapter. This chapter aims at explaining how models of neurons and connected brain nuclei contribute to the understanding of DBS.

Chapter 4
High-Performance Image Reconstruction (HPIR) in Three Dimensions... 121
Olivier Bockenbach, RayConStruct GmbH, Germany
Michael Knaup, University of Erlangen-Nürnberg, Germany
Sven Steckman, University of Erlangen-Nürnberg, Germany
Marc Kachelrieß, University of Erlangen-Nürnberg, Germany

This chapter presents an overview of reconstruction algorithms applicable to medical computed tomography and high-performance 3D image reconstruction. Different families of modern HPC platforms and the optimization methods that are applicable for the different platforms are also discussed in this chapter.

Chapter 5
Compression of Surface Meshes... 163
Frédéric Payan, Université de Nice - Sophia Antipolis, France
Marc Antonini, Université de Nice - Sophia Antipolis, France

The modelling of three-dimensional (3D) objects with triangular meshes represents a major interest for medical imagery. Indeed, visualization and handling of 3D representations of biological objects (like organs for instance) is very helpful for clinical diagnosis, telemedicine applications, or clinical research in general. Today, the increasing resolution of imaging equipments leads to densely sampled triangular meshes, but the resulting data are consequently huge. This chapter presents one specific lossy compression algorithm for such meshes that could be used in medical imagery. According to several state-of-the-art techniques, this scheme is based on wavelet filtering, and an original bit allocation process that optimizes the quantization of the data. This allocation process is the core of the algorithm, because it allows the users to always get the optimal trade-off between the quality of the compressed mesh and the compression ratio, whatever the user-given bitrate. By the end of the chapter, experimental results are discussed, and compared with other approaches.

The improvement on Computer Aided Detection (CAD) systems has reached the point where it is offered extremely valuable information to the clinician, for the detection and classification of abnormalities at the earliest possible stage. This chapter covers the rapidly growing development of self-similarity models that can be applied to problems of fundamental significance, like the Breast Cancer detection through Digital Mammography. The main premise of this work was related to the fact that human tissue is characterized by a high degree of self-similarity, and that property has been found in medical images of breasts, through a qualitative appreciation of the existing self-similarity nature, by analyzing their fluctuations at different resolutions. There is no need to image pattern comparison in order to recognize the presence of cancer features. One just has to compare the self-similarity factor of the detected features that can be a new attribute for classification. In this chapter, the mostly used methods for self-similarity analysis and image segmentation are presented and explained. The self-similarity measure can be an excellent aid to evaluate cancer features, giving an indication to the radiologist diagnosis.

This chapter presents a tutorial on volumetric texture analysis. The chapter begins with different definitions of texture together with a literature review focused on the medical and biological applications of texture. A review of texture extraction techniques follows, with a special emphasis on the analysis of volumetric data and examples to visualize the techniques. By the end of the chapter, a review of advantages and disadvantages of all techniques is presented together with some important considerations regarding the classification of the measurement space.

This chapter describes an integrated view of analysis of Doppler embolic signals using high-performance computing. Fundamental issues that will constrain the analysis of embolic signals are addressed. Major diagnostic approaches to Doppler embolic signals focuses on the most significant methods and techniques used to detect and classify embolic events including the clinical relevancy are presented. The survey includes the main domains of signal representation: time, time-frequency, time-scale and displacement-frequency.

When analyzing the neuronal code, neuroscientists usually perform extra-cellular recordings of neuronal responses (spikes). Since the size of the microelectrodes used to perform these recordings is much larger than the size of the cells, responses from multiple neurons are recorded by each micro-electrode. Thus, the obtained response must be classified and evaluated, in order to identify how many neurons were recorded, and to assess which neuron generated each spike. A platform for the mass-classification of neuronal responses is proposed in this chapter, employing data-parallelism for speeding up the classification of neuronal responses. The platform is built in a modular way, supporting multiple web-interfaces, different back-end environments for parallel computing or different algorithms for spike classification. Experimental results on the proposed platform show that even for an unbalanced data set of neuronal responses the execution time was reduced of about 45%. For balanced data sets, the platform may achieve a reduction in execution time equal to the inverse of the number of back-end computational elements.

Selected Readings

Patient anatomy, biochemical response, as well as functional evaluation at organ level, are key fields that produce a significant amount of multi modal information during medical diagnosis. Visualization, processing, and storage of the acquired data sets are essential tasks in everyday medical practice. In order to perform complex processing that involves or rely on image data a robust as well versatile data structure was used as extension of the Visualization Toolkit (VTK). The proposed structure serves as

Preface

The development of medical imaging brought new challenges to nearly all of the various fields of image processing. Current solutions for image registration and pattern matching need to deal with multiple image modalities since a diagnostic of a patient may need several different kind of imagery (Ferrant 2001, Ferrant 2002, Ino 2003, Samant 2008, Warfield 1998, Warfield 2002). Image registration is also an important part of image guided surgery systems (Grimson 1996, Sugano 2001). Automated recognition and diagnosis require image segmentation, quantification and enhancement tools (BachCuadra 2004, Davatzikos 1995, Freedman 2005, Mcinerney 1996, Savelonas 2009, Wareld 1995, Wells 1996). Particularly, image segmentation and tracking are crucial to cope with the increasing amount of data encountered in medical applications and became crucial for medical image analysis and classification (Hadjiiski 1999, Park 1996, Sahiner 2001). Generation of complex visualizations, like internal organs and brain, became essential in disease diagnosis or patient care. Three-dimensional visualization has proven to be a valuable support tool, especially for the assessment of the shape and position of anatomical structures. A spatial structure is generally easy to comprehend in such view than in a series of cross sections; thus some cognitive load can be taken off the viewer. 3D image reconstruction applications can be used for reporting a diagnostic of a patient avoiding, at least in a first phase, the step to surgery or to provide cross-section slices with information about the tissues contained in the considered slices (Braumann 2005, Chen 1990, Norton 2003, Yagel 1997). In medical imagery, the resolution of 3D representations needs to be high, in order to get the maximum of geometrical details. However such detailed surfaces can be a major drawback for an efficient use of such data. They imply the archival or storage of a large quantity of similar data in a patient database and the communication of large amounts of data during clinical diagnosis or follow-up cares of patients, only to mention the most trivial implications. These facts justify the development of efficient and effective compression methods dedicated to medical imagery. Consequently biomedical diagnostic has been, and still is, greatly improved with all the advances on medical imaging.

The acquisition devices constantly advance towards providing more information in the images, improved resolutions, better repeatability and quality of the acquisitions and faster acquisition. Also the algorithms operating over those images have showed an increasing ability of extracting the information from incomplete and damaged data and incorporate prior knowledge into each acquisition. However, with the constant improvement of the medical scanners, some new challenges have been created for the image processing algorithms.

The images from those devices started to show ever improving quality, resolution and they have been acquired in shorter times. No longer was it necessary to incorporate computational power only towards tasks like denoising or improvement of incomplete data. The amount of data delivered by the medical devices started to grow so significantly that it was necessary to provide more and more computational power in order to properly analyze all the available information in reasonable times. The new interest in medical image processing towards fully 3D processing, which targets improving the information retrieval from the raw image material, also brings new challenges. Three dimensional image acquisition devices like computer tomography (CT), magnetic resonance imaging (MRI), or 3D-ultrasound (3D-US) are increasingly used to support and facilitate medical diagnosis. 3D image processing is a key technique for preoperative surgical planning and intraoperative guidance systems (DiGioia 1998, Ellis 1999, Kawasaki 2004, Kikinis 1996, Liu 2007, Ma 2003). Processing in 3D can capture more of the information in the image data, which can improve the attainable quality of the results. The large amounts of data and the complexity of the 3D methods, obviously, imply long processing times.

The quantity of information started to grow more rapidly than the modern processing units could have keep up with. This has been aligned in time with the turn in the approach for development of modern microprocessors. Until recently we have been witnessing the growing capabilities of new microprocessors in very notable and predictable manner. Their speed has been increasing constantly with the respect to Moore's law, which meant that every algorithm designed at that time would perform better if just executed on more modern processing unit. This trend has changed recently and the producers started to expand the possibilities of their microprocessors by equipping them with several cores and thus giving them the capabilities of parallel processing. Therefore, the concept of parallel processing has migrated from advanced computing centers towards any personal computer (Foster 1998). This fact, together with the growing sizes of medical data, has attracted numerous researchers towards the application of High Performance Computing (HPC) to medical imaging data. Several have been presented above, but others can be found in literature (Kawasaki 2003, Kikinis 1998, Lenkiewicz 2009, Liao 2002, Mizuno-Matsumoto 2000, Ourselin 2002, Rohlfing 2003, Thompson 1997, Warfield 2002).

The most common representatives of the HPC technology have been mainly the computer clusters. A computer cluster is a set of homogeneous computers usually connected through fast local area networks and working together with some network services. Clusters are commonly used to improve performance and/or availability in a cost-effective manner regarding a sole computer with similar computing power or availability (Barbosa 2000, Papadonikolakis 2008). Grid computing goes beyond cluster computing in the sense that nodes can be heterogeneous in terms of hardware and software can be loosely connected across subnets or domains and can be dynamic in terms of the number of nodes that can enter or leave the grid over time. There are several applications for both cluster and grid computing, including biomedical applications (Ataseven 2008, Benkner 2003, Liakos 2005, Mayer 1999). On the other hand, there is an increasing interest on the application of computing technologies to advance biomedical diagnostics and clinical technologies. Computer assisted diagnosis and therapy plays nowadays a key role to decrease young or mid-age mortality, to improve quality of live or to increase life expectancy in aging societies.

In the last three decades computer clusters have served for numerous research centers, government institutions and private enterprises. The technology was rather limited for those institutions as it was expensive and difficult to utilize. The recent progress has turned that trend, as it became relatively inexpensive to obtain a multi-processing unit platform for entities like universities and small enterprises, or virtually any household. This fact of highly increased availability has started a growth in the number of solutions created for this field, namely operating systems, management software and programming tools.

Until recently, medical image analysis has not been a traditional field of application for high performance computing. Furthermore, the amount of data produced by the different scanners has been relatively moderate. Several developments are now moving the field of medical image analysis towards the use of high performance computing techniques. Specifically, this is because of the increase of computational requirements, of the data volume and of the intensity of electronic utilization of the data. It is necessary to further validate and test the robustness of the algorithms by applying them to a larger number of cases, normally to medical databases. The huge volume of data generated by some medical and biological applications may require special processing resources, while guaranteeing privacy and security. Cluster and grid computing become crucial in dealing with huge sensitive data for special medical activities, such as diagnosis, therapy, e-health, tele-surgery, as well as specific domains, such as phylogenetics, genomics and proteomics, or studying virus evolution and molecular epidemiology.

This book explores synergies between biomedical diagnostics and clinical technologies and high-performance cluster and grid computing technologies addressing selected topics in these areas. Special attention is paid to biomedical diagnostics and clinical technologies with critical requirements in terms of processing power, namely 2D/3D medical image segmentation and reconstruction, volumetric texture analysis in biomedical imaging, modeling and simulation in medicine, computer aided diagnosis, analysis of doppler embolic signals, and massive data classification of neural responses.

ORGANIZATION OF THE BOOK

The book is organized into nine chapters focusing some of most important challenges previously presented, namely segmentation, tracking, registration, reconstruction, visualization, compression, classification, and analysis of medical imagery. They are examples on how high performance computing is applied to medical data and bioinformatics in each specific topic.

Two Selected readings were joined for additional reading to complete the book with two important topics: the co-registration and the fusion.

A brief description of each of the chapters follows:

The first chapter provides an overview about most common techniques for 2D/3D medical image segmentation. Most important features, examples of the results that they can bring and examples of application are presented. Promising recent methods are evaluated and compared based on a selection of important features. This chapter is not only an overview but also serves to show which are the directions currently taken by researchers and which of them have the potential to be successful.

The second chapter focuses on 2D/3D medical image segmentation and tracking through statistical region-based active contour models where the region descriptor is selected as the probability density function of an image feature. They focus on active contours or surfaces that are particularly well adapted to the treatment of medical structures since they provide a compact and analytical representation of object shape. Successful applications of this model are described for brain magnetic resonance imaging (MRI), contrast echocardiography, and perfusion MRI.

The third chapter explores modeling and simulation of deep brain stimulation (DBS) in Parkinson disease and intends to explain how models of neurons and connected brain nuclei contribute to the understanding of deep brain stimulation. For that purpose a selection of models capable of describing one or more of the symptoms of Parkinson's disease are presented. A discussion of how models of neurons and connected brain nuclei contribute to the understanding of DBS is presented.

The fourth chapter addresses the problem of high-performance 3D image reconstruction for medical imaging, based on anatomical knowledge, in a time-frame compatible with the workflow in hospitals. The chapter presents an overview of reconstruction algorithms applicable to medical computed tomography and high-performance 3D image reconstruction. Different families of modern HPC platforms and the optimization methods that are applicable for the different platforms are also discussed in this chapter.

The fifth chapter presents a lossy compression algorithm for triangular meshes that may be used in medical imaging. The presented scheme is based on wavelet filtering, and an original bit allocation process that optimizes the quantization of the data. Authors demonstrate that an efficient allocation process allows the achievement of good compression results for a very low computational cost but also present similar visual results when compared to a lossless coder at medium bitrates.

The sixth chapter presents self-similarity models that can be applied to Breast Cancer detection through Digital Mammography. Human tissue is characterized by a high degree of self-similarity, and that property has been found in medical images of breasts, through a qualitative appreciation of the existing self-similarity nature, by analyzing their fluctuations at different resolutions. Authors conclude that self-similarity measure can be an excellent aid to evaluate cancer features, giving an indication to the radiologist diagnosis.

The seventh chapter presents an overview on volumetric texture analysis for medical imaging. Focus was done to the most important texture analysis methodologies, those that can be used to generate a volumetric Measurement Space. The methodologies presented are: *Spatial Domain techniques, Wavelets, Co-occurrence Matrix, Frequency Filtering, Local Binary Patterns and Texture Spectra* and *The Trace Transform*. The chapter ends with a review of the advantages and disadvantages of the techniques and their current applications and present references to where the techniques have been used.

The authors conclude that texture analysis presents an attractive route to analyze medical or biological images and will play an important role in the discrimination and analysis of biomedical imaging.

The eighth chapter describes an integrated view of analysis of Doppler embolic signals using high-performance computing. Fundamental issues that will constrain the analysis of embolic signals are addressed. Major diagnostic approaches to Doppler embolic signals focuses on the most significant methods and techniques used to detect and classify embolic events including the clinical relevancy are presented. The survey includes the main domains of signal representation: time, time-frequency, time-scale and displacement-frequency.

The ninth chapter proposes and assesses experimentally a platform for the mass-classification of neuronal responses using data-parallelism for speeding up the classification of neuronal responses. Authors conclude that a significant computational speed-up can be achieved by exploiting data level parallelism for the classification of the neural response in each electrode.

The next two chapters are two Selected Readings.

The first one is devoted to the development of a framework for image and geometry co-registration by extending the functionality of the widely used Visualization Toolkit (VTK). A real application in stereotactic radiotherapy treatment planning that is based on the particular framework is presented.

The second one is devoted to biomedical image registration and fusion, in order to assist medical knowledge discovery by integrating and simultaneously representing relevant information from diverse imaging resources. An overview on fundamental knowledge and major methodologies of biomedical image registration, and major applications of image registration in biomedicine is presented.

The purpose of this book is to provide a written compilation for the dissemination of knowledge and to improve our understanding about high performance computing in biomedical applications. The book is directed for Master of Science or Doctor of Philosophy students, researchers and professionals working in the broad field of biomedical informatics. We expect that the deep analyses provided inside the book will be valuable to researchers and others professionals interested in the latest knowledge in these fields.

REFERENCES

Ataseven, Y., Akalın-Acar, Z., Acar, C., & Gençer, N. (2008). Parallel implementation of the accelerated BEM approach for EMSI of the human brain. *Medical and Biological Engineering and Computing, 46*(7), 671-679.

BachCuadra, M. (2004). Atlas-Based Segmentation of Pathological MR Brain Images Using a Model of Lesion Growth. *IEEE Transactions on Medical Imaging 23*(10), 1301- 1314.

Barbosa, J., Tavares, J., & Padilha, A. (2001). Parallel Image Processing System on a Cluster of Personal Computers. *Vector and Parallel Processing* (pp. 439-452).

Benkner, S., Dimitrov, A., Engelbrecht, G., Schmidt, R., & Terziev, N. (2003). A Service-Oriented Framework for Parallel Medical Image Reconstruction. *Computational Science,* 691-691.

Braumann, U., Kuska, J., Einenkel, J., Horn, L., Luffler, M., & Huckel, M. (2005). Three- dimensional reconstruction and quantification of cervical carcinoma invasion fronts from histological serial sections. *IEEE Transactions on Medical Imaging, 24*(10), 1286-1307.

Chen, C., Lee, S., & Cho, Z. (1990). A parallel implementation of 3d CT image reconstruction on a hypercube multiprocessor. *IEEE Transactions on Nuclear Science, 37*(3), 1333--1346.

Davatzikos, C., & Prince, J. L. (1995). An Active Contour Model for Mapping the Cortex. *IEEE Transactions on Medical Imaging,* (14), 65-80.

DiGioia, A. M., Jaramaz, B., Blackwell, M., Simon, D. A., Morgan, F., Moody, J. E., Nikou, C., Colgan, B. D., Astion, C. A., Labarca, R. S., Kischell, E., & Kanade, T. (1998). Image guided navigation system to measure intraoperatively acetabular implant alignment. *Clinical Orthopaedics and Related Research,* (355), 8-22.

Ellis, R. E., Tso, C. Y., Rudan, J. F., & Harrison, M.M. (1999). A surgical planning and guidance system for high tibial osteotomy. *Computer Aided Surgery, 4*(5), 264-274.

Ferrant, M., Nabavi, A., Macq, B., Black, P. M., Jolesz, F. A., Kikinis, R., & Warfield, S. K. (2002). Serial registration of intraoperative MR images of the brain. *Medical Image Analysis*, *6*(4), 337-359.

Ferrant, M., Nabavi, A., Macq, B., Jolesz, F. A., Kikinis, R., & Warfield, S. K. (2001). Registration of 3-D intraoperative MR images of the brain using a finite-element biomechanical model. *IEEE Transaction on Medical Imaging*, *20*(12), 1384-1397.

Foster, I. & Kesselman, C. (Ed.). (1998). *The Grid: Blueprint of a New Computing Infrastructure*. San Mateo, CA: Morgan Kaufmann Publishers.

Freedman, D., Radke, R. J., Zhang, T., Jeong, Y., Lovelock, D. M., & Chen, G. T. Y. (2005). Model-based segmentation of medical imagery by matching distributions. *IEEE Transactions on Medical Imaging, 24*(3), 281-292.

Grimson, W., Ettinger, G., White, S., Lozano-Perez, T., Wells, W., & Kikinis, R. (1996). An, Automatic Registration Method for Frameless Stereotaxy, Image Guided Surgery, and, Enhanced Reality Visualization. *IEEE Transactions On Medical Imaging,* (15), 129-140.

Hadjiiski, L., Sahiner, B., Chan, H.P., Petrick, N., & Helvie, M. (1999). Classification of malignant and benign masses based on hybrid ART2LDA approach. *IEEE transactions on medical imaging 18*(12), 1178-87.

Ino, F., Ooyama, K., Kawasaki, Y., Takeuchi, A., Mizutani, Y., Masumoto, J., Sato, Y., Sugano, N., Nishii, T., Miki, H., Yoshikawa, H., Yonenobu, K., Tamura, S., Ochi, T., & Hagihara, K. (2003). A high performance computing service over the Internet for nonrigid image registration. In *Proceedings on Computer Assisted Radiology and Surgery: 17th International Congress and Exhibition* (pp. 193-199).

Kawasaki, Y., Ino, F., Mizutani, Y, Fujimoto, N., Sasama, T., Sato, Y., Tamura, S., & Hagihara, K. (2003). A High Performance Computing System for Medical Imaging in the Remote Operating Room. *High Performance Computing* (LNCS 2913, pp. 162-173). Berlin/Heidelberg: Springer.

Kawasaki, Y., Ino, F., Mizutani, Y., Fujimoto, N., Sasama, T., Sato, Y., Sugano, N., Tamura, S., & Hagihara, K. (2004). High-Performance Computing Service Over, the Internet for Intraoperative Image Processing. *IEEE Transactions On Information Technology In Biomedicine, 8*(1), 36-46.

Kikinis, R., Shenton, M. E., Iosifescu, D. V., McCarley, R. W., Saiviroonporn, P, Hokama, H. H., Robatino, A., Metcalf, D., Wible, C. G., Portas, C. M., Donnino, R. M., & Jolesz, F. A. (1996). A Digital Brain Atlas for Surgical Planning, Model Driven Segmentation, and Teaching. *IEEE Transactions on Visualization and Computer Graphics,* (2), 232-241.

Kikinis, R., Warfield, S. K., & Westin, C. F. (1998). High Performance Computing in Medical Image Analysis at the Surgical Planning Laboratory. *High Performance Computing*, 290-297.

Lenkiewicz, P., Pereira, M. Freire, M. & Fernandes, J. (2009). A New 3D Image Segmentation Method for Parallel Architectures. In *Proceedings of 2009 IEEE International Conference on Multimedia and Expo* (ICME 2009), New York, USA, June 28 - July 3, 2009 (pp. 1813-1816). IEEE Press.

Liakos, K., Burger, A., & Baldock, R. (2005). Distributed Processing of Large BioMedical 3D Images. *High Performance Computing for Computational Science,*142-155.

Liao, H., Hata, N., Iwahara, M., Nakajima, S., Sakuma, I., & Dohi, T. (2002). High-resolution stereoscopic surgical display using parallel integral videography and multi-projector. In *Proceedings of 5th International Conference on Medical Image Computing and Computer-Assisted Intervention* (pp. 85-92).

Liu, W., Schmidt, B., Voss, G, & Muller-Wittig, W. (2007). Streaming Algorithms for Biological Sequence Alignment on GPUs. *IEEE Transactions on Parallel and Distributed Systems, 18*(9), 1270-1281.

Ma, B., & Ellis, R. E. (2003). Robust registration for computer-integrated orthopedic surgery: Laboratory validation and clinical experience. *Medical Image Analysis*, *7*(3), 237-250.

Mayer, A., & Meinzer, H. P. (1999). High performance medical image processing in client/server-environments. *Computer Methods and Programs in Biomedicine, 58*, 207-217.

Mcinerney, T., & Terzopoulos, D. (1996). Deformable Models in Medical Image Analysis: A Survey. *Medical Image Analysis,* (1), 91-108.

Mizuno-Matsumoto, Y., Date, S., Tabuchi, Y., Tamura, S., Sato, Y., Zoroofi, R. A., Shimojo, S., Kadobayashi, Y., Tatsumi, H., Nogawa, H., Shinosaki, K., Takeda, M., Inouye, T., & Miyahara, H. (2000).

Telemedicine for evaluation of brain function by a metacomputer. *IEEE Transaction on Information. Technology. Biomedicine*, *4*(2), 65-172.

Norton, A. & Rockwood, A. (2003). Enabling view-dependent progressive volume visualization on the grid. *IEEE Computer Graphics and Applications*, *23*(2), 22-31.

Ourselin S., Stefanescu R., & Pennec X. (2002). Robust registration of multimodal images: Towards real-time clinical applications. In *Proceedings of 5th International Conference Medical Image Computing and Computer-Assisted Intervention* (pp. 140-147).

Papadonikolakis, M., Kakarountas, A., & Goutis, C. (2008). Efficient high-performance implementation of JPEG-LS encoder. *Journal of Real-Time Image Processing, 3*(4), 303-310.

Park, J., Metaxas, D., Young, A. A., & Axel, L. (1996). Deformable Models with Parameter Functions for Cardiac Motion Analysis from Tagged MRI Data. *IEEE Transactions on Medical Imaging,* 437-442.

Rohlfing, T. & Maurer, C. R. (2003). Nonrigid image registration in shared memory multiprocessor environments with application to brains, breasts, and bees. *IEEE Transaction on Information. Technology in Biomedicine*, *7*(1), 16-25.

Sahiner, B., Petrick, N., Chan, H. P., Hadjiiski, L. M., Paramagul, C., Helvie, M. A., & Gurcan, M. N. (2001). Computer-aided characterization of mammographic masses: accuracy of mass segmentation and its effects on characterization. *IEEE transactions on medical imaging, 20*(12), 1275-84.

Samant, S. S., Xia, J., Muyan-Özçelik P. & Owens J. D. (2008). High performance computing for deformable image registration: Towards a new paradigm in adaptive radiotherapy. *Medical Physics, 35*(8), 3546-3553.

Savelonas, M.A., Iakovidis D. K., Legakis I., & Maroulis, D. (2009). Active Contours Guided by Echogenicity and Texture for Delineation of Thyroid Nodules in Ultrasound Images. *IEEE Transactions on Information Technology in Biomedicine, 13*(4), 519-527.

Sugano, N., Sasama, T., Sato, Y., Nakajima, Y., Nishii, T., Yonenobu, K., Tamura, S., & Ochi, T. (2001). Accuracy evaluation of surface-based registration methods in a computer navigation system for hip surgery performed through a posterolateral approach. *Computer Aided Surgery*, *6*(4), 195-203.

Thompson, P. M., MacDonald, D., Mega, M. S., Holmes, C. J., Evans, A. C., & Toga, A. W. (1997). Detection and Mapping of Abnormal Brain Structures with a Probabilistic Atlas of Cortical Surfaces. *Journal of Computer Assisted Tomography, 21*(4), 567-581.

Wareld, S., Dengler, J., Zaers, J., Guttmann, C. R., Wells, W. M., Ettinger, G. J., Hiller, J., & Kikinis, R. (1995). Automatic identication of Grey Matter Structures from MRI to Improve the Segmentation of White Matter Lesions. *Journal of Image Guided Surgery, 6*(1), 326-338.

Warfield, S. K., Jolesz, F. A., & Kikinis, R. (1998). A high performance computing approach to the registration of medical imaging data. *Parallel Computing*, *24*(9-10), 1345-1368.

Warfield, S. K., Talos, F., Tei, A., Bharatha, A., Nabavi, A., Ferrant, M., Black, P. M., Jolesz, F. A., & Kikinis, R. (2002). Real-time registration of volumetric brain MRI by biomechanical simulation of deformation during image guided surgery. *Computing and Visualization in Science, 5*(1), 3-11.

Wells, W. M.,. Grimson, W.E.L., Kikinis, R., & Jolesz, F. A. (1996). Adaptive Segmentation of MRI Data. *IEEE Transactions on Medical Imaging 15*(4), 429-442.

Yagel, R., Mueller, K., Fredrick Cornhill, J. & Mueller, K. (1997). The Weighted Distance Scheme: A Globally Optimizing Projection Ordering Method for ART. *IEEE Transactions on Medical Imaging*, (16), 223-230.

Chapter 1
Techniques for Medical Image Segmentation:
Review of the Most Popular Approaches

Przemyslaw Lenkiewicz
University of Beira Interior & Microsoft Portugal, Portugal

Manuela Pereira
University of Beira Interior, Portugal

Mário Freire
University of Beira Interior, Portugal

José Fernandes
Microsoft Portugal, Portugal

ABSTRACT

This chapter contains a survey of the most popular techniques for medical image segmentation that have been gaining attention of the researchers and medical practitioners since the early 1980s until present time. Those methods are presented in chronological order along with their most important features, examples of the results that they can bring and examples of application. They are also grouped into three generations, each of them representing a significant evolution in terms of algorithms' novelty and obtainable results compared to the previous one. This survey helps to understand what have been the main ideas standing behind respective segmentation methods and how were they limited by the available technology. In the following part of this chapter several of promising, recent methods are evaluated and compared based on a selection of important features. Together with the survey from the first section this serves to show which are the directions currently taken by researchers and which of them have the potential to be successful.

DOI: 10.4018/978-1-60566-280-0.ch001

INTRODUCTION

Digital image processing applied to the field of medicine offers numerous benefits. They include in particular improvement in the interpretation of examined data, full or nearly full automation of performed tasks, better precision and repeatability of obtained results and also possibility of exploring new imaging modalities, leading to new anatomical or functional insights. One of the most important steps involved in the process of image analysis is the segmentation procedure. This refers to partitioning an image into multiple regions and is typically used to locate and mark objects and boundaries in images. After segmentation the image represents a set of data far more suitable for further algorithmic processing and decision making, which involves tasks like locating tumors and other pathologies, measuring tissue volumes, computer-guided surgery, diagnosis and treatment planning, etc.

Over the last two decades the branch of image processing applied to medicine has evolved significantly and various publications have been presented with the goal of summarizing and evaluating this progress. Several method for assessing the quality of computer aided image segmentation (automatic or not) have been presented in (Chalana & Kim, 1997). An early work published in 1994 by Pun and Gerig (Pun, Gerig, & Ratib, 1994) has presented an outline of typical tasks involved in medical image processing, describing also common problems of such and attempts that had been taken to address them. Approaches that have been presented and discussed include the processing pipeline, image pre-processing (Lutz, Pun, & Pellegrini, 1991), filtering (Frank, Verschoor, & Boublik, 1981), early attempts of image segmentation by edge detection (Margaret, 1992; ter Haar Romeny, Florack, Koenderink, & Viergever, 1991) and region extraction (Jain & Farrokhnia, 1990; Mallat, 1989; Ohanian & Dubes, 1992), matching (Andr, Gu, ziec, & Nicholas, 1994; D. Louis Collins, Terence, Weiqian, & Alan, 1992) and recognition (Kippenhan, Barker, Pascal, Nagel, & Duara, 1992; Pun, Hochstrasser, Appel, Funk, & Villars-Augsburger, 1988). Similar work, published considerably later, has been presented in (James & Nicholas, 2000) by James and Nicholas. Authors have described accurately each step of the segmentation process, with its own difficulties and challenges and with various attempts undertaken by respective researchers to overcome them. They also elaborated on key challenges that are still to be overcame and new possible application areas for the field of computer vision. The document has been structured chronologically and researched efforts characteristic to given time period have been described. Those include in particular: era of pattern recognition and analysis of 2d images until 1984 (Alberto, 1976; Yachida, Ikeda, & Tsuji, 1980), influence of knowledge-based approaches in 1985 – 1991(Carlson & Ortendahl, 1987; Kass, Witkin, & Terzopoulos, 1988) and the development of 3D imaging and integrated analysis in later years, which incorporated more specifically: image segmentation (Chakraborty, Staib, & Duncan, 1996; Malladi, Sethian, & Vemuri, 1995; Staib & Duncan, 1996; Székely, Kelemen, Brechbühler, & Gerig, 1995), image registration, analysis of structure and morphology, analysis of function (including motion and deformation) and physics-based models. In a recent publication by Withey and Koles (Withey & Koles, 2007) the authors have presented their classification of most important medical image segmentation methods in three generations, each showing a significant level of advance comparing to its predecessor. The first generation encapsulated the earliest and lowest-level methods, including very little or none prior information. Algorithms based on image models, optimization methods, and uncertainty models composed the second generation. The third one surrounded in general the algorithms capable of incorporating knowledge.

An interesting approach for image segmentation based on deformable models is gaining a lot of interest in current research and in true medical applications, serving as a medium between low-level computer vision and high-level geometric object representation. The potency of this solution arises from their ability to segment, match, and track images of anatomic structures by exploiting constraints derived from the image data together with *a priori* knowledge about the location, size, and shape of these structures. Deformable models are capable of accommodating the often significant variability of biological structures over time and across different individuals. Furthermore, deformable models support interaction mechanisms that allow medical scientists and practitioners to bring their expertise to bear on the model-based image interpretation task when necessary. The idea was introduced by Kass and Witkin in 1988 with their work about deformable 2D contours, called "snakes" (Kass, Witkin, & Terzopoulos, 1988). Later many authors have proposed their representation models, improvements and significant changes in the original idea, some of the worth mentioning ones being the use of finite element models, subdivision curves and analytical models. Over the last years those methods have been repeatedly summarized and described in survey publications, like (McInerney & Terzopoulos, 1996), (Gibson & Mirtich, 1997) or (Meier, Lopez, Monserrat, Juan, & Alcaniz, 2005).

In (Olabarriaga & Smeulders, 2001) Olabarriaga and Smeulders have focused on the automation property in the medical image segmentation process, discussing on the level of user interaction required by various methods and presenting the progress and trends in this area. This feature is commonly considered to be very important, as one of the main incentives of applying computer image processing to medical solutions is the minimization of need for expert intervention.

In this study we would like to present and evaluate some of the most important image segmentation methods, starting with the ones presented around the year 1980 and followed with the ideas that have emerged in the last few years. Our focus will be directed towards the methods that seem promising to significantly influence the future direction of development for the medical image processing. The methods will be described and their most noteworthy features will be extracted and compared, using a relative scale to grade their effectiveness in terms of those features. This will help to understand better the current needs in this area and possibly predict which directions should be kept and which should be avoided when discussing new ideas for the evolution of medical image segmentation.

PROGRESS IN THE PREVIOUS YEARS

First Generation

Following the classification from (Withey & Koles, 2007), this group refers to the approaches presented in the early 1980s. A particular characteristic of most of the work carried out during this period was that the researchers were primarily thinking in terms of analyzing two-dimensional (2D) image datasets.

Thresholding Methods

This branch describes a group of segmentation methods based on a function that assigns individual pixels to one of two groups based on their intensity value and some predefined threshold value (see Figure 1.). Hence, as a result a binary image is given, whose one state will represent objects of one group of interests and the other state would stand for the second group. This method serves quite well for the tasks in which used images have their intensities clearly distinguished between objects of interest and the rest, usually referred to as the background. From this basic formulation a significant number of ideas has been developed and the thresholding methods have proven to deliver solutions for various medical problems.

Figure 1. Example of applying the thresholding method with three different values for the threshold. Starting from the left: original image, image segmented using low, medium and high threshold values

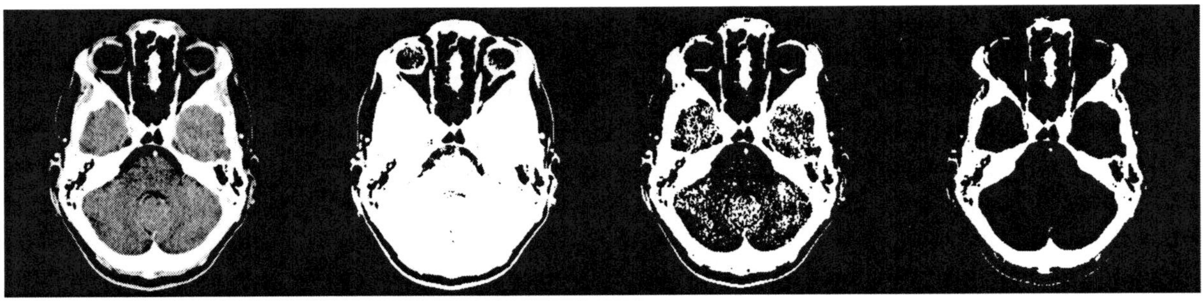

In (Mehmet & Bulent, 2004) we can find the following classification of the threshold methods:

- Methods that analyze the shape properties of the histogram to determine the optimal value for the threshold. In (Weszka & Rosenfeld, 1978) the authors present an example for this method by examining the distance from the convex hull of the histogram, using as the input data a set of infrared images, not related to medicine. In (Sezan, 1985) by Sezan we can see a method based on the analysis of "peaks and valleys" of the histogram.
- Clustering-based methods, where the gray-level samples are subjected to clustering functions with the number of clusters being set always to two. An important example for this method was presented in (Otsu, 1979) where the authors have suggested minimizing the weighted sum of within-class variances of the foreground and background pixels to establish an optimum threshold.
- Entropy-based methods are based on the concept of exploiting the entropy of the distribution of the gray levels in a scene, for example the entropy of the foreground and background regions (Kapur, Sahoo, & Wong, 1985), the cross-entropy between the original and binarized image (Li & Lee, 1993), etc.
- Methods based on attribute similarity search a measure of similarity between the gray-level and the binarized images, such as edge matching shape compactness, gray-level moments, connectivity, texture or stability of segmented objects (Hertz & Schafer, 1988; Ying, 1995).
- The spatial methods use not only gray value distribution but also dependency of pixels in a neighborhood and/or higher-order probability distribution (Kirby & Rosenfeld, 1979).
- Locally adaptive thresholding methods define the threshold value for each pixel according to the local image characteristics, like range, variance or surface-fitting parameters of the pixel neighborhood (Nakagawa & Rosenfeld, 1979).

Region Growing

Region growing segmentation is initiated with a seed location in the image, which is then enlarged gradually with adjacent pixels by checking them against a predefined homogeneity criterion. Pixels that meet the criterion are included in the region. Continuous application of this rule allows the region to grow, defining the volume of an object in the image by identification of similar, connected pixels. Ideas exploiting this method include (Hojjatoleslami & Kittler, 1998), where authors have presented an idea for region growing by pixel aggregation with interesting similarity and discontinuity measures. That method was applied to segmentation of MR images of human brain.

Second Generation

In the middle of 1980s the research subjects started to surround the area of automatic image segmentation, driven from the low level methods with the introduction of uncertainty models and optimization methods as well as a general will to avoid heuristics. Efforts have been taken to overcome the main segmentation problems but segmentation results still remained highly dependent from the input data.

Graph Partitioning

In order to perform segmentation with graph-search methods the image is modeled as a weighted unidirectional graph. The image pixels are used to form nodes of the graph and are interconnected to neighbors using the corresponding pixel associations in the image. The cost value of each interconnection is calculated using the measure of similarity between the pixels. Then, the algorithms from combinatorial optimization are used to obtain minimum-cost solutions. A graph cut is a set of interconnections between nodes in a graph which, when removed, partition the graph into two distinct sets. Fuzzy Connectedness (Udupa & Saha, 2003) and the Watershed Algorithm are examples of graph-search algorithms used in medical image segmentation.

Watershed Algorithm

The watershed transform is a popular segmentation method coming from the field of mathematical morphology. The first attempts to segment images using the watershed segmentation methods (see example in Figure 2.) have been taken in the early 1980s. The algorithm was created by Buecher and Lantuéjoul in their work (Buecher & Lantuéjoul, 1979), where they presented a possible application of watershed to micrography of fractures in steel and bubbles detection in radiography. But its popularity has risen significantly only around the year 1990, because of the work published in (Vincent & Soille, 1991b) (examples of application included segmentation of images of human vertebral column) and also due to significant improvement in computational power of machines available in those days. The idea behind the first implementations of this method can be described as follows: taking a 2D grayscale image as the input let us interpret it as if it was a hypsometric map, with the bright parts being the regions of high

Figure 2. Example of watershed segmentation applied to one-dimensional image. Left image represents the grayscale image. Right image represents the output of the segmentation algorithm: local minima define catchment basins and the local maxima define the watershed lines

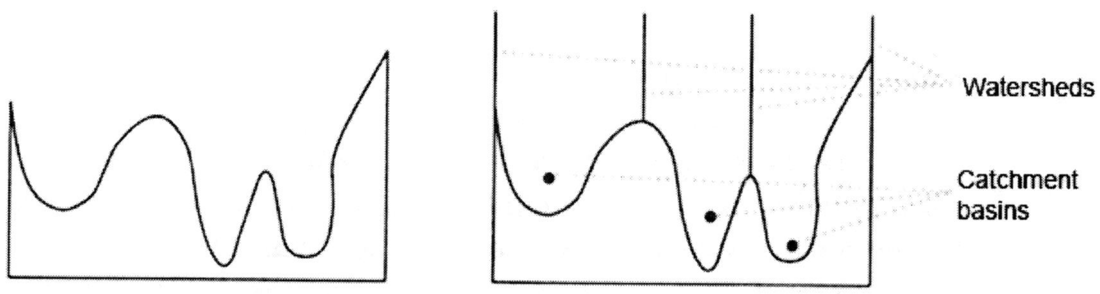

altitude (hills) and the dark parts being the regions of low altitude (valleys). If we now imagined flooding the region with water, we could observe that it gathers in the valleys and rises until it meets one or more neighboring valleys. Now, we would like to prevent the water from flooding from one valley to another, so we construct a dam of one pixel width and high enough to prevent the water from spilling at any point of the process. This process is repeated until the water "rises" until the height of the highest hills of the image. If we now consider the dams that we have constructed during the process, they will be representing the segmentation of our image data. The algorithm has been further developed to include prior knowledge incorporation (Grau, Mewes, Alcaniz, Kikinis, & Warfield, 2004) (algorithm applied to brain MR images) or operate on 3D data (Alan & Ross, 1999) (algorithm applied to household objects, not related to medicine).

Statistical Pattern Recognition (Classifiers-Based Methods)

This family of segmentation methods operates by modeling each of the given image pixels as belonging to one of a known set of classes. The decisions are taken based on a training set, which in most cases needs to be manually created as a prerequisite to the segmentation process itself, thus the classifiers-based techniques are considered as supervised. Application of the training set can be obtain with a number of approaches. The Bayesian classifiers method is among the most commonly used ones, with its functioning based on the Bayes' theorem. Many early approaches to Bayesian image segmentation have used maximum a posteriori (MAP) estimation in conjunction with Markov random fields (like the solution presented in (Thenien, 1983), used for terrain image segmentation) and some of more recent solutions included replacing the MRF model with a novel multiscale random field (MSRF) and the MAP estimator with a sequential MAP (SMAP) estimator derived from a novel estimation criteria (Bouman & Shapiro, 1994) (method applied to a variety of synthetic images). Another commonly encountered classifier is the nearest-neighbor method, where pixels or voxels of the image are grouped in the same classes as a representative of the training set with the most similar intensity. The k-nearest-neighbor (kNN) classifier generalizes this approach, classifying the pixels according to the majority vote of the closest training data.

Clustering

The functioning of clustering methods can be defined as determining the intrinsic grouping in a set of unlabeled data in an unsupervised manner. It is typically carried out by using some measure of difference between individual elements to determine which ones should be grouped into a cluster (Wang, Zheng, Wang, Ford, Makedon, & Pearlman, 2006). As it can be seen, it differs from the classifiers-based methods because it does not require a training set, which it compensates for by iterating between segmenting the image and characterizing the properties of the each class. In a sense, clustering methods train themselves using the available data.

The k-means algorithm (Coleman & Andrews, 1979) performs clustering of the input image pixels or voxels into a given number of groups, with the objective of minimal intra-cluster variance of the attributes. The process is iterative and it is started with the initial division of the input into sets, which can be done either randomly or using some heuristic data. Then, each of the data sets have its mean point (centroid) calculated and the previous step is repeated, meaning the input pixels are reassigned to the groups, which have the calculated mean point the nearest of their own feature value. These steps are usually repeated until a convergence condition is met.

In the fuzzy c-means clustering method the assignment of input pixels to the groups follows a fuzzy-logic formulation, meaning their assignment is expressed with a degree of belonging rather than being assigned completely to one cluster. The segmentation process is performed similarly to the k-means method: each pixel of the input data is assigned randomly to a group, with a random degree of belonging (alternatively, those values can be chosen with some pre-defined method). Then, the centroid for each group is calculated and used to calculate a degree of belonging for each of the pixels, for each of the clusters. The mentioned degree is defined as the inverse of the pixel's distance to the cluster. Similarly as the k-means method, the algorithm continues until convergence, usually defined as the degree of coefficients' change in single iteration. The examples of research around this method include (Wu & Yang, 2002) or (Dunn., 1973), which was applied to heart MRI images.

Neural Networks

We can describe neural networks as massively parallel computing systems constructed from a very large number of processing units of rather big level of simplicity, interconnected with each other with numerous links. The neural network models approach problems presented to them by using organizational principles, namely learning, generalization, adaptivity, fault tolerance and distributed representation, and computation. Those methods are applied in a network of weighted directed graphs in which the nodes are artificial neurons and directed edges (with weights) are connections between neuron outputs and neuron inputs. The main characteristics of neural networks are that they have the ability to learn complex nonlinear input-output relationships, use sequential training procedures, and adapt themselves to the data (Jain, Duin, & Jianchang, 2000). When trained with suitable image data, neural networks can be used for image segmentation. The basic concept of neural networks segmentation can be usually described as an attempt to simulate the human vision skill, which has the benefit of being very robust to noise and corrupted data. The segmentation task itself can be approached as either classification or clustering problems (Boskovitz & Guterman, 2002). Figure 3 presents an example of an auto associative network for finding a three-dimensional subspace.

Deformable Models

The idea of image segmentation using Deformable Models was started by Kass and Witkin in the late 1980s (Kass, Witkin, & Terzopoulos, 1988). The first implementations of that idea included a single contour that was placed in the scene of interests and then subjected to deformations in order to segment the objects present in the scene. The deformations have been constrained by the external and internal energies, which described the features of the scene and of the contour itself, respectively. The external energy was usually calculated using characteristics like image intensities,

Figure 3. Example of an auto associative network for finding a three-dimensional subspace. This network has d inputs and d outputs, where d is the given number of features (Jain, Duin, & Jianchang, 2000)

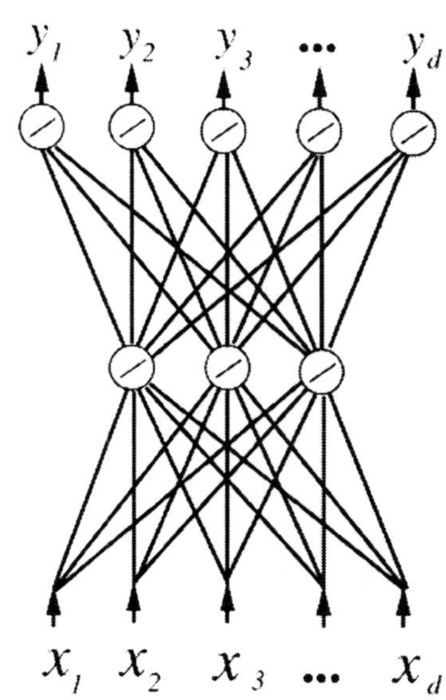

image gradient or edge detection algorithms, while the internal energy was based on the bending and shrinking/growing capabilities of the deforming shape. The publication included tests on pictures not related to medicine. This idea has caused a lot of interest in the field of image segmentation in general and in relation to medicine. An example of deformable model segmentation can be seen in Figure 4. Numerous authors started to propose their improvements and changes to the original formulation, including the geodesic active contours formulation (Caselles, Kimmel, & Sapiro, 1995) (applied to brain MRI images) or active contours for segmentation objects without strictly defined edges (Chan & Vese, 2001) (tested only on artificial images and pictures) among the most noteworthy ones. The former solution introduced a new way to represent the deformable models themselves and to avoid the need for parametric description of their shape. Instead, the authors proposed describing the model as the zero level set of a higher-dimensional function. This implicit representation solution practically eliminated the restrictions to the shape of the models described in an explicit way and allowed segmentation of complex shapes or detection of more than one object in a scene. The drawback was the increased computational demand of the method.

Solutions derived from the original method formulated by Kass in (Kass, Witkin, & Terzopoulos, 1988) used variatonal calculus to determine the solution, more specifically it usually involved solving an Euler differential equation using numerical techniques. A different approach has been presented by Amini and Tehrani in their early publication (Amini, Tehrani, & Weymouth, 1988). The authors started a discussion about some drawbacks of the analytical solution, which included instability of the evolving contour and its tendency to shrink and to distribute unevenly its discretized domain along the contour line. As a new way to approach the subject the authors proposed a solution based on dynamic programming. They argued that it could address successfully some of the mentioned disadvantages, but unfortunately it also suffered from new drawbacks. The method allowed an introduction of new type of constraints, called hard constraints, describing rules that could not be violated. It also guaranteed the numerical stability of the solution, thus addressing a serious disadvantage of the Kass method. Until then, the iterations that formed the intermediate steps of execution showed a large level of instability and for the final solution they had to be considered meaningless. In the Amini method the contour approached the final shape in a smooth manner, introducing a larger level of stability and predictability. As for the drawbacks of new solution, it introduced a big overhead in means of memory requirements and execution times. The complexity of the algorithm was at the level of $O(nm^3)$ where n is the number of points in the discretized domain of the contour and m is the size of the neighborhood of each point which is examined for more optimum position in each step. The authors have tested their methods with

Figure 4. Example of a deformable model segmentation. The left image is a CT scan of a left ventricle. The following images represent consecutive steps of the deformable model evolution (Mcinerney & Terzopoulos, 1995)

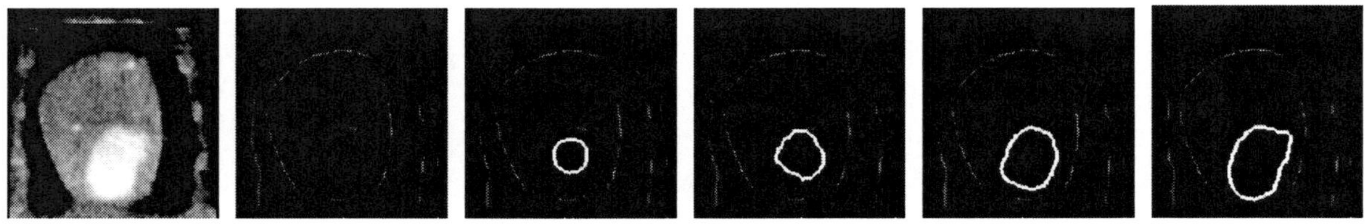

a set of images of household objects, not related to medicine.

The idea of algorithmic approach was further examined by Williams and Shah in (Williams & Shah, 1992). Instead of using dynamic programming they have proposed a greedy algorithm approach and also introduced some advances regarding the energy function estimation. A greedy algorithm delivered a significant improvement in terms of execution time and memory needs, as by the definition it considers only local information in each iteration. Each point representing the contour is placed in a number of positions and using each of these positions a new value of the total contour energy is recalculated. Then the position that corresponds to the lowest value of energy is chosen as the new position of the point. Note that this approach does not guarantee that the resulting solution will be the globally lowest one. However, authors argue that the tests of their method have proven its ability to deliver results very near to those of the dynamic programming version and the performance gain compensates those lacks. The tests have been also performed on images not related to medicine.

Authors have also analyzed the original formulation of the energy function and discussed about possible improvements. In their opinion the continuity terms have been formulated in a way which causes the contour to shrink and to become irregular, because the points tend to gather around specific locations instead of being evenly distributed along the contour. Moreover, when introducing their greedy algorithm to operate on the original formulation they discovered that the unwanted effects tend to become even stronger, because of the nature of the greedy algorithm, namely considering only local information in each iteration. This motivated them to propose a new formulation for the continuity terms, which instead of relying on difference between each two points in the contour, calculated the difference between this distance and the mean distance between all the points in the contour. This introduced a behavior of even distribution of the points and eliminated the shrinking tendency of the contour. To improve the precision of the contour on its sharp edges the authors have introduced new methods of curvature estimation (they propose five different solutions in their paper (Williams & Shah, 1992)) and used them to detect locations to which the points should be attracted. This was achieved by relaxing the second-order continuity constraint at high curvature points. The results of experiments performed by the authors have showed that in terms of execution times the greedy algorithm performs better than the dynamic programming method, reaching execution times near of those of the variational calculus, while maintaining all of the advantages of the Amini method, being stable and flexible for introducing hard constraints.

Third Generation

Atlas-Based Segmentation

Atlas-based segmentation methods applied to medical images take advantage from the similarities between matching anatomical parts of different individuals. However the variation of shapes and sizes exists, still the corresponding organs will always show a set of common features and allow their classification under a single label. This allows describing them with a set of characteristics that would allow in turn recognizing them in medical image data.

Atlas-based segmentation is usually based on a reference set of contours or volumes that roughly represent the objects of interest (see Figure 5.). This atlas data is applied to the image data and subjected to global and local transformations which lead in the end to adjustment of the initial shape to fit the objects present in the medical image data and therefore to segment the desired objects. In the global transformation stage the entire reference data from the atlas is modified using the spatial information (i.e., relative positions) of various parts of an atlas. In this step the similarity (Dawant, Hartmann, Thirion, Maes, Vandermeulen, & Demaerel, 1999) and affine (Rueckert, Lorenzo-Valdes, Chandrashekara, Sanchez-Ortiz, & Mohiaddin, 2002) transformations have been used in previous publications (applied to heart and head MR images). In the local transformations part usually we can encounter iterative optimization of the atlas objects using various types of representation to describe their shape and deformations, like the affine transformations and 2nd-order polynomial transformations published in (Cuisenaire, J.-P., Macq, Michel, de Volder, & Marques, 1996) (segmentation of MR brain images), or the B-splines and thin-plate spline constraints used in (Hyunjin, Bland, & Meyer, 2003) (segmentation of abdominal images). The data represented in the atlas can be described either in a probabilistic or non-probabilistic way. The probabilistic solution can characterize more accurately the variation between the shapes of organs of different individuals but it requires a training set. After the registration step also a classification procedure can be performed, assigning each pixel to a most probable anatomical part, enforcing the overall precision of the segmentation process. This is usually desired, as the registration procedure itself is usually not accurate enough, however some unwanted results can be imposed by the classification procedure, as sometimes in this step it is not possible to distinguish various regions of similar intensity and texture.

Authors in (Ding, Leow, & Wang, 2005) have presented an interesting solution, able in their words to segment 3D CT volume images using a single 2D atlas. Their method used an atlas containing a set of closed contours, representing various human body parts. The atlas was constructed manually, from reference CT scans. The global transformations step was performed by first constructing a target contour with straightforward contour tracing from the acquired image data. Next, the data from the atlas image was

Figure 5. Example of an atlas-based segmentation method. Images present the step of local transformations of the atlas data. The white contours on the left image present the steps of iterative transformations. The right image presents the result after convergence (Ding, Leow, & Wang, 2005). As we can see the segmentation is not complete at this point and further steps are needed to improve the final result

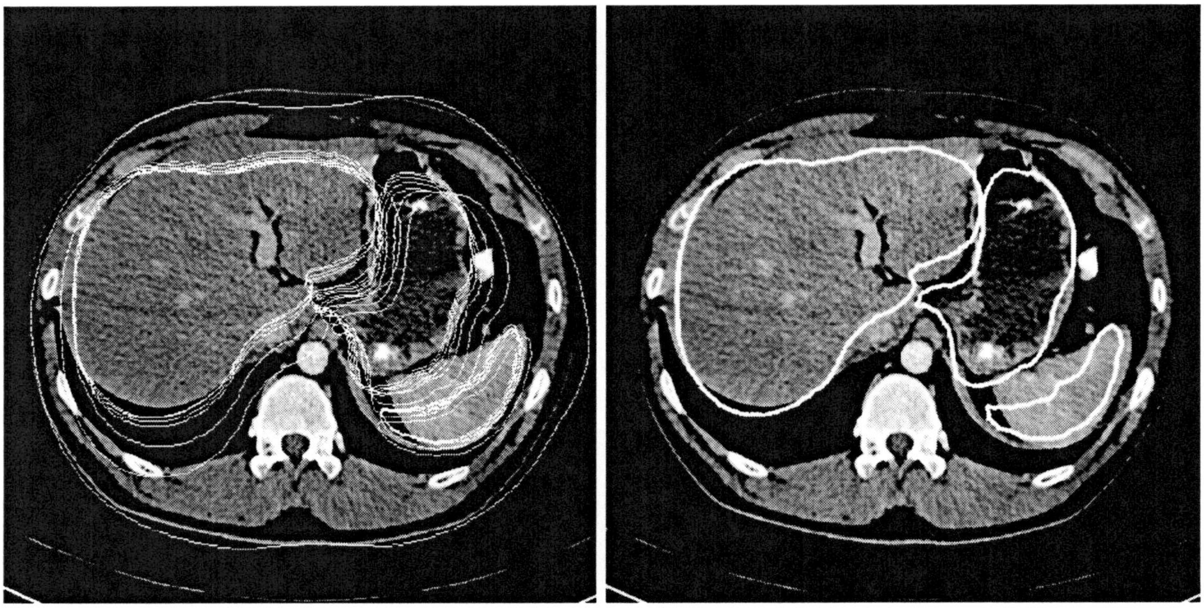

compared with the result, the correspondence between the reference and target shapes was considered and the transformation matrix was computed. Applying this matrix to the target image would transform the target shape in a way making the centers of the reference contours fall within the corresponding body parts in the target image. Then, the local transformation was performed by searching in an iterative manner the local neighborhoods of reference contour points to find possible corresponding target contour points, using features that are invariant to image intensity.

The final step was the contour refinement using the Snakes algorithm (Kass, Witkin, & Terzopoulos, 1988) enriched with Gradient Vector Flow (Chenyang & Jerry, 1997). The results of this three-step segmentation technique are promising, as the authors have stated in their paper. The accuracy of the segmentation was measured in terms of the area of intersection between the target body part (that was obtained manually) and the segmented regions. The results of particular experiments depended on the number of slices participating in the segmentation process and on the part of body that was being segmented, as these two factors can define how much the slice images differ from the reference image present in the atlas. The algorithm executed on liver was showing the similarity index on the level around 0.95 and around 0.9 for the spleen, which proves it to be successful. As for the execution times, the authors have not stated them in their document, but analyzing the construction of the algorithm we can assume with high probability that they showed rather good performance. These results are also very promising when considering the approach that the authors have taken, namely performing segmentation of 3D images with only 2D atlas information. Only single reference shape is required to perform segmentation of a large number of slice images and considering the results published by the authors, it is done with high success rate. The mechanism is constructed in a way that uses the same reference shapes for the initialization step and only differs in the deformations stage to fit to different image slices. Naturally, this means that the success rate will be smaller in those slices, which vary more from the reference images.

Shape Models and Appearance Models

A solution called the active shape model (ASM) was developed on a foundation of deformable models, extending it with a powerful mechanism of prior knowledge incorporation. It takes advantage of the fact that the medical image segmentation task often includes repeating the same processes on very similar sets of input data. For example MRI images of human brain will always show features similar to each other, not regarding the acquisition device or the individual that served as the scanned object. Those similarities will be even stronger if we will consider a single acquisition device used on a number of different individuals. This is why an important possibility to improve the outcome of the segmentation task lies in incorporation of prior knowledge about the expected features of the segmented object.

The methods based on active shape models usually describe the objects of interests by identifying a set of marker points on the edges of an object and examining the differences in their distribution between all the representatives across a set of training images (Timothy, Hill, Christopher, & Haslam, 1993). This process results with creation of a statistical representation of the given object's features, which in turn allows discovering these objects in a scene. Another important advantage is the enforcement of the deformation process, because the shape changes are restrained to the boundaries of the statistical model.

In (Staib & Duncan, 1992) by Staib and Duncan we can find a method of knowledge incorporation with an elliptic Fourier decomposition of the boundary and placing a Gaussian prior on the Fourier coefficients. Their method was tested both on synthetic and on MR cardiac images. In (Leventon, Grimson, & Faugeras, 2000) Leventon proposed incorporating shape information into the evolution process of Casselles' geodesic active contours, what they have applied to segmentation of three dimensional models of seven thoracic vertebrae. Cootes and Beeston (Cootes, Beeston, Edwards, & Taylor, 1999) in turn incorporated the prior knowledge about shape and texture for segmentation of MR brain images via deformable anatomical atlases.

Extending the active shape model with further information, namely not only about the shape of the object, but also about its intensity, the active appearance model (AAM) was created (Timothy, Gareth, & Christopher, 2001). Quite recently an interesting idea was introduced in (Yang & Duncan, 2003) by Yang and Duncan. The authors have examined a rather general feature of 2D MR brain images, namely the gray level variation. The model was based on a MAP framework using the shape-appearance joint prior information and the segmentation was formulated as a MAP estimation of the object shape. The need for finding point correspondences during the training phase was avoided by using level set representation of the shape. Figure 6 contains an example of a training set of human corpus callosum.

In (Grady & Funka-Lea, 2004) Grady and Funka-Lea have presented a semi-automatic method of medical image segmentation using Graph-Theoretic Electrical Potentials applied to CT cardiac data and MR brain images. It assumes that the input information apart from the medical imaging data would include a set of seed points, pre-defined by the user and a set of labels, describing those points. Using this information it would be possible for each unlabelled voxel of the image to estimate a certain value expressed as follows: taking current voxel in account and assuming that a random-walker algorithm would start from this location, what would be the probability that it first reaches each of the labeled seed points? This probability would be obtained with theoretical estimation, with no simulation of random walk. For each voxel of the image a vector of probabilities was then assign, including the above described likelihood for each of the existing labels. The segmentation was performed by assigning each voxel to the label with the highest possibility of encountering. The authors have tested their method on CT cardiac data and MR brain images. The results show that the rather simple assump-

Figure 6. Example of a training set of human corpus callosum outlines (left) and the three primary modes of variance corresponding to it (right) (Leventon, Grimson, & Faugeras, 2000)

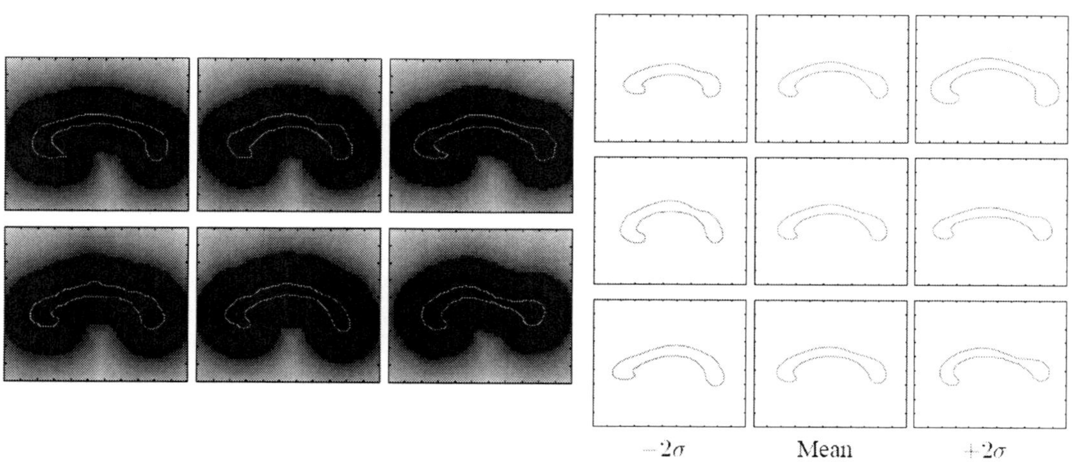

tions taken by the authors when formulating the algorithm have led to a set of very desirable features, like the ability to detect weak object boundaries and respect the medical practitioner's prelabeling choices. Also, the method proved to guarantee that the segmentation will be smooth, with no pixels left out without a classification to one of the existing labels and no discontinuities will be encountered. There was however no information about the execution times of the algorithm.

In (Shen, Shi, & Peng, 2005) Shen and Shi have suggested that the level of precision offered by standard shape models is far from desired and the problem is rooted in its formulation. Because it usually uses a training set of sample segmentations to construct the statistical model, the solution has to apply some type of averaging mechanisms to describe the set of features of our interests. This leads to loss of high-frequency information, like sharp edges and similar details. In order to improve the possibilities of shape models the authors have introduced an algorithm which uses a mean shape template to describe the general features of objects of interest and a separate parametric model to describe high level features, like intensity edges, ridges, and valleys along with information about their location. Performing some experiments on high-contrast CT images of complex organs the authors have obtained a good segmentation, matching in high level the reference samples provided by a human expert. Examples of complex structures in the human spinal column can be seen in Figure 7.

MOST RECENTLY PROPOSED SOLUTIONS

Marker-Based and Knowledge-Based Watershed

The simplicity of the watershed algorithm has been one of its main advantages, as it allowed performing a relatively successful segmentation without the need of any parameters, prior knowledge or user interaction. However, with the growth of demand for precise segmentation the drawbacks of this approach have started to be more noticeable. Since the segmentation process depended strictly on the image data any flaws in those would have to be automatically imposed on the segmentation results, thus the high sensitivity

Figure 7. Examples of complex structures in the human spinal column (top row) and segmentation results obtained by Shen and Shi using separate parametric model to describe high level features (Shen, Shi, & Peng, 2005)

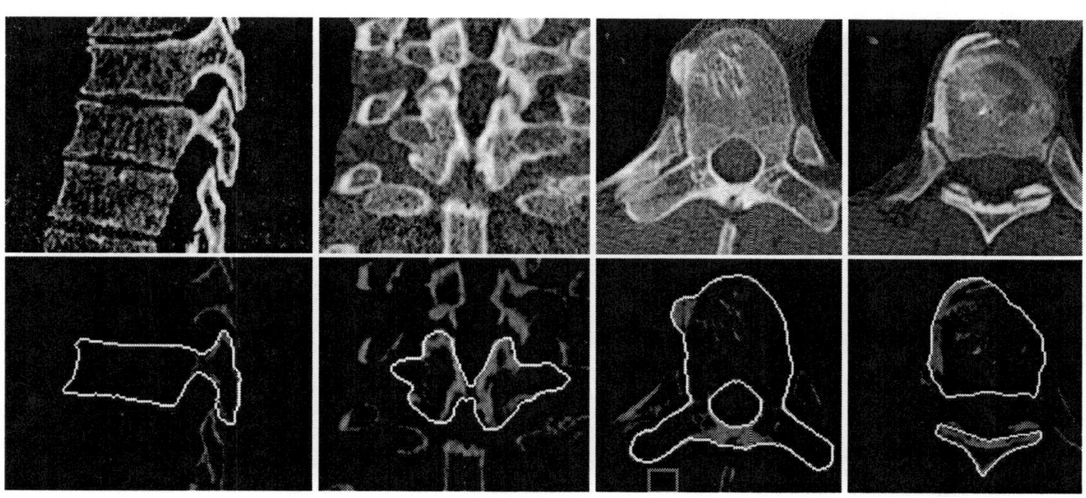

to noise and incomplete image data. Also, the very high tendency for over-segmentation was often criticized. As said before, introducing some level of prior knowledge into the segmentation process can help counter these limits and increase the accuracy of the results.

One of the first successful mechanisms to incorporate knowledge in the Watershed Algorithm was the introduction of markers, resulting in the Marker-Based Watershed. This general name refers to an approach where the user provides information about the desired number and possibly location of regions in the segmented image by placing some markers in the scene (Jean-Francois, Serge, & Delhomme, 1992; Vincent & Soille, 1991a). Further extending the algorithm with spatial prior knowledge resulted with Knowledge-Based Watershed algorithm (Beare, 2006) which introduced a way to constrain the growing of the markers through the use of structuring element-based distance functions. Thanks to these improvements the mentioned methods managed to deal with noisy or incomplete object boundaries. In a recent publication (Lefèvre, 2007) Lefèvre has introduced a new formulation for the marker introduction based on a feature calculation and pixel classification. Their method has s performed well, segmenting color images of size 481×321 pixels in about 15 seconds, with significant improvement in the quality of obtained segmentation comparing to the traditional methods. The tests however are rather poor in their nature, as they have been performed with images not related to medicine, using a portable computer.

Two Stage Methods (Based on a Coarse Approximation and Refinement)

Ardon and Cohen have proposed their segmentation method in (Ardon, Cohen, & Yezzi, 2005) and then further described it and extended it in (Ardon & Cohen, 2006) and (Ardon, Cohen, & Yezzi, 2007). The method is based on minimal paths algorithm used together with 3D deformable models and it targets in improving the performance and segmentation precision of the method.

Following the assumptions of the authors, the method requires some user interaction in the first stage of the process. For each sequence of slice images it is necessary to manually segmented two of them, so the interaction of an expert is required for each case of segmentation. As a simple example the authors have presented in their document a 3D shape of a vase, which was described with two curves – one on the top and one on the bottom (see Figure 8). The possibilities are however wider, for example the two slices can be perpendicular to each other, usually delivering more information about the object to segment and introducing the chance to segment more complex objects. Those two manually segmented slices will deliver then the information to construct the constraining curves for the object to segment. Between those curves a network of paths will be created using gradient descent technique. Those paths will be following the object of the segmentation. To create them the constraining curves are discretized to a finite number of points and for each point in curve c_1 a minimal path between itself and another point in curve c_2 is found. Those paths are minimal with the respect to a potential that takes small values on the object's boundaries(Ardon & Cohen, 2006). The main idea is to produce a path that maintains a balance between reducing its own length and following the points of low values of the cost function (so in fact – following the shape of the object in question). When the search for minimal paths is finished they are then used to construct a surface through interpolation of the network.

As it is possible to see, the above described method assumes a high level of simplification and approximation of the surface in question. It results in good performance and low execution times, but has to result in drawbacks in terms of poor segmentation precision. That is why the authors propose next to adjust the segmentation with the application of level set method. In fact,

Figure 8. Example of application of the 3D Minimal Paths algorithm to an artificial shape. Image on the left shows the original shape with two constraint curves. The middle image shows intersecting slice images, which deliver the information for the minimal paths. Image on the right presents obtained shape approximation (Ardon, Cohen, & Yezzi, 2007)

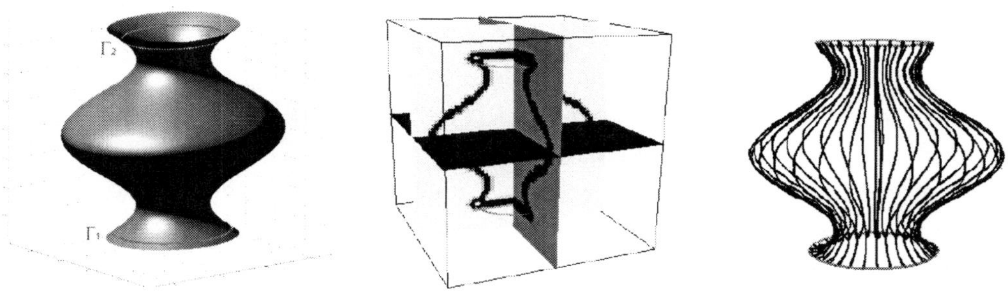

the minimal paths method can be simply perceived as the solution to the initialization problem for deformable models. With its application the resulting model, which will be subjected to the level set method, is already a very near approximation to the final shape. This can improve very significantly both the execution times and the precision of the results comparing to the original idea, which assumed commencing the deformation process from a basic shape, like a sphere or a cylinder. Authors show in their experimental results that in fact both this goals have been obtained – they managed to minimize significantly the number of iterations that were necessary to obtain a stable state of the model and they minimized the chance of obtaining a local minima error, because the model is always initialized very near to its final position. They also managed to successfully segment some scenarios that have failed when subjected to segmentation with a cylinder as the initial shape. This included for example a complex shape consisting of three s-shaped tube objects placed one inside another. The initialization with a single cylinder shape resulted in wrong segmentation, although the level set formulation is capable of topology changes and it detected more than one object in the scene. The result was still quite far from the desired after 150 and after 500 iterations, whereas using the 3D minimal paths solution for the initialization the authors obtained a precise segmentation only after a few iterations of the level set model. Another example of application presented by the authors was segmentation of the left ventricle from the 3D ultrasound images.

The advantages of this initialization method over traditional initialization can be clearly visible. Its main drawback is probably the need to perform two manual segmentations for each scenario. This could be solved by using a 2D automated segmentation method on given slices, thus leading to a complete or near complete automation of the process. 2D segmentation algorithms have received significant interest in the last years and their effectiveness has been severely improved, so it is probable that they would perform well in this situation. However the authors have not suggested or tested that solution in their publications.

Parallel Genetic Algorithm Refinement Method

Work presented in (Fan, Jiang, & David, 2002) by Fan and Jiang introduces a two-stage approach for the segmentation problem, including steps of a quick approximation and then shape refinement with more precise method. As we can see, this is similar to the 3D Minimal Paths approach presented by Ardon and Cohen, although only the general concept is analogous. The quick approximation method involves a using a dynamic equation based on finite differences method. The formulation of the model's energy is enriched with a temporal parameter and thus reconstructed into an evolution equation, in which an estimated surface is used as initial data. Solving that equation results in a fast but coarse descriptor of the object in question. A series of those is then used to generate an initial population to the next step, which is namely surface refinement using a parallel genetic algorithm. Again, we can see a similarity with the idea introduced in (Ibáñez, Barreira, Santos, & Penedo, 2006), although the genetic algorithm is formulated in a slightly different way. Authors have used an idea of a parallel genetic algorithm presented in (MÜHLENBEIN, SCHOMISCH, & BORN, 1991), which is a relatively recent addition to the evolutionary algorithms family. It has however proven to be a strong optimizer, capable of delivering results superior to the traditional genetic algorithm. Broadly speaking its main new feature is the fact that several populations are evolving in an independent manner and migration operator is defined to assure the exchange of information between those populations. The usual scenario assumes that the healthiest individuals are chosen to be transferred to neighboring population and likewise the healthiest are received to replace the worst ones. Experimental results since the introduction of this concept have shown promising abilities of this formulation.

Authors have tested their solution on brain images obtained from the Brainweb project (D. L. Collins, Zijdenbos, Kollokian, Sled, Kabani, Holmes, & Evans, 1998). The implementation was performed in C++ on a 5-PC computer cluster. It is not stated clearly what were the sizes of image used in the research and what exactly were the execution times, but authors state in the conclusions part that the search space was significantly decreased thanks to the two-step approach and that the obtained results show high robustness and steadiness thanks to the parallel genetic algorithm – thus the objectives that authors have set for themselves have been met. This means that the introduced approach has performed in an expectable way.

Hybrid Methods

Numerous solutions proposed by different authors have been based on attempts to combine the possibilities of region-based and boundary-based methods. Those are generally referred to as the hybrid methods and they usually consist of a model formulation to represent the shape and the features of the object in question and of a set of characteristics that have in object to improve the segmentation process (Metaxas & Ting, 2004; O'Donnell, Dubuisson-Jolly, & Gupta, 1998; Rui, Pavlovic, & Metaxas, 2006; Tsechpenakis, Wang, Mayer, & Metaxas, 2007). This is however a generalization, as the attempts to combine the advantages of several segmentation methods have been taken frequently and with many various approaches.

Metaxas and Chen in (Metaxas & Ting, 2004) have pointed out that the integration of region-based and boundary-based methods is usually difficult because the region-based methods developed at that time offered very limited possibility to incorporate the information provided by the boundary-based methods. With their research started in (Chen & Metaxas, 2000) and continued in (Metaxas & Ting, 2004) and (Chen & Metaxas, 2003) they tried to address this issue using the following scheme: a Gibbs Prior Model was prepared from the MR brain image data and default parameters, serving as a base boundary information. Next a 3d mesh was constructed from a series of those 2d masks, using the marching cubes method. Finally, the structure of the 3d mesh was "sculptured" more precisely using the Deformable Models and this final model is used to estimate the parameters for the Gibbs Prior Model, which would replace the default parameters used in the first iteration. This method used a combination of 3D and 2D data to construct its outcome, which could impose some level of inaccuracy because of frequent transitions between two and three dimensional scope. In (Rui, Pavlovic, & Metaxas, 2006) Rui and Metaxas have suggested a new method with a similar idea and the same input medical image data, but using a fully 3D definition of the Deformable Models, which resulted in a much more robust smooth surface segmentation.

Yifei and Shuang in (Yifei, Shuang, Ge, & Daling, 2007) have proposed a solution created from a combination of the morphological watershed transform and fuzzy c-means classifiers. Thus, like most common hybrid solutions, the proposed method integrates the edge-based and region-based techniques. The advantages of the watershed technique applied to medical image segmentation are its simplicity and intuitiveness. It can be also parallelized easily and it always produces a complete segmentation of the image. It is however rather sensitive to noise, it has problems with successful detecting of thin objects and the delivered results are often over-segmented. On the other hand, the FCM algorithm classifies the image by grouping similar data points in feature spaces into clusters. This unsupervised technique that has been successfully applied to feature analysis, clustering, and classifier designs in the fields such as astronomy, geology, medical imaging, target recognition, and image segmentation. Its disadvantage is the fact that it does not deal with the problem of intensity inhomogeneity. The algorithm proposed by the authors operates in three steps. First, the original image is subjected to dilation-erosion contrast enhancement. This allows obtaining well defined object borders, which can help greatly to improve the outcome of the watershed algorithm. Next, the watershed algorithm with internal and external markers is applied. The result returned by it is then subjected to a stage called 'post-processing' by the authors, namely applying a 4-connectness pattern, which helps to get rid of some misleading boundaries. At this point the image represents a set of regions, which are subjected to fuzzy c-means clustering, in order to connect them and eliminate the over-segmentation effect of the watershed transform. The authors have tested their implementation over 80 lung images and compared the results to the ones obtained by the watershed and the c-means algorithms, used apart from each other. The segmentation obtained with the hybrid algorithm has shown a much better level of similarity to the manually performed reference segmentation. There was however no information about the possible overhead in execution times.

Another recent publication presented a slightly different approach to the concept of hybrid methods. The authors in (Hua & Yezzi, 2005) have introduced a two step method of medical image segmentation, which they have applied to MR brain images. In the first step a coarse approximation of the shape would be done using the fast sweeping evolution method based on the image gradient information and the result of this initial segmentation would be enlarged to a local region zone using morphological dilation. In the second step a dual front evolution model would be used to achieve the final boundary.

Implicit and Explicit Deformable Models Representation

As mentioned in the previous chapter, the idea of Deformable Models has been well received amongst the researchers and various ideas about possible improvements have been suggested. One of the most significant subjects has been the discussion about the way in which they are represented. The mechanisms used to describe the segmented shape always influence in big part the segmentation process, as they are responsible (fully or in some part) for features like the ability to perform topological changes, the speed of deformations, the flexibility of the object and some others. In the original formulation of Snakes (Kass, Witkin, & Terzopoulos, 1988) and in other publications (Terzopoulos, Witkin, & Kass, 1988) the parametric representation was introduced, which assumed describing the curve with a set of points, holding information about their coordinates. It was a simple and effective approach but in some solutions the offered possibilities have been not sufficient and representing a shape with a high level of detail required using a big number of points, which was not effective. Different explicit approaches to deformable models representation include the methods based on a B-spline (Precioso & Barlaud, 2002), which allowed describing even shapes of high complexity in a precise and smooth manner and with a limited number of points. That method has been applied to complex scenes segmentation, such as live images from video cameras. A very important effort to improve the possibilities of shape representation has been taken by Caselles and Kimmel in (Caselles, Kimmel, & Sapiro, 1995) by introducing the Geodesic Active Contours. This solution was based on an implicit deformable models representation, namely the levelsets. The implicit representation was later adapted in a number of successor works (Cohen & Kimmel, 1996; Marc, Bernhard, Martin, & Carlo, 2001) and became an important milestone in improving the possibilities offered by the Deformable Models. The features offered by the implicit and explicit representations have been summarized and compared in a number of publications (Gilles, Laure Blanc, & raud, 1999; Montagnat & Delingette, 2000) and in recent publication by Lingrand Montagnat (Lingrand & Montagnat, 2005) a comparative study of implicit and explicit deformable model based methods was performed using authors' own implementations and concrete examples of data, illustrating the differences between the two approaches.

The Active Nets

In contrast to active models based on contour evolution in (Tsumiyama, Sakaue, & Yamamoto, 1989) Tsumiyama and Sakaue have proposed a solution that used active nets. This idea was then further researched and developed by Ansia and Lopez in (Ansia, Lopez, Penedo, & Mosquera, 2000). This solution assumed that instead of evolving a contour the image would be covered with a discrete mesh. The nodes of this mesh would be incorporating the whole image and each node would have the ability to move in a predefined neighborhood, thus evolving the shape of the whole mesh. Based on the boundary information all nodes would be classified into two categories, internal and external. The former ones model the inner topology of the object while the latter perform more similarly to the active contours, trying to fit to the edges of the object in the image. This solution had the goal of combining together the features of region-based and boundary-based segmentation techniques. It managed to give an answer to some fundamental issues of deformable models, like the initialization problem and the ability to change shape topology. The latter feature rose possibilities to segment more than one object in the scene and to detect holes and discontinuities in object bodies. Similarly to the original formulation, the model deformation was controlled by an energy function, which was defined in a way to acquire minimum values when the mesh was placed over the objects of interests. The internal energy depended on first and second order derivatives of the energy function, which controlled contraction and bending features respectively and they were estimated using the finite differences technique. The external energy was described as representation of the features of the scene that guided the deformation process. As a broad outline, in the original formulation the adjustment process consisted of minimizing those functions with a greedy algorithm. The energy of each point of the grid was computed in its current position and its nearest neighborhood; the position with the lowest energy was then chosen as the new position of the point. When no point could be moved to a more optimal position in its nearest neighborhood the algorithm was stopped. As it can be seen using a greedy algorithm to solve the optimum finding problem introduces the risk of stopping at a local minimum instead of the global one. This issue was further examined in (Ibáñez, Barreira, Santos, & Penedo, 2006) by Ibáñez and Barreira and new optimization techniques were introduced, namely a genetic algorithm. Authors have used a standard approach for genetic algorithms presented in (Goldberg, 1989), introducing their own solutions for crossover, mutation, spread and group mutation operators. They also enriched the original energy function with a new term for external energy calculation. It took into consideration the distance of the node from the nearest edge of the object in image. Running experimental segmentations the authors have decided to perform them in a very precise way, using large population sizes, thus the resulting execution times have shown to be very large comparing to the greedy algorithm version. Authors have however obtained a very significant improvement in terms of reliability of their method. It managed to successfully segment objects in scenes (using images of artificial shapes) with which the greedy algorithm has failed completely due to bad initialization, bad parameters for the energy function or to highly noisy images.

Topological Active Volumes

Topological active volumes model was proposed in (Barreira, Penedo, Mariño, & Ansia, 2003) by Barreira and Penedo as an extension of the active nets model into 3D world, applying it to the task of segmenting CT slices of the femur. The authors have again emphasized the valuable features of active nets that solve some inherent problems of deformable models, namely the insensitivity to bad initialization and integration of region and boundary information in the adjustment process. Also the ability to perform topological changes was considered as a valuable feature, allowing the TAVs to detect two or more objects in the scene, model holes and discontinuities in the objects and also adjust themselves to the areas where greater definition is required. With these characteristics the topological active volumes have been a promising solution for the 3-dimensional segmentation. Figure 9 shows an example of an artificial shape segmentation using the Topological Active Volumes.

A topological active volume (TAV) has been defined as a 3D structure composed by interrelated nodes where the basic repeated structure is a cube (Barreira, Penedo, Mariño, & Ansia, 2003). Similarly to the topological active nets, the deformation process was governed by an energy function, with internal and external energies responsible for characteristics of the model and of the scene, respectively. The internal energy estimation has been performed using the finite differences technique in 3D. Also the external energy definition did not change comparing to the topological active nets formulation and also the structure in question was described with internal and external nodes.

The authors have performed their method tests also on artificial noisy images. The behavior of the model was organized as follows: covering the entire 3D structure with the volume; detecting the number of objects of interest; adjustment and description of the objects with energy minimization using local information. In contrast to the active nets model, here each node of the mesh was tested in 26 of its neighbor locations for optimal energy as a natural consequence of operating in a 3D environment. Once the mesh had reached a stable situation, the process of readjustment of the mesh began, the connection breaking was performed and the minimization was repeated. Authors state that the model is fully automatic but on the other hand they formulated its cost function to be dependable from six different parameters, so actually some level user interaction is required. The results

Figure 9. Example of an artificial shape segmentation using the Topological Active Volumes without and with the topology change ability (left and right, respectively) (Barreira, Penedo, Mariño, & Ansia, 2003)

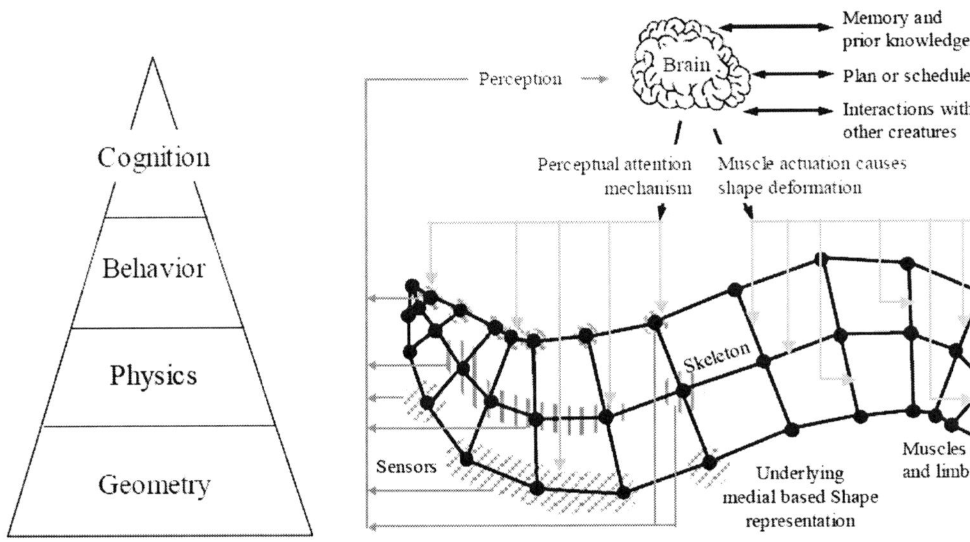

obtained for images with the size of 256x256x80 included about 20 minutes of segmentation time. If we compare it to the results obtained with active nets in (Ibáñez, Barreira, Santos, & Penedo, 2006) we could see that the execution time is significantly larger. The results obtained with active nest using a greedy algorithm, which was also used with active volumes, have varied from 5 seconds to 60 seconds. It is difficult to compare the complexity of the images used in both cases, because in (Ibáñez, Barreira, Santos, & Penedo, 2006) the authors only refer to the images that they have used as simple ones (giving about 5 seconds execution times) and complex ones (giving 30-60 seconds execution times).

As we can see, with the introduction of 3D images we can see a greatly worsened performance. This has source at the fact that not only we need to process significantly larger datasets, but also we have to operate in a 3D environment and perceive the scene as a volume, not a flat image. The result of this can be seen starting with the fact that no longer we operated on 8-pixel environment for each node of the mesh, but 26-pixel one. Also the estimation of the energy of the model becomes more complex, as we need to consider a significantly larger model, with more nodes and more values to calculate. If we take a look at the results obtained in (Ibáñez, Barreira, Santos, & Penedo, 2006) using genetic algorithm, we could predict that probably porting that solution into 3D would result in even larger execution times. Authors have however agreed that future work with their method should include experimenting with more advanced optimization techniques, which should help to shorten the execution times.

Deformable Organisms

As it can be seen in(McInerney & Terzopoulos, 1996)-(Meier, Lopez, Monserrat, Juan, & Alcaniz, 2005) the problem of prior knowledge usability has been addressed in numerous publications. It has been proven that using information about certain features that are common to a group of objects of interest and are know before the segmentation process, can give a broad view over the problem and help in deciding which encountered characteristics are desirable and which are not. This can significantly improve the robustness and

Figure 10. Left: the ALife modeling pyramid (adapted from (Demetri, Xiaoyuan, & Radek, 1994)). Right: a deformable organism model. The brain issues 'muscle' actuation and perceptual attention commands. The organism deforms and senses image features, whose characteristics are conveyed to its brain. The brain makes decisions based on sensory input, memorized information and prior knowledge, and a pre-stored plan, which may involve interaction with other organisms (Hamarneh, McInerney, & Terzopoulos, 2001)

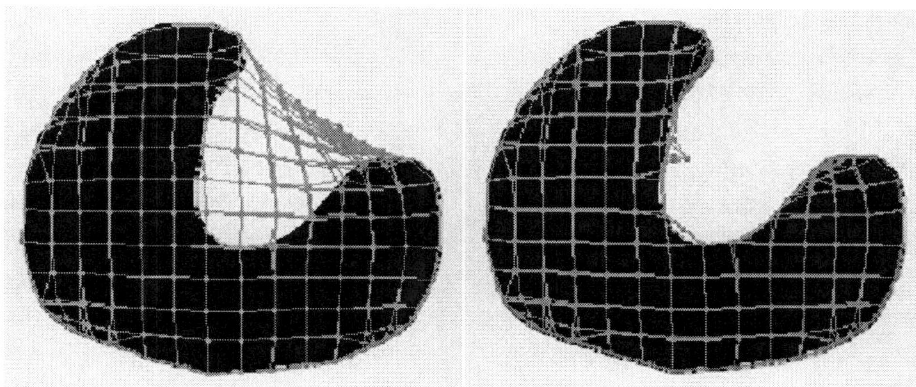

precision of the segmentation process, making it less vulnerable to corrupted or incomplete input data. Typical solutions for prior image incorporation include calculating vectors of characteristics or formulating statistical models describing the features of interest (Montagnat & Delingette, 2000),(Fritscher & Schubert, 2006).

In (Hamarneh, McInerney, & Terzopoulos, 2001) Hamarneh and McInerney have proposed a different perception of how the deformable models can be influenced to behave in a desired way and to take advantage of the prior information about the structures of interest. They have constructed the Deformable Organisms model, which combined the classical approach to deformable models with a decision making mechanism based on the solution of same authors called the Artificial Life (Demetri, 1999) (see Figure 10). The idea was to significantly improve the automation of the segmentation by eliminating the need for human supervision over the whole process.

The model that they proposed was a layer-based architecture, where the higher-level layers had the knowledge about the state and control over the low-level parts. This means that each layer was responsible for some primitive functions, which could be managed by the layer above it. This relation has been repeated recursively over the following layers, resulting in a well-defined and manageable hierarchy between them. At the base of this model authors used a geometric modeling layer to represent the morphology and appearance of the organisms. Following, the physical modeling layer incorporated some principles of biomechanics to control the geometry and simulate biological tissues. Next, the motor control layer, which was responsible for internal muscle actuators in order to synthesize lifelike locomotion. The following layer controlled the behavioral and perceptual capabilities, to provide reactions to environment conditions and other organisms. At the top of the scheme we could find the cognitive layer, responsible for simulating the deliberative behavior, ensuring that the organism is aware about itself and other organisms in the environment, how it acquires and responds to knowledge and how its reasoning and planning processes can help to reach its destination (Hamarneh, McInerney, & Terzopoulos, 2001).

As we can see, the model was defined as far more complex, than in case of traditional deformable models. Comparing these two approaches we can see that the traditional model included only the definition of the geometric and physical modeling layers. In more complex solutions we can see also the introduction of prior knowledge, which can successfully constrain the shape during segmentation process, to better correspond to the actual objects. However, this solution still lacks the awareness ability, meaning the deformable models do not have the knowledge about their position in the scene and also their actions are always guided by local decision making. This means that the decisions cannot be seen as parts of a global intelligence but only as simple choices that do not directly affect the following decisions or the decisions of other models in the scene.

Organisms created by the authors in their study have been called the deformable worms. As the name suggests, they have been imitating simple bodies, described by four medial profiles. Those profiles described respectively: the length, the orientation, the left thickness and the right thickness of the body. Using this features the authors described a way of controlling their shape using the multilevel scheme described above, defining for example the following operators: for the basic geometric representation–bending and stretching; for the motor system–moving a bulge on the boundary, smoothing the boundary, stretching/bending at certain locations; for the perception system–sensing image intensity, image gradient, edge detecting; for the behavioral system–finding specific regions of other organism's body, latching to specific parts of other organisms, thickening right or left side of the body.

Authors have released the deformable worm into a 2D MRI brain image and argued that it progressed successfully to achieve its goal. They present images of the segmented structures and point out that the precision is very satisfying and their framework performed just like it should. Unfortunately, they do not present any execution times, so it is unknown how effective this method is in terms of execution times.

Recent references to this idea include (C. McIntosh & G. Hamarneh, 2006) and (Chris McIntosh & Ghassan Hamarneh, 2006) by McIntosh and Hamarneh. In those publications the authors have introduced artificial life forms called vessel crawlers and spinal crawlers, respectively. Those deformable organisms have been constructed for the purposes of segmentation particular human organism parts, meaning the vasculature system and the spinal column. They were built upon a 4-layer based system for artificial life representation, including the geometrical, physical, behavioral and cognitive levels. Both those solutions have been constructed in a way to incorporate information about the body parts of their interests, namely the geometrical properties of the tubular structures (for the vessel crawlers) and the human spinal cord (for the spinal crawlers). The results produced by those methods has shown that thanks to their high configuration capabilities it is possible to define their behavior in a very precise manner and obtain very promising results in situations where segmentation is a complex procedure (spinal column and vasculature system both fall into this category) (see Figure 11 for results). The spinal column segmentation has been compared to a level-set method and has proven to be more effective, resulting in 10 minutes execution times for a 256x256x60 MRI volume with a very low level of user interaction. The same volume required 30 minutes and a significant level of user interaction using the level-set method. As for the vasculature system segmentation, the authors have focused on presenting the capabilities of their solution to operate with such a complex, branching structure. Comparing to other solutions, the vessel crawlers have presented a great improvement in terms of proper object detection and the precision of results.

EVALUATION OF SELECTED METHODS

Selection of Features

The methods described in section 3 have been characterized using a set of features described below. Those have been selected in a way to allow proper definition and evaluation of the most important characteristics of a given method, which in turn would allow an evaluation of the whole method and provide some level of comparison between different methods.

This selection of features has been performed considering the most common way in which the respective authors describe their algorithms in existing publications. Usually a description of this kind involves a set of experiments and a presentation of the results with careful examination and explanation of the outcome. Observing those we could notice that the features that guarantee the best evaluation are composed from similar to the below presented selection:

- **Sensitivity to parameters:** this describes the reliance of segmentation result from a good selection of parametric values for the algorithm. Those values typically describe the deformable features of the model, like stretching and bending capabilities, its behavior under specific circumstances, etc. High dependability from the parametric values, as well as big number of values to define, are undesirable, as this introduces the need for high level of user interaction.
- **Sensitivity to initialization:** describes the reliance of the result from a good choice of initial shape for the model. Usually the initial stage is assumed to be significantly far from the final, desired shape, being for example a primitive shape, like a circle or cylinder. Ability to perform successful segmentation using such simple initial shape is desirable, because it eliminates the need to perform manual initialization.
- **Sensitivity to noise:** describes the ability of the method to operate on noisy data (ro-

Figure 11. Results of a complex shape segmentation using the vessel crawlers (C. McIntosh & G. Hamarneh, 2006)

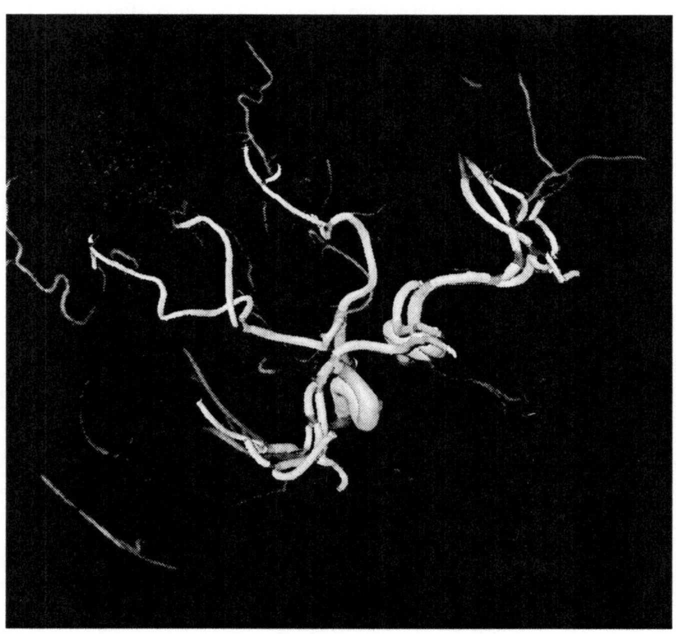

bustness of the method). High sensitivity to noise is not desirable.

- **Topology changes:** describes the ability of the method to successfully detect changes of the model topology during the segmentation process. This allows to detect features like holes and discontinuities in object contour/surface or to detect more than one object in the scene.
- **Segmentation precision:** describes an overall quality of delivered results not considering the errors originating from above described problems (noise, bad parameters, bad initialization), so this feature actually describes how well is the segmentation performed if all the circumstances are advantageous.
- **Execution times:** describes the time necessary to perform the segmentation process, which originates in the complexity of the algorithm.

Each feature has been rated in a comparative scale, choosing values from the following: very low, low, medium, high, and very high. All assumed values are chosen in a relative way, that is to present best their correspondence to each other and they should not be considered as absolute. The results of our evaluation are presented in Table 1.

Comparison

As it can be observed, the effectiveness of image processing applied to computer aided diagnosis has evolved significantly through the last two decades. New possibilities arose with numerous improvements applied to the original ideas of thresholding, graph partitioning or deformable models, but also with the possibility to use computers with radically larger processing power. It is however possible to see that some authors have focused on improving the algorithms' efficiency only together with enlarging its complexity, which in turn diminishes the improvement in processing possibilities of currently available computers and results in ever growing execution times of those algorithms. This is further extended by the fact that modern image processing algorithms operate on massive amounts of image data, acquired from medical scanners offering high resolutions and dimensionality of three or more (for example four-dimensional images, being temporal sequences of three-dimensional images). This is not necessarily a worrying fact, as we are currently witnessing a popularity growth of a new approach to expanding the possibilities of computers, namely parallelization. Distributing the workload of an algorithm between a number of processing units is becoming more popular, delivering new possibilities for algorithms' development, decreasing the need for such a high regard for its complexity.

The solution based on the active nets enriched with genetic algorithm optimization present a set of very impressive features. It seems to be virtually insensitive to bad parameters, bad initialization nor noise (See Table 1). It performs well in complex scenarios thanks to the topology change ability and their segmentation precision proves to be very good. These valuable characteristics take their origin from the formulation of active nets and from the nature of genetic algorithms, which makes them a very powerful optimization tool. Thanks to their ability to automatically favor the best solutions and to self-adapt to different conditions of operation they deliver an answer to a lot of issues of the medical image segmentation problem. Unfortunately, these valuable characteristics result in relatively high execution times. However, as it was mentioned before, the authors in (Ibáñez, Barreira, Santos, & Penedo, 2006) have assumed a very specific approach of high precision and big population sizes for their experiments. The high flexibility of the genetic algorithms promises a large field for improvement for this method and the possibility to reduce the execution times.

Similarly good set of features can be also seen by the solution based on artificial life framework,

Table 1. Comparison of different segmentation methods using a selection of representative features

Method	Sensitivity to parameters	Sensitivity to initialization	Sensitivity to noise	Topology changes ability	Segmentation precision	Execution times
Original snakes by Kass (Kass, Witkin, & Terzopoulos, 1988)	High	High (manual, near the desired contour)	High	Not capable	Low	Low
Amini's dynamic programming method (Amini, Tehrani, & Weymouth, 1988)	High	High	Medium	Not capable	High	High
Williams' greedy algorithm (Williams & Shah, 1992)	High	High	Medium	Not capable	Medium	Low
Methods based on level sets (Caselles, Kimmel, & Sapiro, 1995)	Low	High (similar to original Kass formulation)	Medium	Medium	High	Low
Ardon's 3D Minimal Paths (Ardon, Cohen, & Yezzi, 2005)	Medium	Medium (partial manual segmentation required)	Not tested by the authors, probably Low	High	High	Low
Active Nets (greedy alg.) (Tsumiyama, Sakaue, & Yamamoto, 1989)	Medium	High when combined with noisy images	Medium	Very high	High	Low
Active Nets (genetic alg.) (Ibáñez, Barreira, Santos, & Penedo, 2006)	Very low	Very Low	Low	Very high	Very High	High
Topological Active Volumes (greedy alg.) (Barreira, Penedo, Mariño, & Ansia, 2003)	Medium	High when combined with noisy images	Medium	Very high	High	Very High
Parallel genetic algorithm refinement (Fan, Jiang, & David, 2002)	Low	Low	Not tested by the authors, probably Low	Very high	Very high	Medium
Hybrid methods (Metaxas & Ting, 2004; Yifei, Shuang, Ge, & Daling, 2007)	Low	Low	Medium	Medium	High	Medium
Deformable Organisms (Chris McIntosh & Ghassan Hamarneh, 2006; C. McIntosh & G. Hamarneh, 2006)	High	Low	Low	Very high	Very High	High

the deformable organisms. The approach to the segmentation problem, taken in this case, is quite different from the one described above. Instead of relying on the natural selection mechanisms, authors use a highly configurable, hierarchical model as the base for deformable organisms, thus allowing them to introduce a high amount of knowledge to the model. This information can successfully serve as guidance for the organisms in the segmentation process, defining their actions and responses in specific scenarios. As it is possible to see in our evaluation, this allowed developing a highly-effective segmentation method, which probably is still capable of performing better with the introduction of more research efforts. However, in contrast to the active volumes/genetic algorithms solution, this method lacks the ability of self-adaptation and thus requires a high level of user interaction in terms of method construction and development. The definition of the algorithm and the configuration of the behavioral functions for the organisms have to be precise to obtain optimal results. Also the flexibility of the method is believed to be significantly lower in terms of applying the same method to segmentation of different body parts, different types of scanning devices, etc.

The two-stage solutions, like the 3D minimal paths and the parallel genetic algorithm refinement, benefit richly thanks to a very natural idea of initializing the segmentation process very near its final, desired shape. What is worth noticing is that this solution delivers a very good and effective method to obtain that goal. A quick approximation of the shape to be segmented is performed at the beginning, assuming a high level of simplification and gaining high performance advantage. This step would occupy relatively little time and deliver an initialization position for the deformable model far better than a primitive shape representing absolutely no knowledge about the scene. Because at this point no connection exists between this initialization scheme and further processing with the deformable models method (those steps are independent), we consider this idea strictly as a solution to the initialization problem, which offers significant improvement and can be applied before any other segmentation scenario, not just the one proposed by the authors. It is a good idea, which can possibly bring improvement in segmentation precision and execution time applied to any segmentation solution.

CONCLUSION

In this chapter we have performed a precise study of the trends in medical image analysis, both in the past and at the current time. We have evaluated some of the most interesting work performed in the last few years, which allowed us to see some current tendencies in the field of medical image analysis. One of the most visible is the ever improving quality of segmentation delivered by new methods and new possibilities of those algorithms. As for their execution times, the trends are various. This is a result of a twofold approach for the improvement in algorithms' precision: some of them are constructed to be much more complex than the old ones and that results in ever-growing demand for computational power, the others concentrate on optimization of workflow, which allows obtaining good quality of segmentation while keeping the execution times on a reasonable level. Another important trend is the will to minimize the necessity for human intervention by making the segmentation process less depending from initialization, big number of parameters, which need to be properly selected, and less vulnerable to poor quality data.

REFERENCES

Alan, P. M., & Ross, T. W. (1999). Partitioning 3D Surface Meshes Using Watershed Segmentation. *IEEE Transactions on Visualization and Computer Graphics*, *5*(4), 308–321. doi:10.1109/2945.817348

Alberto, M. (1976). An application of heuristic search methods to edge and contour detection. *Communications of the ACM*, *19*(2), 73–83. doi:10.1145/359997.360004

Amini, A. A., Tehrani, S., & Weymouth, T. E. (1988). *Using Dynamic Programming For Minimizing The Energy Of Active Contours In The Presence Of Hard Constraints.* Paper presented at the Second International Conference onComputer Vision.

Andr, Gu, ziec, & Nicholas, A. (1994). Smoothing and matching of 3-D space curves. *International Journal of Computer Vision, 12*(1), 79–104. doi:10.1007/BF01420985

Ansia, F. M., Lopez, J., Penedo, M. G., & Mosquera, A. (2000). *Automatic 3D shape reconstruction of bones using active nets based segmentation.* Paper presented at the 15th International Conference on Pattern Recognition, 2000.

Ardon, R., & Cohen, L. (2006). Fast Constrained Surface Extraction by Minimal Paths. *International Journal of Computer Vision, 69*(1), 127–136. doi:10.1007/s11263-006-6850-z

Ardon, R., Cohen, L., & Yezzi, A. (2005). A New Implicit Method for Surface Segmentation by Minimal Paths: Applications in 3D Medical Images. In *Energy Minimization Methods in Computer Vision and Pattern Recognition* (pp. 520-535).

Ardon, R., Cohen, L. D., & Yezzi, A. (2007). A New Implicit Method for Surface Segmentation by Minimal Paths in 3D Images. *Applied Mathematics & Optimization, 55*(2), 127–144. doi:10.1007/s00245-006-0885-y

Barreira, N., Penedo, M. G., Mariño, C., & Ansia, F. M. (2003). Topological Active Volumes. In *Computer Analysis of Images and Patterns* (pp. 337-344).

Beare, R. (2006). A Locally Constrained Watershed Transform. *IEEE Transactions on Pattern Analysis and Machine Intelligence, 28*(7), 1063–1074. doi:10.1109/TPAMI.2006.132

Boskovitz, V., & Guterman, H. (2002). An adaptive neuro-fuzzy system for automatic image segmentation and edge detection. *Fuzzy Systems. IEEE Transactions on, 10*(2), 247–262.

Bouman, C. A., & Shapiro, M. (1994). A multiscale random field model for Bayesian image segmentation. *IEEE Transactions on Image Processing, 3*(2), 162–177. doi:10.1109/83.277898

Buecher, S., & Lantuéjoul, C. (1979, September 1979). *Use of watershed in contour detection.* Paper presented at the Int. Workshop Image Processing, Real-Time Edge and Motion Detection/Estimation, Rennes, France.

Carlson, J., & Ortendahl, D. (1987). *Segmentation of Magnetic Resonance Images Using Fuzzy Clustering.* Paper presented at the Proc. Information Processing in Medical Imaging.

Caselles, V., Kimmel, R., & Sapiro, G. (1995). *Geodesic active contours.* Paper presented at the Proceedings of the Fifth International Conference on Computer Vision.

Chakraborty, A., Staib, L. H., & Duncan, J. S. (1996). Deformable boundary finding in medical images by integrating gradient and region information. *IEEE Transactions on Medical Imaging, 15*(6), 859–870. doi:10.1109/42.544503

Chalana, V., & Kim, Y. (1997). A methodology for evaluation of boundary detection algorithms on medical images. *IEEE Transactions on Medical Imaging, 16*(5), 642–652. doi:10.1109/42.640755

Chan, T. F., & Vese, L. A. (2001). Active contours without edges. *IEEE Transactions on Image Processing, 10*(2), 266–277. doi:10.1109/83.902291

Chen, T., & Metaxas, D. (2000). Image Segmentation Based on the Integration of Markov Random Fields and Deformable Models. In *Medical Image Computing and Computer-Assisted Intervention* (pp. 256–265). MICCAI.

Chen, T., & Metaxas, D. (2003). A Hybrid Framework for 3D Medical Image Segmentation. In *Medical Image Computing and Computer-Assisted Intervention - MICCAI 2003* (pp. 703–710). Gibbs Prior Models, Marching Cubes, and Deformable Models. doi:10.1007/978-3-540-39903-2_86

Chenyang, X., & Jerry, L. P. (1997). *Gradient Vector Flow: A New External Force for Snakes*. Paper presented at the Proceedings of the 1997 Conference on Computer Vision and Pattern Recognition (CVPR '97).

Cohen, L. D., & Kimmel, R. (1996). *Global Minimum for Active Contour Models: A Minimal Path Approach*. Paper presented at the Proceedings of the 1996 Conference on Computer Vision and Pattern Recognition (CVPR '96).

Coleman, G. B., & Andrews, H. C. (1979). Image segmentation by clustering. *Proceedings of the IEEE*, *67*(5), 773–785. doi:10.1109/PROC.1979.11327

Collins, D. L., Terence, M. P., Weiqian, D., & Alan, C. E. (1992). *Model-based segmentation of individual brain structures from MRI data.*

Collins, D. L., Zijdenbos, A. P., Kollokian, V., Sled, J. G. A. S. J. G., Kabani, N. J. A. K. N. J., & Holmes, C. J. A. H. C. J. (1998). Design and construction of a realistic digital brain phantom. *IEEE Transactions on Medical Imaging*, *17*(3), 463–468. doi:10.1109/42.712135

Cootes, T. F., Beeston, C., Edwards, G. J., & Taylor, C. J. (1999). *A Unified Framework for Atlas Matching Using Active Appearance Models*. Paper presented at the Proceedings of the 16th International Conference on Information Processing in Medical Imaging.

Cuisenaire, O., J.-P., T., Macq, B. M., Michel, C., de Volder, A., & Marques, F. (1996). Automatic registration of 3D MR images with a computerized brain atlas. *Medical Imaging 1996. Image Processing*, *2710*, 438–448.

Dawant, B. M., Hartmann, S. L., Thirion, J. P., Maes, F., Vandermeulen, D., & Demaerel, P. (1999). Automatic 3-D segmentation of internal structures of the head in MR images using a combination of similarity and free-form transformations. I. Methodology and validation on normal subjects. *IEEE Transactions on Medical Imaging*, *18*(10), 909–916. doi:10.1109/42.811271

Demetri, T. (1999). Artificial life for computer graphics. *Communications of the ACM*, *42*(8), 32–42. doi:10.1145/310930.310966

Demetri, T., Xiaoyuan, T., & Radek, G. (1994). Artificial fishes: autonomous locomotion, perception, behavior, and learning in a simulated physical world. *Artificial Life*, *1*(4), 327–351. doi:10.1162/artl.1994.1.4.327

Ding, F., Leow, W., & Wang, S.-C. (2005). 3D CT Volume Images Using a Single 2D Atlas. In *Computer Vision for Biomedical Image Applications* (pp. 459–468). Segmentation of. doi:10.1007/11569541_46

Dunn, J. C. (1973). A fuzzy relative of the ISODATA process and its use in detecting compact well-sparated clusters. *Journal of Cybernetics*, *3*, 32–57. doi:10.1080/01969727308546046

Fan, Y., Jiang, T., & David, E. (2002). Volumetric segmentation of brain images using parallel genetic algorithms. *IEEE Transactions on Medical Imaging*, *21*(8), 904–909. doi:10.1109/TMI.2002.803126

Frank, J., Verschoor, A., & Boublik, M. (1981). Computer averaging of electron micrographs of 40S ribosomal subunits. *Science*, *214*, 1353–1355. doi:10.1126/science.7313694

Fritscher, K., & Schubert, R. (2006). 3D image segmentation by using statistical deformation models and level sets. *International Journal of Computer Assisted Radiology and Surgery*, *1*(3), 123–135. doi:10.1007/s11548-006-0048-2

Gibson, S., & Mirtich, B. (1997). *A Survey of Deformable Modeling in Computer Graphics*. Cambridge: Mitsubishi Electric Research Lab.

Gilles, A., & Laure Blanc, F., & raud. (1999). Some Remarks on the Equivalence between 2D and 3D Classical Snakes and Geodesic Active Contours. *International Journal of Computer Vision*, *34*(1), 19–28. doi:10.1023/A:1008168219878

Goldberg, D. (1989). *Genetic Algorithms in Search, Optimization, and Machine Learning*. Addison-Wesley Professional.

Grady, L., & Funka-Lea, G. (2004). Multi-label Image Segmentation for Medical Applications Based on Graph-Theoretic Electrical Potentials. In *Computer Vision and Mathematical Methods in Medical and Biomedical Image Analysis* (pp. 230-245).

Grau, V., Mewes, A. U. J., Alcaniz, M., Kikinis, R., & Warfield, S. K. (2004). Improved watershed transform for medical image segmentation using prior information. *Medical Imaging. IEEE Transactions on*, *23*(4), 447–458.

Hamarneh, G., McInerney, T., & Terzopoulos, D. (2001). *Deformable Organisms for Automatic Medical Image Analysis*. Paper presented at the Proceedings of the 4th International Conference on Medical Image Computing and Computer-Assisted Intervention.

Hertz, L., & Schafer, R. W. (1988). Multilevel thresholding using edge matching. *Computer Vision Graphics and Image Processing*, *44*, 279–295. doi:10.1016/0734-189X(88)90125-9

Hojjatoleslami, S. A., & Kittler, J. (1998). Region growing: a new approach. *Image Processing. IEEE Transactions on*, *7*(7), 1079–1084.

Hua, L., & Yezzi, A. (2005). *A hybrid medical image segmentation approach based on dual-front evolution model*. Paper presented at the IEEE International Conference on Image Processing, 2005. ICIP 2005.

Hyunjin, P., Bland, P. H., & Meyer, C. R. (2003). Construction of an abdominal probabilistic atlas and its application in segmentation. *IEEE Transactions on Medical Imaging*, *22*(4), 483–492. doi:10.1109/TMI.2003.809139

Ibáñez, O., Barreira, N., Santos, J., & Penedo, M. (2006). Topological Active Nets Optimization Using Genetic Algorithms. In *Image Analysis and Recognition* (pp. 272-282).

Jain, A. K., Duin, R. P. W., & Jianchang, M. (2000). Statistical pattern recognition: a review. *IEEE Transactions on Pattern Analysis and Machine Intelligence*, *22*(1), 4–37. doi:10.1109/34.824819

Jain, A. K., & Farrokhnia, F. (1990). *Unsupervised texture segmentation using Gabor filters*. Paper presented at the IEEE International Conference on Systems, Man and Cybernetics, 1990.

James, S. D., & Nicholas, A. (2000). Medical Image Analysis: Progress over Two Decades and the Challenges Ahead. *IEEE Transactions on Pattern Analysis and Machine Intelligence*, *22*(1), 85–106. doi:10.1109/34.824822

Jean-Francois, R., Serge, B., & Delhomme, J. (1992). Marker-controlled segmentation: an application to electrical borehole imaging. *Journal of Electronic Imaging*, *1*(2), 136–142. doi:10.1117/12.55184

Kapur, J. N., Sahoo, P. K., & Wong, A. K. C. (1985). A new method for gray-level picture thresholding using the entropy of the histogram. *Graph. Models Image Process.*, *29*, 273–285. doi:10.1016/0734-189X(85)90125-2

Kass, M., Witkin, A., & Terzopoulos, D. (1988). Snakes: Active contour models. *International Journal of Computer Vision*, *1*(4), 321–331. doi:10.1007/BF00133570

Kippenhan, J. S., Barker, W. W., Pascal, S., Nagel, J., & Duara, R. (1992). Evaluation of a Neural-Network Classifier for PET Scans of Normal and Alzheimer's Disease Subjects. *Journal of Nuclear Medicine*, *33*(8), 1459–1467.

Kirby, R. L., & Rosenfeld, A. (1979). A note on the use of ~gray level, local average gray level! space as an aid in threshold selection. *IEEE Transactions on Systems, Man, and Cybernetics*, *SMC-9*, 860–864.

Lefèvre, S. (2007). Knowledge from Markers in Watershed Segmentation. In *Computer Analysis of Images and Patterns* (pp. 579-586).

Leventon, M. E., Grimson, W. E. L., & Faugeras, O. (2000). *Statistical shape influence in geodesic active contours.* Paper presented at the IEEE Conference on Computer Vision and Pattern Recognition, 2000.

Li, C. H., & Lee, C. K. (1993). Minimum cross-entropy thresholding. *Pattern Recognition*, *26*, 617–625. doi:10.1016/0031-3203(93)90115-D

Lingrand, D., & Montagnat, J. (2005). A Pragmatic Comparative Study. In *Image Analysis* (pp. 25–34). Levelset and B-Spline Deformable Model Techniques for Image Segmentation. doi:10.1007/11499145_4

Lutz, R., Pun, T., & Pellegrini, C. (1991). Colour displays and look-up tables: real time modification of digital images. *Computerized Medical Imaging and Graphics*, *15*(2), 73–84. doi:10.1016/0895-6111(91)90029-U

Malladi, R., Sethian, J. A., & Vemuri, B. C. (1995). Shape modeling with front propagation: a level set approach. *IEEE Transactions on Pattern Analysis and Machine Intelligence*, *17*(2), 158–175. doi:10.1109/34.368173

Mallat, S. G. (1989). A Theory for Multiresolution Signal Decomposition: The Wavelet Representation. *IEEE Transactions on Pattern Analysis and Machine Intelligence*, *11*(7), 674–693. doi:10.1109/34.192463

Marc, D., Bernhard, M., Martin, R., & Carlo, S. (2001). *An Adaptive Level Set Method for Medical Image Segmentation.* Paper presented at the Proceedings of the 17th International Conference on Information Processing in Medical Imaging.

Margaret, M. F. (1992). Some Defects in Finite-Difference Edge Finders. *IEEE Transactions on Pattern Analysis and Machine Intelligence*, *14*(3), 337–345. doi:10.1109/34.120328

Mcinerney, T., & Terzopoulos, D. (1995). A dynamic finite element surface model for segmentation and tracking in multidimensional medical images with application to cardiac 4D image analysis. *Computerized Medical Imaging and Graphics*, *19*, 69–83. doi:10.1016/0895-6111(94)00040-9

McInerney, T., & Terzopoulos, D. (1996). Deformable models in medical image analysis: a survey. *Medical Image Analysis*, *1*(2), 91–108. doi:10.1016/S1361-8415(96)80007-7

McIntosh, C., & Hamarneh, G. (2006). *Spinal Crawlers: Deformable Organisms for Spinal Cord Segmentation and Analysis.* Paper presented at the MICCAI (1).

McIntosh, C., & Hamarneh, G. (2006). *Vessel Crawlers: 3D Physically-based Deformable Organisms for Vasculature Segmentation and Analysis.* Paper presented at the Computer Vision and Pattern Recognition, 2006 IEEE Computer Society Conference on.

Mehmet, S., & Bulent, S. (2004). Survey over image thresholding techniques and quantitative performance evaluation. *Journal of Electronic Imaging*, *13*(1), 146–168. doi:10.1117/1.1631315

Meier, U., Lopez, O., Monserrat, C., Juan, M. C., & Alcaniz, M. (2005). Real-time deformable models for surgery simulation: a survey. *Computer Methods and Programs in Biomedicine*, *77*(3), 183–197. doi:10.1016/j.cmpb.2004.11.002

Metaxas, D., & Ting, C. (2004). *A hybrid 3D segmentation framework.* Paper presented at the Biomedical Imaging: Nano to Macro, 2004. IEEE International Symposium on.

Montagnat, J., & Delingette, H. (2000). *Space and Time Shape Constrained Deformable Surfaces for 4D Medical Image Segmentation*. Paper presented at the Proceedings of the Third International Conference on Medical Image Computing and Computer-Assisted Intervention.

Mühlenbein, H., Schomisch, M., & Born, J. (1991). The parallel genetic alghorithm as function optimizer. *Parallel Computing*, *17*(6-7), 619–632. doi:10.1016/S0167-8191(05)80052-3

Nakagawa, Y., & Rosenfeld, A. (1979). Some experiments on variable thresholding. *Pattern Recognition*, *11*(11), 191–204. doi:10.1016/0031-3203(79)90006-2

O'Donnell, T., Dubuisson-Jolly, M. P., & Gupta, A. (1998). *A cooperative framework for segmentation using 2D active contours and 3D hybrid models as applied to branching cylindrical structures.* Paper presented at the Sixth International Conference on Computer Vision, 1998.

Ohanian, P. P., & Dubes, R. C. (1992). Performance evaluation for four classes of tectural features. *Pattern Recognition*, *25*, 819–833. doi:10.1016/0031-3203(92)90036-I

Olabarriaga, S. D., & Smeulders, A. W. M. (2001). Interaction in the segmentation of medical images: A survey. *Medical Image Analysis*, *5*(2), 127–142. doi:10.1016/S1361-8415(00)00041-4

Otsu, N. (1979). A Threshold Selection Method from Gray-Level Histograms. *IEEE Transactions on Systems, Man, and Cybernetics*, *9*(1), 62–66. doi:10.1109/TSMC.1979.4310076

Precioso, F., & Barlaud, M. (2002). B-spline active contour with handling of topology changes for fast video segmentation. *EURASIP Journal on Applied Signal Processing*, (1): 555–560. doi:10.1155/S1110865702203121

Pun, T., Gerig, G., & Ratib, O. (1994). Image analysis and computer vision in medicine.

Pun, T., Hochstrasser, D. F., Appel, R. D., Funk, M., & Villars-Augsburger, V. (1988). Computerized classification of two-dimensional gel electrophoretograms by correspondence analysis and ascendant hierarchical clustering. *Applied and Theoretical Electrophoresis*, *1*(1), 3–9.

Rueckert, D., Lorenzo-Valdes, M., Chandrashekara, R., Sanchez-Ortiz, G. L., & Mohiaddin, R. (2002). *Non-rigid registration of cardiac MR: application to motion modelling and atlas-based segmentation.* Paper presented at the 2002 IEEE International Symposium on Biomedical Imaging.

Rui, H., Pavlovic, V., & Metaxas, D. (2006). *A tightly coupled region-shape framework for 3D medical image segmentation.* Paper presented at the 3rd IEEE International Symposium on Biomedical Imaging: Nano to Macro.

Sezan, M. I. (1985). A peak detection algorithm and its application to histogram-based image data reduction. *Graph. Models Image Process.*, *29*, 47–59.

Shen, H., Shi, Y., & Peng, Z. (2005). 3D Complex Anatomic Structures. In *Computer Vision for Biomedical Image Applications* (pp. 189–199). Applying Prior Knowledge in the Segmentation of. doi:10.1007/11569541_20

Staib, L. H., & Duncan, J. S. (1992). Boundary finding with parametrically deformable models. *IEEE Transactions on Pattern Analysis and Machine Intelligence*, *14*(11), 1061–1075. doi:10.1109/34.166621

Staib, L. H., & Duncan, J. S. (1996). Model-based deformable surface finding for medical images. *IEEE Transactions on Medical Imaging*, *15*(5), 720–731. doi:10.1109/42.538949

Székely, G., Kelemen, A., Brechbühler, C., & Gerig, G. (1995). 3D objects from MRI volume data using constrained elastic deformations of flexible Fourier surface models. In *Computer Vision, Virtual Reality and Robotics in Medicine* (pp. 493–505). Segmentation of. doi:10.1007/BFb0034992

ter Haar Romeny, B., Florack, L., Koenderink, J., & Viergever, M. (1991). Scale space: Its natural operators and differential invariants. In *Information Processing in Medical Imaging* (pp. 239-255).

Terzopoulos, D., Witkin, A., & Kass, M. (1988). Constraints on deformable models: Recovering 3d shape and nonrigid motion. *Artificial Intelligence*, 35.

Thenien, C. (1983). An estimation-theoretic approach to terrain image segmentation. *Computer Vision Graphics and Image Processing*, *22*, 313–326. doi:10.1016/0734-189X(83)90079-8

Timothy, F. C., Gareth, J. E., & Christopher, J. T. (2001). Active Appearance Models. *IEEE Transactions on Pattern Analysis and Machine Intelligence*, *23*(6), 681–685. doi:10.1109/34.927467

Timothy, F. C., Hill, A., Christopher, J. T., & Haslam, J. (1993). *The Use of Active Shape Models for Locating Structures in Medical Images*. Paper presented at the Proceedings of the 13th International Conference on Information Processing in Medical Imaging.

Tsechpenakis, G., Wang, J., Mayer, B., & Metaxas, D. A. M. D. (2007). *Coupling CRFs and Deformable Models for 3D Medical Image Segmentation*. Paper presented at the 11th International Conference on Computer Vision, 2007. ICCV 2007.

Tsumiyama, Y., Sakaue, K., & Yamamoto, K. (1989). Active Net: Active Net Model for Region Extraction. *Information Processing Society of Japan*, *39*(1), 491–492.

Udupa, J. K., & Saha, P. K. (2003). Fuzzy connectedness and image segmentation. *Proceedings of the IEEE*, *91*(10), 1649–1669. doi:10.1109/JPROC.2003.817883

Vincent, L., & Soille, P. (1991a). Watersheds in digital spaces: an efficient algorithm based on immersion simulations. *IEEE Transactions on Pattern Analysis and Machine Intelligence*, *13*(6), 583–598. doi:10.1109/34.87344

Vincent, L., & Soille, P. (1991b). Watersheds in digital spaces: An efficient algorithm based on immersion simulations. *IEEE Transactions on Pattern Analysis and Machine Intelligence*, *13*(6), 583–598. doi:10.1109/34.87344

Wang, Z., Zheng, W., Wang, Y., Ford, J., Makedon, F., & Pearlman, J. D. (2006). Neighboring Feature Clustering. In *Advances in Artificial Intelligence* (*Vol. 3955*, pp. 605–608). Springer Berlin / Heidelberg. doi:10.1007/11752912_79

Weszka, J. S., & Rosenfeld, A. (1978). Threshold evaluation techniques. *IEEE Transactions on Systems, Man, and Cybernetics*, *SMC-8*, 627–629.

Williams, D., & Shah, M. (1992). A Fast algorithm for active contours and curvature estimation. *CVGIP: Image Understanding*, *55*(1), 14–26. doi:10.1016/1049-9660(92)90003-L

Withey, D. J., & Koles, Z. J. (2007). *Medical Image Segmentation: Methods and Software.* Paper presented at the Joint Meeting of the 6th International Symposium on Noninvasive Functional Source Imaging of the Brain and Heart and the International Conference on Functional Biomedical Imaging, 2007. NFSI-ICFBI 2007.

Wu, K.-L., & Yang, M.-S. (2002). Alternative c-means clustering algorithms. *Pattern Recognition*, *35*(10), 2267–2278. doi:10.1016/S0031-3203(01)00197-2

Yachida, M., Ikeda, M., & Tsuji, S. (1980). Plan-Guided Analysis of Cineangiograms for Measurement of Dynamic Behavior of Heart Wall. *Ieee Trans. Pattern Analy. And Mach. Intellig*, *2*(6), 537–542.

Yang, J., & Duncan, J. (2003). 3D Image Segmentation of Deformable Objects with Shape-Appearance Joint Prior Models. In *Medical Image Computing and Computer-Assisted Intervention* (pp. 573–580). MICCAI. doi:10.1007/978-3-540-39899-8_71

Yifei, Z., Shuang, W., Ge, Y., & Daling, W. (2007). *A Hybrid Image Segmentation Approach Using Watershed Transform and FCM.* Paper presented at the Fuzzy Systems and Knowledge Discovery, 2007. FSKD 2007. Fourth International Conference on.

Ying, L. (1995). *Document image binarization based on texture analysis*. State University of New York at Buffalo.

Chapter 2
Medical Image Segmentation and Tracking Through the Maximisation or the Minimisation of Divergence Between PDFs

S. Jehan-Besson
Laboratoire LIMOS CNRS, France

F. Lecellier
Laboratoire GREYC CNRS, France

J. Fadili
Laboratoire GREYC CNRS, France

G. Née
Laboratoire GREYC CNRS, France & General Electric Healthcare, France

G. Aubert
Laboratoire J.A. Dieudonné, France

ABSTRACT

In this chapter, we focus on statistical region-based active contour models where the region descriptor is chosen as the probability density function of an image feature (e.g. intensity) inside the region. Image features are then considered as random variables whose distribution may be either parametric, and then belongs to the exponential family, or non parametric and is then estimated through a Parzen window. In the proposed framework, we consider the optimization of divergences between such PDFs as a general tool for segmentation or tracking in medical images. The optimization is performed using a shape gradient descent through the evolution of an active region. Using shape derivative tools, our work is directed towards the construction of a general expression for the derivative of the energy (with respect to a domain), and the differentiation of the corresponding evolution speed for both parametric and non

DOI: 10.4018/978-1-60566-280-0.ch002

parametric PDFs. Experimental results on medical images (brain MRI, contrast echocardiography, perfusion MRI) confirm the availability of this general setting for medical structures segmentation or tracking in 2D or 3D.

1 INTRODUCTION

Medical structures segmentation or tracking is a key issue to improve medical diagnosis. These steps become crucial to cope with the increasing amount of medical data encountered in medicine. We focus here on active contours or surfaces (Kass, Witkin, & Terzopoulos, 1988; Caselles, Kimmel, & Sapiro, 1997) that are particularly well adapted to the treatment of medical structures because they provide a compact and analytical representation of object shape. The general idea behind active contours model is to apply partial differential equations (PDEs) to deform a curve (in 2D) or a surface (in 3D) towards the boundaries of the objects of interest. Snakes (Kass, Witkin, & Terzopoulos, 1988), balloons (Cohen, 1991) and geodesic active contours (Caselles, Kimmel, & Sapiro, 1997) were pioneering works on active contour models. In these methods, the contour is driven towards image edges. More recently, region-based active contours (i.e. RBAC) were proposed (Cohen, Bardinet, & Ayache, 1993; Ronfard, 1994; Zhu & Yuille, 1996; Chakraborty, Staib, & Duncan, 1996; Paragios & Deriche, 2000; Chan & Vese, 2001). In these approaches, region-based terms can be advantageously combined with boundary-based ones. The evolution equation is generally deduced from a general criterion to minimize that includes both region integrals and boundary integrals. The combination of those two terms in the energy functional allows the use of photometric image properties, such as texture (Paragios & Deriche, 2002; Aujol, Aubert, & Blanc-Féraud, 2003; Rousson, Lenglet, & Deriche, 2004; Karoui, Fablet, Boucher, & Augustin, 2006) and noise (Martin, Réfrégier, Goudail, & Guérault, 2004; Lecellier, Jehan-Besson, Fadili, Aubert, & Revenu, 2006; Galland, Bertaux, & Réfrégier, 2005), as well as geometric properties such as the prior shape of the object to be segmented (Leventon, 2000; Cremers, Tischhäuser, Weickert, & Schnörr, 2002; Tsai, Yezzi, & Wells, 2003; Gastaud, Barlaud, & Aubert, 2003; Foulonneau, Charbonnier, & Heitz, 2003; Lecellier, Jehan-Besson, Fadili, Aubert, Revenu, & Saloux, 2006), see also the review in (Cremers, Rousson, & Deriche, 2007). RBACs have proven their efficiency for a wide range of applications and are widely used in medical image segmentation (see for example Lau & Ozawa, 2004; Cheng, Yang, Fan, 2005; Paragios, 2002; Dydenko, Jamal, Bernard, D'Hooge, Magnin & Friboulet 2006).

As far as the definition of the criterion is concerned, we propose to use, as a region descriptor, the probability density function (PDF) of a given image feature inside the region of interest. Rather than considering the minimization of the anti-log-likelihood for segmentation (Zhu & Yuille, 1996; Chakraborty, Staib, & Duncan, 1996; Paragios & Deriche, 2000; Paragios & Deriche, 2002; Martin, Réfrégier, Goudail, & Guérault, 2004), we focus on the optimization of divergence between PDFs. When considering a segmentation framework, we aim at maximizing the divergence between the PDF of the inside region and the PDF of the outside region. When considering a tracking application, we aim at minimizing the divergence between the PDF of the region of interest and a reference one. The PDF can be considered as parametric (e.g. Gaussian, Rayleigh...) or non parametric (no assumption is made on the law). In the literature, region tracking using non parametric PDFs and active contours has been proposed in (Aubert, Barlaud, Faugeras, & Jehan-Besson, 2003) for video sequences. It has then been developed for cardiac structures tracking in perfusion MRI (p-MRI) sequences in (Rougon, Petitjean, Preteux,

Cluzel, Grenier, 2005). On the other hand some authors (Rathi, Michailovich, Malcolm, & Tannenbaum, 2006; Michailovich, Rathi, & Tannenbaum, 2007) have also proposed to take benefit of the maximization of the Bhattacharya distance between non parametric PDFs for segmentation.

This chapter aims at setting a very general framework for the optimization of divergence between PDFs (maximization for segmentation and minimization for tracking). We propose to give general results for both parametric and non parametric PDFs using shape derivative tools. As far as parametric PDFs are concerned, we pay a particular attention to the random part that contaminates the image coming during its acquisition process, i.e. the noise model as in (Martin, Réfrégier, Goudail, & Guérault, 2004; Lecellier, Fadili, Jehan-Besson, Aubert, & Revenu, 2010; Galland, Bertaux, & Réfrégier, 2005). We then provide a general result for the evolution equation within the framework of multi-parameter exponential family. The rationale behind using the exponential family is that it includes, among others, Gaussian, Rayleigh, Poisson and Bernoulli distributions that have proven to be useful to model the noise structure in many real image acquisition devices (e.g. Poisson for photon counting devices such as X-ray or CCD cameras, Rayleigh for ultrasound images, etc). Our general framework is also specialized to some particular cases, such as the optimization of the Kullback-Leibler (KL) divergence (Kullback, 1959), which gives a very simple expression of the derivative. As far as non parametric PDFs are concerned, the PDF is estimated using the Parzen method. The obtained expression can be derived according to the domain of interest and we then remind a general result for the optimization of the distance between PDFs (Aubert, Barlaud, Faugeras & Jehan-Besson, 2003). This general setting is then applied for the segmentation of medical structures and various examples are taken (brain MRI, p-MRI, Echocardiography) to show the adaptability of such region terms for medical image segmentation and tracking.

2 OPTIMIZATION OF DIVERGENCES BETWEEN PDFS

A natural way of generalizing the use of statistical image features such as the mean and the variance of the intensity for image segmentation is to consider the full probability distribution of the feature of interest within the region, e.g. intensity, color, texture, etc... Such PDFs may be used in a general setting for segmentation and tracking through the optimization of distances or more generally divergences. In this section, we first introduce the functional to optimize and we then remind some general results on shape derivation theory.

2.1 General Setting

Consider a function $y: \mathbb{R}^n \rightarrow \chi \subset \mathbb{R}$ which describes the feature of interest (for example the intensity I). The term $y(\mathbf{x})$ then represents the value of the feature at location x where $x \in \mathbb{R}^n$. Suppose we have learnt the probability density function (PDF) of the feature y within the image region of interest, namely Ω, and let $q(y, \Omega)$ be this PDF. We now assume that we have a function $\Psi: \mathbb{R}^+ \times \mathbb{R}^+ \rightarrow \mathbb{R}^+$ which allows us to compare two PDFs. This function is small if the PDFs are similar and large otherwise. We then introduce the following functional which represents "the distance" or more precisely the divergence between the current PDF estimate $q(y, \Omega)$ and another one $p(y)$:

$$D(\Omega) = \int_{\chi} \psi(q(y,\Omega), p(y))\, dy \tag{1}$$

The distance can be for example the Hellinger distance when:

$$\psi(q(y,\Omega), p(y)) = \frac{1}{2}\left(\sqrt{q(y,\Omega)} - \sqrt{p(y)}\right)^2$$

or the commonly used Kullback-Leibler divergence when:

$$\psi(q(y,\Omega),p(y)) = \frac{1}{2}\left(p(y)\log\frac{p(y)}{q(y,\Omega)} + q(y,\Omega)\log\frac{q(y,\Omega)}{p(y)}\right).$$

Such divergences represent a general setting for both segmentation and tracking in medical images. Indeed in segmentation problems, we generally search for homogeneous regions regarding with a given feature. We may then model the segmentation problem as the maximization of the distance between the PDF of the feature within the inside region and the PDF of the feature within the outside region. In order to fix ideas, let us consider a partition of an image in two regions where Ω is the inside region and Ω^c the complementary outside region. The segmentation may then be formulated as the maximization of the following criterion:

$$D(\Omega,\Omega^c) = \int_{\chi} \psi(q(y,\Omega),p(y,\Omega^c))\,dy \qquad (2)$$

On the other hand, the tracking problem aims at finding a region Ω in a serie of images. We can make the assumption of statistical similarity between the PDFs of the region in two consecutive images. Let us summarize this problem by considering that we have a reference histogram p_{ref} and that we search for the domain that minimizes the following functional:

$$D(\Omega) = \int_{\chi} \psi(q(y,\Omega),p_{ref}(y))\,dy \qquad (3)$$

This last framework may also be applied to supervised segmentation where a reference PDF is learnt on the region of interest. Such a supervised segmentation can be useful in brain MRI for example where the intensity values of the different tissues can be known using an expectation maximisation procedure (Zhang, Brady, & Smith, 2001).

2.2 Evolution Equation and Shape Derivation Tools

In order to find an optimum to these highly non convex optimizations problems, we perform a shape gradient descent using region-based active contours. Indeed, the principle of region-based active contours lies in the deformation of an initial curve (or surface) towards the boundaries of the region of interest. Such a deformation is directed by a geometric partial differential equation (PDE). In order to fix ideas, let us denote by $\Gamma(p,\tau)$ the active contour where p is a parameter of the contour and τ is an evolution parameter. The contour evolves according to the following PDE:

$$\frac{\partial\Gamma(p,\tau)}{\partial\tau} = F\,\mathbf{N} \qquad (4)$$

where F is the velocity of the contour applied in the direction of the unit normal N.

The evolution equation and more particularly the velocity F is computed in order to make the contour evolve towards an optimum of the energy criterion (1). We then have to compute the derivative of the criterion according to the domain which is not trivial. This is mostly due to the fact that the set of regular domains (regular open bounded sets) of R^n does not have the structure of a vector space, preventing us from using in a straightforward way gradient descent methods. To circumvent this problem, we propose to take benefit of the framework proposed in (Jehan-Besson, Barlaud, & Aubert, 2001; Jehan-Besson, Barlaud, & Aubert, 2003; Aubert, Barlaud, Faugeras, & Jehan-Besson, 2003), based on shape derivation principles developed in (Sokolowski & Zolésio, 1992; Delfour & Zolésio, 2001). This framework is particularly well-adapted when dealing with global information of the region such as statistical image features (e.g. mean, variance, entropy, histogram). In this case, one must pay attention to the fact that these features are globally attached to the region and must then be taken into account in the shape derivation framework. Let us now remind some useful definitions and theorems and then explain how we can deduce the evolution equation of an active contour from the shape derivative of the criterion.

2.2.1 Definitions and Theorems for Shape Derivative

Shape derivative theory is developed in (Sokolowski & Zolésio, 1992; Delfour & Zolésio, 2001). Formally, we introduce a mapping T_τ that transforms the initial domain Ω into the current domain $\Omega(\tau)$. For a point $\mathbf{x}\in\Omega$, we denote:

$$\mathbf{x}(\tau)=T(\tau,\mathbf{x}) \; with T(0,\mathbf{x})=\mathbf{x}$$

$$\Omega(\tau)=T(\tau,\Omega) \; with T(0,\Omega)=\Omega$$

Let us now define the velocity vector field V corresponding to $T(\tau)$ as:

$$V(\tau,\mathbf{x}) = \frac{\partial T}{\partial \tau}(\tau,\mathbf{x}) \quad \forall \mathbf{x}\in\Omega, \forall \tau \geq 0$$

We now introduce the main definitions and theorems.

Definition 1: The Eulerian derivative of $J(\Omega) = \int_\Omega k(\mathbf{x},\Omega)\, d\mathbf{x}$ in the direction of V, denoted $<J'(\Omega),\mathbf{V}>$, is equal to

$$< J'(\Omega), \mathbf{V} >= \lim_{\tau\to 0} \frac{J(\Omega(\tau)) - J(\Omega)}{\tau}$$

if the limit exists.

Definition 2: The shape derivative of $k(x,\Omega)$, denoted $k_s(x,\Omega,V)$, is equal to

$$k_s(x,\Omega,V) = \lim_{\tau\to 0} \frac{k(x,\Omega(\tau)) - k(x,\Omega)}{\tau}$$

if the limit exists.

The following theorem gives a general relation between the Eulerian derivative and the shape derivative for region-based terms.

Theorem 1: Let Ω be a C^1domain in R^n and V a C^1 vector field. Let k be a function C^1. The functional $J(\Omega) = \int_\Omega k(\mathbf{x},\Omega)\, d\mathbf{x}$ is differentiable and its Eulerian derivative in the direction of V is the following

$$< J'(\Omega), \mathbf{V} >= \int_\Omega k_s(x,\Omega,V)dx - \int_{\partial\Omega} k(x,\Omega)\big(V(x)\cdot N(x)\big)da(x) \qquad (5)$$

where $\mathbf{N}$ is the unit inward normal to $\partial\Omega$ and da its area element.

The proof can be found in (Sokolowski & Zolésio, 1992; Delfour & Zolésio, 2001) and an elementary one in (Aubert, Barlaud, Faugeras, & Jehan-Besson, 2003). In equation (5), we remark that the shape derivative of a domain integral is composed of two main terms. The first term comes from the variation of the descriptor k with the domain while the second one comes from the variation of the domain itself.

In order to find the shape derivative of criterion (1), we must compute the shape derivative of $k(x,\Omega)=\psi(q(y,\Omega),p(y))$ and so we need an explicit expression of the PDF $q(y,\Omega)$ according to Ω. Both the parametric and the non parametric cases are considered in this chapter. Shape derivation results for parametric PDFs are given in section 3 while shape derivation results for non parametric PDFs are given in section 4.

2.2.2 Computation of the Evolution Equation

From the shape derivative, we can derive the evolution equation that will drive the active contour towards a (local) optimum of the criterion.

Let us suppose that the shape derivative of the criterion $D(\Omega)$ may be written as follows:

$$< D'(\Omega), \mathbf{V} >= -\int_{\partial\Omega} speed(x,\Omega)\left(V(x)\cdot N(x)\right)da(x) \quad (6)$$

In order to fix ideas, let us denote by E(τ) the general criterion D(Ω(τ)). We have E(0) = E(Ω(0)) where Ω(0) is the initial domain. Using a first order Taylor development, we find:

$E(\tau)$=$E(0)$+$\tau E'(0)$+$o(\tau)$=$E(0)$+τ<$D'(\Omega),V$>+$o(\tau)$

Since $\tau \geq 0$, if we want to minimize the criterion E, we must choose a negative shape derivative. As noted in (Debreuve, Gastaud, Barlaud, & Aubert, 2007), interpreting equation (6) as the L^2 inner product on the space of velocities, the straightforward choice is to take **V** = speed(x,Ω) **N**. When minimizing the distance D(Ω), we can then deduce the following evolution equation:

$$\frac{\partial\Gamma}{\partial\tau} = speed(x,\Omega)\,N(x)$$

with $\Gamma(\tau = 0) = \Gamma_0$.

On the contrary, if our goal is to maximize the criterion E, a positive shape derivative must be chosen. When maximizing the criterion, we take:

$$\frac{\partial\Gamma}{\partial\tau} = -\ speed(x,\Omega)\,N(x)$$

Let us now give some general results for shape derivative using parametric or non parametric PDFs and then compute explicitly the evolution equation of the active contour

3 A GENERAL RESULT FOR PARAMETRIC PDFS WITHIN THE EXPONENTIAL FAMILY

In the criterion (1), the current PDF estimate q(y,Ω) is now indexed by a set of parameters $\boldsymbol{\theta} \in \Theta \subset R^{\kappa}$ (e.g. we have $\kappa = 2$ and $\theta = (\mu, \sigma)$ where μ is the mean and σ the variance for the Gaussian distribution when both the location and the scale parameters are unknown). In this chapter, we consider the PDF as a member of the exponential family and it will then be rather indexed by the natural parameter vector η which can be deduced from θ as explained in part 3.1. We then want to optimize:

$$D(\Omega) = \int_{\chi} \Psi(q_{\eta}(y,\Omega), p(y))dy \quad (7)$$

In order to derive the criterion, we must take into account the dependence of the natural parameter with the domain. We then restrict our study to the full rank κ-parameter canonical exponential family (Bickel & Docksum, 2001). For this family, we can establish a 1-1 correspondence between η and Ω and so compute directly the shape derivative of D(Ω).

In the sequel, let us first introduce the exponential family and then explain the computation of the shape derivative. We then specialize our result when parameters are estimated using the ML (Maximum Likelihood) method. We also give some results for the optimization of the Kullback-Leibler (KL) divergence in order to fix ideas.

3.1 The Exponential Family

The multi-parameter exponential family is naturally indexed by a κ-dimensional real parameter vector η and a κ-dimensional natural statistic vector **T**(Y). The Normal, Poisson and Rayleigh distributions exhibit the interesting feature that there is a natural sufficient statistic whose dimension as random vector is independent of the sample size. The class of families of distributions that we introduce in this section was first discovered in statistics by (Koopman, 1936) through investigations of this property. Subsequently, many other properties of these families were discovered and

Figure 1. Some common canonical exponential families

Distribution	θ^T	$\eta(\theta)^T$	$\mathrm{T}(y)^T$	$A(\eta)$	$\mathcal{E}$
Normal	(μ, σ^2)	$(\frac{\mu}{\sigma^2}, \frac{-1}{2\sigma^2})$	(y, y^2)	$\frac{1}{2}\left(-\frac{\eta_1^2}{2\eta_2} - \log\frac{-\eta_2}{\pi}\right)$	$\mathbb{R} \times \mathbb{R}^{-*}$
Gamma	(λ, p)	$(-\lambda, p-1)$	$(y, \log y)$	$-(\eta_2+1)\log -\eta_1 + \log\Gamma(\eta_2+1)$	$\mathbb{R}^{-*} \times]-1, +\infty[$
Beta	(r, s)	$(r-1, s-1)$	$(\log y, \log(1-y))$	$-\log B(\eta_1+1, \eta_2+1)$	$\mathbb{R}^{+} \times \mathbb{R}^{+}$
Poisson	μ	$\log\mu$	y	e^{η}	$\mathbb{R}$
Exponential	λ	$-\lambda$	y	$-\log -\eta$	$\mathbb{R}^{-*}$
Rayleigh	θ^2	$-1/2\theta^2$	y^2	$-\log -2\eta$	$\mathbb{R}^{-*}$

they have become an important class of the modern theory of statistics.

Definition 3: The family of distributions of a Random Variable *(RV)* $Y\{q_{\boldsymbol{\theta}}: \boldsymbol{\theta} \in \Theta \subset \mathrm{R}^{\kappa}\}$ is said a κ-parameter exponential family, if there exist real-valued functions

- $\eta(\theta) = [\eta_1, \ldots, \eta_\kappa]^T \quad with \quad \eta_i : \Theta \subset R^\kappa \rightarrow R$
- $h : R \rightarrow R$
- $B: \Theta \rightarrow R$
- $\mathbf{T} = [T_1, \ldots, T_k]^T : R^k \rightarrow R$

such that the PDF $q_{\boldsymbol{\theta}}(y)$ may be written:

$$q_{\theta}(y) = \mathrm{h}(y)\exp[<\eta(\theta), \mathrm{T}(y)> - \mathrm{B}(\theta)]$$

where $y \in \chi \subset \mathrm{R}$. $\mathbf{T}$ is called the natural sufficient statistic and η the natural parameter vector. The term $< \eta, \mathbf{T} >$ denotes the scalar product.

Letting the model be indexed by the natural parameter η rather than $\boldsymbol{\theta}$, the canonical k-parameter exponential family generated by $\boldsymbol{T}$ and h is defined as follows:

$$q_\eta(y) = h(y)\exp[<\eta(\theta), \mathbf{T}(y)> - A(\eta)] \tag{8}$$

with:

$$A(\eta) = \log \int_{-\infty}^{+\infty} h(y)\exp[< \eta, \mathbf{T}(y) >]\, dy$$

The natural parameter space is defined as $\varepsilon = \{\eta \in \varepsilon \subseteq \mathrm{R}^{\kappa}: -\infty < \mathrm{A}(\eta) < +\infty\}$ (it represents the collection of all η such that $\mathrm{A}(\eta)$ is finite).

We draw the reader's attention to the fact than η is a function of $\theta \in \Theta$ which is the parameter of interest in most applications. Figure 1 provides a synthetic description of some common distributions of the exponential family, with the associated parameters, functions (see Definition 3) and sufficient statistics.

In order to illustrate this figure, let us develop the form of the natural parameters for the Normal law:

$$p(y(x); \mu, \sigma) = \frac{1}{\sigma\sqrt{2\pi}}\exp\left(-\frac{(y(x)-\mu)^2}{2\sigma^2}\right) = \exp\left(-\frac{1}{2}\log(2\pi\sigma^2) - \frac{y^2}{2\sigma^2} + \frac{\mu y}{\sigma^2} - \frac{\mu^2}{2\sigma^2}\right)$$
$$= \exp\left(< \eta, T(y) > - \frac{1}{2}\log(2\pi\sigma^2) - \frac{\mu^2}{2\sigma^2}\right).$$

It follows that:

$$h(y) = 1, \quad T(y) = \begin{bmatrix} y \\ y^2 \end{bmatrix}, \quad \eta = \begin{bmatrix} \frac{\mu}{\sigma^2} \\ -\frac{1}{2\sigma^2} \end{bmatrix},$$

$$A(\eta) = \frac{1}{2}\left(\log(2\pi\sigma^2) + \frac{\mu^2}{2\sigma^2}\right) = -\frac{1}{2}\left(\frac{\eta_1^2}{2\eta_2} + \log\left(\frac{-\eta_2}{\pi}\right)\right).$$

3.1.2 Properties

The following results will be useful for our RBAC scheme based on the exponential family. Their proofs may be found in (Bickel & Docksum, 2001).

Theorem 2. *Let $\{q_\eta : \eta \in \varepsilon\}$ a κ-parameter canonical exponential family with natural sufficient statistic* $\mathbf{T}(Y)$ *and natural parameter space ε, we then have the following properties:*

i. ε is convex.
ii. A: ε→ R is convex
iii. $E[\mathbf{T}(Y)]=\nabla A(\eta)$
iv. $Cov[\mathbf{T}(Y)]=\nabla^2 A(\eta)$

where $\nabla A(\eta) = \left[\frac{\partial A}{\partial \eta_1}(\eta), \ldots, \frac{\partial A}{\partial \eta_\kappa}(\eta)\right]^T$ represents the gradient of A, and $\nabla^2 A(\eta)$ *is the Hessian matrix of A with* $\nabla^2 A(\eta)_{ij} = \frac{\partial^2 A}{\partial \eta_i \partial \eta_j}(\eta)$.

The following theorem establishes the conditions of strict convexity of A, and then those for ∇A to be 1-1 onε. This is a very useful result for optimization (derivation) purposes:

Theorem 3. *Let $\{q_\eta : \eta \in \varepsilon\}$ a full rank (i.e.* $Cov[\mathbf{T}(Y)]$ *is a positive-definite matrix) κ-parameter canonical exponential family with natural sufficient statistic* $\mathbf{T}(Y)$ *and natural parameter space ε, we have (Bickel, 2001):*

i. $\eta \rightarrow \nabla A(\eta)$ is 1-1 on ε.
ii. The family may be uniquely parameterized by $\boldsymbol{\mu}(\eta)=E[\mathbf{T}(Y)]$.
iii. The anti-log-likelihood function is a strictly convex function of η on ε

These results establish a 1-1 correspondence between η and E[**T**(Y)] such that:

$$\boldsymbol{\mu}=\nabla A(\eta)=E[\mathbf{T}(Y)] \Leftrightarrow \eta=\varphi(E[\mathbf{T}(Y)])$$

holds uniquely with ∇A and φ continuous. At this stage, it is interesting to mention that an alternative solution to establish this bijection, is to use the Legendre conjugate (convex analysis) in the same vein as in the work of (Banerjee, Dhillon, Ghosh & Merugu, 2004) which used it to prove the bijection between exponential families and Bregman divergences.

3.1.3 Estimation of the Hyperparameters

In order to estimate the parameters, we replace E[**T**(Y)] by the empirical estimate of the mean $\overline{\mathbf{T}(Y)}$. Indeed, let Y(x) be a continuous random process defined on an homogeneous region Ω, we can suppose that Y(x) is stationary (i.e. the distribution of the random process has certain attributes that are the same everywhere on the region Ω) and ergodic (i.e. the moments of a random process on a finite region approach the moments of the random process on the whole space when the bounds of the region expand towards infinity). By ergodicity, the expectation of any statistic **T**(Y(x)) can then be estimated as:

$$E[\mathbf{T}(Y)] = \lim_{|\Omega| \to \infty} \overline{\mathbf{T}(Y)} = \lim_{|\Omega| \to \infty} \frac{1}{|\Omega|} \int_\Omega \mathbf{T}(y(x))dx$$

Hence, by Weak-Law of Large Numbers (WLLN), the expectation E[**T**(Y)] can be replaced with the empirical estimate of the mean.

Let us note that, in numerical images, the value of the feature y is given only for the discrete points x_i. Using a kernel estimator, the continuous value of **T**(y(x)) can then be estimated using the discrete samples $\tilde{T}(y(x_i))$ as follows (equations are given in one dimension for simplicity reasons): $T(y(x)) = \sum_{i=1}^{N} w_h(x_i, x)\tilde{T}(y(x_i))$ where w_h satisfies $\sum_{i=1}^{N} w_h(x_i, x) = 1$ and $0 \leq w_h(x_i,x) \leq 1$ and h designates the bandwidth of the kernel and N the number of pixels

Let us now express the empirical estimate of the mean, we find:

$$\overline{T(Y)} = \frac{1}{|\Omega|}\int_{\Omega}\sum_{i=1}^{N} w_h(x_i, x)\tilde{T}(y(x_i))dx = \frac{1}{|\Omega|}\sum_{i=1}^{N} \tilde{T}(y(x_i))\int_{\Omega} w_h(x_i, x)dx \tag{9}$$

If the kernel is chosen as a box car function (i.e. $w_h(x_i,x)=1$ if $\boldsymbol{x}\in[-L/2+x_i,L/2+x_i]$) where L is the size of the pixel, we have:

$$\int_{\Omega} w_h(x_i, x)dx = \int_{x_i-\frac{L}{2}}^{x_i+\frac{L}{2}} du = L \tag{10}$$

By replacing (10) in equation (9), and for a regular discrete grid with $|\Omega|$=N.L, we can assume that the continuous empirical mean can be estimated using a discrete sum over the domain (under the WLLN). The error made on the integral estimation depends on the image resolution. For low resolution images, another kernel interpolation term could be easily taken into account in the derivation process. In this chapter, for simplicity reasons, we assume that the continuous empirical mean can be estimated using a discrete sum over the domain.

It is interesting to point out that the obtained discrete estimate coincides with the ML estimator (MLE) of η. Indeed, the MLE of η corresponds to minimizing the anti-log-likelihood score (for independent and identically distributed (iid) data):

$$l(\eta) = -\log\left(\prod_{x_i\in\Omega} p(y(x_i)\right) = -\sum_{x_i\in\Omega}\log(h(y(x_i))) + N\,A(\eta) - \eta\sum_{\Omega}\tilde{T}(y(x_i)).$$

By differentiation according to η, it is obvious that:

$$\nabla A(\hat{\eta}_{MLE}) = \frac{1}{N}\sum_{x_i\in\Omega}\tilde{T}(y(x_i))$$

The MLE is asymptotically unbiased and achieves the Cramer-Rao lower bound when the number of samples tends to infinity.

In order to fix ideas, let us take an example:

Example 1. When dealing with the Rayleigh distribution, we have:

$$\eta = \frac{-1}{2\theta^2}, \quad A(\eta) = -\log(-2\eta) \quad and \quad T(y) = y^2.$$

By computing $A'(\eta) = \overline{T(Y)}$, we find that

$$\frac{-1}{\eta} = \frac{1}{|\Omega|}\int_{\Omega} y(x)^2\,dx,$$

which corresponds to the MLE of the parameter θ^2 given by

$$\hat{\theta}^2_{ML} = \frac{1}{2\mathrm{N}}\sum_{x_i\in\Omega} y(x_i)^2.$$

3.2 Shape Derivative of the Criterion

In the sequel, for the sake of simplicity, we will invariably denote η for the natural parameter and its finite sample estimate over the domain. We are now ready to state our main result:

Theorem 4. *The Gâteaux derivative, in the direction of V, of the functional (9), is:*

$$<D'(\Omega),V>=<\nabla_V\eta,C> \tag{11}$$

where $\nabla_V\eta=[<\eta_1(\Omega)',V>,<\eta_2(\Omega)',V>,\ldots,<\eta_k(\Omega)',V>]^T$ is the Gâteaux derivative of η in the direction of V and <.,.> is the usual scalar product of two vectors and:

$$C=E[\partial_1\Psi(q,p)(\mathbf{T}(Y)-E[\mathbf{T}(Y)])] \tag{12}$$

The term $\partial_1\Psi$ denotes the partial derivative of Ψ according to the first variable.

The proof is detailed in Appendix A.

We then have to compute the shape derivative $\nabla_v \eta$. Such a computation requires an estimation of the expectation $E[\mathbf{T}(Y)]$ as explained in the next section.

Computing the Shape Derivative for the ML Estimator

As mentioned before, the expectation $E[\mathbf{T}(Y)]$ can be replaced with the empirical estimate of the mean $\overline{\mathbf{T}(Y)}$ which is computed over the considered domain Ω. Using such an estimate for the hyperparameter, we can state the following proposition:

Lemma 1. Within the full rank exponential family, and using the MLE estimator for the hyperparameters, the shape derivative $\nabla_v \eta$ can be expressed as:

$$\nabla_v \eta = [\nabla^2 A(\eta)]^{-1} \nabla_v (\overline{\mathbf{T}(Y)}) \tag{13}$$

where *$[\nabla^2 A(\boldsymbol{\eta})]^{-1}$ is the inverse of the Hessian matrix of* $\nabla^2 A$ which is also the Fisher information matrix I. The derivative $\nabla_v(\overline{\mathbf{T}(Y)})$ is given by:

$$\nabla_v(\overline{\mathbf{T}(Y)}). = \frac{1}{|\Omega|} \int_{\partial\Omega} \left(\overline{\mathbf{T}(y)} - \mathbf{T}(y(a))\right) (\mathbf{V} \cdot \mathbf{N}) da(\mathbf{x}), \tag{14}$$

The proof is given in Appendix B.

We can then replace the shape derivative of the natural parameters given in equation (13) in the general equation (11) given in Theorem 4. The corollary that gives the shape derivative then follows:

Corollary 1. The Gâteaux derivative, in the direction of V, of the functional (9), is:

$$
\begin{aligned}
< D'(\Omega), \mathbf{V} > &= \frac{1}{|\Omega|} \int_{\partial\Omega} < \nabla^2 A(\eta)^{-1} (\overline{\mathbf{T}(y)} - \mathbf{T}(y(a))), \mathbf{C} > (\mathbf{V} \cdot \mathbf{N})\, da(\mathbf{x}) \\
&= \frac{1}{|\Omega|} \int_{\partial\Omega} \left(\sum_{i=1}^{\kappa} C_i \sum_{j=1}^{\kappa} \nabla^2 A_{ij}(\eta)^{-1} (\overline{T_j(Y)} - T_j(y(a))) \right) (\mathbf{V} \cdot \mathbf{N})\, da(\mathbf{x})
\end{aligned}
\tag{15}
$$

where the κ components of the vector C are defined as follows:

$$C_i = E\left[\partial_1 \Psi(q, p) \left(T_i(Y) - \overline{T_i(Y)}\right)\right] \quad i \in [1, \kappa]$$

The term $\partial_1 \Psi$ denotes the partial derivative of Ψ according to the first variable.

Example 2. When dealing with the Rayleigh distribution, we have $\kappa = 1$ and:

$A(\eta) = -\log(-2\eta)$, $\nabla^2 A(\eta) = 1/\eta^2$ and $\nabla^2 A(\eta)^{-1} = \eta^2$.

By computing $A'(\eta) = -1/\eta = T_1(Y)$, we find that:

$$C_1 \nabla^2 A(\eta)^{-1} \left(\overline{T_1(Y)} - T_1(y(a))\right) = C_1 \eta^2 \left(-\frac{1}{\eta} - y^2(a)\right)$$

with

$$C_1 = \int_{\mathcal{X}} q(y, \eta(\Omega))\, \partial_1 \Psi(q(y, \eta(\Omega)), p(y)) \left(y^2 + \frac{1}{\eta}\right) dy.$$

And so, replacing η by $-1/2\theta^2$, we find

$$< D'(\Omega), \mathbf{V} > = \frac{1}{|\Omega|} \int_{\partial\Omega} \frac{C_1}{2\theta^2} \left(1 - \frac{y^2(a)}{2\theta^2}\right) (\mathbf{V} \cdot \mathbf{N})\, da(\mathbf{x}).$$

The complete computation of C_1 requires the knowledge of the function ψ as explained in section 3.2.2. Let us now give an example where $\kappa = 2$:

Example 3. When dealing with the Gaussian distribution, we have $\kappa = 2$. We can compute:

$$\nabla^2 A(\eta) = \frac{1}{2\eta_2^2} \begin{bmatrix} -\eta_2 & \eta_1 \\ \eta_1 & 1 - \frac{\eta_1^2}{\eta_2} \end{bmatrix} \quad \textit{and so} \quad \nabla^2 A(\eta)^{-1} = -2\eta_2 \begin{bmatrix} 1 - \frac{\eta_1^2}{\eta_2} & -\eta_1 \\ -\eta_1 & -\eta_2 \end{bmatrix}$$

Using the fact that $T(y) = [y, y^2]^T$ and since we have

$$\eta = \left[\mu / \sigma^2, -1/2\sigma^2\right]^T \quad \textit{and} \quad \bar{y} = \mu \quad \textit{and} \quad \overline{y^2} = \mu^2 + \sigma^2,$$

we find:

$$< D'(\Omega), \mathbf{V} >= \frac{1}{\sigma^2 |\Omega|} \int_{\partial\Omega} \left[-(y(a)-\mu)\left(C_1\left(1+\frac{2\mu}{\sigma^2}\right) - C_2\frac{\mu}{\sigma^2}\right) + (y^2(a)-\sigma^2-\mu^2)\left(C_1\frac{\mu}{\sigma^2} - \frac{C_2}{2\sigma^2}\right)\right](\mathbf{V}\cdot\mathbf{N})da$$

with:

$$C_1 = \int_{\chi} q(y,\eta(\Omega))\,\partial_1\Psi(q(y,\eta(\Omega)),p(y))\left(y-\overline{y}\right)dy,$$
$$C_2 = \int_{\chi} q(y,\eta(\Omega))\,\partial_1\Psi(q(y,\eta(\Omega)),p(y))\left(y^2-\overline{y^2}\right)dy.$$

3.2.2 Shape Derivative Using the Kullback-Leibler Divergence and the ML Estimator

In order to fix ideas, the functional $D(\Omega)$ can be chosen as the Kullback-Leibler and the PDF p belongs to the exponential family with the same parametric law as the PDF q. Let us denote by η_r the parameter of the PDF p. This parameter is supposed to be already computed and so does not depend on the domain. We then have:

$$\Psi(q_\eta(y,\Omega), p_{\eta_r}(y)) = \frac{1}{2}\left(p_{\eta_r}(y)\log\frac{p_{\eta_r}(y)}{q_\eta(y,\Omega)} + q_\eta(y,\Omega)\log\frac{q_\eta(y,\Omega)}{p_{\eta_r}(y)}\right)$$

In this case:

$$\partial_1\Psi(q_\eta(y,\Omega), p_{\eta_r}(y)) = \log q_\eta(y,\Omega) + 1 - \log p_{\eta_r}(y) - \frac{p_{\eta_r}(y)}{q_\eta(y,\Omega)}$$

We then state the following proposition:

Lemma 2. When $p_{\eta r}(y)$ and $q_\eta(y,\Omega)$ are two members of the exponential family that belong to the same parametric law with respective parameters $\boldsymbol{\eta}_r$ and $\boldsymbol{\eta}$, and when the functional $D(\Omega)$ is chosen as the KL divergence, we find for the vector C defined in Theorem 4:

$$\mathbf{C}=\nabla^2 A(\eta)(\eta-\eta_r)+\nabla A(\eta)-\nabla A(\eta_r) \quad (16)$$

The proof is given in Appendix C.

Example 4. When dealing with the Rayleigh distribution, following example 2 with appropriate substitutions, we find:

$$C_1 = 2\theta^2\left(\frac{\theta^2}{\theta_r^2} - \frac{\theta_r^2}{\theta^2}\right) \quad (17)$$

Example 5. When dealing with the Gaussian distribution, following example 3, we find $C=[C_1,C_2]^T$ with:

$$C_1 = \sigma^2\left(\frac{\mu}{\sigma_r^2} - \frac{\mu_r}{\sigma_r^2}\right) + \mu - \mu_r$$
$$C_2 = 2\sigma^2\left(\frac{\mu^2}{\sigma^2} - \frac{\mu\mu_r}{\sigma_r^2}\right) + \sigma^4\left(1+\frac{2\mu^2}{\sigma^2}\right)\left(\frac{1}{\sigma_r^2} - \frac{1}{\sigma^2}\right) + \mu^2 + \sigma^2 - \mu_r^2 - \sigma_r^2 \quad (18)$$

4 A GENERAL RESULT FOR NON PARAMETRIC PDFS

In this section, we focus our attention on non-parametric kernel density estimators which can be useful when the density is unknown or when the region of interest presents several peaks. We want to optimize the following functional:

$$D(\Omega) = \int_{\chi} \Psi(\hat{q}(y,\Omega), p(y))dy, \quad (19)$$

where $\hat{q}(y,\Omega)$ is estimated through the use of a Parzen window as explained in the next subsection.

4.1 Estimation of the PDF

Given a region Ω, we can estimate the PDF of the feature y through the use of the Parzen method (Duda & Hart, 1973): let $K: \chi \rightarrow R^+$ be the Parzen window, a smooth positive function whose integral is equal to 1. For the sake of simplicity but without loss of generality, we assume that K is a Gaussian with 0-mean and variance σ^2, we note:

$$K(y) = \frac{1}{(2\pi\sigma^2)^{1/2}} \exp\left(\frac{-y^2}{2\sigma^2}\right),$$

and, we define:

$$\hat{q}(y,\Omega) = \frac{1}{G(\Omega)} \int_{\Omega} K(y(x) - y)dx,$$

where $y(x)$ is the value of the feature of interest at the point x of Ω and G is a normalizing constant, in general depending of Ω, such that $\int_{\chi} \hat{q}(y,\Omega)dy = 1$. Therefore $G(\Omega)=|\Omega|$.

4.2 Shape Derivative

Using the tools developed in section 2, we compute the shape derivative of the functional (19). We have the following theorem:

Theorem 5. *The shape derivative in the direction V of the functional D defined in (19) is:*

$$< D'(\Omega), \mathbf{V} >= \frac{-1}{|\Omega|} \int_{\partial\Omega} \left(\partial_1 \Psi(\hat{q}(.), p(.)) * K(y(a)) - C(\Omega)\right)(\mathbf{V} \cdot \mathbf{N})da(\mathbf{x}). \quad (20)$$

Where

$$C(\Omega) = \int_{\chi} \partial_1 \Psi(\hat{q}(y,\Omega), p(y)) \ \hat{q}(y,\Omega)\, dy \quad (21)$$

and $\partial_1\Psi(.,.)$ the partial derivative of $\Psi(.,.)$ according to the first variable.

A proof is given in (Aubert, Barlaud, Faugeras, & Jehan-Besson, 2003).

5 MAXIMIZATION OF DISTANCES BETWEEN PARAMETRIC PDFS FOR SEGMENTATION

When considering the segmentation of an image into two regions, namely Ω and its complement Ω^c, we propose here to consider the maximization of the distance between the parametric PDF $q_\eta(y, \Omega))$ which corresponds to the distribution of y inside the region Ω and $q_{\eta c}(y, \Omega^c)$ which corresponds to the distribution of y inside the region Ω^c:

$$D(\Omega, \Omega^c) = \int_{\chi} \Psi(q_\eta(y,\Omega), q_{\eta_c}(y,\Omega^c))dy \quad (22)$$

In this section, we first give the corresponding evolution equation of the active contour and we then propose to experimentally compare the behaviour of such a parametric criterion compared to two other region-based active contour methods, namely the Chan & Vese method (2001) and the minimization of the log-likelihood for a Gaussian distribution proposed by Zhu & Yuille (1996).

5.1 Associated Evolution Equation

We then propose to compute the shape derivative of the criterion (22) as follows:

$$< D(\Omega,\Omega^c), \mathbf{V} >= \int_{\chi} < q'_\eta(y,\Omega), \mathbf{V} > \partial_1 \Psi(q_\eta(y,\Omega), q_{\eta_c}(y,\Omega^c))dy + \int_{\chi} < q'_{\eta_c}(y,\Omega^c), \mathbf{V} > \partial_2 \Psi(q_\eta(y,\Omega), q_{\eta_c}(y,\Omega^c))dy$$

where $\partial_2\psi$ represents the partial derivative of ψ according to the second variable.

We can then apply Theorem 4 and $<D(\Omega,\Omega^c),V>=<\nabla_v\eta,C>+<\nabla_v\eta_c,C^c>$, where C is defined in equation (12) in Theorem 4.

Example 6. When using the KL divergence and the ML estimator for the parameters, and noting that the regions Ω and Ω^c share the same boundary with opposite normals, we find for the Rayleigh distribution:

$$< D(\Omega,\Omega^c)', \mathbf{V} >= \frac{1}{|\Omega|}\int_{\partial\Omega} \frac{C_1}{2\theta^2}\left(1-\frac{y^2(a)}{2\theta^2}\right)(\mathbf{V}\cdot\mathbf{N})\, da(\mathbf{x})$$
$$-\frac{1}{|\Omega^c|}\int_{\partial\Omega} \frac{C_1^c}{2\theta_c^{\,2}}\left(1-\frac{y^2(a)}{2\theta_c^{\,2}}\right)(\mathbf{V}\cdot\mathbf{N})\, da(\mathbf{x})$$

with

$$C_1 = 2\theta^2\left(\frac{\theta^2}{\theta_c^2}-\frac{\theta_c^2}{\theta^2}\right),$$

and

$$C_1^c = -2\theta_c^{\,2}\left(\frac{\theta^2}{\theta_c^2}-\frac{\theta_c^2}{\theta^2}\right).$$

Since we maximize the divergence, we then use the evolution equation (6) which yields:

$$\frac{\partial\Gamma}{\partial\tau} = \left[\left(\frac{\theta^2}{\theta_c^2}-\frac{\theta_c^2}{\theta^2}\right)\left(\frac{1}{|\Omega|}\left(1-\frac{y^2}{2\theta^2}\right)+\frac{1}{|\Omega^c|}\left(1-\frac{y^2}{2\theta_c^2}\right)\right)\right]\mathbf{N} \tag{23}$$

Example 7. When using the KL divergence and the ML estimator for the parameters, we similarly find for the Gaussian distribution:

$$\frac{\partial\Gamma}{\partial\tau} = \frac{1}{\sigma^2|\Omega|}\left[-(y(a)-\mu)\left(C_1\left(1+\frac{2\mu}{\sigma^2}\right)-C_2\frac{\mu}{\sigma^2}\right)+(y^2(a)-\sigma^2-\mu^2)\left(C_1\frac{\mu}{\sigma^2}-\frac{C_2}{2\sigma^2}\right)\right]\mathbf{N}$$
$$-\frac{1}{\sigma_c^{\,2}|\Omega^c|}\left[-(y(a)-\mu_c)\left(C_1^c\left(1+\frac{2\mu_c}{\sigma_c^{\,2}}\right)-C_2^c\frac{\mu_c}{\sigma_c^{\,2}}\right)+(y^2(a)-\sigma_c^{\,2}-\mu_c^{\,2})\left(C_1^c\frac{\mu_c}{\sigma_c^{\,2}}-\frac{C_2^c}{2\sigma_c^{\,2}}\right)\right]\mathbf{N} \tag{24}$$

where C_1 and C_2 are given in equation (18) and C_1^C and C_2^C are computed as C_1 and C_2 by inverting the role of the parameters μ and μ_c and σ and σ_c.

5.2 Experimental Comparison

We propose to experimentally compare the behaviour of our data term based on the maximisation of the symmetrized Kullback-Leibler divergence between parametric PDFs to two other well-known region-based methods (Zhu & Yuille, 1996; Chan & Vese, 2001). The first method is the famous Chan & Vese method who aims at minimizing the following functional

$$D(\Omega,\Omega^c) = \int_{\Omega}\left(y(\mathbf{x})-\mu\right)^2 d\mathbf{x} + \int_{\Omega^c}\left(y(\mathbf{x})-\mu_c\right)^2 d\mathbf{x} + \lambda\int_{\Gamma} ds$$

where the parameters μ and μ_c represent the estimated mean of the feature y within Ω and Ω^c. Such a criterion implies a Gaussian distribution for the feature y with a fixed variance. The corresponding evolution equation can be found in (Chan & Vese, 2001). The second method first proposed by (Zhu & Yuille, 1996) for a Gaussian distribution consists in minimizing the anti log-likelihood as follows

$$D(\Omega,\Omega^c) = -\int_{\Omega}\log(q_{\eta}(y(\mathbf{x}),\Omega)d\mathbf{x} - \int_{\Omega^c}\log(q_{\eta^c}(y(\mathbf{x}),\Omega^c)d\mathbf{x} + \lambda\int_{\Gamma} ds.$$

Let us now compare the behaviour of these criterions for the extraction of an homogeneous region corrupted by a Gaussian noise in an image. We propose to take the example of the segmentation of the White Matter in MRI images. We perform the three evolution equations using the Gaussian assumption for the PDF of the feature y within each region. The feature y is chosen as the intensity of the image. The initial contour is given in Figure 2. The PDF of the intensity within Ω, i.e. inside the contour, $q_{\eta}(I, \Omega)$ is in solid line, the PDF of the intensity within Ω^c, namely $q_{\eta c}(I, \Omega^c)$, is in dotted lines. In Figure 3, we can observe the final active contour obtained using our criterion (22) and the two other criterions mentioned above. We can remark (Figure 3.a) that our criterion acts as an extractor of the most important Gaussian in the initial mixture of Gaussians (see Figure 2.b). The two other criterions separate the mixture without extracting a single Gaussian. So, with our method, we can directly obtain the White Matter

Figure 2. Initial contour and associated PDFs

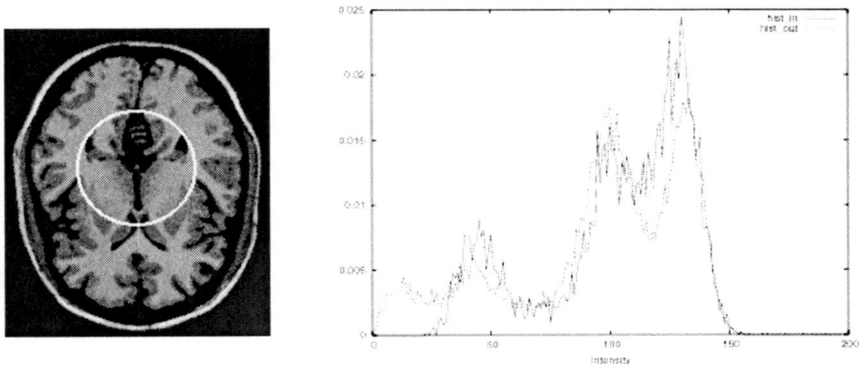

Figure 3. Final active contour and corresponding final PDFs

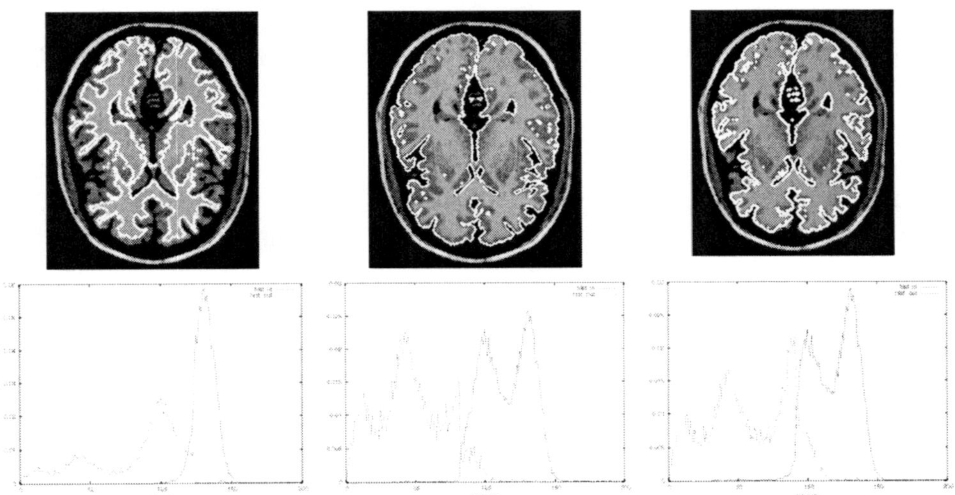

(a) maximisation of the KL divergence

(b) Chan & Vese (2001)

(c) log-likelihood method (Zhu & Yuille, 1996)

of the brain without a multiphase scheme. Some more experimental results for the segmentation of the White Matter are given in section 8.

6 MINIMIZATION OF DISTANCES BETWEEN NON PARAMETRIC PDFS FOR REGION TRACKING

In this section, we consider that there is a statistical similarity between two frames. We then want to minimize the distance between the PDF q and a reference PDF p computed on the previous frame. The region of interest Ω is segmented in a previous frame and the PDF inside this reference region is named p. This region is not necessarily homogeneous which justify the use of non parametric PDFs. We want to minimize the distance between the PDF q and the reference PDF p computed on the previous frame. We also consider the outside PDF q^c whose reference in the previous frame is p^c. The region of interest Ω and its complement region Ω^c share the same boundary, Γ, but with normals pointing in opposite directions. We then look for the partition of the image $\{\Omega, \Omega^c\}$ which minimizes the following criterion

$$J(\Omega,\Omega^c) = D(\Omega) + D(\Omega^c) + \lambda \int_{\Gamma} da\,. \qquad (25)$$

In this criterion, the first two terms are region functionals while the last one is a regularization term weighted by the positive parameter λ which corresponds to the minimization of the curve length. We have of course:

$$D(\Omega) = \int_{\chi} \Psi(\hat{q}(y,\Omega), p(y))dy \quad and$$
$$D(\Omega^c) = \int_{\chi} \Psi(\hat{q}(y,\Omega^c), p^c(y))dy,$$

A straightforward application of Theorem 5 yields:

$$< D'(\Omega), \mathbf{V} >=$$
$$\frac{-1}{|\Omega|}\int_{\partial\Omega}\left(\partial_1\Psi(\hat{q}(.), p(.)) * K(y(a)) - \mathbf{C}(\Omega)\right)(\mathbf{V}\cdot\mathbf{N})da(\mathbf{x})$$

Similar results hold for Ω^c with $N^c = -N$.

From the previous derivatives, we can deduce the evolution of an active contour that will evolve towards a minimum of the criterion J defined in (25). We find the following evolution equation:

$$\frac{\partial\Gamma}{\partial\tau} = \frac{1}{|\Omega|}\left(\partial_1\Psi(\hat{q}(.,\Omega), p(.)) * K(y(\mathbf{x})) - \mathbf{C}(\Omega)\right)\mathbf{N}$$
$$-\frac{1}{|\Omega^c|}\left(\partial_1\Psi(\hat{q}(.,\Omega^c), p^c(.)) * K(y(\mathbf{x})) - \mathbf{C}(\Omega^c) + \lambda\kappa\right)\mathbf{N} \qquad (26)$$

where κ is the curvature of Γ and $\mathbf{C}(\Omega)$, $\mathbf{C}(\Omega^c)$ are given by Theorem 5.

We note that, for each region, two terms appear in the velocity, a local one that compares the two histograms for the intensity of the current point y(x) and a global one C(Ω).

The distance D(Ω) can be for example the Hellinger distance between an estimated PDF $\hat{q}$ and a reference one p. In this case, we have $\partial_1\Psi(q,p) = (\sqrt{q} - \sqrt{p}) / \sqrt{q}$ .Note that the same kind of general results can be found for parametric PDFs through the use of the exponential family using the computation of the shape derivative given in Theorem 4.

7 NUMERICAL IMPLEMENTATION

As far as the numerical implementation is concerned, we use the level set method approach first proposed by Osher and Sethian (1988) and applied to geodesic active contours in (Caselles, Catte, Coll, & Dibos, 1993). The key idea of the level set method is to introduce an auxiliary function U (x,τ) such that Γ(τ) is the zero level set of U. The function U is often chosen to be the signed distance function of Γ(τ). The evolution equations (5) or (6) then becomes $\frac{\partial U(\tau)}{\partial\tau} = F\left|\nabla U\right|$. The velocity function F is computed only on the curve Γ(τ) but we can extend its expression to the whole image domain Ω. To implement the level set method, solutions must be found to circumvent problems coming from the fact that the signed distance function U does not stay a distance function using this PDE (see (Gomes & Faugeras, 2000) for details). In our work, the function U is reinitialized so that it remains a distance function.

8 EXPERIMENTAL RESULTS

In this section, we propose segmentation results on different medical imaging. In all the experiments, the feature y is chosen as the intensity I of the image.

8.1 Segmentation of T1-Weighted MRI Images

In this part, we consider 3D T1-weighted MRI images of the brain. For such images the problem of segmentation is particularly critical for both diagnosis and treatment purposes. It becomes necessary to obtain a robust segmentation of the different tissues (White Matter (WM), Gray Matter (GM), or Cerebrospinal Fluid (CSF)). The applications can be for example the quantification of cortical atrophy for the Alzheimer's disease or the study of brain development. Since the seminal work of Vannier (1988), several segmentation methods have been proposed and evaluated. In (Angelini, Song, Mensh, & Laine, 2007), the authors propose to distinguish two main classes of work: statistical methods (Hashimoto & Kudo, 2000; Marroquin, Vemuri, Botello, Calderon, & Fernandez-Bouzas, 2002; Shattuck & Leahy, 2002; Zavaljevski, Dhawan, Gaskil, Ball, & Johnson, 2000; Ruan, Jaggi, Xue, Fadili, & Bloyet, 2000; Zeng, Staib, Schultz, & Duncan, 1999) and deformables models (Yang & Duncan, 2003; Li, Yezzi, & Cohen, 2006). As far as statistical methods are concerned, comparative studies of different segmentation methods are proposed in (Klauschen, Goldman, Barra, Meyer-Lindenberg, & Lundervold, 2008) with a focus on the variability against noise or non-uniformity in intensity. In (Angelini, Song, Mensh, & Laine, 2007), the authors propose to compare deformable models through the use of the multiphase framework of Chan & Vese (2002) with two other statistical methods and notably an expectation maximisation classification using hidden Markov Random Fields (Zhang, Brady, & Smith, 2001). The results demonstrated the potential of deformable models and especially region-based active contours. Compared to the Chan & Vese method, a distinctive aspect of our approach is that we take into account explicitly the noise model through the use of the PDF of the intensity within a homogeneous region.

8.1.1 Qualitative Results Using Real Data

We propose here an example of CSF segmentation in Figure 4 and an example of WM segmentation in Figure 5 and. In MRI images, the noise model is assumed to be represented by a Rician distribution (Goodman, 1976; Henkelman, 1985; Gubjartsson & Patz, 1995). For large signal intensities the noise distribution can be considered as a Gaussian distribution (this is the case for the WM or the GM) and so the evolution equation (24) can be implemented. Indeed, in (Angelini, Song, Mensh, & Laine, 2007), the authors experimentally demonstrate that the Gaussian assumption is valid in the WM and the GM. In the CSF, this assumption seems less valid due to the low signal intensity in this region. For the CSF which has a low signal intensity, the noise model is then approximated by a Rayleigh noise and in this case, we choose the evolution equation (23). However, let us note that, especially for the CSF, a Rician model would better fit the distribution. In all the experiments, we extract the brain structures manually but we can use a classical skull/scalp stripping method (Smith, 2002). For the segmentation of the CSF, we use a square mask inside the brain to restrict the segmentation area.

Figure 4. Segmentation of the CSF on one slice of a T1 brain MRI

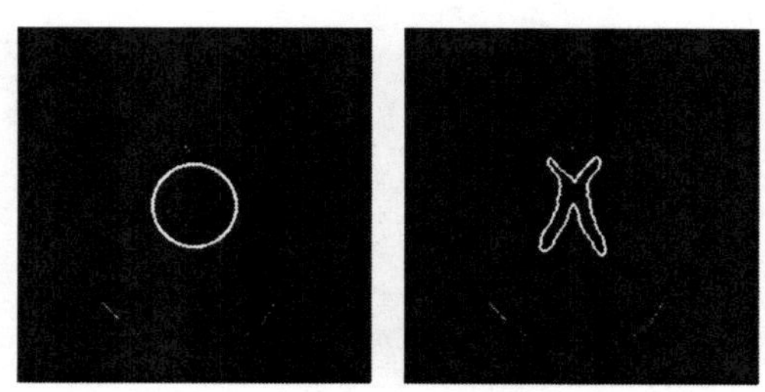

(a) initial contour (b) final contour

8.1.2 Quantitative Results Using Simulated Data

We propose to evaluate the accuracy of our method on simulated brain T1-weighted MRI images provided by the Montreal Neurological Institute Brain Web URL. We perform the segmentation of the WM on a brain MRI image with a noise of 7% (Brain Web offers noise levels ranging from 1 to 9%). In Figure 6, we show our segmentation results and the ground-truth reference segmentation. We also display the misclassified pixels in different colours (red for false positives compared to the reference, green for false negatives). Our method gives a dice coefficient of 0.91, a False Positive Fraction (FPF) of 0.8% and a True Positive Fraction (TPF) of 84%.We also compared quantitatively our results to those obtained using the method developed in (Ruan, Jaggi, Xue, Fadili, & Bloyet, 2000) based on Markov Random Fields. Such a method gives a dice coefficient of 0.92, a FPF of 1.7% and a TPF of 87%. We can remark that our method gives a very small number of false positive voxels, at the price of a higher number of missing voxels. The last point is due to the regularization term which acts by minimizing the curve length.

8.2 Segmentation of Contrast Echocardiography

Contrast echocardiography has proved to be of additional value over conventional two-dimensional echocardiography in the assessment of left ventricular border detection and left ventricular function. Compared to classical echocardiography techniques, a contrast agent is added that provides information about the degree of perfusion and the speed of reperfusion of the myocardium. Due to the addition of this contrast agent which leads the blood to be more reactive, the inside of the left ventricle is shown as a white structure in contrast

Figure 5. 3D Segmentation of WM in a T1-weighted brain MRI

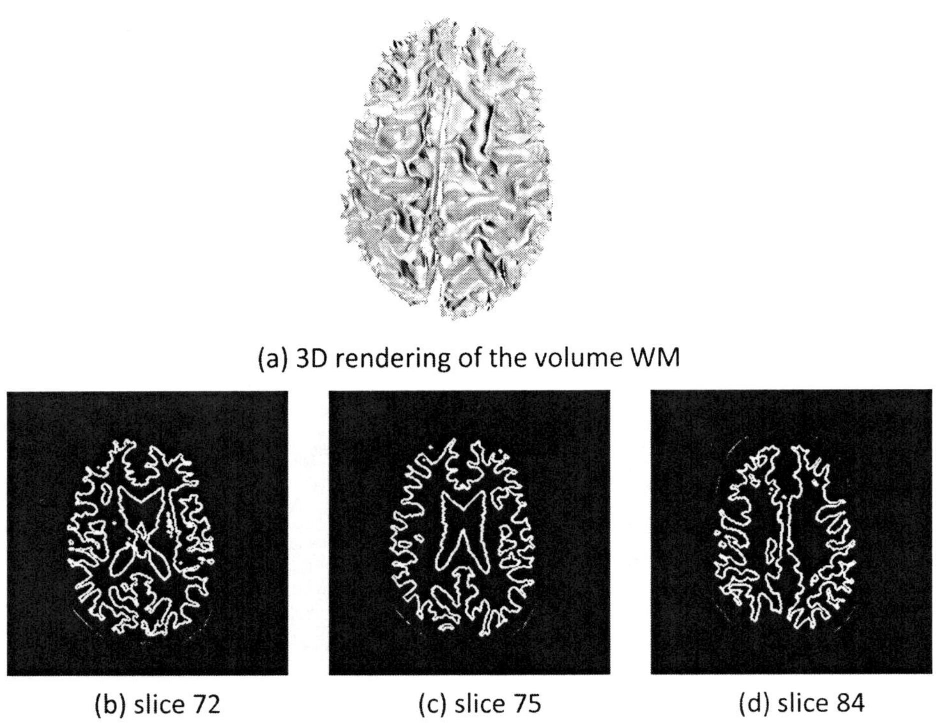

echocardiography. Tracking the boundaries of the left ventricle in such images allow a better quantification of wall motion and perfusion. Since contrast echocardiography is a recent technique (Paelinck & Kasprzak, 1999; Schiller, Shah, Crawford, DeMaria, Devereux, Feigenbaum, et al., 1989), very few papers address such a segmentation issue. As pointed out in (Pickard, Hossack, & Acton, 2006), deformable models are well appropriated due to their adaptability to noise and shape variability. They have also proven their efficiency for classical echocardiography segmentation (Dydenko, Jamal, Bernard, D'Hooge, Magnin, & Friboulet, 2006; Paragios, 2002). The authors of (Pickard, Hossack, & Acton, 2006) propose a segmentation method based on learning shape variability using principal component analysis. In this section, we propose to give some results showing the applicability of our data terms. As the Rayleigh distribution is well suited to model noise in echography (Vannier, Butterfield, Jordan, Murphy, Levitt, & Gado, 1988), this noise model was applied and the evolution equation (23) is used. We segment the left ventricle as shown in Figure 7. The segmentation is accurate all along the sequence. Some more quantitative validation steps are however needed to assess the quality of the results. Our data terms could be mixed with shape prior for more robustness as proposed in (Lecellier, Jehan-Besson, Fadili, Aubert, Revenu, & Saloux, 2006).

8.3 Tracking in p-MRI Sequences

The perfusion MRI (p-MRI) has emerged as a primordial clinical investigation tool in the evaluation of cardiac diseases. Spatio-temporal tracking of myocardial dynamics during the first transit of the contrast bolus allows the identification of hypoperfused or ischemic regions. An automatic quantification tool relies on the accurate segmentation and tracking of the cardiac structures. The main

Figure 6. Difference between the segmented WM tissue and the reference segmentation in T1-weighted Brain MRI simulated images with a noise level of 7%. Each row corresponds to a different slice of the brain volume.

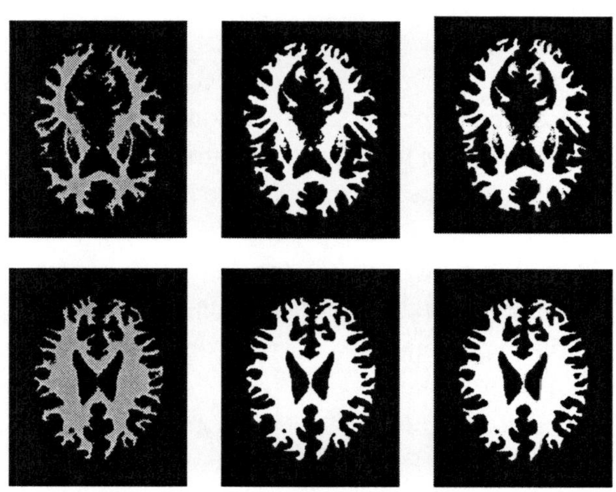

Figure 7. Segmentation of the LV in a contrast echocardiography

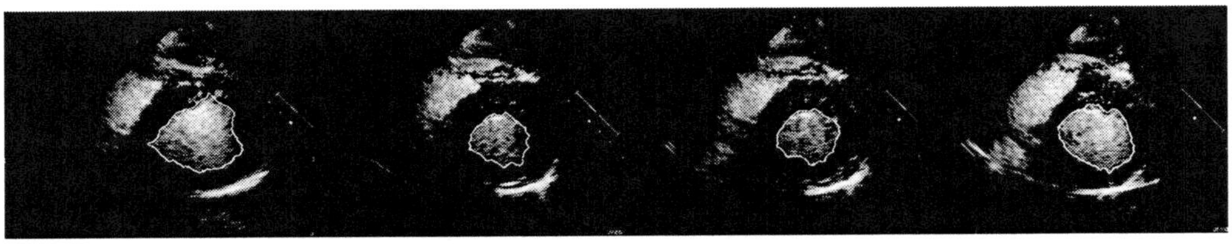

difficulty lies in the fact that the different regions (myocardium, left ventricle) are not homogeneous. Strong variations of intensity appear due to the transit of the contrast agent (Gadolinium). These variations occur inside the regions which makes useless classical segmentation algorithms based on the homogeneous assumption (Chan & Vese, 2001; Lecellier, Jehan-Besson, Fadili, Aubert, & Revenu, 2006). Moreover, regions are sometimes not delimited by a high gradient excluding gradient based methods (Caselles, Kimmel, & Sapiro, 1997). Besides, even if the images are taken at instants corresponding to the same phase of the cardiac cycle, a registration is needed due to the patient breathing (Stegmann, Olafsdottir, & Larsson, 2005; Rougon, Petitjean, Preteux, Cluzel, Grenier, 2005). Instead of a registration of the whole frame, we track the cardiac structures along the sequence as in (Prêteux, Rougon, & Discher, 2006). Following the work proposed in (Aubert, Barlaud, Faugeras & Jehan-Besson, 2003), we use non-parametric PDFs to characterize the distribution of the intensity inside the region. From an initial segmentation of the left ventricle, we track this structure along the sequence by minimizing the distance between the PDF of the intensity of the current region and the PDF of the intensity of the previous one. The evolution equation is given by equation (26). We give here preliminary results on MRI myocardial perfusion sequences acquired on 6 segments in short axis. In Figure 8, we show the evolution of the curve in one frame of the sequence and the joint evolution of the PDF of the inside region. This PDF converges towards the reference PDF as shown in Figure 8.

8.4 Discussion

The experimental results are given in order to prove the applicability of our general setting to medical image segmentation. Indeed, we can observe that various types of noise often contribute to degrade medical images (Gaussian, Poisson, Rayleigh). Our general framework allows the use of these noise models that are covered by the exponential family. As mentioned in (Lecellier, Jehan-Besson, Fadili, Aubert, & Revenu, 2006), the noise model has an influence on the accuracy of the segmentation and on its robustness. The examples show that relevant results are obtained both in MRI and echocardiographic images. Quantitative validation steps still need to be performed for the tested modalities. When dealing with non-homogeneous objects, we propose to rather take full advantage of non parametric PDFs where no assumption is made on the distribution. This has been exploited for tracking the LV in p-MRI sequences.

Medical structures are often really complex and sometimes not very contrasted. In this case maximization of neighbouring PDFs can be problematic and may lead to unsatisfactory local minima. The addition of a shape prior can then be crucial for many applications. In (Lecellier, Jehan-Besson, Fadili, Aubert, Revenu, & Saloux, 2006), we propose to combine our statistical data terms with a shape prior computed using its Legendre Moments based on the work of (Foulonneau, Charbonnier, & Heitz, 2003). Indeed, moments (The & Chin, 1988) give a region-based compact representation of shapes through the projection of their characteristic functions on an orthogonal

Figure 8. Minimization of the distance between the current region PDF (blue) and a reference one (red) corresponding to a reference segmentation given in (a) (the PDFs are the PDFs of the intensity I within each region). The initial and final contours are given in frames (b) and the joint PDFs are given in (c) and (d)

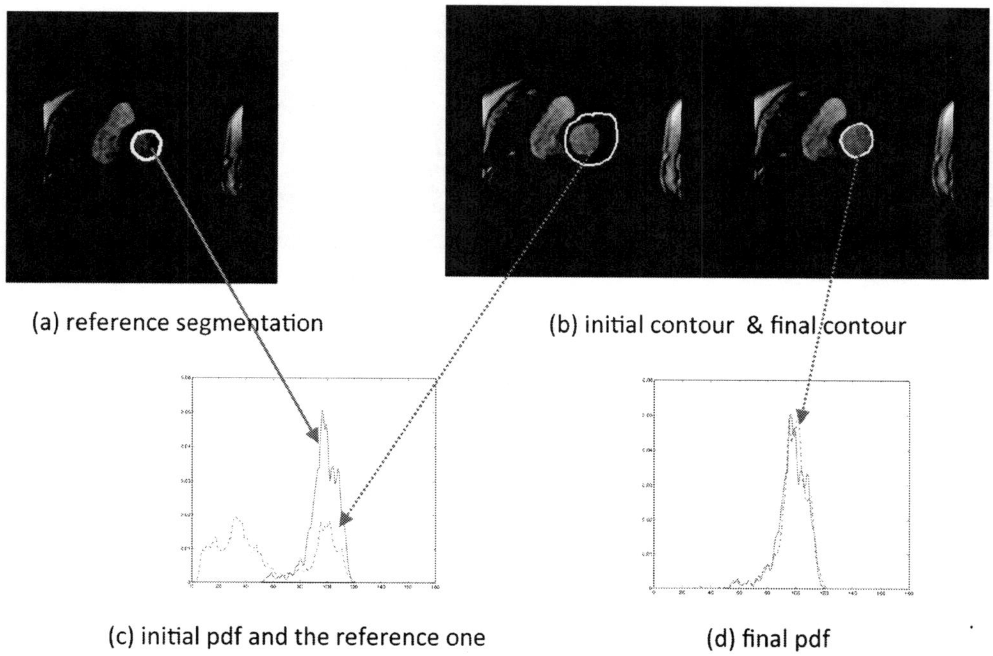

basis such as Legendre polynomials. Scale and translation invariances can be advantageously added as in (Foulonneau, Charbonnier, & Heitz, 2003) for their application to region segmentation, hence avoiding the registration step. To drive this functional towards its minimum, the geometrical PDE is iteratively run without the shape prior, then the shape prior term is updated, and the active contour evolves again by running the PDE with the shape prior. This procedure is repeated until convergence. This extension can be used for the segmentation of the LV in echocardiographic sequences (Lecellier, Jehan-Besson, Fadili, Aubert, Revenu, & Saloux, 2006).

9 CONCLUSION

In this chapter, we propose to give a general setting for the optimization of divergences between PDFs. Such a general setting is valuable for regions segmentation or tracking in medical images or sequences. As far as the segmentation of homogeneous regions is concerned, we propose to maximize the distance between two parametric PDFs belonging to the exponential family. General results are given for the shape derivative and an explicit expression is given when using the KL divergence and the ML estimator of the parameters. On the other hand, we also propose to track non-homogenous regions through the minimization of the distance between the current PDF of the intensity within the region and a reference one. General results are given for the shape derivative using a Parzen kernel estimator of the PDF. Experimental results are given for various modalities (T1-weighted MRI, contrast echocardiography, p-MRI) with different noise models. The generality of this approach is then proven through the accuracy of the segmentation results. This general setting could take benefit of the addition of a shape prior based on the Legendre Moments for the segmentation of very low contrasted regions (e.g echocardiography). Moreover it could be extended to some other parametric laws such as the Rician model which is a better model for low-intensity noise in T1-weighted MRI images.

ACKNOWLEDGMENT

The authors would like to thank Dr. Eric Saloux (CHU Caen) for contrast echocardiography data and Dr. M. Hamon (CHU Caen) for p-MRI sequences. We also want to notice that the part of this work on p-MRI sequences is granted by General Electric Healthcare. The authors also thank Pr. M. Barlaud from Laboratory I3S (France) who contributes to the theoretical work with non parametric PDFs.

REFERENCES

Angelini, E., Song, T., Mensh, B., & Laine, A. F. (2007). Brain MRI Segmentation with multiphase minimal partitioning: a comparative study. *Int.l Journal of Biomedical Imaging.*

Aubert, G., Barlaud, M., Faugeras, O., & Jehan-Besson, S. (2003). Image segmentation using active contours: Calculus of variations or shape gradients? *SIAM Applied Mathematics, 63*(6), 2128–2154. doi:10.1137/S0036139902408928

Aujol, J.-F., Aubert, G., & Blanc-Féraud, L. (2003). Wavelet-based level set evolution for classification of textured images. *IEEE Transactions on Image Processing, 12*(12), 1634–1641. doi:10.1109/TIP.2003.819309

Banerjee, A., Dhillon, I., Ghosh, J., & Merugu, S. (2004). An information theoretic analysis of maximum likelihood mixture estimation for exponential families. In *International Conference on Machine Learning,* 57–64.

Bickel, P. J., & Docksum, K. A. (2001). *Mathematical statistics: basic ideas and selected topics* (2nd ed., *Vol. I*). London: Prentice Hall.

Caselles, V., Catte, F., Coll, T., & Dibos, F. (1993). A geometric model for active contours. *Numerische Mathematik, 66,* 1–31. doi:10.1007/BF01385685

Caselles, V., Kimmel, R., & Sapiro, G. (1997). Geodesic active contours. *International Journal of Computer Vision, 22*(1), 61–79. doi:10.1023/A:1007979827043

Chakraborty, A., Staib, L., & Duncan, J. (1996). Deformable boundary finding in medical images by integrating gradient and region information. *IEEE Transactions on Medical Imaging, 15,* 859–870. doi:10.1109/42.544503

Chan, T., & Vese, L. (2001). Active contours without edges. *IEEE Transactions on Image Processing, 10*(2), 266–277. doi:10.1109/83.902291

Cheng, L., Yang, J., & Fan, X. (2005). A new region-based active contour for object extraction using level set method. *Pattern Recognition and Image Analysis, 3522,* 285–291.

Cohen, L., Bardinet, E., & Ayache, N. (1993). Surface reconstruction using active contour models. *SPIE Conference on Geometric Methods in Computer Vision.*

Cohen, L. D. (1991). On active contour models and balloons. *Computer Vision, Graphics, and Image Processing. Image Understanding, 53*(2), 211–218. doi:10.1016/1049-9660(91)90028-N

Cremers, D., Rousson, M., & Deriche, R. (2007). A review of statistical approaches to level set segmentation: Integrating color, texture, motion and shape. *International Journal of Computer Vision*, *72*(2), 195–215. doi:10.1007/s11263-006-8711-1

Cremers, D., Tischhäuser, F., Weickert, J., & Schnörr, C. (2002). Diffusion snakes: Introducing statistical shape knowledge into the Mumford-Shah functional. *IJCV*, *50*, 295–313. doi:10.1023/A:1020826424915

Debreuve, E., Gastaud, M., Barlaud, M., & Aubert, G. (2007). Using the shape gradient for active contour segmentation: from the continuous to the discrete formulation. *Journal of Mathematical Imaging and Vision*, *28*(1), 47–66. doi:10.1007/s10851-007-0012-y

Delfour, M. C., & Zolésio, J. P. (2001). *Shape and geometries. Advances in Design and Control*. SIAM.

Duda, R., & Hart, P. (1973). *Pattern Classification and Scene Analysis*. John Wiley & Sons.

Dydenko, I., Jamal, F., Bernard, O., D'Hooge, J., Magnin, I. E., & Friboulet, D. (2006). A level set framework with a shape and motion prior for segmentation and region tracking in echocardiography. [Bas du formulaire]. *Medical Image Analysis*, *10*(2), 162–177. doi:10.1016/j.media.2005.06.004

Foulonneau, A., Charbonnier, P., & Heitz, F. (2003). Geometric shape priors for region-based active contours. *In International Conference on Image Processing*.

Galland, F., Bertaux, N., & Réfrégier, P. (2005). Multi-component image segmentation in homogeneous regions based on description length minimization: Application to speckle, Poisson and Bernoulli noise. *Pattern Recognition*, *38*, 1926–1936. doi:10.1016/j.patcog.2004.10.002

Gastaud, M., Barlaud, M., & Aubert, G. (2003). Tracking video objects using active contours and geometric priors, In *IEEE Workshop on Image Analysis and Multimedia Interactive Services*, 170-175.

Gomes, J., & Faugeras, O. (2000). Reconciling distance functions and level sets. *Journal of Visual Communication and Image Representation*, *11*, 209–223. doi:10.1006/jvci.1999.0439

Goodman, J. W. (1976). Some fundamental properties of speckle. *Journal of the Optical Society of America*, *66*, 1145–1150. doi:10.1364/JOSA.66.001145

Gubjartsson, H., & Patz, S. (1995). *The Rician distribution of noisy MRI data*. Magnetic Resonance Medecine.

Hashimoto, A., & Kudo, H. (2000). Ordered-subsets EM algorithm for image segmentation with application to brain MRI. In *IEEE Nuclear Symposium and Medical Imaging Conference*.

Henkelman, R. M. (1985). Measurement of signal intensities in the presence of noise in MR images. *Medical Physics*, 232–233. doi:10.1118/1.595711

Jehan-Besson, S., Barlaud, M., & Aubert, G. (2001). Video object segmentation using eulerian region-based active contours. In *International Conference on Computer Vision*.

Jehan-Besson, S., Barlaud, M., & Aubert, G. (2003). DREAM^{2}S: Deformable regions driven by an Eulerian accurate minimization method for image and video segmentation. *International Journal of Computer Vision*, *53*, 45–70. doi:10.1023/A:1023031708305

Jehan-Besson, S., Barlaud, M., & Aubert, G. (2003). Shape gradients for histogram segmentation using active contours. In *International Conference on Computer Vision*.

Karoui, I., Fablet, R., Boucher, J. M., & Augustin, J. M. (2006). *Region-based image segmentation using texture statistics and level-set methods In*. ICASSP.

Kass, M., Witkin, A., & Terzopoulos, D. (1988). Snakes: Active contour models. *International Journal of Computer Vision*, *1*, 321–332. doi:10.1007/BF00133570

Klauschen, F., Goldman, A., Barra, V., Meyer-Lindenberg, A., & Lundervold, A. (2008). Evaluation of Automated Brain MR Image Segmentation and Volumetry methods. *Human Brain Mapping*, *30*, 1310–1327. doi:10.1002/hbm.20599

Koopman, P. O. (1936). On distributions admitting a sufficient statistic. *Transactions of the American Mathematical Society*, *39*, 399–409.

Kullback, S. (1959). *Information Theory and Statistics*. New York: Wiley.

Lau, P. Y., & Ozawa, S. (2004). A region-based approach combining marker-controlled active contour model and morphological operator for image segmentation. *In IEEE engineering in Medicine and Biology Society, 165–170.*

Lecellier, F., Fadili, J., Jehan-Besson, S., Aubert, G., & Revenu, M. (2010). Region-based active contours with exponential family observations. *International Journal on Mathematical Imaging and Vision*, *36*, 28–45. doi:10.1007/s10851-009-0168-8

Lecellier, F., Jehan-Besson, S., Fadili, J., Aubert, G., & Revenu, M. (2006). *Statistical region-based active contours with exponential family observations*. ICASSP.

Lecellier, F., Jehan-Besson, S., Fadili, J., Aubert, G., Revenu, M., & Saloux, E. (2006). *Region-based active contours with noise and shape priors*. ICIP.

Leventon, M. (2000). *Statistical Models for Medical Image Analysis*. Ph.D. thesis, MIT.

Li, H., Yezzi, A., & Cohen, L.D. (2006). 3D Brain cortex segmentation using dual-front active contours with optional user-interaction. *International Journal of Biomedical Imaging*.

Marroquin, J. L., Vemuri, B. C., Botello, S., Calderon, F., & Fernandez-Bouzas, A. (2002). An accurate and efficient Bayesian method for automatic segmentation of brain MRI. *IEEE Transactions on Medical Imaging*, *21*(8), 934–945. doi:10.1109/TMI.2002.803119

Martin, P., Réfrégier, P., Goudail, F., & Guérault, F. (2004). Influence of the noise model on level set active contour segmentation. *IEEE PAMI*, *26*, 799–803.

Martin, P., Réfrégier, P., Goudail, F., & Guérault, F. (2004). Influence of the noise model on level set active contour segmentation. *IEEE PAMI*, *26*(6), 799–803.

Michailovich, O., Rathi, Y., & Tannenbaum, A. (2007). Image segmentation using active contours driven by the Bhattacharyya gradient flow. *IEEE Trans.s on Image Processing, 16*, 2787-2801.

Osher, S., & Sethian, J. A. (1988). Fronts propagating with curvature-dependent speed: Algorithms based on Hamilton-jacobi formulation. *Journal of Computational Physics*, *79*, 12–49. doi:10.1016/0021-9991(88)90002-2

Paelinck, B. P., & Kasprzak, J. D. (1999). Contrast-enhanced echocardiography: review and current role. *Acta Cardiologica*, *54*(4), 195–201.

Paragios, N. (2002). A Variational Approach for the Segmentation of the Left Ventricle. *International Journal of Computer Vision*, 345–362. doi:10.1023/A:1020882509893

Paragios, N., & Deriche, R. (2000). Coupled geodesic active regions for image segmentation: A level set approach. In *European Conference in Computer Vision*.

Paragios, N., & Deriche, R. (2002). Geodesic active regions and level set methods for supervised texture segmentation. *International Journal of Computer Vision*, *46*(3), 223. doi:10.1023/A:1014080923068

Paragios, N., & Deriche, R. (2002). Geodesic active regions: A new paradigm to deal with frame partition problems in computer vision. *Journal of Visual Communication and Image Representation*, *13*, 249–268. doi:10.1006/jvci.2001.0475

Pickard, J. E., Hossack, J. A., & Acton, S. T. (2006). Shape model segmentation of long-axis contrast enhanced echocardiography. *IEEE Int. Symp. on Biomedical Imaging Nano to Macro*.

Prêteux, F., Rougon, N., & Discher, A. (2006). Region-based statistical segmentation using informational active contours. In *Proceedings SPIE Conference on Mathematics of Data/Image Pattern Recognition, Compression, and Encryption with Applications IX*.

Rathi, Y., Michailovich, O., Malcolm, J., & Tannenbaum, A. (2006). Seeing the unseen: Segmenting with distributions. In *International Conference on Signal and Image Processing*.

Ronfard, R. (1994). Region-based strategies for active contour models. *International Journal of Computer Vision*, *13*(2), 229–251. doi:10.1007/BF01427153

Rougon, N., Petitjean, C., Preteux, F., Cluzel, P., & Grenier, P. (2005). A non-rigid registration approach for quantifying myocardial contraction in tagged MRI using generalized information measures. *Medical Image Analysis*, *9*(4), 353–375. doi:10.1016/j.media.2005.01.005

Rousson, M., Lenglet, C., & Deriche, R. (2004). Level set and region based surface propagation for diffusion tensor MRI segmentation, In *Computer Vision Approaches to Medical Image Analysis nd Mathematical Methods in Biomedical Image Analysis Workshop*.

Ruan, S., Jaggi, C., Xue, J., Fadili, J., & Bloyet, D. (2000). Brain Tissue classification of magnetic resonance images using partial volume modeling. *IEEE Transactions on Medical Imaging*, *19*(12), 1179–1187. doi:10.1109/42.897810

Schiller, N. B., Shah, P. M., Crawford, M., DeMaria, A., Devereux, R., & Feigenbaum, H. (1989). Recommendations for quantitation of the left ventricle by two-dimensional echocardiography. American Society of Echocardiography Committee on Standards, Subcommittee on Quantitation of Two-Dimensional Echocardiograms. *Journal of the American Society of Echocardiography*, *2*(5), 358–367.

Shattuck, D. W., & Leahy, R. M. (2002). BrainSuite: an automated cortical surface identification tool. *Medical Image Analysis*, *6*(2), 129–142. doi:10.1016/S1361-8415(02)00054-3

Smith, S. M. (2002). Fast robust automated brain extraction. *Human Brain Mapping*, *17*(3), 143–155. doi:10.1002/hbm.10062

Sokolowski, J., & Zolésio, J. P. (1992). *Introduction to shape optimization* (Vol. 16 of Springer series in computational mathematics). Springer-Verlag.

Stegmann, M. B., Olafsdottir, H., & Larsson, H. B. W. (2005). Unsupervised motion-compensation of multi-slice cardiac perfusion MRI. *Medical Image Analysis*, *9*(4), 394–410. doi:10.1016/j.media.2004.10.002

The, C. H., & Chin, R. T. (1988). On image analysis by the methods of moments. *IEEE Pattern Analysis and Machine Intelligence*, *10*, 496–513. doi:10.1109/34.3913

Tsai, A., Yezzi, A., & Wells, W. (2003). A shape-based approach to the segmentation of medical imagery using level sets. *IEEE Transactions on Medical Imaging*, *22*, 137–154. doi:10.1109/TMI.2002.808355

Vannier, M. W., Butterfield, R. L., Jordan, S., Murphy, W. A., Levitt, R. G., & Gado, M. (1988). Multispectral analysis of magnetic resonance images. *Radiology, 154*, 221–224.

Vese, L. A., & Chan, T. (2002). A multiphase level set framework for image segmentation using the Mumford and Shah model. *International Journal of Computer Vision, 50*, 271–293. doi:10.1023/A:1020874308076

Yang, J., & Duncan, J. S. (2003). *3D image segmentation of deformable objects with shape appearance joint prior models*. MICCAI.

Zavaljevski, A., Dhawan, A. P., Gaskil, M., Ball, W., & Johnson, J. D. (2000). Multi-level adaptative segmentation of multi-parameter MR brain images. *Computerized Medical Imaging and Graphics, 24*(2), 87–98. doi:10.1016/S0895-6111(99)00042-7

Zeng, X., Staib, L. H., Schultz, R. T., & Duncan, J. S. (1999). Segmentation and measurement of the cortex from 3D MR images using coupled-surfaces propagation. *IEEE Transactions on Medical Imaging, 18*(10), 927–937. doi:10.1109/42.811276

Zhang, Y., Brady, M., & Smith, S. (2001). Segmentation of brain MR images through a hidden Markov random field model and the expectation-maximisation algorithm. *IEEE Transactions on Medical Imaging, 20*(1), 45–57. doi:10.1109/42.906424

Zhu, S., & Yuille, A. (1996). Region competition: unifying snakes, region growing, and bayes/MDL for multiband image segmentation. *IEEE Transactions on Pattern Analysis and Machine Intelligence, 18*, 884–900. doi:10.1109/34.537343

APPENDIX A: PROOF OF THEOREM 1

To compute $< D'(\Omega), \mathbf{V}>$, we must first get the derivative of $q_\eta(y(x))$ with respect to the domain, and apply the chain rule to $\Psi(q_\eta(y(x)), p(y))$. To simplify the notation we write the Eulerian derivative of η as:

$$< \eta'(\Omega), \mathbf{V} >= \nabla_V \eta = [< \eta'_1(\Omega), V >,.., < \eta'_\kappa(\Omega), V >]^T.$$

Using the definition of $q_\eta(y)$ given in (8) and the chain rule applied to $A(\eta(\Omega))$, we obtain:

$$\begin{aligned} < q^{'}(y), \mathbf{V} > &= h(y)\Big(< \nabla_v\eta, \mathbf{T}(y) > - < \nabla_v\eta, \nabla A(\eta) > \exp\big(< \eta(\Omega), \mathbf{T}(y) > -A(\eta)\big)\Big) \\ &= q_\eta(y) < \nabla_v\eta, \mathbf{T}(y) - \nabla A(\eta) > . \end{aligned}$$

By the chain rule applied to $\Psi(q_\eta(y), p(y))$, we get:

$$< \Psi'(q_\eta(y), p(y)), \mathbf{V} >=< q'_\eta(y), \mathbf{V} > \partial_1\Psi(q, p).$$

which gives:

$$< D'(\Omega), \mathbf{V} >= \int_{\chi} q_\eta(y)\, \partial_1\Psi(q,p) < \nabla_v\eta, T(y) - \nabla A(\eta) > dy$$

We introduce:

$$\mathbf{C}(\Omega) = \int_{\chi} q_\eta(y)\, \partial_1\Psi(q,p)\ \big(\mathbf{T}(y) - \nabla A(\eta)\big)\,dy = E\Big[\partial_1\Psi(q,p)\ \big(\mathbf{T}(y) - E[\mathbf{T}(Y)]\big)\Big]$$

which completes the proof.

APPENDIX B: PROOF OF LEMMA 1

When using the MLE, the term $E[\mathbf{T}(Y)]$ can be empirically estimated with $\overline{\mathbf{T}(Y)}$ and so derived easily with respect to the domain Ω. We propose to directly derive the expression $\nabla A(\eta) = \mathbf{T}(y)$. This expression can be written as

$$\frac{\partial A}{\partial \eta_i}(\eta_1,\ldots,\eta_\kappa) = \overline{T_i(Y)} \quad \forall i \in [1,\kappa].$$

We can then compute the shape derivative of this expression, which gives:

$$\sum_{j=1}^{\kappa} < \eta_j', \mathbf{V} > \frac{\partial^2 A}{\partial\eta_i \partial\eta_j}(\eta) =< \overline{T_i(Y)}', V > \quad \forall i \in [1,\kappa],$$

which can be written in the compact form

$$\nabla_V(\overline{\mathbf{T}(Y)}) = \nabla^2 A(\eta)\nabla_v \eta \quad \text{where}$$

$$\nabla_v(\overline{\mathbf{T}(Y)}) = \left[<\overline{T_1(Y)}', \mathbf{V}>, <\overline{T_2(Y)}', \mathbf{V}>, \ldots, <\overline{T_\kappa(Y)}', \mathbf{V}>\right]^T.$$

Restricting our study to the full rank exponential family, where $\nabla^2 A(\eta)$ is a symmetric positive-definite, hence invertible, matrix (Theorem 3), the domain derivative of the parameters η is uniquely determined by $\nabla^2 A(\eta)^{-1}\nabla_V(\overline{\mathbf{T}(Y)}) = \nabla_v \eta$, where $\nabla_v(\overline{\mathbf{T}(Y)})$ is given by

$$\nabla_v(\overline{\mathbf{T}(Y)}) = \frac{1}{|\Omega|}\int_{\partial\Omega}\left(\overline{\mathbf{T}(Y)} - \mathbf{T}(y(a))\right)(\mathbf{V}\cdot\mathbf{N})\, da(\mathbf{x})$$

and the lemma follows.

APPENDIX C: PROOF OF LEMMA 2

Since p and q belongs to the same parametric law, they share the same value for h(y), T(y) and $A(\eta)$ then $\log(q) - \log(p) = <\eta - \eta_\mathbf{r}, T(y)> - A(\eta) + A(\eta_\mathbf{r})$.

The value of $\mathbf{C}$ is then: $\mathbf{C} = s_1 - s_2$, with:

$$s_1 = E\left[\left(<\eta - \eta_\mathbf{r}, T(y)> - A(\eta) + A(\eta_\mathbf{r}) + 1\right)\left(T_i(Y) - E\left[T_i(Y)\right]\right)\right]$$

$$s_2 = E\left[\frac{p}{q}(T_i(Y) - E[T_i(Y)]]E_p\left[T_i(Y) - E(T_i(Y)\right]\right]$$

and

$$E_p[T_i(Y)] = \int_{\chi} p_{n_r}(y)T_i(Y)dy.$$

Developing the expression of the expectation of the second term, we find:

$$s_2 = E_p[T_i(Y) - E[T_i(Y)]] = \nabla A(\mathbf{n}_\mathbf{r}) - \nabla A(\eta)$$

Using the linearity of the expectation, the first term becomes:

$$s_1 = \sum_{j=1}^{\kappa}(\eta_j - \eta_{rj})(E[T_j(Y)T_i(Y)] - E[T_i(Y)]E[T_j(Y)])$$

The term $E[T_j(Y)(T_i(Y)] - E[T_i(Y)]E[T_j(Y)]$ designates the covariance matrix of the sufficient statistics T and can then be replaced by $\nabla^2 A(\eta)_{ij}$= Cov[T(Y)]ij= $\nabla^2 A(\eta)_{j}$, which gives:

$$s_1 = \sum_{j=1}^{K} (\eta_j - \eta_{rj}) \nabla^2 A(\eta)_{ij}$$

and then:

$$\mathbf{C} = \nabla^2 A(\eta)(\eta - \eta_{\mathbf{r}}) + \nabla A(\eta) - \nabla A(\eta_{\mathbf{r}}).$$

Chapter 3
Modeling and Simulation of Deep Brain Stimulation in Parkinson's Disease

T. Heida
University of Twente, The Netherlands

R. Moroney
University of Twente, The Netherlands

E. Marani
University of Twente, The Netherlands

ABSTRACT

Deep Brain Stimulation (DBS) is effective in the Parkinsonian state, while it seems to produce rather non-selective stimulation over an unknown volume of tissue. Despite a huge amount of anatomical and physiological data regarding the structure of the basal ganglia (BG) and their connections, the computational processes performed by the basal ganglia in health and disease still remain unclear. Its hypothesized roles are discussed in this chapter as well as the changes that are observed under pathophysiological conditions. Several hypotheses exist in explaining the mechanism by which DBS provides its beneficial effects. Computational models of the BG span a range of structural levels, from low-level membrane conductance-based models of single neurons to high level system models of the complete BG circuit. A selection of models is presented in this chapter. This chapter aims at explaining how models of neurons and connected brain nuclei contribute to the understanding of DBS.

INTRODUCTION: PARKINSON'S DISEASE (PD)

Detection of MPTP

In 1982 in northern California, a young male, age 29, used a new synthetic heroin, injecting approximately 20 g of the drug intravenously during a 1-week period. "He had a long history of drug abuse beginning at age 22, including heroin, cocaine, marijuana, lysergic acid diethylamide (LSD) and amphetamine. Toward the end of the binge he experienced increasing slowness and rigidity. This culminated in admission to a local hospital where profound and unremitting Parkin-

DOI: 10.4018/978-1-60566-280-0.ch003

sonism was observed" (Langston et al. 1999). His brother, who had injected approximately the same drug in the same amounts, developed an identical clinical condition. Treatment with carbidopa/L-dopa resulted in marked improvement. In 1982, a group of approximately 300 young addicts in northern California may have been exposed to this substance; several of them developed severe Parkinsonism after intravenous injection of this new synthetic heroin that was being sold on the streets at the time.

A missing textbook on organic synthesis from the university library of San Francisco University led to a student engaged in the synthesis of designer drugs.The chemical modification of existent, often naturally occurring psychoactive drugs, i.e., "everything a kitchen chemist can engineer", are exempt from legal control because of their unique chemical structure. In this case Meperidine (Demerol, Pethidine) was used. Normally Meperidine relieves moderate to severe pain and belongs to the narcotic analgetics, a group of pain medications similar to morphine (see Langston et al. 1983). From this analgetic substance a new synthetic heroine was produced from Meperidine (ethyl ester of 1-methyl-4-phenyl-piperidine-carboxylic acid) into MPPP, the "designer heroin" (1-methyl-4-phenyl-4-propionoxypiperidine). Based on the samples obtained from his supplier the drug contained not only MPPP but also 2.5 to 2.9% of MPTP (1-methyl-4-phenyl-1,2,3,6-tetrahydropyridine) by weight, a byproduct in the synthesis of MPPP. Biotransformation produces from MPTP the 1-methyl-4-phenylpyridinium ion (MPP^+), which is taken up by the dopamine (DA) transporter of the substantia nigra neurons, where it blocks the mitochondrial respiratory chain (see Langston et al. 1999 and references herein).

An experimental monkey model was developed. MPTP was quickly shown experimentally to selectively destroy nerve cells in the substantia nigra after systemic administration. The resulting striatal dopamine depletion explained most, if not all of the clinical features of Parkinson's disease (PD) (for an extensive overview see: Langston et al. 1983, Langston et al. 1999, and an earlier report by Davis et al. 1979).

Although an experimental animal model is present and enormous efforts have been carried out to detect the cause of Parkinsonism, what initiates the disease still remains unknown. Moreover, human studies have an ethical drawback and a case as described above is seldom found in literature. Therefore, experimental results from animals, often not possible to translate to the human situation, especially rat and mouse results, is what scientists have to relay on. Consequently, model studies based on systems theory and neuroanatomical and neurophysiological data are of the utmost importance in the study of Parkinson's disease and are significant in their contribution to the understanding of Parkinson's disease and the mechanism(s) of Deep Brain Stimulation (DBS), nowadays mainly carried out in the subthalamic nucleus (Benabid et al. 2000).

Short History

The appreciation that the motor disorder of Parkinson's syndrome results from the degeneration of the extrapyramidal system and especially the degeneration of the substantia nigra came slowly (see Usunoff et al. 2002 and references herein). Parkinson's description in 1817 of the disease - "shaking palsy", "paralysis agitans"- "Involuntary tremulous motion, with lessened muscular power, in parts not in action and even when supported; with a propensity to bend the trunk forwards, and to pass from a walking to a running pace: the senses and intellects being uninjured." speculated on a disease state of the spinal cord and medulla oblongata. Although a tuberculoma was found in the substantia nigra in a patient with hemiparkinsonism around 1819 (see Usunoff et al. 2002 for references) the primary importance of the substantia nigra escaped for a further quarter of a century scientific notice. Lewy (1912, 1914) directed the attention to the globus pallidus and putamen.

He proposed a dysfunction of the thyroid gland. Attracted by the results of Von Economo (1917, 1918), the special involvement of the substantia nigra in encephalitis lethargica (with the same clinical picture as paralysis agitans), brought Tetriakoff (1919) to study the pathological anatomy of the substantia nigra. He found in a series of "Parkinsonian" patients lesions in the substantia nigra. These results were repeatedly reported in the nineteen twenties (see Usunoff et al. 2002 for references). Finally, it was Hassler (1937, 1938, and 1939) who by his cytoarchitectonic studies illuminated the problem. He found that large parts of the substantia nigra degenerated, but not all. The most spared areas are in the lateral rostral and medial caudal substantia nigra (for an atlas of the substantia nigra and the parts that degenerates see Usunoff et al. 2002).

Still scientists opposed the results (Meyers 1958, Denny-Brown 1962, and others). Mettler (1944, 1964) resisted the results, since primate lesions in the substantia nigra did not brought forward the clinical symptoms known in Parkinson's disease. Now in the "dopaminergic era" it is firmly established that Parkinson's disease in humans is due to substantia nigra degeneration, causing a depletion of dopamine in the striatum.

Norepinephrine and Acetylcholine

One should note that Hassler (1938) already reported that other catecholaminergic nuclei are also involved in Parkinson's disease. The locus coeruleus, for example, is also injured, indicating that other than the dopaminergic system of the catecholaminergic systems are damaged by the disease. This noradrenergic nucleus undergoes degeneration in the rostral direction: caudal parts heavily degenerate, while rostral parts are seemingly spared. Strange enough this is not reported in the three post-mortem studied MPTP patients (see Langston et al. 1999), indicating that MPP^+ directs itself exclusively to the substantia nigra dopamine transporter.

The pedunculopontine nucleus (PPN) has been found to degenerate also during Parkinsonism, at the same time as the substantia nigra (Braak et al. 2004). A serious reduction in the acetylcholine producing enzyme choline acetyl transferase mRNA has been found in MPTP treated cynomolgus monkeys (Gomez-Gallego et al. 2007).

Neuromelanin

Most catecholaminergic areas in the brain are characterized by the presence of neuromelanin which is a by-product of the catecholaminergic metabolism. The amount of cells loaded with neuromelanin is differential. The highest amount of neuromelanin positive cells is found in the substantia nigra (80-90%). Degeneration of the substantia nigra releases the "black substance" from its blackness, due to the inherent removal of neuromelanin by the degeneration. However, catecholaminergic areas in the central grey only contain 3% of neurons loaded with neuromelanin. Therefore, disappearance of neuromelanin does not give an indication of the severity of the degeneration in most nuclei, except in the substantia nigra (Usunoff et al. 2002 and references herein).

Lewy Bodies

In neuropathology it was found that Lewy bodies (Lewy, 1913) are invariable present in a portion of the surviving neurons in the substantia nigra. Lewy bodies are eosinophilic, round, 5-20 μm in diameter balls with a central core, surrounded by a pale-staining halo. Lewy bodies are considered the hallmark of Parkinson's disease in the substantia nigra. If no Lewy bodies are found the diagnosis is not Parkinson's disease. In fact an absolute diagnosis therefore is always made after death by the neuropathologist (see Usunoff et al. 2002 for references and for more information). In MPTP patients Lewy bodies were not found (Langston et al. 1999).

Types of Parkinson's Diseases

The types of Parkinson's diseases are based on neuropathological evidence. The main subdivision is: Idiopathic Parkinsonism and Multisystem degenerations, also called "Parkinson-plus syndromes". Parkinson-plus syndromes are Parkinson's diseases in combination with degenerations of other parts of the central nervous system. To these multisystem degenerations belong: progressive supranuclear palsy, Parkinsonism-dementia complex (better known as Guam Parkinsonism-dementia disease), corticobasal degeneration, multiple system atrophy (MSA), Pick's disease, and early-onset Parkinsonism. Other diseases can also be involved in the degeneration of the substantia nigra: Huntington's disease, Hallervorden-Spatz disease and even Alzheimer's disease. There are some rare neuronal degenerative disorders that also involve the substantia nigra (for an extensive overview see Usunoff et al. 2002). It should be made clear here that all models concerning Parkinson's disease concern idiopathic Parkinsonism. Moreover in these models the inherent supposition is that the whole substantia nigra pars compacta is degenerated, which is only partially true (see above).

Parkinson Symptoms

PD motor symptoms are classically discerned in rhythmic tremor of resting muscles (present in 70-100% of the patients) and (associated to it) stiffness (rigidity; present in 89-99% of the patients), and slowness of movement (bradykinesia: slow movement, hypokinesia: reduced movements; present in 77-98% of the patients) or absence or loss of voluntary movements (akinesia). There is no deterioration in sensation. Swallowing or digestion as well as sphincter function is not affected. Speech becomes blurred in later stages if the movements of tongue, jaw and larynx muscles are slowed, which can be so impaired by muscular rigidity and akinesia that the patient is virtually mute.

Tremor concerns rhythmic alternating contractions of opposing muscular groups at a frequency of 3-8 Hz. Fingers and thumb show this in the so-called "pill rolling" phenomenon. There is irregular fluctuation in the amplitude of the movements, going over from the fingers to the wrist or elbow and afterwards returning back to the fingers. It also may occur in the ankle or knee with the same fluctuations. It can be present in the lips and the eyelids, when lightly closed or in the relaxed tongue and palate. It is rarely found in the trunk musculature or extra-ocular muscles. Strong contractions, sleep and total relaxation of axial musculature damp the tremor. Tremor increases during stress and anxiety.

Rigidity and hypokinesia: Rigidity is present in the affected limbs at each joint. As a reaction to movement (passive or active) plastic resistance occurs and is more intense in flexors than in extensors. This relaxing resistance shows rhythmic fluctuations named the "cogwheel phenomenon". The rigidity is more widespread than the tremor, influencing spine and neck too. This results in the "stooped" posture with slightly flexed upper limb and hip joints. Dyskinesia and dystonia comprise the persistent maintenance of a posture by exaggerated muscle tone. In dystonia the posture is not an intermediate between flexion or extension as dyskinesia is in Parkinson's disease. Power and contraction of muscles, as the reflexes, are not impaired, only movement is. Reflexes can be submerged due to the rigidity of the muscles. Facial musculature is also involved, affecting the facial expression with an unnatural immobility. Together with the absence of smaller movements of the face, this gives the "Parkinsonian mask". In Parkinson's disease gait is also disturbed. The limitation of movement results in small steps in walking (marche à petits pas) and initiation of movement is retarded. The slowness in compensatory movements results in difficulty to maintain balance. A few steps backward (retropulsion) or forward (propulsion), turning or maintaining balance is difficult. Micrographia is common; the writing becomes progressively smaller and may trail away to nothing (partially taken from Brain and Walton 1969).

BACKGROUND: COMPUTATIONAL MODELING OF BASAL GANGLIA (BG) FUNCTION

The basal ganglia (BG) exert a critical influence over the control of voluntary movement, and a wide range of movement disorders arise due to BG dysfunction. An abundance of computational models have been developed in an attempt to explain the role of the BG in health and disease. The starting point for modeling is the interpretation the researcher gives to the function of the BG. Since there are such diverse thoughts on BG function, inherently various approaches have been chosen, resulting in computational models that differ in a number of ways:

- Level of analysis (system vs. cellular level)
- Incorporation of anatomical and/or physiological data
- Capability of explaining PD symptoms
- Role assigned to the BG
- Inclusion of effects of DBS or medication

System level models use a comparatively high level of abstraction, in which the BG are decomposed into functional units, with each nucleus being modelled as a single equation, representing the combined actions of all neurons or a set of neurons within the nucleus. The advantage of system-level models is that they allow the exploration of the role of the BG in the global control of voluntary movement, within the context of the complete BG-thalamocortical circuit. They also allow the investigation of the effect on the circuit's behaviour caused by an additional path or component. However, as systems-level models are based on the mean firing rates of nuclei, the nature of the firing pattern (bursting, oscillatory, irregular) is obscured. For example a regular tonic activity level may result in the same average firing rate as a bursty firing pattern with intervals of quiet.

Cellular level models, which are based on detailed cell activity at the membrane level, can provide more detailed firing pattern information. The nature of the firing pattern, which underlies the mean firing rate outputs of system-level models, can be explored. The recent emphasis on the importance of changes in firing pattern in the normal and abnormal functioning of the BG may indicate a need to model nuclei at a more detailed level. However, cellular-level models typically look only at the activity of single nuclei, or the interactions of relatively few nuclei, and the number of cells included in the models is limited.

The sequence generation and selection model of Berns et al. (1998) proposes that the BG is capable of learning sequences of actions by reinforcement mechanisms and of reproducing the learned action sequences. Reinforcement learning specifies how a sequence of actions can be learned through reward signals provided at the conclusion of the sequence. Most computational models demonstrating reinforcement learning in the BG are based on the Actor-Critic model, for example the model of Suri and Schultz (1998), which demonstrates the learning of long sequences of pattern associations, or the computational model of working memory based on the prefrontal cortex and basal ganglia of O'Reilley and Frank (2006). In addition, Frank (2005) presented a theoretical basis for cognitive procedural learning functions of basal ganglia that provides a mechanistic account of cognitive deficits observed in Parkinson's patients.

As reinforcement learning models are based more on the learning of sequences of actions than the facilitation of actions, these models are not treated in this chapter. The models in this chapter are restricted to BG motor functions.

Before discussing a number of selected computational models at different levels, the connections in basal ganglia, their hypothesized roles and the changes observed in Parkinson's disease are described.

THE CONNECTIONS IN BASAL GANGLIA

The classic view of the pathways through the basal ganglia (BG) was first proposed by Alexander et al. (1986), Albin et al. (1989), and De Long (1990). According to these authors, two major connections link the BG input nucleus (striatum) to the output nuclei (globus pallidus internus/ substantia nigra pars reticulata: GPi/SNr), namely the "direct" and "indirect" pathways (Figure 1 and Figure 10). Normal motor behaviour depends on a critical balance between these two pathways. The BG output nuclei have a high rate of spontaneous discharge, and thus exert a tonic, GABA-mediated, inhibitory effect on their target nuclei in the thalamus. The inhibitory outflow is differentially modulated by the direct and indirect pathways, which have opposing effects on the BG output nuclei, and thus on the thalamic targets of these nuclei. The spiny projection neuron is the major projection neuron of the striatum and therefore can be subdivided in two subpopulations that constitute the direct and indirect pathways. The spiny neurons make up 95% of all the striatal projection neurons (Gerfen and Wilson 1996)

It should be noted that the classical definition of the basal ganglia (BG) as: putamen, nucleus caudatus, globus pallidus internus (entopeduncular nucleus in rats) and externus together with substantia nigra and subthalamic nucleus (STN) (Nieuwenhuys et al. 2008) has been extended by Heimer et al. (1982), in which both the ventral pallidum (within it the accumbens nucleus) and

Figure 1. Schematic overview of the connections involved and their relative connection strengths in the corticothalamic-basal ganglia motor loop for A) the normal situation, and B) the Parkinsonian situation. blue lines indicate inhibitory pathways; red lines indicate excitatory pathways. In the Parkinsonian situation an imbalance exists between direct and indirect pathway, the excitatory input from STN is increased while the inhibitory effect of the direct pathway is decreased, resulting in overactivity in the output nuclei of the basal ganglia causing a strong inhibition of the thalamus

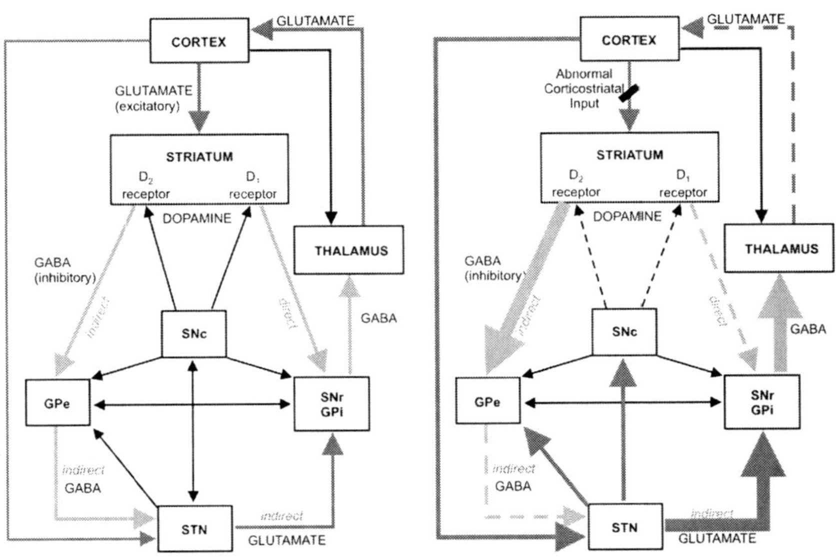

A) B)

certain olfactory areas are added, explaining emotional or motivational stimuli (called the associative module). Kelley et al. (1982) developed a comparable concept for the amygdala, explaining limbic aspects of the system. Therefore, motor, limbic and associative striatal circuits are discerned (for an overview see: Nieuwenhuys et al. 2008, Temel et al. 2005, and Gerfen and Wilson 1996). In this chapter only the motor circuitry is considered.

Terminology of the basal ganglia is inconsequent and frequently misused (Mettler, 1968). Therefore, in this chapter the following definitions are used: striatum contains putamen and caudate nucleus, corpus striatum encompasses putamen, caudate nucleus and globus pallidus, while lentiform nucleus is the globus pallidus and the putamen.

The pedunculopontine nucleus (initiator of movements, the automatic regulation of postural muscle tone and gait or rhythmic limb movements) is by various authors added to the basal ganglia (e.g. Gerfen and Wilson, 1996) and by others considered a brain stem nucleus (Marani et al. 2008).

Direct and Indirect Pathway

The direct pathway arises from spiny inhibitory striatal efferents that contain GABA, dynorphin and substance P and projects directly to the output nuclei: globus pallidus internus (GPi) and pars reticulata of the substantia nigra (SNr). It is transiently activated by increased phasic excitatory input from the substantia nigra pars compacta (SNc) to the striatum. Activation of the direct pathway briefly suppresses the tonically active inhibitory neurons of the output nuclei, disinhibiting the thalamus, and thus increasing thalamocortical activity (Figure 1 and Figure 10).

The indirect pathway arises from spiny inhibitory striatal efferents that contain both GABA and enkephalin. These striatal neurons project to the globus pallidus externus (GPe) (but also to the GPi). The GPe projects to the STN, via a purely GABAergic pathway, which finally projects to the output nuclei via an excitatory, glutamatergic projection. The indirect pathway is phasically activated by decreased inhibitory input from the SNc to the striatum, causing an increase in striatal output. Activation of the indirect pathway tends to suppress the activity of GPe neurons, disinhibiting the STN, and increasing the excitatory drive on the output nuclei, thereby decreasing thalamocortical activity (Figure 1 and 9).

During the execution of specific motor acts, movement-related neurons within the BG output nuclei may show either phasic increases or phasic decreases in their normally high rates of spontaneous discharge. Voluntary movements are normally associated with a graded phasic reduction of GPi discharge mediated by the direct pathway, disinhibiting the thalamus and thereby gating or facilitating cortically initiated movements. Phasic increases in GPi discharge may have the opposite effect (Alexander and Crutcher 1990).

There is still debate as to the exact role of the direct and indirect pathways in the control of movement. Two hypotheses have been put forward (Alexander and Crutcher 1990):

1. *Scaling hypothesis*: Both the direct and indirect inputs to the BG output nuclei may be directed to the same set of GPi neurons, whereby the temporal interplay between the activity of direct and indirect inputs allows the BG to influence the characteristics of movements as they are carried out. With this arrangement, the direct pathway facilitates movement, and then, after a delay, the indirect pathway "brakes" or "smoothes" the same cortically initiated motor pattern that was being reinforced by the direct pathway.
2. *Focusing hypothesis*: The direct and indirect inputs associated with a particular motor pattern could be directed to separate sets of GPi neurons. In this configuration, the motor circuit would play a role in reinforc-

ing the currently selected pattern via the direct pathway and suppressing potentially conflicting patterns via the indirect pathway. Overall, this could result in the focusing of neural activity underlying each cortically initiated movement in a centre-surround fashion, favouring intended and preventing unwanted movements.

Nigrostriatal dopamine projections exert contrasting effects on the direct and indirect pathways. Dopamine is released from the SNc into the synaptic cleft, where it binds to the receptors of the striatum. The effect of dopamine is determined by the type of receptor to which it binds. Striatal spiny neurons projecting in the direct pathway (containing GABA, dynorphin + substance P) have D1 dopamine receptors which cause excitatory post-synaptic potentials, thereby producing a net excitatory effect on striatal neurons of the direct pathway. Those spiny neurons projecting in the indirect pathway (containing GABA + enkephalin) have D2 receptors which cause inhibitory post-synaptic potentials, thereby producing a net inhibitory effect on striatal neurons of the indirect pathway. The facilitation of transmission along the direct pathway and suppression of transmission along the indirect pathway leads to the same effect – reducing inhibition of the thalamocortical neurons and thus facilitating movements initiated in the cortex. Thus, the overall influence of dopamine within the striatum may be to reinforce the activation of the particular basal ganglia-thalamocortical circuit which has been initiated by the cortex (Gerfen and Wilson 1996).

A second receptor type is restricted to the spiny neurons of the indirect pathway. The purinergic receptor adenosine A2a is exclusively present on these spiny neurons and is totally absent on the direct spiny projecting neurons. This is in contrast to the dopamine receptors, where each of the pathways still contains 5% spiny neurons with the other dopamine receptor (Gerfen and Wilson 1996). Activation of D2 receptor or of adenosine A2a receptor show antagonistic effects. "This suggests that these two receptor systems, acting on an individual neuron, may modulate the responsiveness of these neurons to activation of the other receptor" (Gerfen and Wilson 1996). A2a agonist treatment reduces the binding affinity of D2 receptors for dopamine.

Hyperdirect Pathway

The cortico-STN-GPi "hyperdirect" pathway has recently received a lot of attention (Nambu et al. 2000/2002/2005, Brown 2003, BarGad et al. 2003, and Squire et al. 2003). The hyperdirect pathway conveys powerful excitatory effects from the motor-related cortical areas to the globus pallidus internus, bypassing the striatum. The hyperdirect pathway is therefore an alternative direct cortical link to the BG, possibly as important to motor control as the corticostriatal-GPi pathway, which is typically considered to be the main cortical relay in the BG. However, recently doubt on the existence of the presence of the cortico-STN connection in *humans* has been brought forward (Marani et al. 2008).

Anatomical studies have shown that STN-pallidal fibres arborize more widely and terminate on more proximal neuronal elements of the pallidum than striato-pallidal fibres. Thus, the striatal and STN inputs to GPi form a pattern of fast, widespread, divergent excitation from the STN, and a slower, focused, convergent inhibition from the striatum (Squire et al. 2003). A point-to-point relation is favored by Shink et al. (1996), in which a reciprocal connection is present between the same neuronal populations in the STN and GPi. The same STN population also has a reciprocal connection with a population of neurons in the GPe, indicating that recurrent loops are present in the indirect pathway. In Figure 1 only the GPe-STN loop is indicated.

Furthermore, cortico-STN neurons and cortico-striatal neurons belong to distinct populations. Thus, signals through the hyperdirect pathway may broadly inhibit motor programs; then signals through the direct pathway may adjust the selected motor program according to the situation.

Nambu et al. (2000/2002/2005) propose a dynamic centre-surround model based on the hyperdirect, direct and indirect pathways to explain the role of the BG in the execution of voluntary movement. When a voluntary movement is about to be initiated by cortical mechanisms, a corollary signal is transmitted from the motor cortex to the GPi through the hyperdirect pathway, activates GPi neurons and thereby suppresses large areas of the thalamus and cerebral cortex that are related to both the selected motor program and other competing programs (Figure 2A, top). Next, another corollary signal through the direct pathway is conveyed to the GPi, inhibiting a specific population of pallidal neurons in the centre area, resulting in the disinhibition of their targets and release of the selected motor program (Figure 2A, middle). Finally, a third corollary signal through the indirect pathway reaches the GPi, activating neurons therein and suppressing their targets in the thalamus and cerebral cortex extensively (Figure 2A, bottom). This sequential information processing ensures only that the selected motor program is initiated, executed and terminated at the selected timing. In Parkinson's disease the indirect and hyperdirect pathway show elevated activity levels, while activity in the direct pathway is reduced (see also Figure 1B), resulting in reduced disinhibition in thalamus leading to hypokinesia (bradykinesia and/or akinesia) (Figure 2B; see also previous section).

During voluntary limb movements, the GPi displays an increase in activity in the majority of neurons, with movement-related increases tending to occur earlier than decreases. In addition, onset of activity in the subthalamic nucleus (STN) occurs earlier than that in the pallidum (Mink 1996). Based on these observations, it is likely that the increased pallidal activity during voluntary limb movements is mediated by the net excitatory, faster hyperdirect pathway, while the decreased pallidal activity is mediated by the net inhibitory, slower direct pathway. It has been observed that the hyperdirect pathway requires about 5 to 8 ms for a cortical signal to propagate through the BG,

Figure 2. Dynamic centre-surround model explaining the function of basal ganglia in motor control. Activity changes in the thalamus (Th) and/or cortex (Cx) resulting from sequential inputs from the hyperdirect (top), direct (middle) and indirect (bottom) pathways in both the normal case (A) and the Parkinsonian case (B). (Adapted from Nambu 2005)

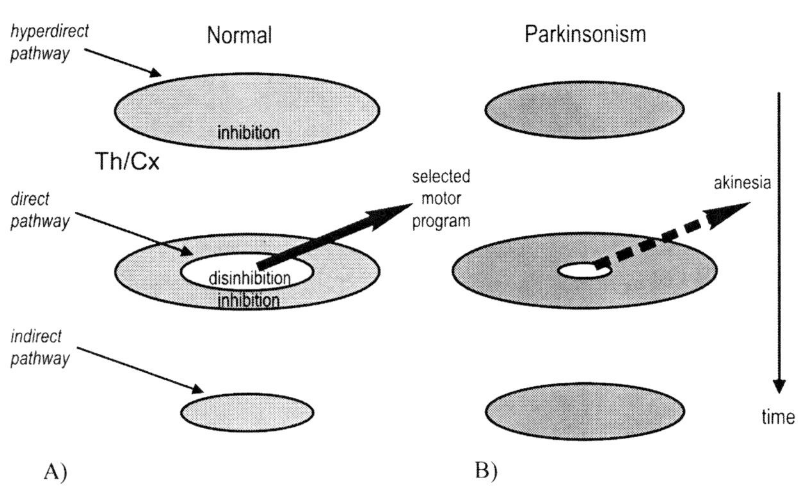

while the direct route takes about 15 to 20 ms, and the indirect pathway approximately 30 ms (Suri et al. 1997, Squire et al. 2003). Pallidal neurons with increased activity may represent those in the surrounding area of the selected motor program, while pallidal neurons with decreased activity may represent those in the centre area, whose number should be much smaller than that in the surrounding area.

Integration vs. Segregation in Basal Ganglia

There is ongoing debate among BG experts on the subject of integration versus segregation of information within the basal ganglia. On the one hand, Percheron et al. (1991) maintain that a substantial amount of synaptic convergence and functional integration exists within the basal ganglia-thalamocortical circuitry, due to the fact that the axons of striatal projection neurons cross the dendritic fields of many pallidal regions before terminating in a particular pallidal area.

On the other hand, Alexander and Crutcher (1990) maintain that a high degree of segregation exists at many levels within the motor circuit. They emphasize the parallel distributed processing architecture of the basal ganglia, with the many parallel loops which pass sequentially through the basal ganglia nuclei remaining largely segregated. Anatomical and physiological studies have confirmed that functional segregation exists along parallel somatotopic channels. The two opposing views are illustrated in Figure 3.

Based on the well-known estimates that the total population of striatal neurons outnumber all of the pallidal and nigral neurons combined by two to three orders of magnitude, Percheron et al. (1991) believe that individual neurons within the basal ganglia output nuclei must receive convergent inputs from a large number of striatal neurons and insist that their findings provide strong evidence against the concept of parallel, functionally segregated basal ganglia-thalamocortical circuits. Squire et al. (2003) also support the convergence-theory, based on 1) a reduction of the number of neurons at each level from the cortex to striatum to GPi, 2) the large number of synapses on each striatal neuron, 3) the large dendritic trees of striatal and GPi neurons, and 4) the interaction across circuits mediated by SNc and GPe neurons.

Figure 3. Conflicting views of information processing within the basal ganglia: integration (convergence) of information (A) vs. segregated parallel processing (B). Approximate numbers of neurons in the cortex, striatum and GPi in the monkey brain are listed in the centre. (Adapted from Bergman et al. 1998)

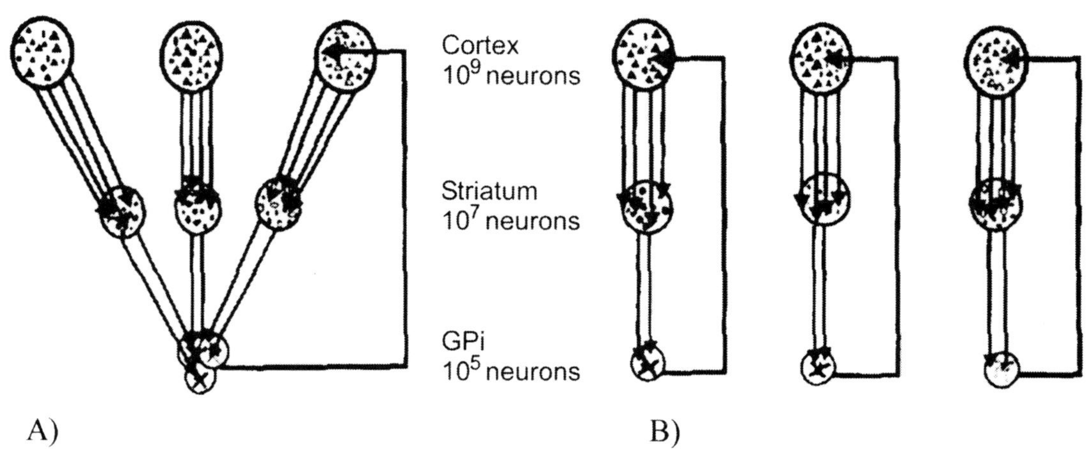

Alexander and Crutcher (1990) maintain that a high degree of segregation exists at many levels within the motor circuit. They emphasize the parallel distributed processing architecture of the basal ganglia, with the many parallel loops which pass sequentially through the basal ganglia nuclei remaining largely segregated. Anatomical and physiological studies have confirmed that functional segregation exists along parallel somatotopic channels, as described in Romanelli et al. (2005) and Strafella et al. (2005). Alexander and Crutcher (1990) also found that separate populations of neurons within the supplementary motor area (SMA), motor cortex and putamen in monkeys discharged selectively in relation to:

- target-level variables (reflecting the location of the target in space);
- trajectory/kinematics-level variables (reflecting the direction of limb movement, independent of muscle pattern or limb dynamics);
- dynamics/muscle-level variables (reflecting movement force and/or muscle pattern).

This suggests that within each of the somatotopic channels of the motor circuit (leg, arm, orofacial) there may well be a deeper level of organisation represented by functionally specific sub-channels that encode selectively, but in parallel, information about distinct functional levels of motor processing, such as target location, limb kinematics and muscle pattern.

In agreement with Percheron, Alexander and Crutcher (1991) acknowledge that convergence of information does exist within circuits, but suggests that the important question is whether or not it is based on convergence of inputs from closely grouped and functionally related striatal neurons, thus maintaining functional specificity along the basal ganglia-thalamocortical pathways.

Although anterograde tracers have shown that a single striatal axon may contact several target neurons in passing, it finally ensheaths a single neuron with a dense termination, suggesting that the physiological effect is more focused. Alexander et al. (1991) propose that as these striatal neurons are myelinated, they do not necessarily affect the regions which they pass. Mink (1996) found that anterograde tracers injected into two nearby but non-adjacent sites in the putamen had little overlap of their termination zones in GPi, providing further that evidence exists to support the view of segregation. Squire et al. (2003) also provides plentiful evidence in support of parallel segregated loops, including:

- the preserved somatotopy in the cortex and BG;
- relative preservation of topography through the BG (e.g. the motor cortex–putamen–GPi–VLo thalamus (oral part of the ventrolateral nucleus)–motor cortex loop and the prefrontal cortex–caudate–SNr–VA thalamus (ventral anterior nucleus)–prefrontal cortex loop);
- the finding that separate groups of GPi neurons project via the thalamus to separate motor areas of the cortex.

Alexander and Crutcher (1990) conclude that structural convergence and functional integration are more likely to occur *within* rather than *between* the separate basal ganglia-thalamocortical circuits, and that integration may be based on the temporal coincidence of processing within pathways whose functional segregation is rather strictly maintained than on the spatial convergence of functionally disparate pathways.

The Role of the Basal Ganglia

It is widely accepted that the basal ganglia play a crucial role in the control of voluntary movement. However, what exactly the BG do for voluntary movement is still under debate. Many clues as to the function of this complex group of subcortical structures have been obtained by examining the deficits that occur following disorders of the BG, such as Parkinson's disease and Huntington's disease, animal models of MPTP-induced Parkinsonism, single-cell microelectrode recordings of neuronal activity, as well as imaging studies of blood flow and metabolism. However, despite extensive research on the subject, the function of the BG within the cortico-BG-thalamocortical circuit is still unclear. The wide variety of roles attributed to the BG in the control of movement is described below.

Focused Selection & Inhibition of Competing Programs

A large number of motor programs may act through common descending pathways in the brainstem and spinal cord. Simultaneous activation of competing motor programs could result in ineffective action and cause inappropriate muscular co-contraction and abnormal postures and movements (Mink 1996). Therefore, during any given movement, a multitude of potentially competing motor mechanisms must be inhibited to prevent them from interfering with the desired movement. The tonically active inhibitory output of the internal part of the globus pallidus (GPi) normally acts as a "brake" on motor patterns. When a movement is initiated, GPi neurons projecting to the parts of the thalamus involved in the desired movement decrease their discharge, removing the tonic inhibition of the thalamus, and thus reinforcing appropriate patterns of cortical activity and facilitating movement of the desired motor pattern. At the same time, GPi neurons projecting to competing motor patterns increase their firing rate, thereby increasing inhibition of the thalamus and suppressing unintended movements. Focusing of movements enables and reinforces the currently selected movement and inhibits competing motor mechanisms, preventing them from interfering with the intended movement. It is believed that the initiatory mechanisms in the cortex may be intact in PD, but the mechanical onset of movement is delayed due to a reduced disinhibition of the thalamus by the GPi, preventing release of the brake from desired motor programs (Mink 1996).

Movement Gating & Velocity Regulation

The BG gate the initiation of motor actions that have been initiated in the cortex, allowing desired movements to proceed. Excitatory input from the cortex results in a smoothly varying phasic disinhibition of the thalamus, providing the "GO" signal for the motor command and setting the overall velocity of the movement. The time taken to execute movements is inversely proportional to the magnitude of cortical input. The presence of dopamine reinforces the desired movement, facilitating conduction through the direct pathway and suppressing conduction through the indirect pathway (Contreras-Vidal 1995, Alexander and Crutcher 1990).

Action Selection

The BG act to resolve conflicts between sensorimotor systems competing for access to the final common motor path (motorneurons and muscles). One or more actions are selected out of a multitude of such actions presented to the basal ganglia by the cortex. The selection is based on the assumption that cortical signals to the striatum encode the salience of requests for access to the motor system. The BG selects the most salient action and enables clean and rapid switching between movements. The nature of the actions selected may be low-level "simple" motor actions or high-level "complex" behavioural schemes (Gurney 2001a/2001b, Prescott 2002).

Sequence Generation

The BG facilitates action sequencing by learning and reproducing sequences of actions. Multimodal information is filtered in the BG by selecting previously learned optimal actions. Memory of the sequence of actions may be maintained within the BG or the cortex. The BG then project to cortical areas that implement these actions, aiding in the production of optimal action sequences. Sequence generation depends on the presence of local working memory within the BG and a dopamine reinforcement signal in response to rewards (Berns and Sejnowski 1998).

Reinforcement Learning

The role of the BG in reward mediated learning is based on long-term reward-related enhancement of corticostriatal synapses. By reinforcement learning, the BG learns to generate or select actions that maximise reward. The reward is based on a reinforcement signal provided by dopaminergic inputs from the SNc. The presence of low dopamine levels is a valid reinforcement signal or a less binding activity to the dopamine receptor as can be initiated by the adenosine receptor for the D2 receptor. A suppression of dopamine activity is a negative reinforcement signal, making the action less likely to be selected in future (Brown et al. 1999, Suri and Schultz 1998, Bar-Gad et al. 2003).

Regulation of Muscle Tone

The BG output to the brainstem motor networks, mainly via the pedunculopontine nucleus (PPN), could be involved in locomotion induction, the automatic regulation of postural muscle tone and rhythmic limb movements that accompany voluntary movements. The PPN, located in the brainstem, consists of the glutamatergic pars dissipatus (PPNd) and the cholinergic pars compacta (PPNc). The PPN receives glutamatergic inputs from the STN, and GABAergic inputs from the GPi and SNr. The PPN is an important relay nucleus between the BG and the spinal cord. Inhibitory GABAergic axon collaterals from the GPi appear to terminate preferentially on the glutamatergic neurons of the PPNd, which provide descending projections to the spinal cord. These projections are thought to be important in muscle tone control and movement initiation. Cholinergic projections from the PPN to the dopamine-containing neurons of the SNc have been observed in rats and non-human primates. A significant projection to the STN has also been documented, along with a less dense innervation of the pallidum (for an overview see Garcia-Rill 1991, and Marani et al. 2008).

An excessive GABAergic inhibition of the PPN may increase the level of muscle tone (hypertonus), and play a role in the axial symptoms of PD, such as gait disorders and postural instability and induce gait starting problems (Takakusaki et al. 2004, Breit et al. 2004, Pahapill and Lozano, 2000). Blocking the GABA-ergic inhibitory input to the PPN indeed reduces akinesia in MPTP treated monkeys (Nandi et al. 2002a).

Unlikely Roles of the BG

Disorders of the basal ganglia in humans (e.g., Parkinson's disease), suggest that higher, organisational aspects of motor control may be more affected than the elemental properties of movement. Parkinson's disease patients can control the kinematic and dynamic features of movement, such as force and direction, while their ability to perform sequences of movements is impaired (Aldridge et al. 2004). Thus, it appears that the basal ganglia are not involved in the control of the kinematic and dynamic features of voluntary movement control. The fact that most movement-related BG neurons fire after the agonist muscles become active argues against movement initiation by the BG (Mink 1996), which is rather directed to the PPN (Garcia-Rill 1991).

PATHOPHYSIOLOGY OF PARKINSON'S DISEASE

Degeneration of Nigrostriatal Pathway

The primary pathological feature of Parkinson's disease (PD) is a progressive degeneration of midbrain dopaminergic neurons in the SNc. The affected area of the SNc gives rise to most of the dopaminergic innervation of the sensorimotor region of the striatum. Thus a loss in dopamine (DA) mainly affects the nigrostriatal pathway (Calabresi et al. 2000, Usunoff et al. 2002). The resulting loss of DA-mediated control of striatal neuronal activity leads to an abnormal activity of striatal neurons, which is generally considered to be the origin of PD motor symptoms.

Using the direct / indirect pathway model, PD and its symptoms are explained as an imbalance between the direct and indirect pathways which transmit information from the striatum to the BG output nuclei (Figure 1 and 9). The model predicts that dopaminergic denervation of the striatum ultimately leads to an increased firing rate of BG output nuclei, which acts as a brake on the motor cortex via the inhibitory projection to the thalamus. Due to the differential effects of dopamine on the D1 and D2 dopamine receptors of the striatum, a loss of striatal DA results in a reduction in transmission through the direct pathway and an increase in transmission through the indirect pathway. In the direct pathway, a reduction in inhibitory input to the output nuclei occurs. Within the indirect pathway, an excessive inhibition of GPe leads to disinhibition of the STN, which in turn provides an excessive excitatory drive to the GPi. The overall effect of such imbalances would lead to increased neuronal discharge in the GPi. The enhanced activity of the output nuclei results in an excessive tonic and phasic inhibition of the motor thalamus. The subsequent reduction of the thalamic glutamatergic output to the motor cortex would cause a reduction in the usual reinforcing influence of the BG motor circuit upon cortically initiated movements. The reduced excitation of the motor cortex might lessen the responsiveness of the motor fields that are engaged by the motor circuit, leading to the hypokinetic symptoms of bradykinesia and akinesia as seen in Parkinson's disease.

In the Parkinsonian state, when a voluntary movement is about to be initiated by cortical mechanisms, signals through the hyperdirect and indirect pathways expand and suppress larger areas of the thalamus and cortex than in the normal state. Signals through the direct pathway are reduced. Thus, smaller areas of the thalamus and cortex are disinhibited for a shorter period of time than in the normal state, resulting in bradykinesia. In addition, not only the unwanted motor program, but also the selected motor program, cannot be released, resulting in akinesia of Parkinson's disease (see Figure 2 and Nambu 2005).

Changes in Neuronal Firing Rate

Changes in neuronal firing rate induced by depletion of striatal DA in PD include increased firing rates in the striatum, GPi and STN and a minimally decreased discharge in the GPe. The tonic firing rates of BG nuclei in the normal and Parkinsonian case are summarised in Table 1.

Relatively little data are available on the human pedunculopontine nucleus (PPN), as most studies to-date have been performed on non-human primates. Evidence suggests that the PPN may potentially have an important role in explaining some of the symptoms of PD. Akinesia may be attributable, in part, to the increased inhibitory action of descending pallidal projections to the PPN rather than pallidal inhibition of thalamocortical neurons, as lesions of the thalamus have not been found to produce akinesia. Thus, it has been suggested that DBS of the PPN may be of therapeutic value in the treatment of PD.

A conflicting view exists on the changes in PPN firing rate that occur in PD patients. Decreased firing rates of PPN neurons have been demonstrated in Parkinsonian rats, consistent with increased inhibition from BG outputs (Pahapill and Lozano 2000). However, Wichmann et al. (1996) have reported an overactive PPN in Parkinsonian animals, consistent with a major increase of input from the STN. Neuropathological studies on humans have reported a significant loss of the large cholinergic neurons of the PPNc in Parkin-

Table 1. Tonic firing rates of basal ganglia (BG) nuclei

Nucleus	Tonic activity (Hz)		Species	Reference
	Normal	Parkinsonian		
Striatum (projection neurons)	0.1 – 1	9.8 ± 3.8	Human Human	(Squire 2003) (Magnin 2000)
Striatum (TANs)	2 – 10 5.52		Human Human	(Squire 2003) (Bennett 1999)
STN	20 18.8 ± 10.3	42.3 ± 22.0 41.4 ± 21.3 35 ± 18.8 37 ± 17 25.8 ± 14.9	Human Human Human Monkey	(Squire 2003) (Benazzouz 2002) (Magnin 2000) (Bergman 1994)
GPi	60 – 80 78 ± 26 53	91 ± 52.5 89.9 ± 3.0 95 ± 32 60 / 76	Human Human Human Monkey Monkey	(Squire 2003) (Magnin 2000) (Tang 2005) (Filion 1991) (Bergman 1994)
GPe	70 76 ± 28 62.6 ± 25.8	60.8 ± 21.4 51 ± 27	Human Human Monkey Monkey	(Squire 2003) (Magnin 2000) (Filion 1991) (Kita 2004)
SNc	2		Human	(Squire 2003)

GPi - globus pallidus internus; GPe - globus pallidus externus; SNc - substantia nigra pars compacta; STN - subthalamic nucleus; TAN - tonically active neuron.

son's disease patients, the magnitude of which is similar to the neuronal loss within the SNc. This raises the possibility that PPN neurons may be susceptible to the same degenerative mechanisms as nigral dopaminergic neurons, and that PPN dysfunction may be important in the pathophysiology of locomotor and postural disturbances of Parkinsonism. Pahapill and Lozano (2000) and Mena-Segovia et al. (2004) also propose that the PPN may partly contribute to SNc degeneration through the excitotoxic effect of its glutamatergic synaptic contacts on the SNc.

Changes in Neuronal Firing Pattern

The pattern of discharge of basal ganglia neurons is thought to be equally as important as the *rate* of discharge in the execution of smooth movements. Several alterations in the discharge pattern have been observed in neurons of the BG in PD subjects, which suggest that the firing pattern may play an important role in the pathophysiology of this disease. These alterations include a tendency of neurons to discharge in bursts, increased correlation and synchronization of discharge between neighboring neurons, rhythmic and oscillatory behaviour, and a more irregular firing pattern. An abundance of literature exists detailing the changes in firing pattern which occur in the striatum, GPi, STN and thalamus of the PD patient. A summary is given here.

Bennett et al. (2000) found that the tonic firing of striatal cholinergic neurons or tonically active neurons (TANs) in rat brain slices was replaced by persistent oscillatory activity following MPTP-induced Parkinsonism. This suggests that spike timing in cholinergic cells is critically involved in both the normal functioning of the striatum and the pathophysiological processes that occur in Parkinsonian states.

Burst discharges increased from 78% to 89%, and the average burst duration decreased from 213

± 120 to 146 ± 134 ms, with no significant change in the average number of spikes per burst in *GPi* neurons of African green monkeys following MPTP-induced Parkinsonism. The percentage of cells with 4- to 8-Hz periodic oscillatory activity increased significantly from 0.6% to 25% after MPTP treatment (Bergman et al. 1994). During episodes of rest tremor, 19.7% of the GPi cells of Parkinsonian patients fired periodically at a frequency of 4.7 Hz (Magnin 2000). Increased synchrony and correlated activity between the firing of GPi output neurons has also been found by Bergman et al. (1998), Lozano et al. (2002) and Tang et al. (2005). Oscillatory basal ganglia output may drive oscillatory activity in thalamic neurons that are already more prone to develop rhythmic bursts because their membrane potential is lowered by the overall increased inhibition by GPi under Parkinsonian conditions.

The percentage of STN cells that discharged in bursts increased from 69% to 79% in African green monkeys following MPTP treatment, and the average burst duration decreased from 121 ± 98 to 81 ± 99 ms (Bergman et al. 1994). Periodic oscillatory activity at low frequency, highly correlated with tremor, was detected in 16% of cells in STN after MPTP treatment, as opposed to 2% before, with an average oscillation frequency of 5.1 Hz (Bergman et al. 1994). Benazzouz et al. (2002), examined the firing pattern of STN cells of Parkinsonian patients using single unit microelectrode recordings and found two types of discharge pattern: a population of cells characterised mainly by tonic activity with an irregular discharge pattern and occasional bursts (mixed pattern); and a population of cells with periodic oscillatory bursts synchronous to resting tremor (burst pattern). Benazzouz et al. (2002) propose that a high level of STN neuronal activity with an irregular and bursty pattern (mixed pattern) may contribute to akinesia and rigidity, whereas the periodic oscillatory bursts (burst pattern) may contribute to tremor.

Excessive correlations between thalamic neurons were found in vervet monkeys following MPTP intoxication in both the symptomatic and asymptomatic states (Pessiglione et al. 2005). Magnin et al. (2000) found four different types of firing patterns within the thalamus of Parkinsonian patients: sporadic activity (with a mean frequency of 18.8 ± 17.7 Hz); random bursting activity; rhythmic bursting activity; and tremor-locked activity.

Loss of Functional Segregation

Hyperactivity of Corticostriatal Transmission

Due to the close anatomical proximity of cortical glutamatergic and nigral dopaminergic terminals on the dendritic spines of striatal projection neurons, interactions occur between these two neurotransmitter systems. It has been found that the degeneration of nigrostriatal dopaminergic fibres induces an increased concentration and excessive release of glutamate from corticostriatal terminals. In individuals with PD, there is a significant increase in the percentage of glutamatergic synapses, resulting in a hyperactivity of corticostriatal glutamate-mediated transmission, with increased numbers of striatal neurons responding to cortical stimulation. In vitro experiments revealed that chronic denervation of the striatum caused an abnormality in corticostriatal transmission, accounting for the increased excitability of striatal neurons recorded in vivo (Calabresi et al. 2000).

Enlarged Area of Dopamine Release

Strafella et al. (2005) found that, following cortical stimulation, the amount of striatal DA release in the Parkinsonian brain of early PD patients was, as expected, less than in the normal case. However, the size of the significant cluster of DA release in the Parkinsonian brain was found to be 61.4% greater than the more focal release of DA observed in healthy subjects, who have a very spatially confined area of DA release. Residual DA terminals may have a larger field of influence, as the released DA diffuses out to more distant regions due to the loss of re-uptake sites. The abnormal release of glutamate in PD subjects may contribute to the enlarged area of DA release, by activating larger areas of dopaminergic terminals (Calabresi et al. 2000). The spatially enlarged area of DA release following cortical stimulation may reflect a functional reorganization of the cortical inputs and a loss of neuronal functional segregation of cortical information to the striatum, and thus of striatal neurons, in PD patients. Abnormalities in glutamate-DA interactions are believed to have important functional implications in the pathogenesis of PD motor symptoms (Strafella et al. 2005).

Bergman et al. (1998) hypothesize that DA modulates the cross-connections between corticostriatal projections of different sub-circuits, facilitating independent action of striato-pallidal modules, as shown in Figure 4A. However, following DA depletion, the segregation of afferent channels to the striatum is lost and the networks of the basal ganglia lose their ability to keep the corticostriatal projections of the various sub-circuits independent, resulting in a greater coupling between sub-circuits (Figure 4B). This results in the previously inhibited cross-connections between "parallel" subcircuits becoming more active, which can be seen in the increased correlations between the firing of GPi output neurons.

Enlargement of Receptive Fields

Abnormally large somatosensory receptive fields and a severely reduced selectivity of pallidal neurons to passive limb movements have been observed in MPTP-treated monkeys. In intact monkeys, pallidal responses were typically related to movement about a single contralateral joint and in only one direction. In the Parkinsonian monkey, the proportion of neurons responding to passive limb movement quadrupled in GPi (from 16 to 65%) and nearly doubled in GPe (from 18 to 30%), compared to the intact animal, with neurons responding to more than one joint, to both upper

Figure 4. Dopamine modulation of corticostriatal projections. Bergman et al. 1998 hypothesize that the main action of dopamine is to regulate the coupling level between the different subcircuits of the basal ganglia resulting in segregated channels in the normal state (A); broken lines indicate a reduced efficacy of cross-connections between channels. In case of dopamine depletion this segregation is lost (B), resulting in synchronized activation of pallidal (GPi) neurons. (Adapted from Bergman et al. 1998) GPi - globus pallidus internus

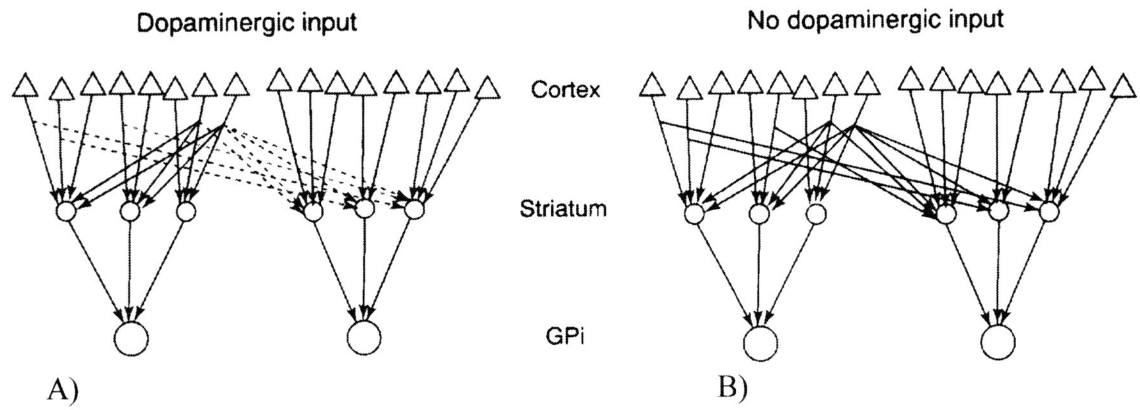

and lower limbs, bilaterally, and to more than one direction of movement. In some cases, a single neuron responded to 9 joints (Filion 1988). In the STN, less specific responses to passive limb manipulation have also been observed: in patients with long-standing PD, 12% of the movement-related STN neurons of PD patients responded to stimulation of arm and leg and approximately 25% of neurons responded to stimulation of multiple joints, compared to no movement-related neurons responding to stimulation of both arm and leg and 9% of neurons responding to stimulation of multiple joints in the control case (Romanelli et al. 2005). In the thalamus, specificity of receptive fields, following MPTP intoxication of monkeys, was found to be markedly decreased from 69% in the normal state, to 15% in the Parkinsonian case, with neurons frequently responding to manipulation of several joints and even several limbs (Pessiglione et al. 2005).

The above data suggest that functional abnormalities of the basal ganglia, produced by PD, are likely to affect the internal organisation of the body map. In pathological conditions there is an enlargement of the receptive fields and consequent loss of specificity. In the absence of DA the control of excitatory influences mediated by corticostriatal inputs and cholinergic interneurons is largely reduced. A larger number of striatal efferent neurons are therefore more easily activated by any excitatory input without selectivity. It has been suggested that the reduced specificity observed in pallidal neurons might be a consequence of widened receptive fields in the striatum (Alexander and Crutcher 1991).

The well-defined somatotopic organisation in the sensorimotor regions of the basal ganglia nuclei is an essential feature of physiologic sensorimotor processing and is important for the selection of movements. It is likely that a blurring of the body maps may affect the selection and focusing of movements and the balance between agonist and antagonist muscle groups. The inability to select the appropriate input signals, and to attenuate unwanted signals, means that the basal ganglia are unable to facilitate the execution of complex, learned behaviours, hence the akinesia. Pessiglione et al. (2005) propose that the impaired functional segregation between striatopallidal pathways, caused by DA depletion, could explain both the loss of specificity and the excess of correlations within cortico-BG circuits. Within the motor circuit, the loss of functional segregation could lead to co-selection of antagonist motor programs, resulting in both akinesia/bradykinesia and muscular rigidity. The inability to de-correlate motor sub-circuits may explain why PD patients have difficulty in performing two simultaneous movements.

Several models of basal ganglia function assign to it a role of focused selection and surrounding inhibition, whereby the activity of corticostriatal loops involved in the desired current task is enhanced, and competing motor networks are suppressed. The loss of functional segregation in PD may lead to an impaired inhibition of competing motor patterns, causing some of the motor symptoms observed in PD (Strafella et al. 2005).

Changes in Neurotransmitter Content

Extrastriatal Dopamine

Studies have demonstrated a significant dopaminergic innervation of the GPi. The STN, which also contains DA receptors, is thought to receive direct projections from the SNc (see Marani et al. 2008). It is hypothesized that the dopaminergic deficit in the basal ganglia might influence the hyperactivity and oscillatory bursting of the STN and GPi directly, in addition to the increased tonic disinhibition of these structures by an under-active GPe, following DA loss in the striatum (Blandini et al. 2000, Bergman et al. 1994). However, contradictory results have also been found: Zhu et al. (2002) found, in a study of rat brain slices, that the STN mainly expresses D2-type DA receptors and concluded that dopaminergic input has an excitatory effect on the STN. Thus, direct dopaminergic denervation of the STN would cause a hypoactivity of STN firing.

Moderate loss of DA has also been observed in many sub-cortical limbic regions of the forebrain, in several limbic cortical and neocortical areas, and in the tegmental area. However, changes in extrastriatal DA neurons are much less pronounced than the nigrostriatal DA loss, and it remains uncertain whether the comparatively mild degree of DA reduction in extrastriatal regions is sufficient to produce overt clinical deficits (Hornykiewicz 1989).

Non-Dopaminergic Systems

Changes in the non-dopaminergic systems are small in comparison with the profound striatal DA loss. They may be fully compensated by the remaining neurons and thus fail to produce any observable functional clinical deficits. However, it is worth noting the changes that occur in non-DA systems, which may contribute to PD symptoms (Hornykiewicz 1989):

- As L-dopa (Levodopa) is converted to norepinephrine, it is thought that norepinephrine may enhance the effectiveness of DA. The reduction of norepinephrine observed in the substantia nigra of PD patients may, therefore, further aggravate the motor deficits.
- Striatal DA activity normally exerts a tonic inhibitory influence on the activity of striatal cholinergic neurons. The loss of dopaminergic inhibitory influence in PD results in cholinergic overactivity and a corresponding aggravation of PD symptoms. However, compensatory mechanisms in the body may act to reduce striatal acetylcholine synthesis, thereby minimizing the adverse consequences of relative cholinergic overactivity. This may explain the modest therapeutic effect of anticholinergic medication.
- The interaction between DA and GABA is vitally important in the normal functioning of the basal ganglia. The levels of GABA in the Parkinsonian striatum have been found to be elevated, in inverse proportion to the severity of DA loss. GABA may exert an inhibitory influence on striatal cholinergic activity, which may explain why GABAergic drugs potentiate the anti-Parkinsonian effect of the L-dopa treatment.
- The treatment of purinergic adenosine receptor A2a with agonists reduces the binding affinity of D2 receptors for dopamine. Moreover, A2a antagonists are thought to reduce L-dopa induced dyskinesia in PD and gives improvement of motor disabilities in MPTP treated monkeys. On more arguments than given here, adenosine antagonists are considered to induce anti-Parkisonian activity. Caffeine belongs to the xanthine chemical group and can block adenosine receptors and can be considered to induce adenosine antagonistic activity. Indications are present that coffee drinkers are better protected towards PD. The extra-effect is that protection of the dopaminergic substantia nigra neurons occurs by adenosine antagonists and by xanthines, giving a lower risk on PD (for a review see Xu et al. 2005).

DEEP BRAIN STIMULATION (DBS)

The most effective neurosurgical procedure to date in the treatment of PD is based on the electrical stimulation of small targets in the basal ganglia, a procedure known as Deep Brain Stimulation (DBS). High-frequency electrical stimulation (>100Hz) is delivered by means of electrodes implanted deep in the brain. A constant stimulation is delivered by a pacemaker-like pulse generator. The positioning of the implanted electrode leads and pulse generator is illustrated in Figure 5. The most popular targets for DBS are:

- motor thalamus (thalamic ventral intermedius nucleus or Vim)
- globus pallidus internus (GPi)
- subthalamic nucleus (STN)

A comparison between lesions of the Vim and GPi with DBS in the same structures shows a rather equal beneficial result for the main symptoms in Parkinson's disease. Such a comparison is not possible for the STN, since lesions of the STN produces hemiballism (for an overview see Marani et al. 2008). Nevertheless DBS of the STN produces better overall results than lesions or DBS in Vim and GPi (Table 2).

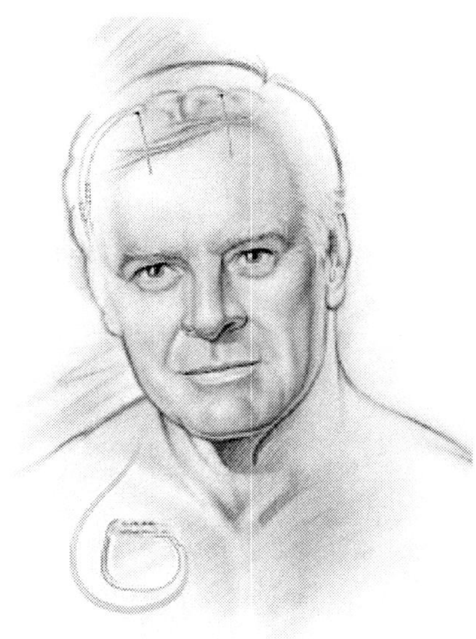

Figure 5. Configuration of the DBS system. The drawing shows the positioning of the implanted bilateral DBS electrode leads, the extension wires and the pulse generator (pacemaker). (Courtesy Medtronic)

DBS of the STN is currently done with monopolar cathodic stimulation at a frequency of 120-180 Hz, and amplitude of 1-5 V with a pulse duration of 60-200 μs. In most patients the most optimal settings are found by trial and error. An average reduction is obtained in akinesia of 42%, rigidity of 49%, and tremor of 27% (Benabid et al. 2002, and reference herein).

DBS of the thalamus is used to treat essential tremor and other forms of tremor (Schuurman et al. 2000). Thalamic DBS can produce an 80% improvement in PD tremor. DBS of the GPi and STN is used to treat the symptoms of PD. Stimulation of these targets has been shown to produce an 80% improvement in PD tremor and dyskinesias, more than 60% improvement in bradykinesia and rigidity, and approximately 40-50% improvement in gait and postural dysfunction. GPi or thalamus is targeted for the treatment of dystonia (Lozano et al. 2002).

Deep brain stimulation of the pedunculopontine nucleus (PPN) has recently been carried out in PD patients (for an overview see Kenney et al. 2007). Earlier studies in monkeys showed that lesions of the PPN produce akinesia. Low fre-

Table 2. Comparison of the effects of lesions and DBS in Vim, GPi and DBS of STN

Symptom	Thalamotomy Vim	DBS Vim	Pallidotomy GPi	DBS GPi	DBS STN
Tremor	++	++	0 - +	++	++
Rigidity	+	+	++	++	++
Hypokinesia	0	0	+	+	++
Dyskinesia	+	+	++	++	0 - ++
Dystonia	+	0	++	+	++

GPi - globus pallidus internus; STN - subthalamic nucleus; Vim - thalamic ventral intermedius nucleus. 0: no effect; +: moderate effect; ++: good effect quency stimulation reduced akinesia, while high frequency stimulation causes akinesia in monkeys (Nandi et al 2002b) These results were confirmed in MPTP treated monkeys by Jenkinson et al. (2004), indicating also that low frequency stimulation increases, while high frequency stimulation decreases motor activity. This caused renewed interest in the PPN (for reviews see Pahapill and Lozano 2000).

In PD patients gait disturbance and postural instability are difficult to manage clinically especially in patients in advanced stages. Bilateral DBS of the PPN in combination with STN-DBS showed that PPN-DBS was effective on gait and postural instability at low frequency stimulation (Stefani et al. 2007; for bipolar contacts; 60 μs pulse width, 25 Hz, 1.5-2V). The same was already found by Plaha and Gill in a short term study (2005; also 20-25 Hz), confirming the results found in monkeys. PPN implantation in PD are claimed to be safe (Mazzone et al. 2005). Motor effects of PPN-DBS are mainly caused by changing the spinal cord excitability (Pierantozzi et al. 2008) while the interaction between PPN and STN is kept responsible for the BG change in firing patterns (Florio et al. 2007).

The topography and localization of the PPN is still a matter of discussion (see for an overview Marani et al. 2008), that leads to uncertainties on optimal electrode placing (Zrinzo et al. 2007). Moreover, it cannot be stated that the PPN stimulation effect is a pure cholinergic effect, since the cholinergic PPN neurons are dispersed between other neurochemical types of neurons (see Jenkins et al. 2006; Marani et al. 2008).

There is little argument that DBS, high frequency electrical stimulation (120-180 Hz), of the STN, GPi and thalamus has been an effective tool in the treatment of the various symptoms of Parkinson's disease, as well as other movement disorders. However, therapeutic stimulation parameters for DBS (polarity, pulse amplitude, pulse width, frequency) have been derived primarily by trial and error for all three brain areas. There remains considerable debate concerning the methods underlying the beneficial effect of DBS and its mechanisms of action are still unknown: "DBS produces a non-selective stimulation of an unknown group of neuronal elements over an unknown volume of tissue" (Grill et al. 2001).

Due to the comparable effects of high frequency stimulation to a lesion of the nucleus, it appears that DBS of the STN or GPi induces a functional inhibition of the stimulated region, and thus to decreased neuronal activity. However, on the basis of physiological principles, one would expect that the effects of DBS are due to excitation of the neural elements (axons, soma) surrounding the tip of the electrode, and thus to increased firing of the axons projecting away from the stimulated region (see e.g. Ashby et al. 1999, and Hashimoto et al. 2003). This contradiction could be called the explanatory gap of DBS.

So, does DBS excite or inhibit its target nucleus? To answer this question it is necessary to examine a number of differential effects which are likely to occur due to stimulation, some or all of which may contribute to the overall observable effect.

Which Neuronal Elements are Influenced by DBS?

At a physiological level, DBS can have multiple effects on its targets due to the wide range of neuronal elements that may be stimulated by the electrode's current field (Breit et al. 2004, Lozano et al. 2002, Grill and McIntyre 2001, Holsheimer et al. 2000). It is known that axons are much more excitable than cell bodies, and that large myelinated fibres are more excitable than unmyelinated axons. Current density decreases with distance from the electrode tip and axons near the cathode are more likely to be activated than axons near the anode. Electrical stimulation is more likely to activate fibres oriented parallel to the current field than fibres oriented transversely (Ranck 1975). Furthermore, electrodes for DBS may be placed in regions with heterogeneous populations of neuronal elements. The applied current may affect several neuronal components in the proximity of the stimulation electrode, with each being subject to both depolarizing and hyperpolarizing effects. Stimulation may influence afferent (axon or axon terminal) and efferent projection neurons, as well as local interneurons. Differential effects may occur in the cell body and axon of the same neuron, due to the possibility of a stimulation-induced functional decoupling between cell body and efferent projections. It was found that the firing of the cell body of directly stimulated neurons is not necessarily representative for the efferent output of the neuron (McIntyre et al. 2004b). Extracellular stimulation may also excite or block axons of passage, and fibre activation will result in both antidromic and orthodromic propagation.

The Explanatory Gap, Intrinsic vs. Extrinsic Factors: Hypotheses

Various hypotheses on the mechanisms of action of DBS exist:

Depolarisation Block

High-frequency stimulation may lead to a depolarisation block of neuronal transmission by inactivation of voltage-gated sodium and calcium ion channels. A prolonged depolarisation of the membrane causes the voltage-gated sodium channels to be trapped in their inactivated state, thus prohibiting the initiation of new action potentials, inducing a powerful inhibition in the stimulated structure (McIntyre et al. 2004a, Breit et al. 2004, Benabid et al. 2002, Lozano et al. 2002, Grill and McIntyre 2001).

Activation of Afferent Inputs

The threshold for activation of axons projecting to the region around the electrode is lower than the threshold for direct activation of local cell bodies. Therefore DBS may excite inhibitory afferent axons projecting to the target nucleus, increasing inhibition of the target and thus playing a role in the suppression of somatic firing. Stimulation may also activate excitatory afferents. The overall effect on the target structure would therefore be the summation of excitatory and inhibitory afferent inputs (McIntyre et al. 2004a, Breit et al. 2004, Benabid et al. 2002, Dostrovsky and Lozano 2002). In the case of the GPi, DBS may activate inhibitory afferent fibres from the GPe and striatum and excitatory afferent fibres from the STN. As the inhibitory afferents are more numerous, the overall effect is an increased inhibition of the GPi.

Activation of Efferent Axons

High frequency stimulation may activate the efferent projection axons leaving the target structure, directly influencing the output of the stimulated nucleus.

Synaptic Failure

Stimulation-induced synaptic transmission failure may occur due to an inability of the stimulated neurons to follow a rapid train of electrical stimuli. Neurotransmitter depletion or receptor desensitisation could result from continuous long-term stimulation. This synaptic depression would lead to the neurons activated by the stimulus train being unable to sustain high-frequency synaptic action on their targets, resulting in reduced efferent output (McIntyre et al. 2004a, Breit et al. 2004, Dostrovsky and Lozano 2002, Lozano et al. 2002).

"Jamming" of Abnormal Patterns

Stimulation-forced driving of efferent axons (jamming) may impose a high-frequency regular pattern of discharge on the axons, which is time-locked to the stimulation. Insufficient time between DBS pulses may prevent the neurons from returning to their spontaneous baseline activity. DBS disrupts the normal functioning of neurons including any pathological patterns, erasing the bursty, synchronous firing observed in PD patients, so that the system cannot recognise a pattern. According to this hypothesis, DBS does not reduce neural firing, but instead induces a modulation of pathological network activity causing network-wide changes (McIntyre et al. 2004a, Breit et al. 2004, Benabid et al. 2002, Garcia et al. 2005a, Garcia et al. 2005b, Montgomery and Gale 2005).

Activation of Nearby "Large Fibre" Systems

Many fibres of passage run close by the structures targeted by DBS. It is possible that direct activation of these fibre tracts may contribute to DBS effectiveness. For example, dopaminergic pathways to the globus pallidus and the striatum pass through the STN, and the axon bundles of pallidothalamic and nigrothalamic pathways also pass close-by. These pathways may be activated directly by STN stimulation (Grill and McIntyre 2001, Vitek 2002).

Neurotransmitter Release

Stimulation may excite axon terminals on the pre-synaptic neurons which project to the target nucleus. In response to each stimulus, these axon terminals release inhibitory or excitatory neurotransmitters, which diffuse across the synaptic cleft to activate receptors on the target neurons. The release of glutamate induces an excitatory postsynaptic potential (EPSP), whereas the release of GABA induces an inhibitory postsynaptic potential (IPSP) (Grill and McIntyre 2001, Lozano et al. 2002).

In the case of DBS of the GPi, stimulation may evoke the release of the inhibitory neurotransmitter GABA from the pre-synaptic terminals of the putamen and GPe, and the excitatory neurotransmitter glutamate from STN neurons. GABAergic synaptic terminals are far more numerous than glutamatergic terminals in the GPi, accounting for about 90% of the total synapses (Wu et al. 2001), so the excitatory effect is masked by the inhibitory effect, resulting in an overall inhibition of the post-synaptic neurons by summation of IPSPs. In contrast, the thalamus contains more excitatory synapses than inhibitory ones, so the effect is one of excitation.

Antidromic Effects

Electrical stimulation of an axon causes impulses to travel both antidromically as well as orthodromically. Neurons may therefore be activated antidromically via stimulation of their afferent inputs to the target structure. In this way, stimulation of the STN or thalamus could potentially "backfire" to the cortex by stimulation of cortical inputs to the target structure (Lozano et al. 2002).

High and Low Frequency Effects

The statement that DBS works by high frequency modulation of the neuronal areas involved, is now denied, due to the effect of low frequency stimulation needed for PPN effects. The manner in which low frequency PPN stimulation works is unknown.

Akinesia is thought to be caused by high frequency stimulation of the PPN, because it inhibits the nucleus, producing its effects by its descending spinal cord pathway to the spinal motor centres.

PPN low frequency stimulation reduces gait disturbances and postural instability. However PPN hypoactivity also reduces the discharge of the dopaminergic substantia nigra neurons. On the other hand hypoactivity caused by PPN degeneration in Parkinsonism, transmitted by the PPN-spinal bundle, is held responsible for rigidity (see discussion in Gomez-Gallego et al. 2007).

Others indicate a hyperactivity of the PPN in Parkinsonism, especially in rat studies (Orieux et al. 2000; Breit et al. 2005). In short, literature shows controversial results for the explanation of the effect of low frequency DBS in the PPN. As a consequence modeling the DBS effect of PPN stimulation is hard to perform, also because different types of neurons and various neurotransmitter inputs (ACh, GABA and substance P) are involved.

In summary, most authors agree that the overall effect of DBS is an inhibition of the target structure, although the stimulation may cause either activation or inhibition of individual neuronal elements in the vicinity of the electrode. Vitek (2002) suggests a possible explanation for the conflicting observations on the effects of DBS – inhibition or excitation. Although DBS may inhibit cellular activity in the stimulated structure via activation of inhibitory afferent fibres projecting to that site, the output from the stimulated structure may be increased, due to the activation of projection axons leaving the target structure, which discharge independently of the soma. The underlying mechanisms of DBS appear to differ depending on the type of nucleus being stimulated and the exact location of the electrode within the nucleus.

The observed effect of stimulation is probably a combination of several of the mechanisms described above. It is important to determine exactly which neuronal elements are affected by DBS in order to obtain a better understanding of the mechanisms by which DBS provides its beneficial effects.

Adverse Effects of DBS

In a review paper (Temel et al. 2005) the involvement of the STN in the limbic and associative circuitries is studied. Cognitive disorders like altered verbal memory and fluency, altered executive functioning, changed attention behaviour such as disturbed working memory, mental speed and response inhibition are reported to result from DBS. The same holds for the limbic involvement of the STN. Changes in personality, depression, (hypo) mania, anxiety, and hallucinations are reported. These adverse effects are thought to be related to the limbic and associative circuits that loop also the BG and in which the STN is an important relay station too (see Nieuwenhuys et al. 2008).

COMPUTATIONAL MODELING OF PARKINSON'S DISEASE AND DBS AT A CELLULAR LEVEL

Neurons can be modeled using the properties of the ion channels in the membrane. There are several methods that use Hodgkin and Huxley type equations (Hodgkin and Huxley 1952) describing ion channel dynamics. The single cell models considered here are (subthalamic nucleus (STN) as well as thalamus, and the internal and external part of the globus pallidus (GPi and GPe)), are mainly made for understanding DBS effects in the STN. Therefore, some properties of the subthalamic neurons are briefly summarized in the next session, in order to understand the significance of these models.

Subthalamic Nucleus Neuron Model

For most neurons, including the STN, only limited information regarding the presence, types and properties of ion channels in human neurons is available. Consequently (STN) models are mostly based on information obtained from studies on rats. A comparison between two single compartment models of STN neurons is described taken into consideration their spontaneous activity and the transformation of this activity into a bursting pattern as observed under Parkinsonian conditions (dopamine depletion) and recorded in brain slices (for an overview see Heida et al. 2008).

Single Spike Mode, Plateau Potentials, and Bursting

From in vivo experimental studies in monkeys it was found that the neurons of the subthalamic nucleus perform a dual function: 1) they discharge continuously and repetitively at low frequencies (10-30 Hz) in awake resting state, and 2) they discharge bursts of high-frequency spikes (up to several hundred per second), which can last up to hundred millisecond preceding, during, and after limb or eye movements in awake state.

In vitro brain slice studies show that tonic discharges of single spikes were recorded in subthalamic neurons in a regular manner when no additional inputs were applied. Spontaneous firing rates of 5-40 spikes/s were recorded. Nakanishi et al. (1987) reported that spontaneous firing occurred at membrane potentials between -40 and -65 mV, while Beurrier et al. (1999) discovered a mean discharge frequency of 22 Hz at membrane potentials ranging between -35 and -50 mV. The cycle of the resting oscillation of STN neurons consisted of single action potentials with a duration of 1 ms (Nakanishi et al. 1987), which is followed by an afterhyperpolarization that contains three phases: 1) a fast afterhyperpolarization, 2) a slow afterhyperpolarization (sag), and 3) a subsequent slow-ramp depolarization. Other studies (for an overview see Heida et al. 2008) on single spikes demonstrated:

- Rhythmic firing is an inherent property of STN neurons;
- Recurrent excitatory connections within the STN were ruled out to be involved in spontaneous firing and its periodicity;
- N inward current is activated in the voltage range of the depolarization phase of spontaneous activity;
- TTX abolished all activity, proving that voltage dependent sodium currents are required for oscillatory mechanisms of STN cells;
- A powerful calcium dependent potassium current is present based on the large afterhyperpolarization present.

Beurrier et al. (1999) found that about 46% of the neurons that were looked at were also able to fire in bursts while no input was applied. Burst firing was present in the membrane potential range of -42 to -60 mV, which is somewhat lower than the membrane potentials that were found in neurons showing single spike activity. According to Beurrier et al. (1999) STN neurons were able to switch from one mode to the other depending on membrane potential. However, for rhythmic bursting activity to occur in STN cells, it is expected, as investigated in explant cultures, that (part of) the STN-GP network is intact (Plenz and Kitai 1999, Song et al. 2000).

A possible explanation for the observed oscillatory bursting activity can be found in the involvement of synaptic inputs involving T-type channels. T-type channels were thought to be important in the generation of oscillatory behaviour, and in STN neurons these channels have a preferential distribution in dendritic processes (Song et al. 2000). This was found from acutely isolated STN neurons in which dendritic processes are lost during dissociation. No low-voltage-activated channels were found in these neurons, suggesting that the low-threshold T-type channels are located within the dendritic processes.

At hyperpolarized state long-lasting depolarizing potentials, so called plateau potentials, were generated in STN cells in response to depolarizing or hyperpolarizing current pulses which clearly outlasted the duration of the applied current pulses and could trigger repetitive firing in which the firing rate increased along with the development of the slow depolarization. Two phases in the plateau potential can be discerned when TTX is added suppressing sodium currents: 1) a slow depolarization triggered by the depolarizing current pulse (50 pA, 200 ms), and 2) an after-depolarization triggered at the break of the current pulse. The slow depolarizing potential was thus TTX-resistant, but was Ca^{2+}-dependent.

The early phase of the plateau potential was found to be insensitive to membrane perturbations; the stability index, defined as the ratio of the peak potential after a perturbing current pulse during a plateau potential to the potential immediately before the current, was one or close to one during the initial phase of the plateau potential (Otsuka et al. 2001). This robustness gradually decreased toward the end of the plateau potential as was tested by the injection of negative current pulses.

Neurons in which a plateau potential could be evoked by a depolarizing current pulse at hyperpolarized states also generated a plateau potential after termination of a hyperpolarizing current pulse. Nevertheless, plateau potentials were triggered within a narrow range of membrane potentials: Beurrier et al. (1999) found a range between -50 and -75 mV; Otsuka et al. (2001) reported a threshold hyperpolarization level at which a plateau potential was first induced of -74.98 ± 1.96 mV. All these results show that plateau potentials are induced by the activation of voltage-dependent conductances. The results from whole-cell recordings using different types of Ca^{2+} channel blockers suggested that both Ca^{2+} entry through L-type Ca^{2+} channels and intracellular free Ca^{2+} ions are involved in the generation of plateau potentials.

Similar to the increase in spontaneous firing rate with increasing temperature, the occurrence of action potentials in combination with a plateau potential was also found to be dependent on temperature. A plateau potential that did not evoke action potentials at 20°C did evoke action potentials even at its late phase at 25 °C. Raising the temperature also appeared to increase the duration of the plateau potential.

According to Otsuka et al. (2001) plateau-generating neurons tend to be located in the lateral part of the nucleus. However, although the morphology of plateau-generating neurons did not appear to differ from that of nonplateau-generating neurons, the input resistance at resting membrane potentials of plateau-generating neurons was found to be significantly larger than that of nonplateau-generating neurons (813±70 vs. 524±50 MΩ).

Channels that were found to be present and to be important for the functioning of the subthalamic neurons (for references see Heida et al. 2008):

- A high-threshold L-type Ca^{2+} channel which has slow inactivation dynamics that depends both on the membrane potential and Ca^{2+}, plateau potential induction;
- Low-voltage activated T-type Ca^{2+} currents, responsible for fast inactivation, and generation of low threshold spikes (LTS);
- High voltage activated subtypes N, Q and R types, of which the N type causes Ca^{2+} entry after neurotransmission.

In this section two single compartment models will be described. A comparison of the two models as well as a comparison with experimental data is given (see also Heida et al. 2008).

Single Compartment STN Model of Terman (2002) and Rubin (2004)

The membrane potential v of the single compartment model of the STN according to Terman and Rubin (Terman et al. 2002, and Rubin and Terman 2004) is described by

$$C_m \frac{dv}{dt} = -I_{Na} - I_K - I_{Ca} - I_T - I_{AHP} - I_{leak}$$

In which the incorporated ionic currents are described as follows:

- $I_{Na} = g_{Na} m_\infty^3 h (v - v_{Na})$ Na^+ current, with instantaneous activation variable m_∞ and inactivation variable h;

- $I_K = g_K n^4 (v - v_K)$ delayed rectifier K^+ current (high activation threshold, fast activation time constant), with activation variable n;
- $I_{Ca} = g_{Ca} s_{\infty}^2 (v - v_{Ca})$ high-threshold Ca^{2+} current with instantaneous activation variable s_{∞};
- $I_T = g_T a_{\infty}^3 b_{\infty}^2 (v - v_{Ca})$ low-threshold T-type Ca^{2+} current, with instantaneous activation variable a_{∞} and inactivation variable b_{∞}; by using this equation the T-type current includes the effects of a hyperpolarization-activated inward current, the sag;
- $I_{AHP} = g_{AHP} (v - v_K) \dfrac{[Ca^{2+}]_{in}}{[Ca^{2+}]_{in} + k_1}$ Ca^{2+}-activated, voltage-independent "afterhyperpolarization" K^+ current, with $[Ca^{2+}]_{in}$ the intracellular concentration of Ca^{2+} ions, and k_1 the dissociation constant of this current;
- $I_{leak} = g_{leak}(v - v_{leak})$ leak current.

Gating kinetics of the ionic conductances were calculated according to $\dfrac{dw}{dt} = \dfrac{w_{\infty} - w}{\tau_w}$ with $w = n, h, r$. Steady state activation and inactivation functions are $w_{\infty} = \dfrac{1}{1 + \exp\left[-(v - \theta_w)/k_w\right]}$ with $w = n, m, h, a, r, s$, and θ_w and k_w the half-inactivation/activation voltage and slope, respectively.

The inactivation function b_{∞} of the T-type current is determined according to

$$b_{\infty} = \frac{1}{1 + \exp\left[(r - \theta_b)/k_b\right]} - \frac{1}{1 + \exp\left[-\theta_b/k_b\right]}$$

Activation time constants used are described as $\tau_w = \tau_w^0 + \dfrac{\tau_w^1}{1 + \exp\left[-(v - \theta_w^{\tau})/\sigma_w\right]}$ for $w = n, h, r$. The intracellular Ca^{2+} concentration is determined by

$$\frac{d}{dt}[Ca^{2+}]_{in} = \varepsilon\left(-I_{Ca} - I_T - k_{Ca}[Ca^{2+}]_{in}\right)$$

in which the constant ε combines the effects of buffers, cell volume, and the molar charge of calcium; k_{Ca} is the Calcium pump rate constant. All currents are expressed in pA/μm², conductances in nS/μm², the capacitance of the cells is normalized to 1 pF/μm². Parameter values can be found in Terman et al. 2002, Rubin and Terman 2004, and Heida et al. (2008).

Terman et al. (2002) have used the model of the STN neuron in combination with a GPe cell model (8 to 20 neurons of each type) to explore the arrangement of connections among and within the nuclei and the effective strengths of these connections that are required to generate the oscillatory activity that has been observed in patients with Parkinson's disease.

The outcome of the model single STN neuron of Terman (2002) and Rubin (2004) showed:

- *Spontaneous activity:* The model neuron generates a spontaneous firing rate of 3 Hz. The duration of a single spike is about 2.5 ms, which is longer than those found experimentally (~1 ms). A resting membrane potential of -57 mV was present that varied between -70 to 50 mV during an action potential. During spontaneous activity no slow afterhyperpolarization nor a slow-ramp depolarization was found. The TTX sodium current with negative slope was according to the experimental curves. Applying depolarizing currents with increasing amplitude produces increasing spike frequencies.
- *Bursts:* Rebound bursts could be induced at the break of applied hyperpolarizing currents resulting from the low-threshold T-type current, with a maximum rebound burst length

of about 200 ms as shown in Figure 6A. Terman et al. (2002) do not mention plateau potentials and also do not indicate to have tested the response of the STN neuron model when the membrane potential was kept at a hyperpolarized state. As described by Heida et al. (2008), the model is not able to generate plateau potentials.

Single Compartment STN Model of Otsuka (2004)

The STN neuron model of Otsuka et al. (2004) is based on the dynamics involved in the voltage-dependent generation of a plateau potential. According to Otsuka et al. (2004), single compartment models are justified because experimental studies suggested that the subcellular origin of a plateau potential (the cause of bursting activity) is the soma and/or proximal dendrites. The responses of the model to injection of depolarizing current pulses at the resting and hyperpolarized membrane potentials were judged against recordings from plateau-generating neurons in brain slices.

The membrane potential v of the single compartment model of the STN is described by:

$$C_m \frac{dv}{dt} = -I_{Na} - I_K - I_A - I_T - I_L - I_{Ca-K} - I_{leak}$$

in which:

- $I_{Na}=g_{Na}m^2h(v-v_{Na})$ Na$^+$ current, with activation variable m and inactivation variable h;
- $I_K=g_K n^4(v-v_K)$ delayed rectifier K$^+$ current (high activation threshold, fast activation time constant), with activation variable n;
- $I_A=g_A a^2 b(v-v_K)$ A-type K$^+$ current (low activation threshold, fast activation and inactivation time constants), with activation variable a and inactivation variable b;
- $I_T=g_T p^2 q(v-v_{Ca})$ low-threshold T-type Ca^{2+} current with activation variable p and inactivation variable q;
- $I_L=g_L c^2 d_1 d_2(v-v_{Ca})$ L-type Ca^{2+} current with activation variable c, voltage-dependent inactivativation variable d_1, and Ca^{2+}-dependent inactivation variable d_2.
- $v_{Ca} = \frac{RT}{zF}\frac{[Ca^{2+}]_{ex}}{[Ca^{2+}]_{in}}$ Nernst equation for Calcium, with $[Ca^{2+}]_i$the intracellular Calcium-concentration, $[Ca^{2+}]_{ex}$ the extracellular Calcium-concentration (2 mM), R the gas constant, T absolute temperature (of which no indication is given by Otsuka et al. (2004) other than a temperature of 30°C during the experiments), and z the valence which in this case is 2; reversal potentials of other ionic channels were assumed constant;
- $I_{Ca-K}=g_{Ca-K}r^2(v-v_K)$ Ca^{2+}-activated K$^+$ current with Ca^{2+}-dependent inactivation variable r;
- $I_{leak}=g_{leak}(v-v_{leak})$ leak current.
- $\frac{d[Ca]_i}{dt} = -\alpha I_{Ca} - K_{Ca}[Ca]_i$ intracellular Ca^{2+} concentration, depends on the total Ca^{2+} current, K_{Ca} is the removal rate (ms^{-1}), $\alpha = \frac{1}{zF}$ with z the valence of Calcium, and F Faraday's constant.

C_m is the membrane capacitance and is set at 1 μF/cm^2. Currents are expressed in μA/cm^2; conductances are expressed in mS/cm^2.

Calcium channels of N-, P-, and Q-types as indicated by Song et al. (2000), are not included since these channels have not been found to be involved in plateau potentials. The types and dynamics of the ionic channels included in the model were identified by patch clamp and whole cell recordings from slices (Otsuka et al. 2000; Beurrier et al. 1999; Song et al. 2000; Wigmore and Lacey 2000; Do and Bean 2003; Rudy and McBain 2001). Gating kinetics of the ionic conductances were calculated using the following equation $\frac{dw}{dt} = \frac{w_\infty - w}{\tau_w}$, with $w = a, b, c, d_1, d_2, h, m, n, p, q, r$. Steady state activation and inactivation functions are described by

$$w_\infty = \frac{1}{1 + \exp\left[\left(v - \theta_w\right)/k_w\right]}$$

with θ_w and k_w the half-inactivation/activation voltage and slope, respectively. Activation time constants used are expressed by

$$\tau_w = \tau_w^0 + \frac{\tau_w^1}{1 + \exp\left[\left(v - \theta_w^\tau\right)/\sigma_w\right]}$$

for $w = a, m$, and

$$\tau_w = \tau_w^0 + \frac{\tau_w^1}{\exp\left[-\left(v - \theta_w^{\tau 1}\right)/\sigma_w^1\right] + \exp\left[-\left(v - \theta_w^{\tau 2}\right)/\sigma_w^2\right]}$$

for $w = b, c, d_1, d_2, h, n, p, q, r$. Parameter values can be found in Otuska et al. (2004), and Heida et al. (2008).

The results of the model of Otsuka (2004) can be summarized as follows (see Heida et al. 2008):

- *Spontaneous activity:* The reproduction of the model of the STN neuron without additional inputs showed a spontaneous spiking rate of about 5 Hz. According to Otsuka et al. 2004, the model neuron fires at about 10 Hz, while from Figure 1A in the paper a frequency of about 6 Hz can be estimated. The produced wave form of a single action potential is similar to the one presented by Otsuka et al. 2004. The duration of a single action potential is about 2 ms; the resting membrane potential is about -58 mV with membrane potentials varying from -65 to 40 mV during action potentials. A fast afterhyperpolarization can be discerned followed by a slow afterhyperpolarization phase, however, the membrane subsequently remains at around a resting membrane potential of -57 mV in contrast to the slow-ramp depolarization (the third phase) as observed by Bevan and Wilson (1999). A (TTX-sensitive) sodium current with a negative slope conductance was found. With depolarizing input currents the firing rate of the STN neuron model increases.
- *Bursts:* A hyperpolarizing current pulse is able to induce burst firing in the neuron model. No additional inputs were needed, and after the burst the neuron regains its spontaneous activity. A gradual decrease in firing rate is observed during the last phase of the burst in comparison to the experimental observations of Beurrier et al. (1999). No clear "long-lasting depolarizing potential" is seen in this situation, which would indicate that this is not a plateau potential. However, at the break of a hyperpolarizing input current while in addition a constant hyperpolarizing current is applied that maintains the membrane at a hyperpolarized state, a clear elevation of the membrane potential, i.e., a plateau potential, is induced at the break of the pulse in combination with the generation of a burst.
- *Plateau potentials:* The model is able to produce plateau potentials and burst firing when from a hyperpolarized state a depolarizing or hyperpolarizing input current is applied (Figure 6B). For membrane potentials below about -70 mV a plateau potential was induced with burst spiking that outlasted the current injection in comparison to experimental data (lower two graphs in Figure 6B). Although in the paper of Otsuka et al. (2001) plateau potentials have been defined to have a minimum half-decay time of 200 ms, the paper of Otsuka et al. (2004) does not mention this definition. A clear "long-term" elevation of membrane potential during the bursting activity can be

discerned which will be used here to indicate the presence of a plateau potential.

Heida et al. (2008) concluded from their computer simulations that deinactivation of the T-type current ($q \rightarrow 0.6$) during the current pulse, and the activation of the T-type current ($p \sim 1$) and deinactivation of I_{CaK} ($r \sim 1$) at the break of the current pulse with slow deactivation and inactivation, respectively, seem to be responsible for the generation of a plateau potential.

Figure 6. Comparison of the results from the Terman/Rubin (A) and Otsuka (B) STN model. Settings A) hyperpolarizing inputs of -25, -30, and -45 pA/μm² for upper, middle and lower graph, respectively, during 300 ms starting at t=2500 ms. Settings B) upper graph: hyperpolarizing input current of -2 μA/cm² for 300 ms starting at t=1300 ms; middle graph: the membrane is kept at a hyperpolarized state by application of a constant input current of -5 μA/cm² while an additional hyperpolarizing current of -3 μA/cm² is applied for 300 ms starting at t=1300 ms; lower graph: the membrane is kept at a hyperpolarized state by application of a constant input current of -7.5 μA/cm² while an additional depolarizing current of 7.5 μA/cm² is applied for 50 ms starting at t=1300 ms. The middle and lower graph of B) show the generation of a plateau potential

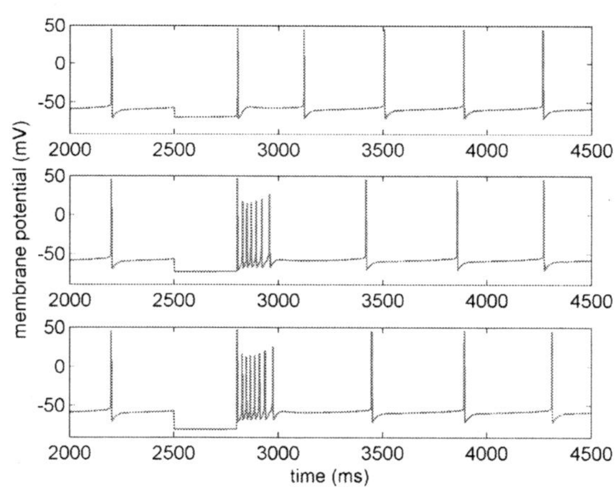

A)

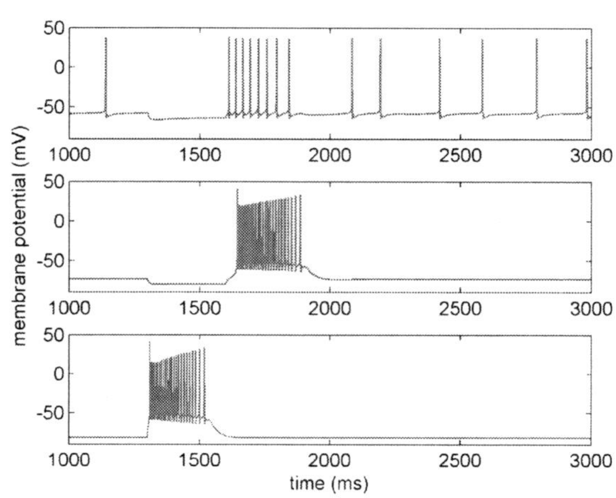

B)

Comparison of Single Compartment STN Models

Comparison of the Terman and Rubin model versus the Otsuka model (Figure 6) brings forward several differences:

1. The equations and parameter values, dimensions and scaling are completely different. For example, Otsuka et al. (2004) describe currents in $\mu A/cm^2$ ($=A/m^2$) while Terman et al. (2002) express currents in $pA/\mu m^2$ ($=10^{-2}$ A/m^2).
2. Both models show spontaneous activity that may be explained by a negative slope conductance in the range associated with the resting phase (at around -58 mV) as observed in both models in their steady-state *I-V* curves.
3. Rubin and Terman's model gives rise to spontaneous activity at nearly 3 Hz, while Otsuka's model arrives at nearly 5 Hz. These firing rates are at the lower limit of those observed in experimental studies in which firing rates of 5-40 spikes/s have been found. Rubin and Terman (2004) apply an additional constant current of 25 $pA/\mu m^2$ in order to increase the firing rate.
4. The shape of the action potential is more realistic in the model of Otsuka et al. (2004), however, in both situations peak duration is longer than those observed experimentally.
5. Both models demonstrate bursting activity at the break of hyperpolarizing inputs.
6. The model of Otsuka et al. (2004) does show the ability to generate rebound potentials without generating a plateau potential, however, duration of this burst is comparable to the burst duration generated in combination with a plateau potential. Terman and Rubin (Terman et al. 2002, and Rubin and Terman 2004) expect the ability to generate bursting activity to represent the Parkinsonian condition. No additional hyperpolarization was applied. In addition, no clear long-lasting depolarization, i.e., a plateau potential, was present during this bursting activity.

Decrease in firing rate during rebound bursts as well as the duration of rebound responses in relation to the amplitude and duration of the input current pulse are more realistically simulated by the model of Otsuka et al. (2004, see Heida et al. 2008). It may therefore be concluded that the Otsuka model shows the best comparison to the results obtained from the experimental studies.

Multi-Compartment STN Model

Gillies and Wilshaw (2006) made a multi-compartment model of a STN neuron including morphological parameters like soma size, dendritic diameters and spatial dendritic configuration (Figure 7), taken from Afsharpour et al. (1985), and Kita et al. (1983), in combination with their electrical properties. Channel dynamics of STN neurons are scarcely found in literature, therefore these were borrowed from thalamic and cortical neurons.

The distribution and density of ion channels in the model were organized by four parameters: 1) the soma channel density; 2) the overall density across all the dendritic trees; 3) the amount of density that is uniform across the dendritic trees; 4) specification of the linear distribution ranging between -1 (maximally distal) and 1 (maximally proximal).

Passive membrane properties are described according to

$$C_{m,i}\frac{dv_i}{dt} = \frac{v_{i-1} - v_i}{r_{i-1,i}} - \frac{v_i - v_{i+1}}{r_{i,i+1}} - I_{ion,i}$$

with for each compartment i, $C_{m,i}$ the membrane capacitance, v_i the membrane potential, and $r_{i-1,i}$ and $r_{i,i+1}$ the axial resistance between compartment i and its previous and following compartment.

Figure 7. Dendritic tree morphology as implemented in the multi compartment model of Gillies and Wilshaw. (Adapted from Gillies and Wilshaw 2006)

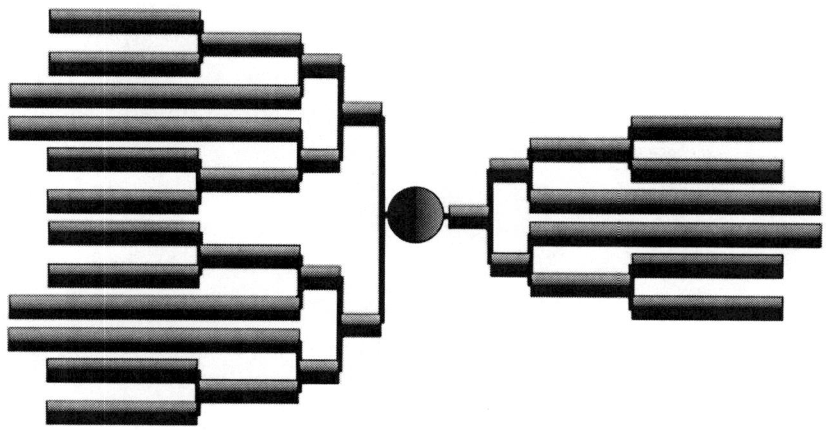

$I_{ion,i}$ is the combination of the ionic currents in the compartment, which in case of a passive membrane consists of a leak current only.

Active membrane properties are described as follows

$$I_{ion,i}=I_{Na,i}+I_{NaP,i}+I_{KDR,i}+I_{Kv31,i}+I_{sKCa,i}+I_{h,i}+I_{CaT,i}+I_{CaL,i}+I_{CaN,i}+I_{leak,i}$$

The ionic channels included in this model are: I_{Na} a fast-acting Na^+ channel, I_{NaP} a persistent Na^+ channel, I_{KDR} a delayed rectifier K^+ channel, I_{Kv31} a fast rectifier K^+ channel, I_{sKCa} a small conductance Ca^{2+}-activated K^+ channel, I_h hyperpolarization-activated cation channel, I_{CaT} a low-voltage-activated T-type Ca^{2+} channel, I_{CaL} a high-voltage-activated L-type Ca^{2+} channel, I_{CaN} a high-voltage-activated N-type Ca^{2+} channel, and I_{leak} a leak current (details can be found in Gillies and Willshaw 2006).

Although several channels were implemented only a restricted amount of channels were needed to produce STN neuronal behaviour. Several experimental studies showed that the T-type Ca^{2+} channel was found necessary as a trigger of many of the behaviours, which was also found in the modeling approach. Other channels that play an important role in mimicking STN neuronal behaviour were also determined by the model: a low-voltage-activated L-type Ca^{2+} channel and a small conductance Ca^{2+}-activated K^+ channel.

The exact values and the density and distribution of the channels into the multi-compartment model of a STN neuron are difficult to determine and are based on approximations. An overview of this multi-compartment model can be found in Heida et al. (2008).

In producing a multi-compartment model the localization of the receptors in the postsynaptic thickening over the dendritic tree is important. Several neurons in the BG circuitry contain a specialized localization of afferents on their dendritic shafts, determining the input-output transformation. The integration of postsynaptic potentials (PSP) occurs over the dendrite and soma. The specific membrane resistivity, the specific membrane capacitance and the intracellular resistivity govern the passive propagation of the synaptic potentials over the dendritic tree. Summation of excitatory PSP's and inhibitory PSP's determine the outcome at the axon hillock. However, the outcome of excitatory summation is not only determined by the factors mentioned above. The morphology of the dendritic tree is as important for the summation in passive neurons Spruston et al. (2008): "1) the presence of dendrites accelerates the excitatory PSP decay near the synaps, 2) cable filtering of dendritic excitatory PSP slows their time course as measured at the soma, thus increasing temporal summation at the soma, 3) sublinear summation is expected for synapses located electrotonically close together, but is minimal for electrotonically separated inputs."

Rules governing the excitation-inhibition interactions are also well known (see Spruston et al. 2008). The creation of multi-compartment models, therefore, need a sound base in the three dimensional structure of the neuron type studied and in the topography of the localization of ionic channels that are guided by neurotransmission.

Cagnan et al. (2009) used a multi-compartment model to test the effects of GABA-ergic GPi projection on thalamic neurons. Adding the nigro-thalamic (dopaminergic) and the cortico-thalamic (glutamatergic) projection by modeling dopaminergic and glutamatergic receptors could have demonstrated the overall effects of the most important connections (GABA, glutamate, and dopamine) on the thalamo-cortical relay neurons, especially if the different localizations of these receptors had been introduced in the three dimensional constructed model of the thalamo-cortical relay neuron.

Network Models of Parts of the Basal Ganglia

As observed in experimental studies, for rhythmic bursting activity to occur in STN cells, a (partially) intact STN-GP network is required. In this situation two features of STN plateau potentials may be relevant:

1. Because a plateau potential can be evoked as a rebound potential, a short train of spikes in GP neurons would hyperpolarize STN neurons and a plateau potential would then occur as a rebound potential, evoking a train of spikes in STN neurons;
2. STN activity would cause immediate feedback inhibition from the GP, but this inhibition might not immediately terminate STN spiking activity because the early part of plateau potentials appears to be resistant to inhibitory perturbations.

In this case, a hyperpolarization of the STN membrane as required for a plateau potential to occur, is caused by inhibitory inputs from GP neurons. Another option for the generation of a hyperpolarization may be the opening of K^+ channels by metabolic signaling pathways (Otsuka et al. 2001).

Terman et al. (2002) studied the dynamic interactions of the network of the subthalamic nucleus and the external segment of the globus pallidus by conductance-based computational models. Similarly, the membrane potential v of the single compartment model of the GPe is described by

$$C_m \frac{dv}{dt} = -I_{Na} - I_K - I_{Ca} - I_T - I_{AHP}$$
$$-I_{leak} + I_{app} - I_{GPe \to GPe} - I_{STN \to GPe}$$

in which the incorporated ionic currents are similar to the equations used for the STN cell except for the T-type current, for which a simpler equation is used, $I_T = g_T a_\infty^3 (v) r (v - v_{Ca})$ with r satisfying a first-order differential equation (dw/dt) with τ_r constant. I_{app} is a constant hyperpolarizing current representing the input from striatum which is assumed a common input to all GPe cells. Without any inputs GPe cells are spontaneously active with a spiking frequency of about 29 Hz.

$I_{GPe \to GPe}$ represents the synaptic input from recurrent connections in GPe

$$I_{GPe \to GPe} = g_{GPe \to GPe} \left(v - v_{GPe \to GPe}\right) \sum_{i=1}^{n} s_i \ ,$$

while the synaptic input from STN to GPe is described by

$$I_{STN\to GPe} = g_{STN\to GPe}\left(v - v_{STN\to GPe}\right)\sum_{i=1}^{n} s_i .$$

Similarly, the STN receives input from GPe according to

$$I_{GPe\to STN} = g_{GPe\to STN}\left(v - v_{GPe\to STN}\right)\sum_{i=1}^{n} s_i ;$$

$g_{GPe\to GPe}$, $g_{GPe\to STN}$, and $g_{STN\to GPe}$ are the synaptic conductance from GPe to GPe, from GPe to STN, and from STN to GPe, respectively. The (GABAergic) synaptic coupling from GPe to STN is inhibitory with a reversal potential of -85 mV, while the reversal potential for the inhibitory recurrent connections in GPe is -100 mV. The (glutamatergic) synaptic coupling from STN to GPe is excitatory with a reversal potential of 0 mV. The summation is taken over the presynaptic neurons according to synaptic variables described as $\frac{ds_i}{dt} = \alpha H_\infty\left(vg_i - \theta_g\right)\left[1 - s_i\right] - \beta s_i$ with vg_i the membrane potential of the presynaptic neuron nr. *i*, and the function

$$H_\infty\left(v\right) = \frac{1}{1 + \exp\left[-\left(v - \theta_g^H\right)/\sigma_g^H\right]} .$$

Networks of 8-20 neurons are constructed in which various organizational levels are produced. This had to be done since the anatomical construction of the GPe-STN network was hardly labored upon in neuroanatomy, neurotransmitter receptor differentiation was not incorporated, and interconnectivity between STN neurons was omitted. Moreover, the channels present were taken from slice preparations that differ presumably from those in vivo.

Simulation results show that the cellular properties of STN and GPe neurons can give rise to a variety of rhythmic or irregular self-sustained firing patterns, depending on the arrangement of connections among and within the nuclei and change in the connection strengths. In the *random, sparsely connected architecture* each GPe cell sends inhibitory input to a small proportion of the STN, and each STN cell sends excitatory input to a small proportion of the GPe. Depending on the strength of the connections this architecture may show 1) irregular firing for a weak connection from STN to GPe or a strong inhibition from GPe to GPe, 2) episodic firing, or 3) continuous uncorrelated firing for strong excitatory connections from STN to GPe and weak inter-GPe connections. The *structured, sparsely connected architecture* creates an off-center architecture that avoids direct reciprocal connections between GPe and STN resulting in clustered activity with variable subsets of highly correlated neurons. Simulating *structured, tightly connected architecture* and several related architectures revealed that propagating waves may occur in the network.

Globus pallidus-STN connections are determined by small neuronal groups in squirrel monkeys (Smith et al. 1994). GPe and STN populations innervate the same groups in the GPi. Medial and lateral parts of the GPi and GPe project to lateral and medial parts of the STN respectively. Moreover "individual neurons in the GPe project via collaterals to both GPi and STN and similarly, that neurons in the STN project to both the GPi and GPe" (Shink et al. 1996; see Figure 8). These reciprocal connections are considered the anatomical substrate for the complex sequences of excitation and inhibition in the STN (Smith et al. 1994/1998). For the projections of the GPe towards the STN as described by Terman et al. (2002) a group of GPe neurons inhibit a group within the STN, while the same population of STN neurons excites the same population GPe neurons responsible for the STN inhibition. Therefore, from the proposed networks by Terman et al. (2002) only the first architecture compares to the anatomical reality as described by Shink et al. (1996).

Terman et al. (2002) conclude that, although the model contained a simplified representation of the cellular properties of STN and GPe cells and the influences that act upon them, the dependence on network architecture requires detailed knowledge of the anatomy, which is lacking. Model simulations may aid in the prediction of likely connectivity architectures under specific physiological and pathophysiological conditions.

The simulation results showed that increasing the (constant) striatal input I_{app} into GPe neurons (as should occur after dopaminergic denervation), and a weakened intrapallidal (inhibitory) coupling, i.e., a decreased $g_{GPe \rightarrow GPe}$, may shift the network into an oscillatory Parkinsonian-like mode. The increased STN activity results in an increased inhibitory output from basal ganglia to thalamus, causing the hypokinetic symptoms associated with Parkinson's disease.

Simulating DBS at the Cellular Level

As indicated, experimental data reveal that the output nuclei of the basal ganglia (GPi) become overactive in Parkinson's disease, increasing the level of inhibition in thalamus. High frequency stimulation was found to increase activity even more in stimulated areas, from which the beneficial effect is hard to grasp.

Basal Ganglia Network Activity Resulting from STN DBS

Rubin and Terman (2004) extended their GPe-STN network and developed a network model of part of the basal ganglia based on single-compartment models of GPi, GPe, STN and thalamocortical

Figure 8. Globus pallidus: subthalamic nucleus (GP-STN) network structures based on tracing studies performed by Shink et al. 1996: "Small groups of interconnected neurons in the associative (A), and sensorimotor (B) territories of the GPe and STN innervate, via axon collaterals a common functionally-related region in the GPi." GPi –globus pallidus internus; GPe–globus pallidus externus; STN–subthalamic nucleus

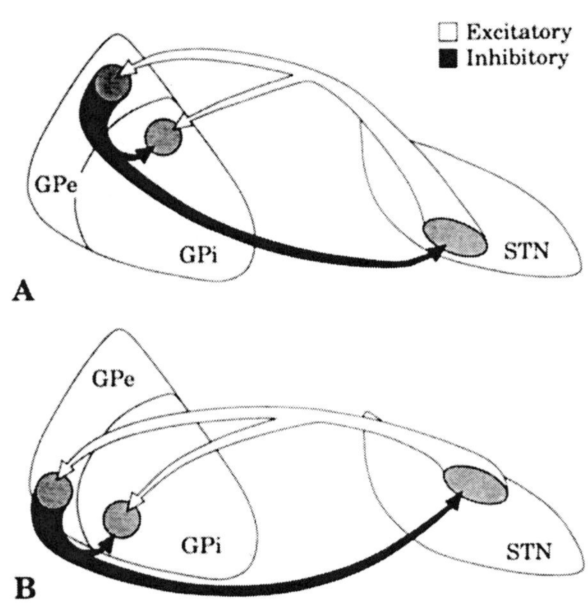

relay neurons. The network is schematically shown in Figure 9. This model is capable of showing an irregular and uncorrelated output from GPi comparable to the "normal" state, allowing the thalamus to relay depolarising cortical signals such as sensorimotor signals, accurately. In contrast, in a "Parkinsonian" state in which GPi and STN neurons fire bursts of action potentials at a tremor frequency of 3-8 Hz, the model showed that bursts are synchronised among subpopulations of neurons. The rhythmic inhibition from GPi to the thalamus disrupts the thalamic ability to relay cortical information.

Excitatory input to the STN, provided by DBS, leads to increased activity of the STN neurons which in turn excites inhibitory GPi neurons, increasing their activity by inducing them to fire tonically at high frequency. Thus DBS replaces the phasic, synchronous firing pattern of STN and GPi neurons associated with Parkinsonian conditions, with a high frequency, tonic, asynchronous activity. Although the firing rate of GPi neurons is increased, the rhythmic pattern is eliminated, restoring the ability of the thalamus to relay its sensorimotor input faithfully.

STN and GPe neuron types are described using equations similar to the ones already described. GPi neurons were modeled exactly as the GPe neurons, however, in order to match firing frequencies with in vivo data instead of in vitro data, additional depolarizing constant inputs were applied to STN (25 pA/μm^2), GPe (2 pA/μm^2), and GPi (3 pA/μm^2).

In the network two thalamic neurons are modeled. They are described according to

$$C_m \frac{dv}{dt} = -I_{Na} - I_K - I_{Ca} - I_T - I_{leak} - I_{GPi\to Th} + I_{SM}$$

These cells are supposed to act as a relay station of incoming sensorimotor signals I_{SM}, which are represented by periodic step functions, $I_{SM}=i_{SM}H(\sin(2\pi t/\rho_{SM}))[1-H(\sin(2\pi(t+\delta_{SM})/\rho_{SM}))$ with H the Heaviside step function as defined ($H(x)=0$ for $x<0$, and $H(x)=1$ for $x\geq 0$) and ρ_{SM} the period, and i_{SM} the amplitude of the signal, and δ_{SM} the duration of the positive phase. They also receive input from the basal ganglia via GPi, $I_{GPi\to Th}$. Further model details can be found in Rubin and Terman (2004).

Figure 9. Part of the basal ganglia network as modeled by Rubin and Terman (2004). (Adapted from Rubin and Terman 2004) GPi: globus pallidus internus; GPe: globus pallidus externus; STN: subthalamic nucleus

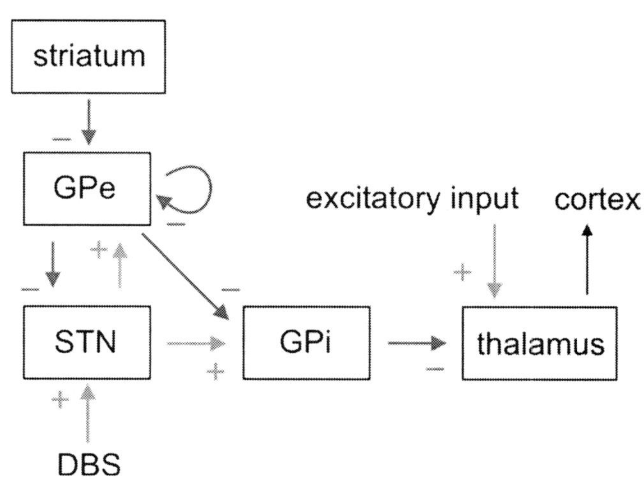

The DBS signal driving the STN is modelled similar to the pulsed signal of the sensorimotor signal. Stimulation in STN leads to increased activity of the STN neurons which in turn excites inhibitory GPi neurons, increasing their activity by inducing them to fire tonically at high frequency. Thus DBS replaces the phasic, synchronous firing pattern of STN and GPi neurons associated with parkinsonian conditions, with a high frequency, tonic, asynchronous activity. Although the firing rate of GPi neurons is increased, the rhythmic pattern is eliminated; stimulation with an amplitude of 200 pA/μm^2, a stimulation period of 6 ms (i.e., about 167 Hz), and a pulse duration of 0.6 ms, completely restores the thalamic ability to relay the sensorimotor signal.

TC relay reliability was further investigated by driving a slightly modified version of the model TC cell by GPi spike trains recorded extracellularly from monkeys rendered Parkinsonian by injection of MPTP (Guo et al., 2008) while also a DBS system was implanted in the STN region with a scaled-down stimulation lead. The simulations reveiled a significant improvement in the ability of the TC cell to relay excitatory stimuli when it is exposed to GPi signals recorded under therapeutically effective DBS, relative to GPi signals that were recorded under therapeutically ineffective DBS or in absence of DBS. The same results were found in a heterogeneous population of model TC cells. In addition, based on a computational approach, relay reliability was gradually lost when the burstiness and correlation of inhibitory spike trains was increased, i.e., the transition from normal to Parkinsonian conditions.

PD and DBS as Synaptic Input from GPi to Thalamocortical Relay Neuron

Cagnan et al. (2009) studied the GPi projection on the thalamocortical (TC) relay neuron. Based on the study of Rubin and Terman (2004), investigating the oscillatory behaviour in basal ganglia as received by the thalamus may clarify why some activity patterns induced in the BG network are associated with pathophysiology while others are associated with treatment. Initially, a multi-compartment model with 3D reconstructed morphology was used (Huguenard and Prince 1992, Destexhe et al. 1998), which was systematically reduced into a single compartment model representing the soma of the thalamic projection neuron (McIntyre et al. 2004b, Destexhe et al. 1998, Huguenard and McCormick 1992, and McCormick and Huguenard 1992). The single-compartment model is described by:

$$C_m \frac{dv}{dt} = -I_{Na} - I_K - I_T - I_h - I_{Ks}$$
$$-I_{Na,leak} - I_{K,leak} - I_{GPi-Th} - I_{DBS}$$

with spike generating currents I_{Na} and I_K, a low threshold calcium current I_T, which plays a vital role in generation of action potentials in response to hyperpolarizing input, a hyperpolarization activated cation current I_h, a slowly activating potassium current I_{Ks}, and sodium and potassium leak currents I_{Naleak} and I_{Kleak}, which determine the resting membrane potential of the TC relay neuron. I_T is described according to the Goldman-Hodgkin-Katz current equation while all other currents I_{Naleak}, I_{Kleak}, I_{Na}, I_K, I_h, I_{Ks} are described using the Hodgkin-Huxley formalism.

The main objectives in this study are to investigate the effect of low frequency synchronized activity associated with Parkinson's disease, and the effect of DBS induced high frequency activity including the study on the functional basis of the inverse relationship that has been reported between DBS stimulus frequency and amplitude, i.e., the therapeutic window for frequency and amplitude combinations (Benabid et al. 1991). The effect of the high frequency effect of DBS is studied from the perspective that DBS will not influence the thalamic neuron itself, but its (inhibitory and excitatory) connections.

The GABAergic GPi input is described as $I_{GPi-Th}(t)=g_{GPi-Th}(1+\alpha\sin(\varphi(t)))(V_m-E_{GABA})$ with E_{GABA} the synaptic reversal potential (-85 mV), g_{GPi-Th} the mean synaptic conductance, α the modulation depth ($0 \leq \alpha \leq 1$, with α=0 meaning uncorrelated input, and $\alpha > 0$ meaning correlated input), and $\varphi(t)$ representing the phase of the oscillatory behaviour of the synaptic conductance, which is described as

$$\phi\left(t+dt\right)=\phi\left(t\right)+2\pi f dt+N\left(0,\sigma\right)\sqrt{dt}$$

with f the frequency of the oscillatory signal, and $N(0,\sigma)$ Gaussian random noise of mean 0 and variance σ.

In order to investigate the effect of DBS on the oscillatory pathological behaviour, an additional synaptic input is defined, according to $I_{DBS}(t)=g_{DBS}(syn_{DBS}(t,f_{DBS}))(V_m-E_{DBS})$ with E_{DBS} the reversal potential, which is 0 mV when this input is assumed to be excitatory, and -85 mV when representing an inhibitory (GABAergic) input. The function $syn_{DBS}(t,f_{DBS})$ is a periodic exponential decay with a decay rate of 10 ms describing the synaptic conductance change resulting from DBS, i.e., the presynaptic neurons show a highly correlated activity pattern at the frequency of stimulation.

The results of the model simulations show that (Cagnan et al. (2009)):

1. the thalamocortical relay neuron preferentially responds to correlated inhibitory GPi input within the theta and beta bands (i.e., a frequency range of 3-10 Hz, and 15-30 Hz, respectively, which may induce the motor symptoms associated with Parkinsons's disease);
2. DBS input parameters, required to arrest the response of the TC relay neuron to correlated GPi input, follow the clinically observed inverse relationship between pulse amplitude and DBS frequency;
3. DBS modulates the neuronal response to low frequency oscillatory BG activity at the thalamic level.

An even more reduced version of the thalamocortical relay neuron is described by Meijer et al. (in prep.). In this paper the single compartment model of Cagnan et al. (2009) is reduced to a three-dimensional model:

$$C_m\frac{dv}{dt}=-I_{Na,t}-I_{K,DR}-I_T-I_{Na,leak}-I_{K,leak}-I_P-I_{DBS}$$

$$\frac{dk}{dt}=\frac{k_\infty\left(V\right)-k}{\tau_k\left(V\right)}$$

$$\frac{dh}{dt}=\frac{h_\infty\left(V\right)-h}{\tau_h\left(V\right)}$$

with v the membrane potential, k and h are the inactivation variables of the sodium and T-type current, respectively. Ionic currents include $I_{x,leak}$ representing the sodium and potassium leak currents, $I_{K,DR}$ the fast and $I_{K,s}$ the slow potassium currents, $I_{Na,t}$ the sodium current, I_T a low-threshold T-type Ca^{2+} current, I_h a hyperpolarization-activated current. The synaptic input from GPi, I_P, represents an oscillatory Parkinsonian signal and I_{DBS} the stimulation signal also received via GABAergic synaptic input from GPi, and are described as $I_P=g_P(t)S(t,T_P)(V-E_{GABA})$ and $I_{DBS}=g_{DBS}(t)S(t,T_{DBS})(V-E_{GABA})$, respectively, where $S(t,T)=Y(\sin(2\pi t/T))Y(\sin(2(t\pi/T+0.5)))$, a periodic step function with period T and a pulse length equal to half a period; $Y(u)=1/(1+\exp(-u/0.001))$. This three-dimensional model which still shows subthreshold oscillations and spikes, enables to work out the geometric mechanism behind the existence and the properties of the frequency-amplitude curve of the effectiveness of DBS, similar to the "Benabid-curve" (Benabid et al. 1991). From this simulation study it can be concluded that the effect of DBS via a synaptic pathway can be to reduce the inactivation of calcium and thereby preventing the membrane potential to reach the firing threshold.

SYSTEM LEVEL MODELS OF BASAL GANGLIA

Neuroanatomical Models

System models are described classically in neuroanatomy (Figure 10 is a good example). In Parkinson's disease these "box and arrow" overviews, describing interactions between nuclei of the basal ganglia and the cortex, are mainly used. The main output of the basal ganglia is via the cortical pyramidal tract. Although included in Figure 10 it often is missed in these models. The model of Albin et al. (1989) and DeLong (1990) is called the "classic" model and was constructed to explain the pathological functioning of the basal ganglia in movement disorders present in the Parkinsonian state.

Cell groups or cell masses determine the basal ganglia. However, these basal ganglia cell groups are functionally determined rather than morphologically (Nieuwenhuys et al. 2008). Still morphology mirrors itself in the nomenclature of the basal ganglia. The striatum (caudate and putamen) contain the same structural elements: medium spiny projection neurons and aspiny interneurons (large and small to medium interneurons). In the rat a subdivision in caudate nucleus and putamen is impossible, due to the fact that the corticofugal system is dispersed over the whole striatum, while in primates the bundling of corticofugal fibers in the capsula interna organizes the bipartition of the striatum. In the models in this section the expression of striatum in direct and indirect circuit will be used.

The direct striatal circuit is subdivided in a subcircuitry that passes over the GPi (A) and one that passes over the substantia nigra pars reticulata (B) (see Nieuwenhuys et al. 2008).

A. Subcircuitry over GPi: Cortex (+ *excitatory*) → Striatum (- *inhibitory*) → GPi (-) → Thalamus (+) (nucleus ventralis anterior and ventralis lateralis pars anterior; and centre median and parafascicular nucleus) → which projects back to the striatum (centre median and parafascicularis nuclei) and the cortex (all thalamic nuclei mentioned).
B. Subcircuitry over pars reticulate: Cortex (+ *excitatory*) → Striatum (- *inhibitory*) → pars reticulata (-) → Thalamus (+) (ventralis anterior and paralaminar part of mediodorsal thalamic nucleus) → all thalamic parts project back to the cortex.

Comparison with Figure 1 shows, that in the direct circuitry, the neuroanatomical data provide more subtle relations. The recurrent information back to the striatum is missing (1) and the single block representing the thalamus concerns different nuclei of that cell mass (2) of which some specifically receive brainstem input. Furthermore:

1. "Interestingly, the cortical efferents from these various parts of the centre median-parafascicular complex project specifically to the cortical areas that have the same striatal targets as the direct thalamostriatal projections from these parts" (Nieuwenhuys et al. 2008). There is a point-to-point relation in the striatum for the cortical areas projecting to that striatal area and the thalamic neurons that project to the same cortical areas, which also project to that striatal area belonging to that part of the cortex. This loop "provides the second-largest source of excitatory input to the striatum" (Nieuwenhuys et al. 2008).
2. Although there are reciprocal connections between the cortex and the specific nuclei of the thalamus (ventralis anterior, ventralis lateralis and medial dorsal nucleus) the so-

Figure 10. Neuroanatomical schemes for basal ganglia input and output and the direct and indirect striatal output pathways (Courtesy Prof. Dr. H.J. Groenewegen, see Groenewegen and Van Dongen 2008). GPI - globus pallidus internus; GPE - globus pallidus externus; SNC - substantia nigra pars compacta; SNR - substantia nigra pars reticulata; Striatum: Put - putamen, Caud - Caudate nucleus, Acb - nucleus accumbens; STN - subthalamic nucleus; Thalamus: ML - medial lemniscus, IL - intra-laminar nucleus, VA - ventral anterior, VL - ventral lateral, MD - medio dorsal nucleus, VTA - ventral tegmental area; VP - ventral pallidum; sc - central sulcus; SP - substance P; ENK - enkephalin; DYN - dynorphin; GABA - gamma amino butyric acid

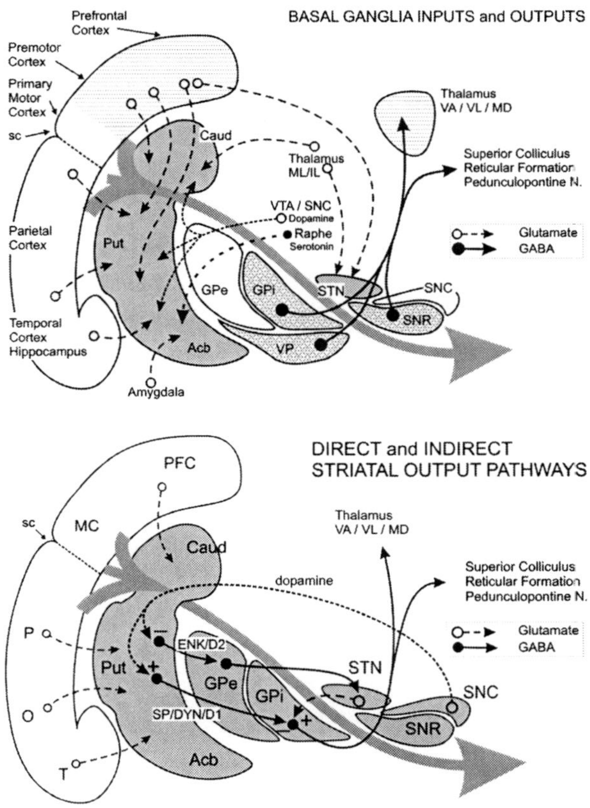

called midline nuclei of the thalamus are non-specific nuclei. Although these non-specific nuclei have a reciprocal relation with their part of the cortex (centre median and primary sensory and motor cortex; parafascicular nucleus and association cortical areas), their projections to the cortex are more widespread. These non-specific nuclei receive ascending projections of a large variety of brainstem nuclei including the pedunculopontine nucleus. So the sub-circuitry over the GPi of the direct pathway seemingly is also under "input control" of the brainstem.

For modeling the block representing the thalamus in the direct pathway should be divided in three parts based on neuroanatomical data: one for the loop over the substantia nigra pars reticulata (it concerns the ventral anterior and paralaminar part of the medial dorsal thalamic nuclei), another for the GPi loop over the ventralis anterior and ventralis lateralis pars anterior, and a third part, also for the GPi loop, in which brainstem input can be relayed to the striatal parts that also receive cortical input from those cortical areas these thalamic nuclei project to. Seemingly this last thalamic part can modulate the striatal input in the direct pathway via brainstem information or in other words the basal ganglia direct pathway is not a closed loop as pretended in modeling.

The indirect striatal circuit contains one main circuit: Cerebral cortex (+ *excitatory*) → Striatum (- *inhibitory*) → GPe (-) → STN (+) → (GPi (-) and SNr) → Thalamus (+) → Cortex. However, next to this circuitry there is a striato- nigro- striatal circuit (see Nieuwenhuys et al. (2008) for details) that is related to the indirect striatal circuitry by the projection of the subthalamic-substantia nigra pars reticulata connection. Via the internal relation between the pars reticulata and pars compacta of the substantia nigra and the inhibiting effects of the striatum on both nigra parts, the nigra effects back on the striatum are hard to predict (Nieuwenhuys et al. 2008). In Figure 1 only the striatal-nigro connection is brought up; the feed back towards the striatum is missing. Via the striato-nigro-striatal circuitry the connection with the limbic and associative striatal circuitry is also maintained (Joel and Weiner, 1997).

Action Selection

Action selection is the resolution of conflicts between requests for behavioural expression that require a common motor resource. The notion that the basal ganglia could play a role in solving the problem of action selection brought forward a "biological plausible system level model".

The most recent example of a computational model based on the concept of action selection is the model of Gurney et al. (1998/2001a/2001b). This model reinterprets the functional anatomy of the BG in which the direct/indirect classification is replaced by selection and control circuits, as shown in Figure 11. The focused D1 inhibitory pathway from striatum to GPi (originally the direct pathway), together with a diffuse excitatory pathway from STN to GPi (indirect pathway), form a primary feed-forward selection circuit. A second group of intrinsic connections centred on the GPe acts as a control circuit to regulate the performance of the main selection mechanism by reducing the output of the GPi and STN, although the full significance of this signal scaling is unclear at present.

Figure 11. Selection/control architecture of basal ganglia (Gurney et al. 1998). GPi - globus pallidus internus; GPe - globus pallidus externus; STN - subthalamic nucleus; D1 - type 1 dopamine receptor; D2 - type 2 dopamine receptor

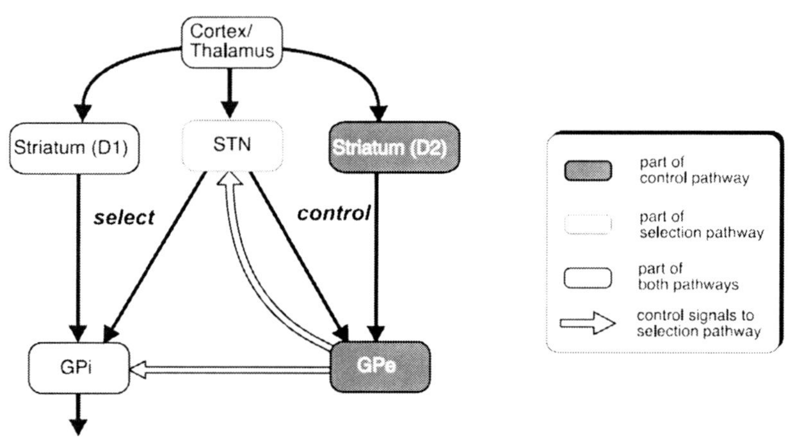

Cortical input to the striatum is described in terms of "channels" where each channel refers to a competing resource or action. Channels are assumed to carry salience or urgency information. Local competition between a group of channels competing for a common motor resource is carried out via lateral inhibition within the striatum, leaving a single channel active. Global competition is carried out via the striatum-GPi selection pathway, in which the striatum of each channel inhibits the GPi in proportion to the salience of the channel. The output of the model is an inhibition of GPi firing in the selected channel.

Within each channel, each nucleus of the BG is modelled as a single equation, the output of which is a normalised mean firing rate between 0 and 1:

$$y_i=(a_i-\varepsilon_i)H(a_i-\varepsilon_i)$$

where a_i is the activation equation of the neuron (see eqns. below) consisting of the sum of the weighted excitatory and inhibitory afferent inputs to the nucleus, ε_i is the threshold for activation of the neuron, and $H(x)$ is a heaviside step function.

The tonic concentration of dopamine (DA) is modelled as a parameter, λ that ranges between 0 and 1, with 0 signifying no DA and 0.2 signifying normal DA levels. In agreement with Albin et al. (1989), DA inhibits the D2-mediated (control) pathway and facilitates the D1-mediated (selection) pathway. Thus, a reduction of DA enhances the control mechanisms and suppresses the selection mechanisms. DA is included in the model as an additional weight on the afferent inputs to the striatum. Thus, the weight on the selection pathway is increased by $(1+\lambda)$:

$$a_i^s=\left(1+\lambda\right)\left(\sum w_m y_m-\sum w_k y_k\right)$$

whereas the weight on the control pathway is decreased by $(1-\lambda)$:

$$a_i^c=\left(1-\lambda\right)\left(\sum w_m y_m-\sum w_k y_k\right)$$

where y is the normalised firing rate of the excitatory/inhibitory input to the striatum and w is the weight of the input. The subscript m represents the mth excitatory input and the subscript k represents the kth inhibitory input.

The authors have demonstrated that reduced DA results in a "stiffer" competition in which there are fewer winners and a reduced disinhibition of the thalamus by the GPi, consistent with bradykinesia. Very low levels of DA result in a failure to select any channel, consistent with akinesia. High DA levels result in simultaneous channel selection even for low salience inputs, possibly consistent with hyperkinesia.

Tremor Model

Haeri et al. (2005) developed a system model of the basal ganglia describing the relationships between the striatum, external part of the globus pallidus (GPe), subthalamic nucleus (STN), internal part of the globus pallidus (GPi) and subtantia nigra pars compacta (SNc), as illustrated in Figure 12. The design of this model is based on the assumption that the input-output relation of a single neuron can be seen as a first-order dynamic system. Furthermore, in each nucleus a lot of neurons are working in parallel, and therefore, each block in the model, and thus each nucleus, is represented as a first-order system with inhibitory and excitatory characteristics included in its transfer function. Parameter values are selected considering the output of the system to resemble Parkinsonian tremor. As substantia nigra pars compacta is considered to be the main component in generating tremor, all non-linearities (such as threshold effects) are included in this block (G_1).

The GPi output of the model illustrates the tremor frequency. The quantity of DA (and other neurotransmitters) is modelled as a connection strength or gain g between the blocks, with a

Figure 12. Basal ganglia model of Haeri et al. (2005), where g and 1/g represent the quantity of neurotransmitter along the pathways. The output (OUT) is considered to be correlated with tremor

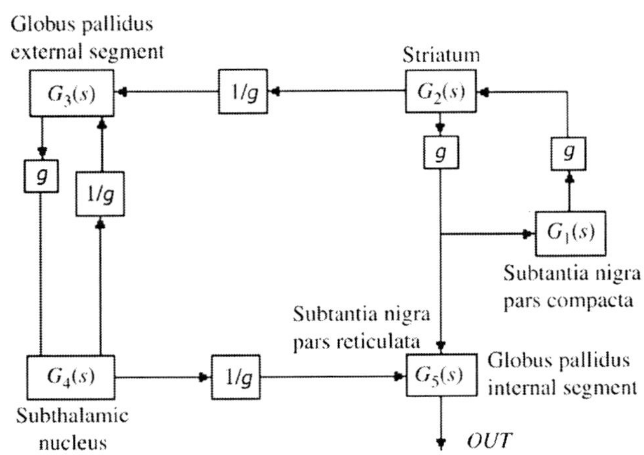

value of 1 representing normal levels. The relationship is taken as inverse, so a decrement of neurotransmitter is modelled as a gain of g and an increase is modelled as a gain of $1/g$. In PD, g is given a value of 10 in contrast to a value of 1 for the normal situation.

Administration of Levodopa was modeled as a second-order dynamic system including a delay time for drug effect initiation, according to

$$G\left(s\right) = \frac{k\exp\left(-T_0 s\right)}{\left(1+sT_1\right)\left(1+sT_2\right)}$$

with T_0 the delay time, T_1 and T_2 time constants in hours, and k an amplification factor. In order to model the drug effect on tremor the input of this system is plasma drug concentration and the output is the gain of dopamine change, g.

DBS is assumed to control the parameter g, according to the equation:

$$g_{(t\to\infty)} = g(0) - \frac{A}{e^{\tau/tc} - 1}$$

where $g(0)$ is the initial value of g, A is the stimulation amplitude, τ is the stimulation period and tc is a time constant, which is dependent on the patient. Thus, DBS causes an increase in the level of DA and a related increase (g) or decrease ($1/g$) of other neurotransmitters along each pathway. The model has demonstrated the presence of tremor during PD conditions and the elimination of tremor during DBS.

Although the idea of modeling drug administration and DBS via a gain that describes the level of neurotransmitter present in the basal ganglia is interesting but debatable for the latter aspect, a considerable defect of the model lies in the fact that eliminating the indirect pathway does not influence the simulation. Therefore, the general idea that Parkinson's disease causes an imbalance between the two pathways is not included in this model. Furthermore, as graphically presented by the authors, the connection strength of the direct pathway is decreased in the Parkinsonian situation in comparison to the normal situation, and thus the increased connection strengths in the indirect pathway should be expected to influence the system's behaviour.

Figure 13. Two modules of the BG-thalamocortical circuit for simulating complex movements; '-' indicate inhibitory pathways; '+' indicate excitatory pathways. Each module contains premotor and supplementary motor areas (SMA), basal ganglia circuitry providing the input to thalamus, which drives the central pattern generator of the parietal and primary motor cortex which is represented by the vector-integration-to-endpoint (VITE) model. DA - dopamine; GPi - globus pallidus internus; GPe - globus pallidus externus; SMA - supplementary motor area; SNc - substantia nigra pars compacta; STN - subthalamic nucleus; TPV - target position vector; PPV - present position vector; VITE - vector-integration-to-endpoint

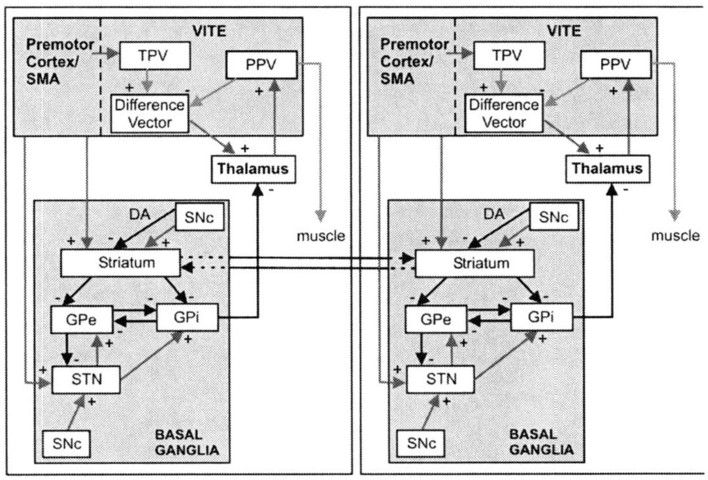

Bradykinesia Model

The model presented by Moroney et al. (2008) attempts to describe bradykinesia and is based on the model developed by Contreras-Vidal & Stelmach (1995), and Bullock & Grossberg (1988), which provides a systems-level mathematical description of basal ganglia-thalamocortical relations in normal and Parkinsonian movements. This model was extended by introducing realistic firing rates, realistic striatal and STN activities resulting from cortical inputs, addition of the hyperdirect pathway, and inclusion of delay times according to experimentally determined time required for a cortical signal to propagate through the basal ganglia and thalamus and back to the cortex. The most important extension to the basic model to enable the simulation of complex movements was the inclusion of multiple BG-thalamocortical circuits. Each degree-of-freedom, e.g. shoulder flexion, shoulder extension, elbow pronation, is controlled by a separate circuit, called a "module". This implies that separate modules control each individual muscle group. The idea of separate circuits is strongly supported by the somatotopic organization and its interconnections present in both cortex, striatum, GPi and GPe, and the STN as based on neuroanatomical tracing results (for an overview see Nieuwenhuys et al. 2008, more specific Alexander et al. 1990, and Romanelli et al. 2005)

The "active module refers to the circuit corresponding to the currently executing motor program, while "inactive" modules refer to surrounding circuits that are not involved in the current movement. To simulate the simultaneous movement of several joints, two or more modules would be activated at the same time. To simulate sequential movements, a second module would be activated immediately after the first has finished. The model was initially extended to include two modules that represent elbow flexion and extension, as shown in Figure 13, but more modules can be added.

The model contains three parts in each modules: 1) the cortex producing motor programming and sequencing by the premotor and supplementary motor areas (SMA), 2) the basal ganglia circuitry, responsible for movement gating and modulation, and 3) a part that constitutes central pattern generation by the parietal and primary motor cortex (VITE model), all coupled together. The exchange of information between the modules relays over the striatum, which is also strongly supported by neuroanatomical tracer studies (for an overview see Nieuwenhuys et al. 2008).

The general description of the mean firing rate of a part of a nucleus in the basal-ganglia circuit is given by

$$\frac{d}{dt}N_k = -A_k N_k + \left(B_k - N_k\right)\sum_{i=1}^{n} W_{exc,i} Y_{exc,i} - \left(N_k - D_k\right)\sum_{i=1}^{m} W_{inh,i} Y_{inh,i}$$

with A_k is the passive decay rate of neural activity, B_k is the upper bound and D_k the lower bound of neural activity, $Y_{exc,i}$ and $Y_{inh,i}$ represent the excitatory and inhibitory inputs that are received via connections with strengths $W_{exc,i}$ and $W_{inh,i}$, respectively; k represents the nucleus (i.e. k=*Sr*, *Gi*, *Ge*, *Stn* or *Th*).

The Vector-Integration-To-Endpoint or VITE model was developed by Bullock and Grossberg (1988) to model the desired kinematics of point-to-point arm movements to a stationary object with no unexpected external forces. The VITE circuit models motor cortical operations performed during arm pointing movements; it generates an outflow signal, representing the desired arm trajectory, which is sent to the lower brainstem and spinal centers to guide muscle contractions.

The inclusion of the VITE circuit in the model has the advantage of allowing the actual movement trajectory to be observed, rather than just the firing rates of the nuclei.

Parkinson's disease was simulated as a reduction in the level of dopamine, as well as a loss of functional segregation between the two modules. The dynamics of neurotransmitter levels in the striatum are modeled using non-linear differential equations to account for the accumulation and depletion processes that occur during movement. The modulation has a medium-term effect on neural activity in the BG, which is consistent with the metabotropic action of DA. The neurotransmitter dynamics on the direct (GABA, substance P and dynorphin) and indirect (GABA and enkephalin) pathways respectively are:

$$\frac{d}{dt}Nd = b\left(B_{SP/DYN}\left(DA\right) - Nd\right) - c * Sr * Nd,$$

and

$$\frac{d}{dt}Ni = b\left(B_{ENK}\left(DA\right) - Ni\right) - c * Sr * Ni$$

where: *Nd* / *Ni* is amount of neurotransmitter available for signaling in the direct / indirect pathway, respectively, *b* is the re-accumulation rate of neurotransmitter, *c* is the depletion constant of neurotransmitter, $B_{SP/DYN}(DA)$ / $B_{ENK}(DA)$ is the maximum amount of neurotransmitter in direct / indirect pathway ($B_{SP/DYN}(DA)=DA^2$, $B_{BNK}(DA)=1+e^{-4.6DA}$), and *Sr* is the striatal activity.

There is evidence for inhibitory recurrent connections among striatal projection neurons, and Tunstall et al. (2002) believe that inhibitory interactions between spiny projection neurons may be a key determinant of the signal processing operations performed in the striatum. These connections form an opponent circuit through mutual inhibition which occurs laterally between groups of neurons of the same nucleus. This lateral inhibition is mediated by axon collaterals from projection neurons in neighbouring motor modules. It is proposed that lateral inhibition among medium spiny neurons of the striatum serves to focus striatal activity. During movement, increased striatal activity in the active channel should serve to inhibit striatal neurons in neighbouring modules, thus reducing the activity of unwanted modules, and suppressing undesired movements.

In the present model, lateral inhibition has been implemented at the level of the striatum only. The implementation of lateral inhibition involved the inclusion of an additional inhibitory input to the striatum. As seen in the equation below, the striatum is inhibited by axon collaterals from neurons in neighbouring motor channels according to the following equation that gives the mean firing rate of the striatal projection neurons (*Sr*):

$$\frac{d}{dt}Sr(t) = -A_{Sr}Sr(t) + \left(B_{Sr} - Sr(t)\right)$$
$$\left(I_{CorSr}\left(t - \tau_{CorSr}\right) + I_{tonicSr}\right) - \left(Sr(t) - D_{Sr}\right)\sum_{\substack{x \neq current \\ module}} Sr_x(t)$$

where I_{CorSr} is an excitatory input from the cortex, $I_{tonicSr}$ represents the level of tonic activity within the striatum, and $\Sigma Sr_x(t)$ represents the inhibition by axon collaterals from striatal neurons in neighbouring motor modules, i.e., lateral inhibition.

The Parkinsonian state was introduced by changing the dopamine "concentration" (DA=0.8) in the basal ganglia model and comparing the results to the "normal" dopamine concentration (DA=1). The primary deficits in movement resulted directly from dopamine loss. However, loss of functional segregation contributed to the bradykinetic symptoms, due to interference from competing motor modules on the currently executing movement, and a reduced ability to suppress unwanted movements. Loss of segregation also led to excessive neurotransmitter depletion, affecting the performance of sequential movements. The results of the simulation of elbow flexion of 90° indeed show an increase of the GPi activity that should reduce thalamus activity in the Parkinsonian state. The activity of GPi and thalamus for the Parkinsonian situation in comparison to the normal (control) situation is given in the figure below.

DA loss resulted in a slight decrease in GPe activity and an increase in STN activity of PD patients compared to controls (not shown), leading to an increase in GPi activity. The reduction in neurotransmitter along the direct path caused a reduction in the inhibition of the GPi by the striatum, leading to a disinhibition of the GPi. The increased GPi activity due to changes in both the direct and indirect paths produced a smaller disinhibition of the thalamus in PD patients, and thus a reduced thalamic activity in the active channel, as seen in Figure 14.

Figure 14. Elbow flexion performed by module 1 (active module) under normal and Parkinsonian conditions. GPi activity is increased in the active module in PD (A), resulting in reduced disinhibition of the thalamus (B), and thus resulting in inhibition of the desired movement, i.e., bradykinesia

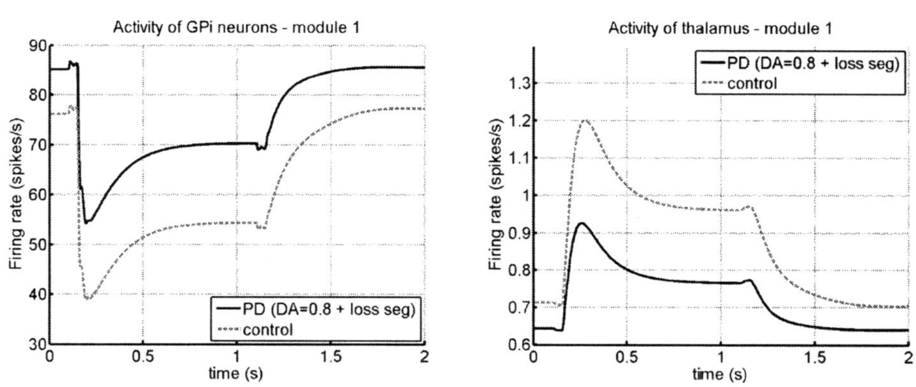

A) B)

The effect of lateral inhibition and loss of functional segregation is shown in Figure 15A. Due to the cortical input to module 1 to perform elbow flexion, striatal activity in module 2 is reduced below tonic levels due to the increased inhibition from active striatal neurons in module 1. Changes in striatal activity propagated through the circuit to the GPi, where a further increase in GPi activity was observed for the normal situation, on top of the already increased activity due to the fast action of the hyperdirect pathway, as illustrated in Figure 15B. The resulting increased inhibition of the thalamus would act to inhibit movement in the undesired channel, adding to the focusing effect, whereby desired movements are facilitated while undesired movements are inhibited more strongly. This supports the benefit of lateral inhibition within the striatum, which is the focusing effect which it provides to the desired movement, via inhibition of movement in the channels representing undesired movements.

Due to loss of functional segregation as occurs in PD, module 2 also received an input from cortex that overruled the effect of lateral inhibition as indicated in Figure 15A. GPi activity decreased thereby disinhibiting the thalamus, and thus undesired movements or cocontractions resulted.

The model also can be used to study DBS. One of the possible mechanisms suggested for the beneficial effects of DBS of the STN in improving the symptoms of PD is an inhibition of the STN nucleus. DBS was implemented in the model as a direct inhibitory input to the STN (other possible mechanisms are described by Moroney et al. (2008) however, these will not be discussed here). In case of DBS Parkinsonian symptoms are generally severe, and thus a strongly reduced dopamine level was assumed (i.e., DA=0.7).

The increased inhibitory input to the STN caused a large reduction in the output firing rate of the STN nucleus, which was far below normal levels, as can be seen in Figure 16. Note that normal neural activity as well as PD activity (DA=0.8) are shown in the following figures for comparison. The reduced STN activity caused a reduction in the activity of the GPi to slightly below normal levels, as well as a reduction in GPe activity far below the normal firing rate, as seen in Figure 17.

Figure 15. Direct effect of striatal lateral inhibition and the loss of functional segregation in Parkinson's Disease (PD) on striatal neurons (A) and downstream effects on GPi activity (B) of the inactive module. In the control situation striatal lateral inhibition results in an increased activity in GPi thereby inhibiting the thalamus and preventing movement in the accompanying muscle group. Under Parkinsonian conditions GPi activity is decreased resulting in disinhibition of the thalamus creating cocontractions

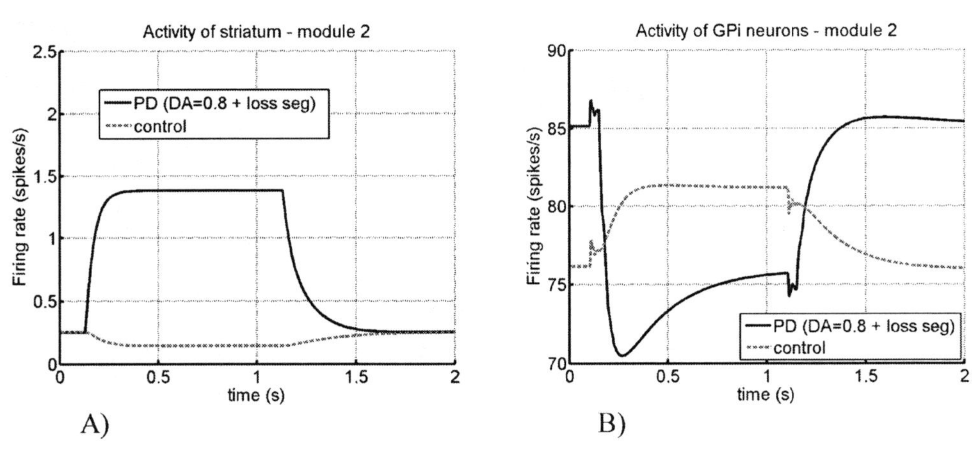

The reduced GPi activity resulted in a greater disinhibition of the thalamus, causing an increase in thalamic activity to almost normal levels, greatly improving the symptoms of bradykinesia. The movement parameters from the VITE were significantly improved. The results of the experimental study of Benazzouz et al. (2000) show that high-frequency stimulation of the subthalamic nucleus induces a net decrease in activity of all cells recorded around the site of stimulation in the subthalamic nucleus. As a consequence, the reduction of the excitatory glutamatergic output from the subthalamic nucleus deactivates substantia nigra pars reticulata neurons and thereby induces a disinhibition of activity in the ventrolateral motor thalamic nucleus, which

Figure 16. A large reduction in STN activity results from direct inhibition of the STN cell body, one of the hypothesized mechanisms of DBS.

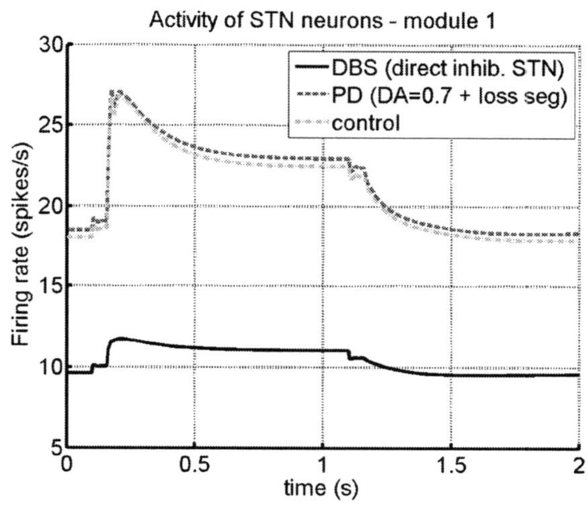

Figure 17. If DBS causes inhibition of STN activity, the model shows that the indirect result of stimulation is a reduction in GPi activity (A) to a normal level, and a reduction in GPe activity (B) to below the normal level.

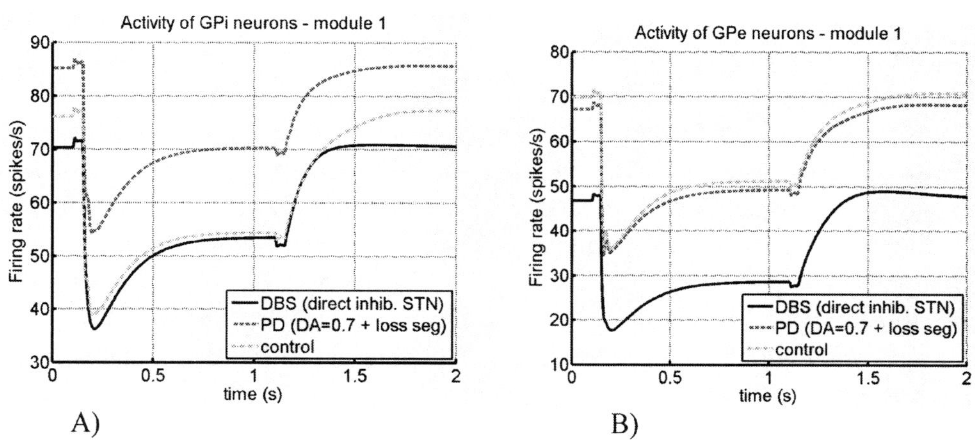

should result in activation of the motor cortical system.

The elbow flexion and extension as simulated by the model of Moroney et al. (2008) was compared to analogous measurements in Parkinson patients, showing large similarities.

CONCLUSION

The reviewed models presented in this chapter are capable of describing one or more of the symptoms of PD, although no model has been found in literature that incorporates all the symptoms. The lack of morphometric and electrophysiological information hampers the description of models of BG and therefore hinders the verification of hypothesized BG function and explaining the mechanism(s) of DBS. For example, the incorporated ionic channels in single and multi-compartment models of neuronal cells and their injected current are only partially based on parameters found in vivo.

The neuroanatomical system schemes on BG motor connections as found in literature are in accordance with each other. Refinement is still going on, especially towards the existence of various channels or modules working in parallel or sequentially for separate muscle actions. Although re-entrant cortical and subcortical loops are described in literature (see e.g. Groenewegen and Van Dongen 2008), such a re-entrant input in the models is missing totally.

Only one model directly coupled output from basal ganglia neurons via thalamus to the function of muscle groups involved. All other models predict on their best a thalamic output that hardly can be converted into dysfunction of muscle groups, explaining Parkinsonian symptoms like tremor, bradykinesia, rigidity or hypokinesia.

Multi-compartment models of neurons allow to bring in the three dimensional topography of the cell body, dendrites and axon. However, it is impossible to determine all parameters that describe the neuron, like the density and distribution of the various synaptic and ionic channels. Thus, in order to develop a multi-compartment model one has to collect experimental data both on cellular morphology and on the distribution and kinetics of membrane channels. Fitting of experimental data into parameter values that cause the model to reproduce the firing behaviour of the particular neuron is often required. This process may then also allow the development of a single-compartment model that produces similar behaviour.

The most astonishing fact regarding modeling Parkinson's disease and DBS is that, while PD is caused by depletion of dopamine, only a few models incorporate this depletion directly as base for inducing Parkinsonian behaviour in the models studied.

FUTURE RESEARCH DIRECTIONS

The motor signs of Parkinson's disease are mainly hypokinetic such as akinesia/bradykinesia, rigidity and loss of normal postural reflexes. The most identifiable sign of Parkinson's disease, however, is resting tremor, which is a hyperkinetic symptom. Although substantia nigra degeneration and dopamine depletion are the hallmark of PD, the pathophysiology of the Parkinsonian symptoms and especially of Parkinsonian tremor are still under debate. Abnormal synchronous oscillating neuronal activity produced by the weakly coupled neural networks of the basal ganglia-thalamo-cortical loops is expected to underly the PD symptoms. The mechanism of Deep Brain Stimulation may be the suppression of this synchronous oscillating behaviour or by rendering the circuit insensitive to oscillatory activity. However, it is important to know which circuits are actually influenced by DBS, since the stimulation may reach neuronal elements outside the nucleus that is expected to be stimulated. Furthermore, present evidence supports the view that the basal ganglia loops are influenced by other neuronal structures and systems.

With improving computer technology calculation times are considerably reduced creating the opportunity to increase the complexity of the models as described in this chapter. But, considering the complexity of biological and (electro-) physiological reality, computational models will always have their limitatations. One must, however, realize that animal models or laboratory preparations are also often imperfect representations of reality.

Investigating and mimicking the behaviour of a single neuron or a network of neurons and/or nuclei with the use of computational models requires detailed morphological data including three-dimensional measurements of the neurons, the dimensions and (membrane) properties of the different compartments, their connections, and the density, distribution and chemical and electrical properties of the synapses. Therefore, to improve future models, experimental research is essential. While models may generate testable predictions and may help to formulate new hypotheses, experiments are required to reject or accept the hypotheses. With respect to Parkinson's disease the ultimate goal is to link the symptoms of the disease with the neuronal behaviour of basal ganglia in motor control, and to discover the exact mechanism, or combination of mechanisms, of deep brain stimulation that alter this behaviour and thereby reduce the symptoms.

REFERENCES

Afsharpour, S. (1985). Light microscopic analysis of Golgi-impregnated rat subthalamic neurons. *The Journal of Comparative Neurology*, *236*, 1–13. doi:10.1002/cne.902360102

Albin, R. L., Young, A. B., & Penney, J. B. (1989). The functional anatomy of basal ganglia disorders. *Trends in Neurosciences*, *12*, 366–375. doi:10.1016/0166-2236(89)90074-X

Aldridge, J. W., Berridge, K. C., & Rosen, A. R. (2004). Basal ganglia neural mechanisms of natural movement sequences. *Canadian Journal of Physiology and Pharmacology*, *82*, 732–739. doi:10.1139/y04-061

Alexander, G., & Crutcher, M. (1991). Reply: letter to the editor. *Trends in Neurosciences*, *14*, 2.

Alexander, G. E., DeLong, & M. R., Strick, P. L. (1986). Parallel organization of functionally segregated circuits linking basal ganglia and cortex. *Annual Review of Neuroscience*, *9*, 357–381. doi:10.1146/annurev.ne.09.030186.002041

Alexander, G. E., & Crutcher, M. D. (1990). Functional architecture of basal ganglia circuits: neural substrates of parallel processing. *Trends in Neurosciences*, *13*, 266–271. doi:10.1016/0166-2236(90)90107-L

Ashby, P., Kim, Y. J., Kumar, R., Lang, A. E., & Lozano, A. M. (1999). Neurophysiological effects of stimulation through electrodes in the human subthalamic nucleus. *Brain*, *122*(Pt 10), 1919–1931. doi:10.1093/brain/122.10.1919

Bar-Gad, I., Morris, G., & Bergman, H. (2003). Information processing, dimensionality reduction and reinforcement learning in the basal ganglia. *Progress in Neurobiology*, *71*, 439–473. doi:10.1016/j.pneurobio.2003.12.001

Benabid, A., Benazzous, A., & Pollak, P. (2002). Mechanisms of Deep Brain Stimulation. *Movement Disorders*, *17*, S73–S74. doi:10.1002/mds.10145

Benabid, A. L., Krack, P., Benazzouz, A., Limousin, P., Koudsie, A., & Pollak, P. (2000). Deep brain stimulation of the subthalamic nucleus for Parkinson's disease: Methodologic aspects and clinical criteria. *Neurology*, *55*, S40–S44.

Benabid, A. L., Pollak, P., Gervason, C., Hoffman, D., Gao, D. M., & Hommel, M. (1991). Long-term suppression of tremor by chronic stimulation of the ventral intermediate thalamic nucleus. *Lancet*, *337*, 403–406. doi:10.1016/0140-6736(91)91175-T

Benazzouz, A., Breit, S., Koudsie, A., Pollak, P., Krack, P., & Benabid, A. (2002). Intraoperative Microrecordings of the Subthalamic Nucleus in Parkinson's Disease. *Movement Disorders*, *17*, S145–S149. doi:10.1002/mds.10156

Benazzouz, A., Gao, D. M., Ni, Z. G., Piallat, B., Bouali-Benazzouz, R., & Benabid, A. L. (2000). Effect of high-frequency stimulation of the subthalamic nucleus on the neuronal activities of the substantia nigra pars reticulate and ventroalteral nucleus of the thalamus in the rat. *Neuroscience*, *99*, 289–295. doi:10.1016/S0306-4522(00)00199-8

Bennett, B., & Wilson, C. (1999). Spontaneous Activity of Neostriatal Cholinergic Interneurons In Vitro. *The Journal of Neuroscience*, *19*, 5586–5596.

Bergman, H., Feingold, A., Nini, A., Raz, A., Slovin, H., Abeles, M., & Vaadia, E. (1998). Physiological aspects of information processing in the basal ganglia of normal and parkinsonian primates. *Trends in Neurosciences*, *21*, 32–38. doi:10.1016/S0166-2236(97)01151-X

Bergman, H., Wichmann, T., Karmon, B., & De Long, M. R. (1994). The Primate Subthalamic Nucleus II. Neuronal Activity in the MPTP Model of Parkinsonism. *Journal of Neurophysiology*, *72*, 507–520.

Berns, G. S., & Sejnowski, T. J. (1998). A Computational Model of How the Basal Ganglia Produce Sequences. *Journal of Cognitive Neuroscience*, *10*(1), 108–121. doi:10.1162/089892998563815

Beurrier, C., Congar, P., Bioulac, B., & Hammond, C. (1999). Subthalamic nucleus neurons switch from single spike activity to burst-firing mode. *The Journal of Neuroscience*, *19*, 599–609.

Bevan, M. D., & Wilson, C. J. (1999). Mechanisms underlying spontaneous oscillation and rhythmic firing in rat subthalamic neurons. *The Journal of Neuroscience*, *19*, 7617–7628.

Bezard, E., Gross, C. E., & Brotchie, J. M. (2003). Presymptomatic compensation in Parkinson's disease is not dopamine-mediated. *Trends in Neurosciences*, *26*, 215–221. doi:10.1016/S0166-2236(03)00038-9

Blandini, F., Nappi, G., Tassorelli, C., & Martignoni, E. (2000). Functional changes of the basal ganglia circuitry in Parkinson's disease. *Progress in Neurobiology*, *62*, 63–88. doi:10.1016/S0301-0082(99)00067-2

Braak, H., Ghebremedhin, E., Rub, U., Bratzke, H., & Del Ttredici, K. (2004). Stages in the development of Parkinson's disease-related pathology. *Cell and Tissue Research*, *318*, 124–134. doi:10.1007/s00441-004-0956-9

Brain Lord, & Walton, J.N. (1969). *Brain's Diseases of the nervous system*. London: Oxford University Press.

Breit, S., Lessmann, L., Benazzouz, A., & Schulz, J. B. (2005). Unilateral lesion of the pedunculopontine nucleus induces hyperactivity in the subthalamic nucleus and substantia nigra in the rat. *The European Journal of Neuroscience*, *22*, 2283–2294. doi:10.1111/j.1460-9568.2005.04402.x

Breit, S., Schulz, J. B., & Benabid, A. (2004). Deep brain stimulation. *Cell and Tissue Research*, *318*, 275–288. doi:10.1007/s00441-004-0936-0

Brown, J., Bullock, D., & Grossberg, S. (1999). How the Basal Ganglia Use Parallel Excitatory and Inhibitory Learning Pathways to Selectively Respond to Unexpected Rewarding Cues. *The Journal of Neuroscience*, *19*(23), 10502–10511.

Brown, P. (2003). Oscillatory nature of human basal ganglia activity: relationship to the pathophysiology of Parkinson's disease. *Movement Disorders*, *18*, 357–363. doi:10.1002/mds.10358

Bullock, D., & Grossberg, S. (1988). Neural Dynamics of Planned Arm Movements: Emergent Invariants and Speed-Accuracy Properties During Trajectory Formation. *Psychological Review*, *95*, 49–90. doi:10.1037/0033-295X.95.1.49

Cagnan, H., Meijer, H. E., van Gils, S. A., Krupa, M., Heida, T., Rudolph, M., Wadman, W. J., & Martens, H. C. F. (2009). Frequency-selectivity of a thalamocortical relay neuron during Parkinson's disease and Deep Brain Stimulation: a computational study. *European Journal of Neuroscience*, 30,1306-1317 (DOI:10.1111/j.1460-9568.2009.06922.x)Calabresi, P., Centonze, D., & Bernardi, G. (2000). Electrophysiology of dopamine in normal and denervated striatal neurons. *Trends in Neurosciences, 23*, S57-S63.

Contreras-Vidal, J. L., & Stelmach, G. E. (1995). A neural model of basal ganglia-thalamocortical relations in normal and Parkinsonian movement. *Biological Cybernetics*, *73*, 467–476. doi:10.1007/BF00201481

Davis, G. C., Williams, A. C., & Markey, S. P. (1979). Chronic parkinsonism secondary to intravenous injection of meperidine analogues. *Psychiatry Research*, *1*, 249–254. doi:10.1016/0165-1781(79)90006-4

DeLong, M. R. (1990). Primate models of movement disorders of basal ganglia origin. *Trends in Neurosciences*, *13*, 281–285. doi:10.1016/0166-2236(90)90110-V

Denny-Brown, D. (1962). *The Basal Ganglia and their relation to disorders of movement*. Oxford: Oxford University Press.

Destexhe, A., Neubig, M., Ulrich, D., & Huguenard, J. (1998). Dendritic low-threshold calcium currents in thalamic relay cells. *The Journal of Neuroscience*, *18*, 3574–3588.

Do, M. T. H., & Bean, B. P. (2003). Subthreshold sodium currents and pacemaking of subthalamic neurons: modulation by slow inactivation. *Neuron*, *39*, 109–120. doi:10.1016/S0896-6273(03)00360-X

Dostrovsky, J., & Lozano, A. (2002). Mechanisms of Deep Brain Stimulation. *Movement Disorders*, *17*(3), S63–S68. doi:10.1002/mds.10143

Filion, M., & Tremblay, L. (1991). Abnormal spontaneous activity of globus pallidus neurons in monkeys with MPTP-induced parkinsonism. *Brain Research*, *547*, 142–151.

Filion, M., Tremblay, L., & Bedard, P. J. (1988). Abnormal influences of passive limb movement on the activity of globus pallidus neurons in parkinsonian monkeys. *Brain Research*, *444*, 165–176. doi:10.1016/0006-8993(88)90924-9

Florio, T., Scarnati, E., Confalone, G., Minchella, D., Galati, S., & Stanzione, P. (2007). High frequency stimulation of the subthalamic nucleus modulates theactivity of pedunculopontine neurons through direct activation of excitatory fibers as well as through indirect activation of inhibitory pallidal fibers in the rat. *The European Journal of Neuroscience*, *25*, 1174–1186. doi:10.1111/j.1460-9568.2007.05360.x

Frank, M. J. (2005). Dynamic dopamine modulation in the basal ganglia: a neurocomputational account of cognitive deficits in medicated and nonmedicated Parkinsonism. *Journal of Cognitive Neuroscience*, *17*, 51–72. doi:10.1162/0898929052880093

Garcia, L., D'Alessandro, G., Bioulac, B., & Hammond, C. (2005b). High-frequency stimulation in Parkinson's disease: more or less? *Trends in Neurosciences*, *28*, 4. doi:10.1016/j.tins.2005.02.005

Garcia, L., D'Alessandro, G., Fernagut, P., Bioulac, B., & Hammond, C. (2005a). Impact of High-Frequency Stimulation Parameters on the Pattern of Discharge of Subthalamic Neurons. *Journal of Neurophysiology*, *94*, 3662–3669. doi:10.1152/jn.00496.2005

Garcia-Rill, E. (1991). The pedunculopontine nucleus. *Progress in Neurobiology*, *36*, 363–389. doi:10.1016/0301-0082(91)90016-T

Gerfen, C. R., & Wilson, C. J. (1996). The basal ganglia. In L. W. Swanson (Ed.) *Handbook of Chemical Neuroanatomy vol 12: Integrated systems of the CNS, Part III* (pp. 371-468).

Gillies, A., & Willshaw, D. (2006). Membrane channel interactions underlying rat subthalamic projection neuron rhythmic and bursting activity. *Journal of Neurophysiology*, *95*, 2352–2365. doi:10.1152/jn.00525.2005

Gomez-Gallego, M., Fernandez-Villalba, E., Fernandez-Barreiro, A., & Herrero, M. T. (2007). Changes in the neuronal activity in the pedunculopontine nucleus in chronic MPTP-treated primates: an in situ hybridization study of cytochrome oxidase subunit I, choline acetyl transferase and substance P mRNA expression. *Journal of Neural Transmission*, *114*, 319–326. doi:10.1007/s00702-006-0547-x

Grill, M. W., & McIntyre, C. C. (2001). Extracellular excitation of central neurons: implications for the mechanisms of deep brain stimulation. *Thalamus & Related Systems*, *1*, 269–277.

Groenewegen, H. J., & Van Dongen, Y. C. (2008). Role of the Basal Ganglia. In Wolters, E. C., van Laar, T., & Berendse, H. W. (Eds.), *Parkinsonism and related disorders*. Amsterdam: VU University Press.

Guo, Y., Rubin, J., McIntyre, C., Vitek, J., & Terman, D. (2008). Thalamocortical relay fidelity varies across subthalamic nucleus deep brain stimulation protocols in a data driven computational model. *Journal of Neurophysiology*, *99*, 1477–1492. doi:10.1152/jn.01080.2007

Gurney, K., Prescott, T. J., & Redgrave, P. (2001a). A computational model of action selection in the basal ganglia. I. A new functional anatomy. *Biological Cybernetics*, *84*, 401–410. doi:10.1007/PL00007984

Gurney, K., Prescott, T. J., & Redgrave, P. (2001b). A computational model of action selection in the basal ganglia. II. Analysis and simulation of behaviour. *Biological Cybernetics*, *84*, 411–423. doi:10.1007/PL00007985

Gurney, K., Redgrave, P., & Prescott, A. (1998). *Analysis and simulation of a model of intrinsic processing in the basal ganglia (Technical Report AIVRU 131)*. Dept. Psychology, Sheffield University.

Haeri, M., Sarbaz, Y., & Gharibzadeh, S. (2005). Modeling the Parkinson's tremor and its treatments. *Journal of Theoretical Biology*, *236*, 311–322. doi:10.1016/j.jtbi.2005.03.014

Hashimoto, T., Elder, C. M., Okun, M. S., Patrick, S. K., & Vitek, J. L. (2003). Stimulation of the subthalamic nucleus changes firing pattern of pallidal neurons. *The Journal of Neuroscience*, *23*, 1916–1923.

Hassler, R. (1937). Zur Normalanatomie der Substantia nigra. *Journal für Psychologie und Neurologie*, *48*, 1–55.

Hassler, R. (1938). Zur Pathologie der Paralysis agitans und des postencephalitischen Parkinsonismus. *Journal für Psychologie und Neurologie*, *48*, 387–476.

Hassler, R. (1939). Zur pathologischen Anatomie des senilen und des parkinsonistischen Tremor. *Journal für Psychologie und Neurologie*, *49*, 193–230.

Heida, T., Marani, E., & Usunoff, K. G. (2008). The subthalamic nucleus: Part II, Modeling and simulation of activity. *Advances in Anatomy, Embryology, and Cell Biology*, 199.

Heimer, L., Switzer, R. D., & Van Hoesen, G. W. (1982). Ventral striatum and ventral pallidum. Components of the motor system? *Trends in Neurosciences*, *5*, 83–87. doi:10.1016/0166-2236(82)90037-6

Hodgkin, A., & Huxley, A. F. (1952). A quantative description of membrane current and its application to conduction and excitation in nerve. *The Journal of Physiology*, *117*, 500–544.

Holsheimer, J., Demeulemeester, H., Nuttin, B., & De Sutter, P. (2000). Identification of the target neuronal elements in electrical deep brain stimulation. *The European Journal of Neuroscience*, *12*, 4573–4577.

Hornykiewicz, O. (1989). The Neurochemical Basis of the Pharmacology of Parkinson's Disease. Handbook of Experimental Pharmacology 88. *Drugs for the Treatment of Parkinson's Disease* (pp. 185-204). Calne, D.B.: Springer-Verlag.

Huguenard, J. R., & McCormick, D. A. (1992). Simulation of the currents involved in rhythmic oscillations in thalamic relay neurons. *Journal of Neurophysiology*, *68*, 1373–1383.

Huguenard, J. R., & Prince, D. A. (1992). A novel T-type current underlies prolonged calcium-dependent burst firing in GABAergic neurons of rat thalamic reticular nucleus. *The Journal of Neuroscience*, *12*, 3804–3817.

Jenkins, N., Nandi, D., Oram, R., Stein, J. F., & Aziz, T. Z. (2006). Pedunculopontine nucleus electric stimulation alleviates akinesia independently of dopaminergic mechanisms. *Neuroreport*, *17*, 639–641. doi:10.1097/00001756-200604240-00016

Jenkinson, N., Nandi, D., Miall, R. C., Stein, J. F., & Aziz, T. Z. (2004). Pedunculopontine nucleus stimulation improves akinesia in a Parkinsonian monkey. *Neuroreport*, *15*, 2621–2624. doi:10.1097/00001756-200412030-00012

Joel, D., & Weiner, I. (2000). The connections of the dopaminergic system with the striatum in rats and primates: an analysis with respect to the functional and compartmental organization of the striatum. *Neuroscience*, *96*, 451–474. doi:10.1016/S0306-4522(99)00575-8

Kelly, A. E., Domesick, V. B., & Nauta, W. J. H. (1982). The amygdalostriatal projection in the rat – an anatomical study by anterograde and retrograde tracing methods. *Neuroscience*, *7*, 615–630. doi:10.1016/0306-4522(82)90067-7

Kenney, C., Fernandez, H. H., & Okum, M. S. (2007). *Role of deep brain stimulation targeted to the pedunculopontine nucleus in Parkinson's disease* (pp. 585-589). Editorial in: Future Drugs Ltd.

Kita, H., Chang, H. T., & Kitai, S. T. (1983). The morphology of intracellularly labeled rat subthalamic neurons: a light microscopic analysis. *The Journal of Comparative Neurology*, *215*, 245–257. doi:10.1002/cne.902150302

Kita, H., Nambu, A., Kaneda, K., Tachibana, Y., & Takada, M. (2004). Role of Ionotropic Glutamatergic and GABAergic Inputs on the Firing Activity of Neurons in the External Pallidum in Awake Monkeys. *Journal of Neurophysiology*, *92*, 3069–3084. doi:10.1152/jn.00346.2004

Langston, J. W., Ballard, P., Tetrud, J., & Irwin, I. (1983). Chronic parkinsonism in humans due to a product of meperidine-analog synthesis. *Science*, *219*, 979–980. doi:10.1126/science.6823561

Langston, J. W., Forno, L. S., Tetrud, J., Reeves, A. G., Kaplan, J. A., & Karluk, D. (1999). Evidence of active nerve cell degeneration in the substantia nigra of humans years after 1-Methyl-4-phenyl- 1,2,3,6- tertahydropyridine exposure. *Annals of Neurology*, *46*, 598–605. doi:10.1002/1531-8249(199910)46:4<598::AID-ANA7>3.0.CO;2-F

Lewy, F. H. (1912). Paralysis agitans. I Pathalogische Anatomie. In Lewandowsky, M. H. (Ed.), *Handbuch der Neurologie* (*Vol. 3*, pp. 920–933). Berlin: Springer.

Lewy, F. H. (1913). Zur pathologischen Anatomie der Paralysis agitans. *Deutsch Zeitschr Nervenheilk*, *50*, 50–55.

Lozano, A., Dostrovsky, J., Chen, R., & Ashby, P. (2002). Deep brain stimulation for Parkinson's disease: disrupting the disruption. *The Lancet Neurology*, *1*, 225–231. doi:10.1016/S1474-4422(02)00101-1

Magnin, M., Morel, A., & Jeanmonod, D. (2000). Single-unit analysis of the pallidum, thalamus and subthalamic nucleus in parkinsonian patients. *Neuroscience*, *96*(3), 549–564. doi:10.1016/S0306-4522(99)00583-7

Marani, E., Heida, T., Lakke, E. A. J. F., & Usunoff, K. G. (2008). The subthalamic nucleus: Part I, Development, cytology, topography and connections. *Advances in Anatomy, Embryology, and Cell Biology*, 198.

Mazzone, P., Lozano, A., Stanzione, P., Galati, S., Scarnati, E., Peppe, A., & Stefani, A. (2005). Implantation of human pedunculopontine nucleus: a safe and clinically relevant target in Parkinson's disease. *Neuroreport*, *16*, 1877–1881. doi:10.1097/01.wnr.0000187629.38010.12

McCormick, D. A., & Huguenard, J. R. (1992). A model of the electrophysiological properties of thalamocortical relay neurons. *Journal of Neurophysiology*, *68*, 1384–1400.

McIntyre, C. (2001). Extracellular excitation of central neurons: implications for the mechanisms of deep brain stimulation. *Thalamus & Related Systems*, *1*, 269–277.

McIntyre, C. C., Grill, W. M., Sherman, D. L., & Thakor, N. V. (2004b). Cellular effects of Deep Brain Stimulation: Model-Based Analysis of Activation and Inhibition. *Journal of Neurophysiology*, *91*, 1457–1469. doi:10.1152/jn.00989.2003

McIntyre, C. C., Savasta, M., Kerkerian-Le Goff, L., & Vitek, J. L. (2004a). Uncovering the mechanism(s) of action of deep brain stimulation: activation, inhibition, or both. *Clinical Neurophysiology*, *115*, 1239–1248. doi:10.1016/j.clinph.2003.12.024

Meijer, H. G. E., Krupa, M., Cagnan, H., Heida, T., Martens, H., & Van Gils, S. A. (in prep.). Mathematical studies on the frequency response of a model for a thalamic neuron. *Journal of Computational Neuroscience*.

Mena-Segovia, J., Bolam, J. P., & Magill, P. J. (2004). Pedunculopontine nucleus and basal ganglia: distant relatives or part of the same family? *Trends in Neurosciences*, *27*, 585–588. doi:10.1016/j.tins.2004.07.009

Mettler, F. A. (1944). Physiologic consequences and anatomic degeneration following lesions of primate brain stem. *The Journal of Comparative Neurology*, *80*, 69–148. doi:10.1002/cne.900800107

Mettler, F. A. (1946). Experimental production of static tremor. *Proceedings of the National Academy of Sciences of the United States of America*, *89*, 3859–3863.

Mettler, F. A. (1968). Anatomy of the basal ganglia. In Vinken, P. J., & Bruyn, G. W. (Eds.), *Handbook of Clinical Neurology* (*Vol. 6*, pp. 1–55). Amsterdam: North Holland Publ. Co.

Meyers, R. (1968). Ballismus. In Vinken, P. J., & Bruyn, G. W. (Eds.), *Handbook of Clinical Neurology* (pp. 476–490). Amsterdam: North Holland Publ. Co.

Mink, J. W. (1996). The basal ganglia: focused selection and inhibition of competing motor programs. *Progress in Neurobiology*, *50*, 381–425. doi:10.1016/S0301-0082(96)00042-1

Montgomery, E., & Gale, J. (2005). *Mechanisms of Deep Brain Stimulation: Implications for Physiology, Pathophysiology and Future Therapies*. 10th Annual Conference of the International FES Society.

Moroney, R., Heida, T., & Geelen, J. A. G. (2008). Modeling of bradykinesia in Parkinson's disease during simple and complex movements. *Journal of Computational Neuroscience*, *25*, 501–519. doi:10.1007/s10827-008-0091-9

Nakanishi, H., Kita, H., & Kitai, S. T. (1987). Electrical membrane properties of rat subthalamic neurons in an in vitro slice preparation. *Brain Research*, *437*, 35–44. doi:10.1016/0006-8993(87)91524-1

Nambu, A. (2005). A new approach to understand the pathophysiology of Parkinson's disease. *Journal of Neurology 252*, IV/1-IV/4.

Nambu, A., Tokuno, H., Hamada, I., Kita, H., Imanishi, M., & Akazawa, T. (2000). Excitatory cortical inputs to pallidal neurons via the subthalamic nucleus in the monkey. *Journal of Neurophysiology*, *84*, 289–300.

Nambu, A., Tokuno, H., & Takada, M. (2002). Functional significance of the cortico-subthalamo-pallidal 'hyperdirect' pathway. *Neuroscience Research*, *43*, 111–117. doi:10.1016/S0168-0102(02)00027-5

Nandi, D., Aziz, T. Z., Giladi, N., Winter, J., & Stein, F. (2002a). Reversal of akinesia in experimental parkinsonism by GABA antagonist microinjections in the pedunculopontine nucleus. *Brain*, *123*, 2418–2430. doi:10.1093/brain/awf259

Nandi, D., Liu, X., Winter, J. L., Aziz, T. Z., & Stein, J. F. (2002b). Deep brain stimulation of the pedunculopontine region in the normal non-human primate. *Journal of Clinical Neuroscience*, *9*, 170–174. doi:10.1054/jocn.2001.0943

Nieuwenhuys, R., Voogd, J., & van Huijzen, C. (2008). *The human central nervous system*. Berlin: Springer.

O'Reilly, R. C., & Frank, M. J. (2006). Making working memory work: a computational model of learning in the prefrontal cortex and basal ganglia. *Neural Computation*, *18*, 283–328. doi:10.1162/089976606775093909

Orieux, G., Francois, C., Féger, J., Yelnik, J., Vila, M., & Ruberg, M. (2000). Metabolic activity of excitatory parafascicular and pedunculopontine inputs to the subthalamic nucleus in a rat model of Parkinson's disease. *Neuroscience*, *97*, 79–88. doi:10.1016/S0306-4522(00)00011-7

Otsuka, T., Abe, T., Tsukagawa, T., & Song, W. J. (2000). Single compartment model of the voltage-dependent generation of a plateau potential in subthalamic neurons. *Neuroscience Research. Supplement*, *24*, 581.

Otsuka, T., Abe, T., Tsukagawa, T., & Song, W.-J. (2004). Conductance-based model of the voltage-dependent generation of a plateau potential in subthalamic neurons. *Journal of Neurophysiology*, *92*, 255–264. doi:10.1152/jn.00508.2003

Otsuka, T., Murakami, F., & Song, W. J. (2001). Excitatory postsynaptic potentials trigger a plateau potential in rat subthalamic neurons at hyperpolarized states. *Journal of Neurophysiology*, *86*, 1816–1825.

Pahapill, P. A., & Lozano, A. M. (2000). The pedunculopontine nucleus and Parkinson's disease. *Brain, 123*, 1767–1783. doi:10.1093/brain/123.9.1767

Percheron, G., & Filion, M. (1991). Parallel processing in the basal ganglia: up to a point (letter to the editor). *Trends in Neurosciences, 14*, 55–56. doi:10.1016/0166-2236(91)90020-U

Pessiglione, M., Guehl, D., Rollard, A., Francois, C., Hirsch, E., Feger, J., & Tremblay, L. (2005). Thalamic neuronal activity in dopamine-depleted primates: evidence for a loss of functional segregation within basal ganglia circuits. *The Journal of Neuroscience, 25*, 1523–1531. doi:10.1523/JNEUROSCI.4056-04.2005

Pieranzotti, M., Palmieri, M. G., Galati, S., Stanzione, P., Peppe, A., & Tropepi, D. (2008). Pedunculopontine nucleus deep brain stimulation changes spinal cord excitability in Parkinson's disease patients. *Journal of Neural Transmission, 115*, 731–735. doi:10.1007/s00702-007-0001-8

Plaha, P., & Gill, S. S. (2005). Bilateral deep brain stimulation of the pedunculopontine nucleus for Parkinson's disease. *Neuroreport, 16*, 1883–1887. doi:10.1097/01.wnr.0000187637.20771.a0

Plenz, D., & Kitai, S. T. (1999). A basal ganglia pacemaker formed by the subthalamic nucleus and external globus pallidus. *Nature, 400*, 677–682. doi:10.1038/23281

Prescott, T. J., Gurney, K., Montes-Gonzalez, F., Humphries, M., & Redgrave, P. (2002). The robot basal ganglia: action selection by an embedded model of the basal ganglia. In Nicholson, L., & Faull, R. (Eds.), *Basal Ganglia VII*. Plenum Press.

Ranck, J. B. (1975). Which elements are excited in electrical stimulation of mammalian central nervous system? *Annual Review Brain Research, 98*, 417–440.

Romanelli, P., Esposito, V., Schaal, D. W., & Heit, G. (2005). Somatotopy in the basal ganglia: experimental and clinical evidence for segrated sensorimotor channels. *Brain Research. Brain Research Reviews, 48*, 112–128. doi:10.1016/j.brainresrev.2004.09.008

Romo, R., & Schultz, W. (1992). Role of primate basal ganglia and frontal cortex in the internal generation of movements. III. Neuronal activity in the supplementary motor area. *Experimental Brain Research, 91*, 396–407. doi:10.1007/BF00227836

Rubin, J., & Terman, D. (2004). High frequency stimulation of the subthalamic nucleus eliminates pathological rhythmicity in a computational model. *Journal of Computational Neuroscience, 16*, 211–235. doi:10.1023/B:JCNS.0000025686.47117.67

Rudy, B., & McBain, C. J. (2001). Kv3 channels: voltage-gated K^+ channels designed for high-frequency repetitive firing. *Trends in Neurosciences, 24*, 517–526. doi:10.1016/S0166-2236(00)01892-0

Schuurman, P. R., Bosch, A. D., Bossuyt, P. M. M., Bonsel, G. J., van Someren, E. J. W., & de Bie, R. M. A. (2000). A comparison of continuous thalamic stimulation and thalatomy for suppression of severe tremor. *The New England Journal of Medicine, 342*, 461–468. doi:10.1056/NEJM200002173420703

Shink, E., Bevan, M. D., Bolam, J. P., & Smith, Y. (1996). The subthalamic nucleus and the external pallidum: two tightly interconnected structures that control the output of the basal ganglia in the monkey. *Neuroscience, 73*, 335–357. doi:10.1016/0306-4522(96)00022-X

Smith, Y., Bevan, M. D., Shink, E., & Bolam, J. P. (1998). Microcircuitry of the direct and indirect pathways of the basal ganglia. *Neuroscience, 86*, 353–387.

Smith, Y., Wichmann, T., & DeLong, M. R. (1994). Synaptic innervation of neurons in the internal pallidal segment by the subthalamic nucleusand the external pallidum in monkeys. *The Journal of Comparative Neurology*, *343*, 297–318. doi:10.1002/cne.903430209

Song, W.-J., Baba, Y., Otsuka, T., & Murakami, F. (2000). Characterization of Ca^{2+} channels in rat subthalamic nucleus neurons. *Journal of Neurophysiology*, *84*, 2630–2637.

Spruston, N., Stuart, G., & Häusser, M. (2008). Dendritic integration. In Stuart, G. (Ed.), *Dendrites* (pp. 351–399). Oxford University Press.

Squire, L. R., Bloom, F. E., McConnell, S. K., Roberts, J. L., Spitzer, N. C., & Zigmond, M. J. (2003). The Basal Ganglia. In *Fundamental Neuroscience* (2nd ed., pp. 815–839). Academic Press.

Stefani, A., Lozano, A. M., Peppe, A., Stanzione, P., Galati, S., & Tropepi, D. (2007). Bilateral deep brain stimulation of the pedunculopontine and subthalamic nuclei in severe Parkinson's disease. *Brain*, *130*, 1596–1607. doi:10.1093/brain/awl346

Strafella, A., Ko, J. H., Grant, J., Fraraccio, M., & Monchi, O. (2005). Corticostriatal functional interactions in Parkinson's disease: a rTMS/[11C] raclopride PET study. *The European Journal of Neuroscience*, *22*, 2946–2952. doi:10.1111/j.1460-9568.2005.04476.x

Suri, R. E., Albani, C., & Glattfelder, A. H. (1997). A dynamic model of motor basal ganglia functions. *Biological Cybernetics*, *76*, 451–458. doi:10.1007/s004220050358

Suri, R. E., & Schultz, W. (1998). Learning of sequential movements by neural network model with dopamine-like reinforcement signal. *Experimental Brain Research*, *121*, 350–354. doi:10.1007/s002210050467

Takakusaki, K., Saitoh, K., Harada, H., & Kashiwayanagi, M. (2004). Role of the basal ganglia-brainstem pathways in the control of motor behaviours. *Neuroscience Research*, *50*, 137–151. doi:10.1016/j.neures.2004.06.015

Tang, J., Moro, E., Lozano, A., Lang, A., Hutchison, W., Mahant, N., & Dostrovsky, J. (2005). Firing rates of pallidal neurons are similar in Huntington's and Parkinson's disease patients. *Experimental Brain Research*, *166*, 230–236. doi:10.1007/s00221-005-2359-x

Temel, Y., Blokland, A., Steinbusch, H. W., & Visser-Vandewalle, V. (2005). The functional role of the subthalamic nucleus in cognitive and limbic circuits. *Progress in Neurobiology*, *76*, 393–413. doi:10.1016/j.pneurobio.2005.09.005

Terman, D., Rubin, J. E., Yew, A. C., & Wilson, C. J. (2002). Activity patterns in a model for subthalamopallidal network of the basal ganglia. *The Journal of Neuroscience*, *22*, 2963–2976.

Tretriakoff, C. (1919). *Contribution a l'étude de l'anatomie pathologique du locus niger de Soemmering avec quelques déductions relatives a la pathogenie des troubles du tonus musculaire et de la maladie du Parkinson.* Thesis No 293, Jouve et Cie, Paris.

Tunstall, M. J., Oorschot, D. E., Kean, A., & Wickens, J. R. (2002). Inhibitory interactions between spiny projection neurons in the rat striatum. *Journal of Neurophysiology*, *88*, 1263–1269.

Usunoff, K. G., Itzev, D. E., Ovtscharoff, W. A., & Marani, E. (2002). Neuromelanin in the Human Brain: A review and atlas of pigmented cells in the substantia nigra. *Archives of Physiology and Biochemistry*, *110*, 257–369. doi:10.1076/apab.110.4.257.11827

Vitek, J. (2002). Mechanisms of Deep Brain Stimulation: Excitation or Inhibition. *Movement Disorders*, *17*, S69–S72. doi:10.1002/mds.10144

Von Economo, C. J. (1917). Neue Beitrage zur Encephalitis lethargica. *Neurologisches Zentralblatt*, *36*(21), 866–878.

Von Economo, C. J. (1918). Wilsons Krankheit und das "Syndrome du corpse strie". *Zentralblatt für die gesamte. Neurologie et Psychiatrie*, *44*, 173–209.

Wichmann, T., & DeLong, M. R. (1996). Functional and pathophysiological models of the basal ganglia. *Current Opinion in Neurobiology*, *6*, 751–758. doi:10.1016/S0959-4388(96)80024-9

Wigmore, M. A., & Lacey, M. G. (2000). A Kv3-like persistent, outwardly rectifying, Cs^{+}-permeable, K^{+} current in rat subthalamic nucleus neurones. *The Journal of Physiology*, *527*, 493–506. doi:10.1111/j.1469-7793.2000.t01-1-00493.x

Wu, Y., Levy, R., Ashby, P., Tasker, R., & Dostrovsky, J. (2001). Does Stimulation of the GPi Control Dyskinesia by Activating Inhibitory Axons? *Movement Disorders*, *16*, 208–216. doi:10.1002/mds.1046

Xu, K., Bastia, E., & Schwarzschild, M. (2005). Therapeutic potential of adenosine A2A receptor antagonists in Parkinson's disease. *Pharmacology & Therapeutics*, *105*(3), 267–310. doi:10.1016/j.pharmthera.2004.10.007

Zhu, Z., Bartol, M., Shen, K., & Johnson, S. W. (2002). Excitatory effects of dopamine on subthalamic nucleus neurons: in vitro study of rats pretreated with 6-hydroxydopamine and levodopa. *Brain Research*, *945*, 31–40. doi:10.1016/S0006-8993(02)02543-X

Zrinzo, L., Zrinzo, L. V., & Hariz, M. (2007). The pedunculopontine and peripeduncular nuclei: a tale of two structures. *Brain*, *130*, E73. doi:10.1093/brain/awm079

Chapter 4
High-Performance Image Reconstruction (HPIR) in Three Dimensions

Olivier Bockenbach
RayConStruct GmbH, Germany

Michael Knaup
University of Erlangen-Nürnberg, Germany

Sven Steckmann
University of Erlangen-Nürnberg, Germany

Marc Kachelrieß
University of Erlangen-Nürnberg, Germany

ABSTRACT

Commonly used in medical imaging for diagnostic purposes, in luggage scanning, as well as in industrial non-destructive testing applications, Computed Tomography (CT) is an imaging technique that provides cross sections of an object from measurements taken from different angular positions around the object. CT, also referred to as Image Reconstruction (IR), is known to be a very compute-intensive problem. In its simplest form, the computational load is a function of $O(M \times N^3)$, where M represents the number of measurements taken around the object and N is the dimension of the object. Furthermore, research institutes report that the increase in processing power required by CT is consistently above Moore's Law. On the other hand, the changing work flow in hospital requires obtaining CT images faster with better quality from lower dose. In some cases, real time is needed. High Performance Image Reconstruction (HPIR) has to be used to match the performance requirements involved by the use of modern CT reconstruction algorithms in hospitals. Traditionally, this problem had been solved by the design of specific hardware. Nowadays, the evolution of technology makes it possible to use Components of the Shelf (COTS). Typical HPIR platforms can be built around multicore processors such as the Cell Broadband Engine (CBE), General-Purpose Graphics Processing Units (GPGPU) or Field Programmable Gate Arrays (FPGA). These platforms exhibit different level in the parallelism required to implement CT reconstruction algorithms. They also have different properties in the way the computation can be carried

DOI: 10.4018/978-1-60566-280-0.ch004

out, potentially requiring drastic changes in the way an algorithm can be implemented. Furthermore, because of their COTS nature, it is not always easy to take the best advantages of a given platform and compromises have to be made. Finally, a fully fleshed reconstruction platform also includes the data acquisition interface as well as the vizualisation of the reconstructed slices. These parts are the area of excellence of FPGAs and GPGPUs. However, more often then not, the processing power available in those units exceeds the requirement of a given pipeline and the remaining real estate and processing power can be used for the core of the reconstruction pipeline. Indeed, several design options can be considered for a given algorithm with yet another set of compromises.

1 INTRODUCTION

1.1 The 3D Image Reconstruction Problem

Also referred to as Computed Tomography (CT), 3D image reconstruction is an imaging technique that provides cross sections of an object from measurements taken from different angular positions around the object (Figure 1). Sound descriptions of the principles and underlying mathematics have been the topic of numerous books and publications (Kak 1988, Herman 1980, Kalender 2005, Natterer 1989). CT is commonly used in medical imaging for diagnostic purposes, in luggage scanning, as well as in industrial non-destructive testing applications. Since Hounsfield (1972) patented the first CT scanner, new X-ray source-detector technologies have made a revolutionary impact on the possibilities of Computed Tomography.

From the pure mathematical point of view, the solution to the inverse problem of image reconstruction had been found for the two dimensional case by Johann Radon in 1917 (Radon 1986). Nevertheless, the use of an ever-improving technology fuels the research community. As a result, there seems to be an endless stream of new reconstruction algorithms.

Image reconstruction is known to be a very compute-intensive problem. In its simplest form, the computational load is a function of $O(M \times N^3)$[1], where M represents the number of measurements taken around the object and N is the dimension of the object. Both values typically lie in the range between 500 and 1500. Only through the use of High Performance Computing (HPC) platforms the reconstruction can be performed in a delay that is compatible with the requirements of the above-mentioned applications. Moreover, CT scanners have entered the stage of wide deployment, and the requirements for processing power for implementing the new algorithms has steadily been above Moore's law. As a consequence, one cannot expect to run modern reconstruction algorithms on commonly available computers. Therefore, high-performance computing solutions are commonly used to solve the computational problem of image reconstruction.

Nevertheless, there are significant variations in the size of the reconstruction problem. Even for a given application, e.g. medical imaging, the selected values for M and N can vary depending on several factors, such as the region of interest and the desired image quality. By nature, the reconstruction problem exhibits inherent independence between subsets of input samples and between subparts of the reconstructed volume, making it suitable for parallelization techniques. Indeed the ultimate HPC platforms, as they are required for high-performance image reconstruction (HPIR), must provide powerful processing blocks that allow for parallelization. In addition, HPC platforms also need to remain flexible enough to enable the architecture to scale to address the different problem sizes without undue reduction in the efficiency.

The quality of a given CT implementation is also measured against the quality of the recon-

Figure 1. Principle of Computed Tomography. The object to be reconstructed is illuminated from different angles by a fan beam of X-ray photons. The absorption of X-ray photons is measured from every angle

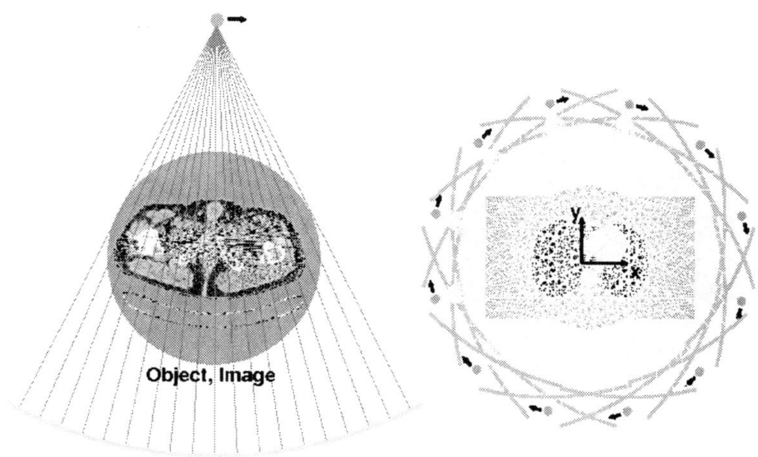

structed volume. The quality is evaluated against gold reference standards. It largely depends on the reconstruction algorithm and, for a given algorithm, on the accuracy and the precision at which the different processing steps have been carried out. Inaccurate and imprecise operations can introduce all kinds of reconstruction artifacts, easily recognizable in the resulting volume.

In order to reach the desired image quality, several factors need to be considered when implementing the different processing steps. Firstly, the quality of the measured samples plays an important role. Although the analysis of the samples' quality is beyond the scope of this chapter, it is worth noticing that they influence the complexity of the de-noising algorithms, which in turn influence the selection of the HPC platform for running the appropriate de-noising algorithms. Secondly, the precision at which the computation has to be carried out also depends on the size of the problem, i.e. the number of voxels to reconstruct as well as the desired spatial resolution. Since a big part of the problem consists in computing coordinates, one must ensure that the computation uses enough bits to accurately compute those coordinates.

Due to the large variety in the type of reconstruction problems, there is also a wide spectrum of possible HPC platforms to consider. However, considering the inherent properties of the problem, there are only a few families of devices which can be used for solving the problem in a time and cost effective way. Firstly, the size of the problem is fairly large, but the individual data sets are also independent from each other. This naturally calls for a high degree of parallelism. Secondly, the size of the problem and the desired resolution influence the number of bits at which the computation has to take place. Ideally this number should be variable. Thirdly, the performance requirements of the final application also dictate the number of processing elements needed to meet the processing time.

There are several families of devices that can be looked at to efficiently design an HPC platform: the Application Specific Integrated Circuit (ASIC), the Field Programmable Gate Array (FPGA), the multicore processor architecture and General-Purpose Graphics Processing Units (GPGPUs). All these devices exhibit, to a certain extent, the desired properties for building at least a part of the HPC reconstruction platform. They all have been successfully used in existing designs. Furthermore, significant hardware design is in progress for these device families. They all have a dense roadmap so that one can trustfully consider designing future

HPC platforms for 3D reconstruction using future versions of those devices.

1.2 Chapter Structure

This chapter concentrates on 3D image reconstruction for medical imaging. This application is based on anatomical knowledge that most readers have learned. Readers can best understand the implications of image quality on the reconstruction algorithm. Nevertheless, the same HPIR principles used for clinical imaging, can be used as well for non-destructive material testing, security scanning applications, micro-CT imaging or any other related tomographic technique.

This chapter is organized as follows: Section 3 describes the scanner technologies used in hospitals along with the most common scan protocols. The scanner technology puts strong requirements on the speed at which the raw data needs to be acquired and the typical workflow in hospitals imposes a pace at which this data must be processed.

Section 4 describes the reconstruction algorithms applicable to medical CT and HPIR. The way data is processed and the required processing steps for reconstructing a volume are detailed in this section. The type of computation (e.g. integer, floating point) is also given since it influences the selection of the processing device that should be selected for each processing step.

The different families of modern HPC platforms are presented in section 5. This section discusses the optimization methods that are applicable for the different platforms along two axes: a) how to take advantage of the accelerating features of a given processing device and b) how to take advantage of geometrical properties of the scanner to remove performance bottlenecks. The impact of the different optimization methods differs depending on the target platform.

Since the various HPC platforms have different advantages and shortcomings, one is forced to consider tradeoffs when selecting a specific device for a given processing step. Section 5 also discusses various aspects that may influence decision making such as floating-point computation capability, ease of integration, roadmap and life-cycle management.

1.3 Conventions and Notations

1.3.1 Geometry

Several geometrical conventions and definitions shall be used in this chapter. Although there are strong similarities between a C-arm and a CT scanner, different symbols shall be used because they are commonly found that way in existing literature.

Figure 2 represents a diagram of a C-arm CT scanner.

θ projection angle,
γ cone angle in the v-direction,
κ cone angle in the u direction,
SO source to object distance,
SI source to detector distance,
ξ, η voxel coordinates in source-detector reference system.

Figure 3 represents a diagram of a gantry-based CT scanner. It is worth noticing that all detector elements are equidistant to the focal spot.

β fan angle,
θ projection angle,
R_F distance from the focal spot to the center of rotation,
R_D distance from the detector to the center of rotation,
R_{FD} distance from the focal spot to the detector: $R_{FD} = R_F + R_D$.

1.3.2 Performance Measure

Since this chapter is dedicated to evaluating HPC platforms for 3D image reconstruction, it is

Figure 2. Geometry definition for a C-arm based scanner

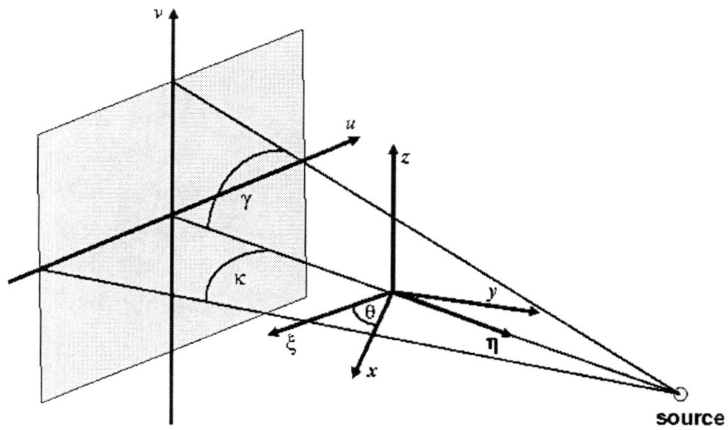

convenient to introduce the metrics that place all platforms on a common ground. In addition, this chapter concentrates on the filtered backprojection methods which consist of two major processing steps: the fast convolution and the backprojection. In other words, the metrics of interest are the speed at which the fast convolution can take place and how fast the backprojection can be done.

The fast convolution is performed detector row per detector row. Most of the detectors considered in this chapter are made of several detector rows, with each row having in the order of 1024 detector elements. The performance of a given platform shall be measured as a number of memory updates per second. When N is the total number of detector lines to convolve and M is the number of detector elements per line (assuming M is a power of 2), the number of memory updates is proportional to $N \times 2M \times \mathrm{lb}(2M)$. We define the number of 1024^3 memory updates per second as Giga Convolution Updates per second (GC/s). For example, convolution of 512 projections of size 1024^2 requires 11 GC.

Figure 3. Geometry definition of a gantry-based CT scanner

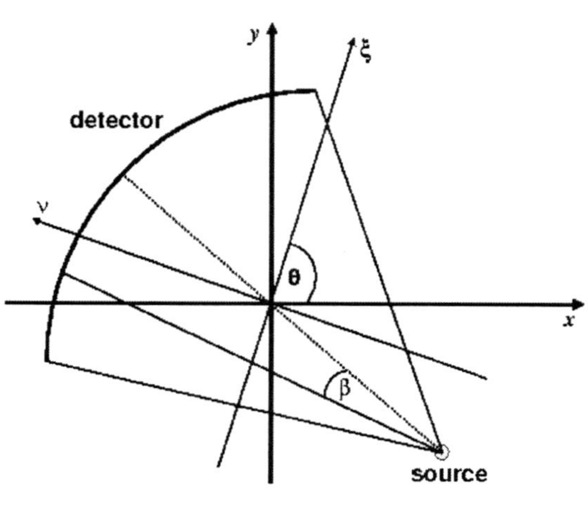

The backprojection is a matter of updating all voxels in the volume of interest from all available projections. When N is the number of projections and $N_x \times N_y \times N_z$ is the number of voxels of the volume, we require $N \times N_x \times N_y \times N_z$ memory updates for backprojection. Again, we define the number of 1024^3 memory updates per second as Giga Voxel Updates per second (GU/s). For example, the backprojection of 512 projections into a 512^3 volume requires 64 GU.

2 CT RECONSTRUCTION IN HOSPITALS

Numerous CT applications can be used for establishing a diagnostic of a patient without making the step to surgery. The ultimate goal of CT for medical imaging is to provide cross-section slices with information about the tissues contained in the considered slices through values given as Hounsfield Units (HU), or more recently, atomic numbers.

3D CT reconstructions are routinely performed in hospitals and mainly use two types of devices: C-arm based scanners (Figure 4) and gantry-based scanners (Figure 5). In both cases, the source and the detector are mounted on opposite sides of the object to scan. The major differences between the two devices can be summarized as follows:

- Coverage: the C-arm uses a flat detector panel that is usually large enough to cover the area of interest. In comparison, the medical CT scanner has a thinner collimation and performs continuous rotation around the object while the table moves in one direction to offer the desired coverage through a spiral scan.
- Length of acquisition: a C-arm is mechanically limited to perform a scan of typically less than 360°. Due to slipring technology, the clinical CT gantry can perform a virtually unlimited number of rotations in order to acquire the relevant data.
- Speed: a typical sweep of a C-arm rotates at about 40° per second. A modern clinical CT performs three rotations per second.
- Reconstructed volume: the C-arm typically enables reconstructing a volume that is completely included in the cone of the X-ray beam. The CT gantry enables reconstructing the object on a slice-by-slice basis.

Both types of scanners achieve spatial-resolution values of far below 1 mm. In order to reach the desired image quality, modern scanners acquire in the order of 1000 projections per full rotation.

A modern flat panel has 1024^2 pixels, each sample is represented on 12 to 14 bits. Detectors for the high end CT gantries count 64 rows of about 1024 detector elements, each sample encoded on 20 to 24 bits; recent detectors even have 320 detector rows. This gives the first important metric for the definition of the HPC platform: the bandwidth required to face the incoming stream of raw data. A C-arm based scanner generates in the order of 300 MB/s and modern CT gantries produce an excess of 800 MB/s. It is also worth

Figure 4. C-arm CT scanner. The source and detector are mounted on a C-shaped arm that rotates around the object. (Courtesy of Ziehm Imaging GmbH, Nürnberg, Germany)

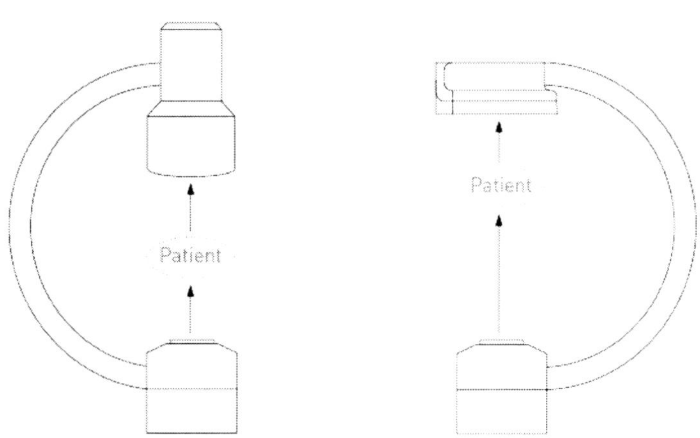

noticing that while the data flow from a C-arm stops once the sweep is completed, the acquisition time for a CT gantry is virtually endless. In addition, due to the spiral trajectory, it is possible to start the reconstruction of the first slices while the acquisition for the subsequent ones is still taking place[2].

CT scanners are routinely used in hospitals for clinical diagnostics. The scan protocol has been decided in advance by the radiologist and the only thing that remains to be done is to bring the patient on the table, perform the scan and the CT reconstruction. In larger hospitals, there is a continuous stream of patients, calling for a time efficient use of the scanner. An efficient organization leads to higher-patient throughput, up to one patient every few minutes. However, operators like to ensure that the CT scan was successful before the patient leaves the table. This can be done only through CT reconstruction, at least for a subset of the volume of interest. Therefore, in order to sustain a high-patient throughput, it is desirable to perform the CT reconstruction as fast as possible, ideally in real time.

To give a first sense of the level of performance required to perform a CT reconstruction, let us consider the example of a C-arm with a detector of 1024×1024 elements, taking 512 projections. In addition, the size of the volume to reconstruct is 512^3. This problem requires 11 GC and 64 GU. This represents quite an impressive task as shall be seen in the following sections.

3 RECONSTRUCTION ALGORITHMS

There is an ever increasing number of reconstruction algorithms. Reconstruction algorithms can be grouped in larger families depending on the approach they follow. The first dichotomy consists in separating the analytical methods from the iterative approaches (Figure 6). Analytical methods mainly rely on a mathematical approach where the solution to the reconstruction problem can be expressed by a closed formula.

In the family of analytical methods, the second dichotomy consists in separating exact from approximate algorithms. Exact algorithms have a mathematical proof while all others approximate

Figure 5. The word's first dual-source scanner, the Siemens Somatom Definition as an example for a Gantry-based scanner. The source and detector are mounted on a ring that rotates around the patient. The coverage in the z-dimension is given by a constant motion of the table. The image was taken at the Institute of Medical Physics (IMP), Erlangen, Germany

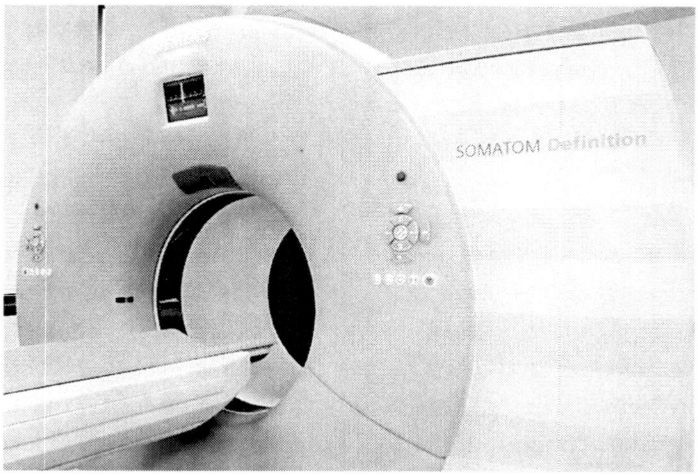

Figure 6. Classification of reconstruction algorithms. Further decomposition of these categories can be carried out depending on the properties of the methods

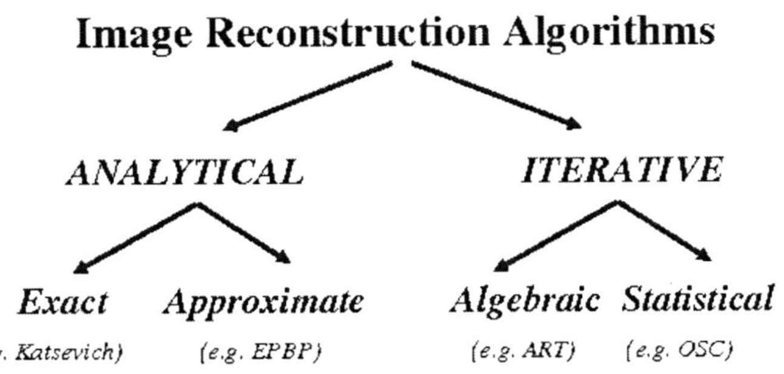

the exact solution to some extent[3]. There are good reasons to select approximate algorithms for a given application. For example, Fourier space reconstruction algorithms (Schaller 1998, Grangeat 1987) are exact methods that require a scan of the whole object to provide a result. For reasons related to reducing the X-ray exposure, it is not desirable to scan the full body of the patient when the Region of Interest (ROI) is limited to a given area. There are ways to overcome this problem and perform exact image reconstruction when only a region of interest has been scanned. Those, however, do not make use of all detector data and therefore are less-dose efficient. This makes the whole method less attractive.

Finally, it is a pitfall to believe that the use of an exact method inherently produces perfect images. The implementation of the mathematical formulas implies a discretization step that can introduce severe artifacts if coded without precautions. Nevertheless, provided the discretization step is properly carried out, it is likely that the exact method provides better results when compared to approximate algorithms.

In contrast to the analytical reconstruction algorithms whose solution can be expressed as a closed analytical formula and that perform discretization as the last step, iterative approaches start by discretizing the problem and formulate the image reconstruction problem as a huge system of linear equations[4]. The reconstruction formula is therefore not a closed equation, but rather a recursive description of how to iteratively improve the image. Common to almost all iterative reconstruction algorithms is the forward- and backprojection step. The forward projection step takes an estimate of the image as input and computes line integrals through the image to come up with a virtual raw data set that corresponds to the estimated image. This virtual raw data set is then compared to the measured raw data. In the simplest case, this is done by a simple subtraction. The result of this comparison, i.e. the residual error in the virtual raw data, is then backprojected into the image to get another, better image estimate. The procedure is repeated until the image estimate meets the user's image-quality criteria. It is never repeated until full convergence since this would take an infinite number of iterations. Depending on the type of iterative image reconstruction algorithm and depending on the type of initialization the numbers of iterations reported lie between 2 and 500 iterations.

A disadvantage of iterative reconstruction is its rather long computation time. Every iteration requires at least one forward- and at least one backprojection. Thereby, it is more than twice as slow as analytical image reconstruction techniques that require only a single backprojection operation. In addition, iterative algorithms cannot reconstruct small portions of the object. Rather, they need to reconstruct the whole object; otherwise those parts of the object that are not covered by the image would not contribute to the forward projection operation. In clinical CT, where the typical image size is 512^2 and the typical image covers only a small part of the patient, this has the consequence that images of size 1024^2 need to be reconstructed if an iterative image reconstruction algorithm is used. Hence, each forward- and backprojection step is four times slower than one backprojection step of analytical image reconstruction. Summarizing, the iterative reconstruction requires at least 16 times more update steps (per iteration!) than analytical algorithms.

The advantage of iterative image reconstruction is that the physics of the measurement can be directly modeled into the forward projection step. This implies that images of better quality, i.e. better spatial resolution, lower image noise and less artifacts, can be reconstructed.

3.1 Analytical Methods

Analytical methods are based on a mathematical approach of the physics. The most common method is called the filtered backprojection (FBP). There are many flavors of filtered backprojection algorithms, but they all share the same common approach. The projection data are first corrected from acquisition and geometrical inaccuracy, such as the non linearity of the detector elements, then they are filtered and backprojected onto the volume. From the programming point of view, these methods have an important and appealing property: they make it possible to take the projections one by one, to backproject them individually onto the volume and to discard them after use. One can consider that the input-projection stream undergoes a transformation to produce the output slices. If we take the example of a 64-detector row CT scanner, it acquires in the order of 3000 projections per second and under specific scanning protocols, can produce 192 slices, each typically represented on a 512^2 matrix.

This method has a direct impact on the way the algorithm is implemented. The most obvious way to write the program puts at the outer loop the handling of individual projections and into the inner loops the indexing of individual voxels.

Listing 1

```
void reconstruction (unsigned int N_proj,
                     unsigned int Nx,
                     unsigned int Ny,
                     unsigned int N)
{
  unsigned int p_idx, i_idx, j_idx, k_idx;
  for (p_idx = 0; p_idx < N_proj; p_idx++)
  {
    /*
      Read the projection data
      pre process the data
      filter the projection
      Also, get the projection angle theta
    */
    for (i_idx = 0; i_idx < Nx; i_idx++)
    {
      for (j_idx = 0; j_idx < Ny; j_idx++)
      {
        for (k_idx = 0; k_idx < Nz; k_idx++)
        {
          /*
            Compute the coordinates of the projection point of
            voxel r(x, y, z) for angle theta.
            backproject the value read
```

```
on the detector
                    onto the considered pixel.
                */
            }
        }
    }
  }
}
```

Listing 1 shows a reference implementation of a reconstruction algorithm. The first step consists in correcting the data for geometrical discrepancies of the scanner (e.g. the trajectory is not circular) and non homogeneity of the detector elements (e.g. detector gain and offset corrections). Most common methods use very simple conditioning and correction of the data. However, sophisticated methods for noise reduction such as adaptive filtering (Kachelriess 2001, Bockenbach 2007, Haykin 2002) can also be applied on the projection data. Those corrections are aimed at increasing the quality of the reconstructed volume, but cannot correct inherent approximations of the reconstruction algorithms.

The approximations during reconstruction are generally introduced at the filtering and backprojection phases. The approximations made during the filtering step are nicely visible in spiral-CT algorithms based on the Tam-Danielsson window and the PI-line concepts (Turbell 2001)[5].

The approximations during backprojection are related to the way the coordinates of the point projection and the contribution of the projection to the volume, are computed. The accuracy of the computation is a key factor for limiting the approximations done during backprojection. They are the topic of the following sections.

3.1.1 Feldkamp-Davis-Kress (FDK) Algorithm

Considering the case of a FDK algorithm (Feldkamp 1984), applied to a C-arm device (Figure 2 and Figure 4), the reconstruction process consists of three major steps. First, the samples need to be weighted to account for the cone angle along both axes u and v, i.e. by the cosine of angles γ and κ. The cone angle can be computed as:

$$\cos\kappa\cos\gamma = \frac{SO}{\sqrt{SO + u^2 + v^2}} \tag{1}$$

The weighted projection must be filtered row wise with a convolution kernel. The selection of the **convolution** kernel influences the smoothness of the reconstruction volume. Most commonly used kernels are based on Ram-Lak (Ramachandran 1971) or Shepp-Logan (Shepp 1974) filters. The filtering of projection taken at angle ϑ is given by the equation (Kalender 2005):

$$\tilde{p}^{P}(\vartheta,u,v) = \left(\frac{SO}{\sqrt{SO + u^2 + v^2}}\,p^{P}(\vartheta,u,v)\right) * h^{P}(u) \tag{2}$$

The filtered projections can then be used for performing the backprojection step.

$$f(x,y,z) = \int_0^{2\pi} \frac{SO^2}{\left(SO + x\cos\vartheta + y\sin\vartheta\right)^2}\,\tilde{p}^{P}\left(\vartheta, u(x,y,\vartheta), v(x,y,\vartheta)\right)d\vartheta \tag{3}$$

In other words, the reconstruction of the voxel at coordinates $r(x,y,z)$ consists in taking the contributions from all pre-weighted and filtered projections. The contribution is the value read on a specific location on the detector. This location is given by the point where the ray from the source passing through the considered voxel hits the detector. The projection of voxel (x,y,z) for projection angle ϑ is given by coordinates(u,v):

$$u = \eta\frac{SI}{SO - \xi} \tag{4}$$

$$v = z\frac{SI}{SO - \xi} \tag{5}$$

Where ξ and η are given by:

$$\xi = x\cos\vartheta + y\sin\vartheta \tag{6}$$

$$\eta = -x\sin\vartheta + y\cos\vartheta \tag{7}$$

The coordinates (u,v) usually do not hit the detector on one detector cell. Therefore, interpolation is used for computing the weighted contribution of the pixels surrounding the coordinates. Bilinear interpolation is the most commonly used technique[6].

Using a straight implementation of the algorithm shown in Listing 1, we can measure the execution time on any standard PC. For the reconstruction of the example system described in section 3 (11 GC and 64 GU) on the selected reference PC platform, the filtering of the data took 0.2 hours and the backprojection took 0.95 hours. This performance meets 0.016 GC/s and 0.018 GU/s.

3.1.2 Extended Parallel Backprojection (EPBP)

There is a wide variety of analytical algorithms available for dealing with the spiral CT problem (Figure 3 and Figure 5). The EPBP (Kachelriess 2004) belongs to the approximate reconstruction methods and is one of the most interesting for his capabilities in addressing medical CT applications, such as cardiac imaging combined with full-dose usage. Being an analytical method, EPBP shares its foundations with the FDK algorithm, and specifically the filtered backprojection approach. The major difference between FDK and EPBP is the geometry of the scan and the acquisition of the raw-projection data. Instead of following a circular arc, the source and detector may also follow a spiral trajectory with a horizontal displacement of d in the z-dimension. The position $\vec{s}$ of the source for a given rotation angle α is:

$$\vec{s}(\alpha) = \begin{pmatrix} R_F \sin\alpha \\ -R_F \cos\alpha \\ d\frac{\alpha}{2\pi} + o \end{pmatrix} \tag{8}$$

where R_F is the radius of the circle followed by the source and o is the start offset of the source at angle α=0.

Every detector element can be located according to its fan angle β and offset b from the normal ray in the z-dimension. Indeed, the position of a specific detector element on the helix is given by:

$$\vec{r}(\alpha,\beta,b) = \vec{s}(\alpha) + \begin{pmatrix} -R_{FD}\sin(\alpha+\beta) \\ R_{FD}\cos(\alpha+\beta) \\ b \end{pmatrix} \tag{9}$$

where R_{FD} represents the length of the normal ray from the source to the detector.

For performing the backprojection, one needs to find the point projection (β, b) of the considered voxel (x,y,z) on the detector for a projection angle ϑ. Using the intersection theorem, the coordinates of this point projection are given as:

$$\begin{pmatrix} \beta \\ b \end{pmatrix} = \begin{pmatrix} -\arcsin\frac{\xi}{R_F} \\ \frac{R_{FD}}{\sqrt{R_F^2 + \xi^2} + \eta}\left(z - d\frac{\alpha}{2\pi} - o\right) \end{pmatrix} \tag{10}$$

Here, ξ is the distance of voxel (x,y,z) from the isocenter (i.e. rotation axis) as defined in equation (6).

The major advantage of EPBP over other types of spiral-image reconstruction algorithms, be it exact or approximate spiral cone-beam image reconstruction algorithms, is the capability to fully use the acquired data and thereby to achieve full-dose usage. EPBP does this by applying a voxel-specific weighting approach. Each voxel "sees" the x-rays under different ranges of projection angles. The illumination of a voxel by x-rays may even be interrupted, depending on the position of the voxel in the field of measurement (FOM). EPBP takes fully account of these subtleties and backprojects all data into the voxel that actually contribute. Other approaches, such as the exact-image reconstruction algorithms available (Katsevich 2002) make use of the detector data only in a certain data window. Detector pixels outside this window (that is closely correlated to the so-called Tam-window) are not used for image reconstruction although they contain valid projection data. Hence, EPBP achieves a better-dose usage and a lower-image noise compared to other algorithms at the same level of spatial resolution.

3.2 Iterative Image Reconstruction

Originally developed by Gordon, Bender, Herman in 1970 (Gordon 1970), iterative methods usually do not try to solve the problem based on underlying mathematic formulas. Instead, they solve the reconstruction problem in an iterative refinement of a guessed volume until a given convergence criteria is met. Unlike analytical methods, the reconstruction cannot take the projections one by one and discard them after they have been used. Instead, the input projections must remain available to the reconstruction algorithm until it has converged.

In methods like Kaczmarz (Kaczmarz 1937), each iteration consists of a forward projection of the guessed volume, resulting in a collection of projection data. This data set is compared to the captured projection set. The general formula is given by:

$$f_j^{i+1} = f_j^i + N_B \qquad (11)$$

Where f_j^i represents the voxel j of the volume to reconstruct at iteration i and N_B is the result of the backprojection followed by the normalization:

$$N_B = \lambda \frac{F}{\sum_{n=1}^{N} w_{in}^2} \qquad (12)$$

Where λ represents a relaxation factor influencing the contribution of the current iteration on the volume, w_{ij} the weights affecting the individual voxels for a given ray and F is the correction of the forward projection step:

$$F = (p_i - \sum_{n=1}^{N} w_{in} f_n^k) w_{ij} \qquad (13)$$

As can be taken from the formulas, iterative algorithms such as the Algebraic Reconstruction Technique (ART) (Gordon 1974) can be implemented in a very flexible way. Although the selection of the relaxation factor and the accuracy of the weights can improve the performance, iterative approaches suffer from long processing times when compared to analytical methods.

It is also worth mentioning that the forward projection step is critical to obtain good image quality (Figure 7). The forward projection consists in weighing the effect of the voxel at coordinates $f(x,y)$ to projection p_i. The selection of the weights defines the contribution of the voxels in the neighborhood of the considered ray. Depending on the selection of those weights, the forward projection turns into well-known methods such as (Joseph 1982, Siddon 1985). In addition, sophisticated methods perform an over-sampling of the detectors, i.e. trace several rays between the source and a given detector element or model the ray profile.

Figure 7. The forward projection problem. For a given object to reconstruct, the algorithm needs to generate synthetic projections from the guessed object. Those estimated projections are compared to the actual ones

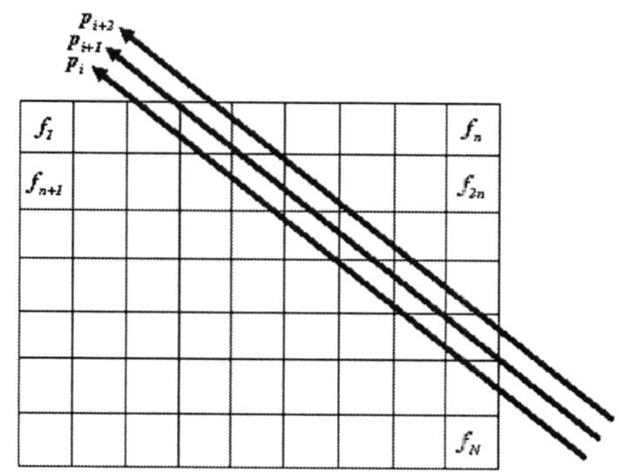

$$\sum_{j=1}^{N} w_{ij} f_j = p_i$$

3.3 Comparing Analytical and Iterative Methods

All in all, the compromise that a designer for a HPC platform has to make is to:

- obtain prior knowledge of how applicable analytical methods are for the scan methods in terms of angular coverage and numbers of projections, and
- evaluate the level of noise in the projections that the scanner will produce.

Once those parameters are accessible, one can decide between analytical and iterative methods and set other parameters according to the desired image quality. The overall processing time will be a function of the number of voxels to reconstruct and of the number of projections available. For analytical methods, the computational cost is dominated by the backprojection. In the iterative case, the price to pay for backprojection is the same as in the analytical case, but one has to pay the price for the forward projector. The forward projection is generally a critical component of iterative reconstruction. In order to achieve good image quality, one has to pay attention to this processing step. Many methods perform an oversampling during this step. This oversampling consists in casting several rays from the source to the same detector element at a finer-grained stepping that the spacing of the detector elements.

Therefore, the processing cost of an iterative approach is $(T_{BP}+N_s T_{FP})N_{iter}$ where T_{BP} is the processing time of the backprojection, T_{FP} the processing time of the forward projection, linearly increasing with the over-sampling ratio N_s, N_{iter} represents the number of iteration required for convergence. Consequently, since iterative methods by definition require several iterations, the processing time of such methods is also inherently higher than for analytical approaches.

4 HIGH PERFORMANCE COMPUTING PLATFORMS

4.1 Selected Platforms

There is a broad variety of HPC solutions available and capable of tackling the reconstruction problem. Since the nature of the reconstruction problem exhibits a significant level of independence among the projection data, among part of the reconstructed volume and between the volume and the projections, platforms that are inherently built for a high level of parallelism are more suitable for higher performance. Typical technologies that can be considered are:

- Symmetric or asymmetric multiprocessor and multicore architectures. This type of architecture connects several processors or cores together to main memory and I/O devices through elaborate interconnect fabrics, such as trees and rings. The Intel multi-core architectures and the Cell Broadband Engine (CBE) processor have been selected for this category,
- General-Purpose Graphics Processing Units (GPGPUs). Their original intention is to address all the volume rendering problems common to graphics display. Since their ultimate goal is to properly render a large number of individual pixels, their internal architecture offers a higher degree of parallelism than multiprocessor and multicore approaches,
- Field Programmable Gate Arrays (FPGAs). They are built around a large collection of elementary compute elements and a reconfigurable interconnect network. A typical implementation offers tens of thousands of compute elements within one chip.

This section compares several different platforms against performance. Their architecture and performance levels are so different that it becomes difficult to get a comprehensive understanding of their relative performance, advantages and shortcomings without a point of reference.

4.1.1 Reference Platform

At the moment of writing, all computer users have had the opportunity to make acquaintance with Personal Computers (PC) based on Intel or AMD processors and to get an idea about the performance for most commonly used applications such as text editors and games. In 2008, dual-core processors like the Intel Core 2 Duo (Figure 8) are commonly used for laptop computers, and one or multiple quad-core processors are commonly used for desktop PCs. Reconstruction can be optimized

Figure 8. Block diagram of the Intel Dual-Core processor. It consists of a duplication of two fully populated processor cores, sharing the L2 cache and the system bus

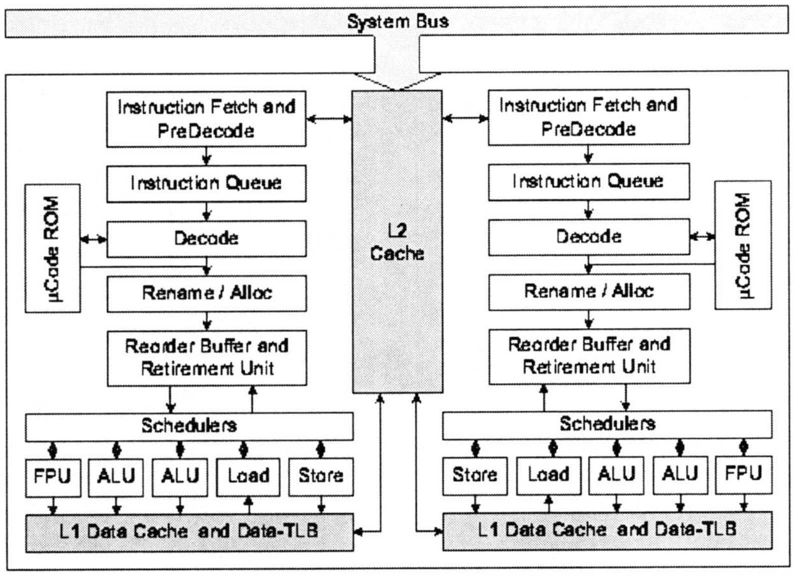

to work efficiently on this kind of platforms as demonstrated by Yu (2001).

The Intel Core 2 Duo is the easiest expression of symmetric multicore architecture: there are actually two processors on the same chip with dedicated resources like the Arithmetic and Logical Unit (ALU) and the level 1 (L1) data caches.

On the other hand, the two cores share the L2 cache for data and instructions as well as the system bus. Indeed, dealing with the memory accesses from two separate cores put increased stress on the bus management. Moreover, PC architectures are facing an increasing number of memory bandwidth-hungry devices. In order to be capable of sustaining the numerous bus transactions without impacting the performance of the cores, the architecture of the motherboard is becoming more and more complex with the involvement of complex bridges (Figure 9).

Modern processors commonly implement data and/or instruction caches. Caches isolate the core processing from other data transactions originated from peripheral devices and enable the processor to perform at maximum speed without being disturbed by memory transaction originated by peripheral devices. They also provide fast access to recently used instructions and data items, and are intended to take best advantages of the temporal and spatial locality of memory and instruction accesses. The ideal case appears when all the instructions and data items needed for a given computation step are present in the cache. To get closer to this ideal case, a given program must be adapted in such a way that it exhibits the proper temporal and spatial locality in data[7].

The program given in Listing 1 does not take spatial nor temporal locality for data accesses into consideration and walks through the complete volume in the inner loops for every projection. Figure 10 shows the projection of one specific slice on the detector. For the considered projection angle, accessing the projection points of two consecutive voxels makes large jumps in memory (the offset between sequential voxels is even

Figure 9. Block diagram of a typical motherboard for the Intel Core2 Duo processor. All data transactions are handled by the MCH and ICH bridges

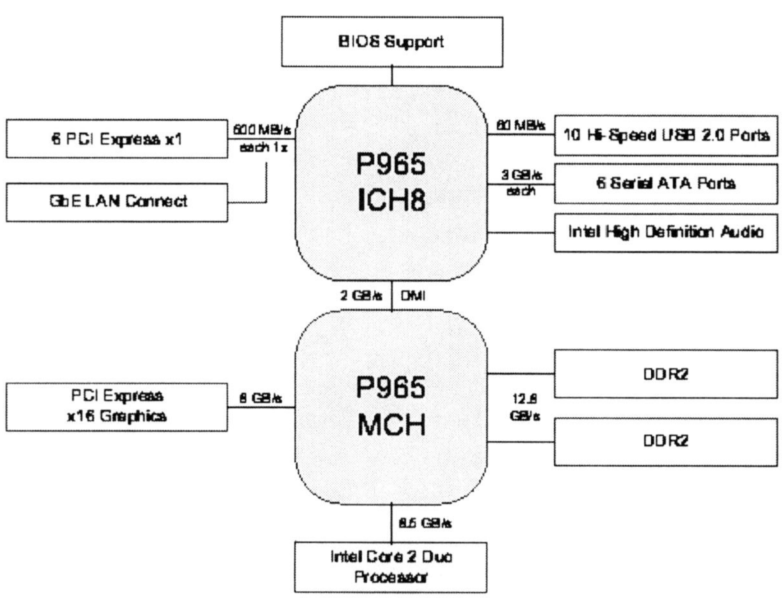

Figure 10. Projection of slice at z_0=0.0 and o=0.0 onto the detector at angle $-\pi/8$ and a table displacement of 1.0. R_F is set to 570 mm and R_{FD} to 1140 mm. The size of the slice is 512×512 pixels

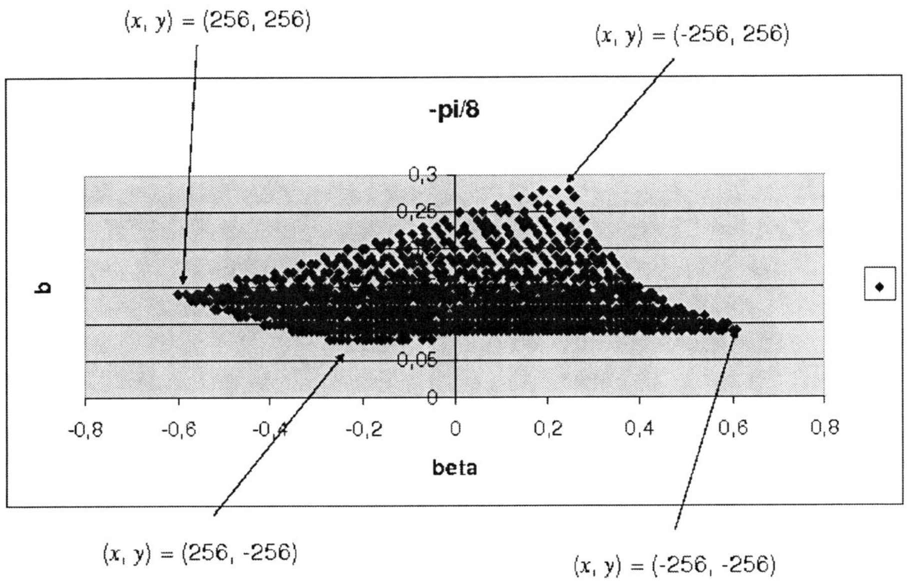

negative in this case), and hence does not show the locality required for best cache performance.

In order to take advantage of the data caches, the program exposed in Listing 1 must be reorganized. As already stated, all the volume needs to be updated by the contributions from all the projections. This means that however much the code is optimized, the complete volume has to be read from main memory, updated with the contributions of all projections and written back to memory. The projection data needs only to be read, and can then be discarded. Indeed, the projection data requires only one memory operation while the volume data requires two. For optimal performance, it is preferable to keep the volume data into the caches and read the projection data on demand[8].

512^3 is a typical volume size in CT reconstruction. Each voxel is commonly in single-precision, floating-point representation. The volume takes 512 MB of memory. Because today's technology doesn't propose processors with caches large enough to hold this amount of data, it is most convenient to subdivide the problem into sub-volumes as shown in Figure 11. Selecting the sub-volume size in accordance with the cache size can allow reading and writing the whole volume only once[9]. To fully measure the performance difference, let us consider the example of the backprojection of 512 projections on a 512^3 volume on the reference platform, and more specifically, the data movement costs. The reference platform can sustain ~3GB/s for reading and writing. The execution of the program in Listing 1 requires 85 seconds! Using sub-volumes of size 32^3 brings this time down to 13s, indeed significantly reducing the reconstruction time. This cranks the performance up to 0.1 GC/s and 0.11GU/s.

4.1.2 The CBE Processor

The CBE processor (Figure 12) can be considered as a multicomputer on a chip (Flachs 2005, Hofstee 2005, Pham 2005). It has been used for implementing several reconstruction algorithms (Kachelriess 2007, Knaup 2006). The CBE re-

Figure 11. Decomposing the reconstruction of the volume into sub-volumes allows reducing the amount of projection data necessary for the update of the considered sub-volume

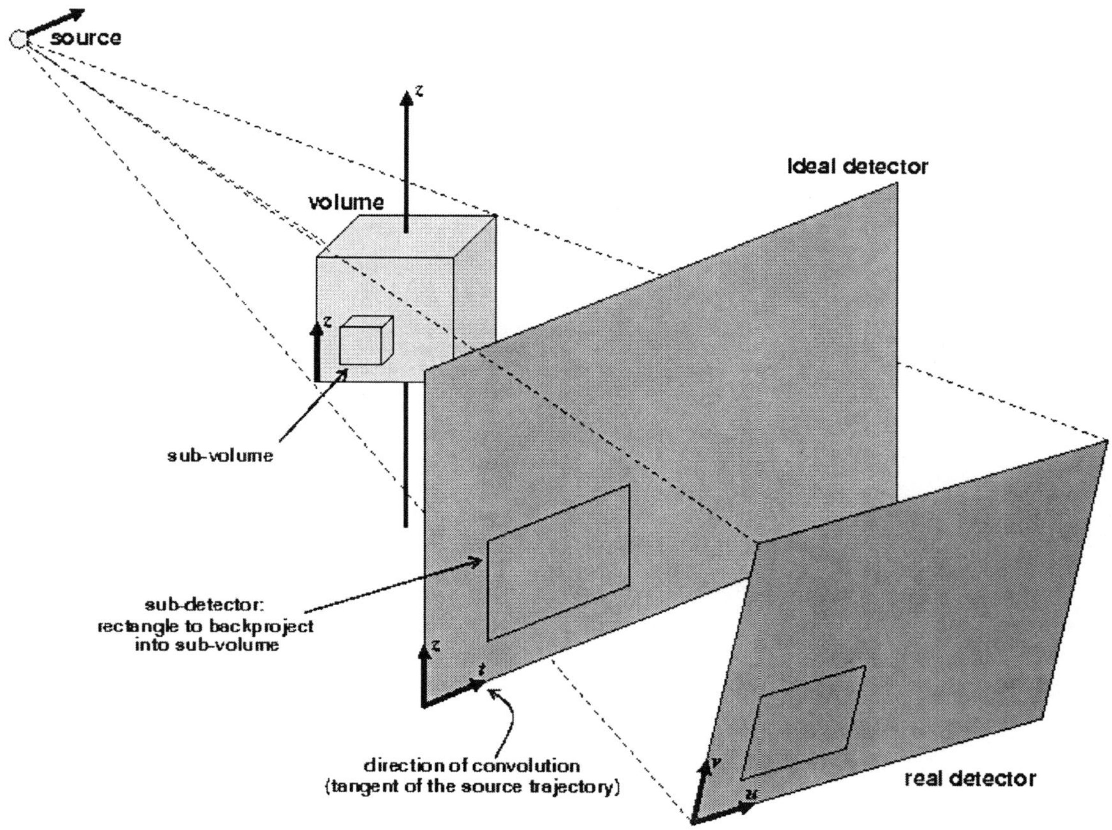

quires individually programming the PowerPC Processing Element (PPE) and all eight Synergistic Processing Elements (SPEs).

The processing elements are connected together and with the external devices (e.g. memory, the Southbridge) over the Element Interconnect Bus (EIB). The EIB provides an aggregate bandwidth of ~200 GB/s. For the reference design at 3.2 GHz, the CBE offers a RamBus interface (XDR) with a peak bandwidth of 25 GB/s. The Coherent Interface is designed for building system with two CBE processors in Symetric Multi Processing (SMP) mode.

Since all processors and devices are directly tapped on the EIB, all participants can access all available resources. For instance, data transfers originated by peripheral devices can target the XDR without disturbing the computation taking place in the PPE and SPEs, except for the bandwidth used for the transfer. Conversely, assuming memory translations have been properly set up, the PPE and the SPEs (using Direct Memory Access, DMA) can transparently access all XDR-memory and peripheral-memory spaces.

The PPE is a dual-threaded, 64-bit Power Architecture with included integer, floating-point and VMX functional units as well as 32 KB L1 caches for code and data. The PPE also has a 512 KB L2 cache and a Memory Management Unit (MMU) for memory protection and translation purposes.

An SPE (Figure 13) is based on a Reduced Instruction Set Computer (RISC) architecture and

Figure 12. Block diagram of the Cell Broadband Engine Processor. A Power PC processor and eight synergistic processing units are connected together through the high-speed Element Interconnect Bus. The EIB also allows for structured and arbitrated access to memory

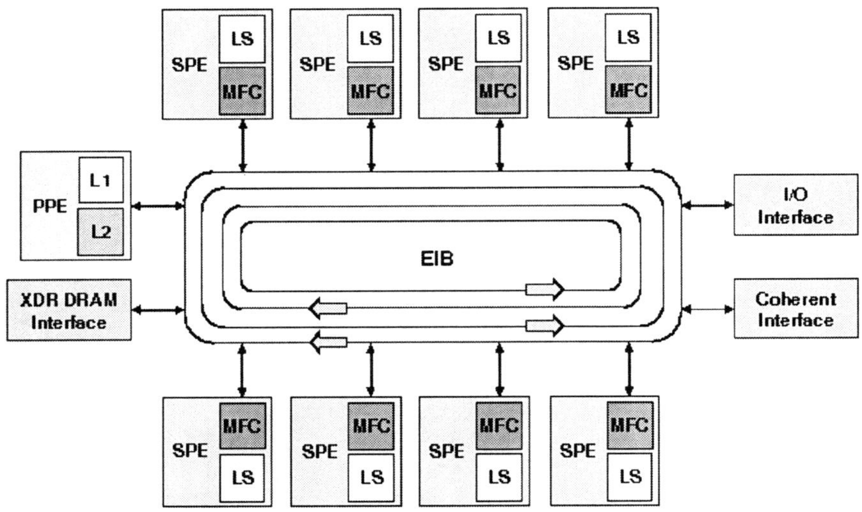

consists of a dual-issue core with 256 KB of Local Store (LS). Every SPE also implements DMA capabilities with data coherency management in the Memory Flow Controller (MFC). The SPE core is a 128-bit Single Instruction Multiple Data (SIMD) ALU which allows performing the same instruction on four floating-point numbers, or four 32-bit integer numbers, or eight 16-bit integers, or sixteen 8-bit integers in a single blow.

The 256 KB of LS have to hold all program segments[10], i.e. code, stack and data. It is rather small for handling complex problems such as CT reconstruction. Static RAM provides fast access for the core but doesn't automatically fill like a cache does when the core requests a data item not already present. Instead, data must be moved manually with the DMA engines.

Using the same optimization techniques as for the reference platform, the LS is already half full with a cube of 32^3 voxels in floating-point format. In the case of flat panels, each projection requires several MB of memory space and high-end CT scanners with 64 detector rows or more, a full projection represents 256 KB. Therefore, on the CBE processor, it is compulsory to load only the relevant part of the projection into LS. Given the scanner geometry, the coordinates of the sub-volume and the projection angle, one can compute the coordinates of the minimum rectangle that holds the shadow of the considered sub-volume on the projection. For typical scanner geometries, this shadow represents only a few KB worth of projection data.

In order to take advantage of the common optimization technique that consists in hiding the data-transfer time behind the computation time with the DMA engine, double buffering of the projection data must be implemented. Listing 2 gives an example of the implementation of the algorithm on the SPE. The spe_reconstruction() function is called once per sub-volume. It is assumed that the coordinates and sizes of the shadows are known in advance and stored in local store.

Listing 2

```
void spe_reconstruction (unsigned int
N_proj,
```

Figure 13. Block diagram of the Synergistic Processing Element. The core is a 128- bit SIMD architecture that accesses 256 KB of Local Store. Data can be exchanged with main memory through DMA

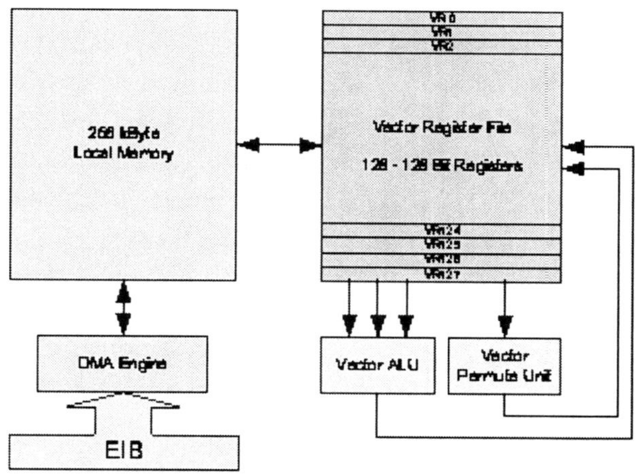


```
                    unsigned int Nx,
                    unsigned int Ny,
                    unsigned int Nz)
{
  unsigned int p_idx, i_idx, j_idx,
k_idx;
  /*
          For the first 2 projection
angles,
          get the coordinates and
size of the shadow
          start to DMA the shadow in
the projection data
  */
  for (p_idx = 0; p_idx < N_proj; p_
idx++)
  {
    /*
    */
    for (i_idx = 0; i_idx < Nx; i_
idx++)
    {
      for (j_idx = 0; j_idx < Ny; j_
idx++)
      {
        for (k_idx = 0; k_idx < Nz;
k_idx++)
        {
          /*
            Compute the coordinates
of the projection point of
            voxel (x, y, z) for angle
theta.
            backproject the value
read on the detector
            onto the consider pixel
          */
        }
      }
    }
    /*
      Wait for the DMA of the (p_
idx+1) to finish,
      get the coordinates and size of
the shadow for (p_idx+2)
      start the DMA for the shadow in
the projection data
    */
  }
}
```

This data-mining technique not only enables the program to run on the CBE processor, but also provides good performance for the FDK algorithm.

As described later in this section, there are other optimizations that can be implemented on the CBE. Jumping ahead, it is possible to perform the backprojection of 512 projections onto a 512^3 volume in about 15 s on one CBE processor.

Taking this number to a higher level, it means that the CBE processor is capable of "digesting" 512/15 projections and producing 512/15 slices per second. For instance, let's suppose that the projections are 1024^2 pixels large and that the slices are 512^2 matrices. If the data is coded on a single-precision floating point, the CBE can consume ~136MB/s of input projections and output 34MB/s. Even though these numbers remain modest, it starts to stress common communication links, in terms of latency or throughput or both. It is even more true for spiral-CT reconstruction algorithms. With elaborate optimization techniques, it is possible to reconstruct 240 slices/second, for a total of ~250MB/s.

As a consequence, as for many HPC solutions, the use of a high-density solution puts hard constraints on the acquisition system to bring the data to the processors and to get the results to the downstream processing steps.

Mercury Computer Systems, Inc. has implemented the CBE processor on the Cell Accelerator Board (CAB). The CAB (Figure 14) is a PCI Express (PCIe) board, aimed at being inserted into high-end PCs. The architecture of the CAB is articulated around the Southbridge (SB). The SB binds together the Cell, the DDR2 memory extension and the devices on the PCIe bus into one single address space that the CBE can exploit for complex applications. The SB is designed as a crossbar capable of simultaneously sustaining data transactions between any pair of source-destination. For example, the SB allows for a transfer between PCIe and DDR2 to happen at the same time as DDR2-to-XDR transfer. Those transfers are handled by several DMA engines built inside the SB and dealt with at the speed of the slowest of the involved endpoints.

The PCIe bus offers a peak bandwidth of several GB/s in each direction. This bandwidth can easily accommodate the data rates required for the backprojection performance that can be achieved with the CBE processor. So, provided the backprojection performance matches the requirements of the overall application, one can build a HPC solution based on a standard PC. One needs to rearrange the code in such a way that all the preprocessing and filtering is done on the host processor; the filtered projections are sent to the

Figure 14. Block diagram of the Cell Accelerator Board (CAB). For 3D image reconstruction, it is important that the input and output data can be efficiently conveyed to and from the processor

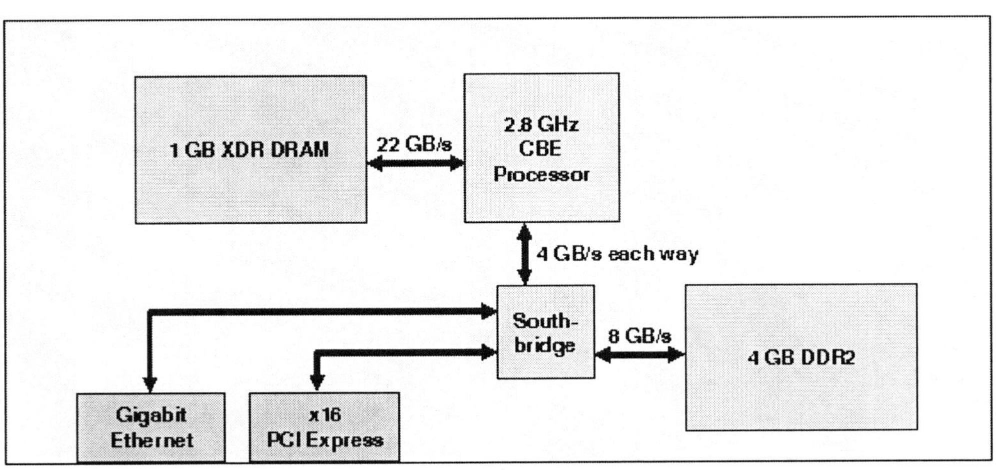

CAB and the reconstructed slices post processed on the host before visualization.

4.1.3 The FPGA Platform

FPGAs are based on a collection of elementary building blocks belonging to a reduced number of different types, connected together with a grid network (Figure 15). The building blocks can perform simple operations and range in different categories: the Configurable Logic Blocks (CLBs), internal block RAM (BRAM), multipliers and for the most sophisticated devices, small ALUs. Those building blocks are tied together with a configurable interconnect fabric, making it possible to propagate the output of one CLB to any other on the chip.

A modern FPGA also includes two other kinds of elements on the chip. Firstly, there are several Distributed Clock Manager (DCM) implanted at strategic locations on the chip. Because every element inside the FPGA can be operated at a given rate, the FPGA chip includes several DCMs to generate the appropriate clock signals and to keep those clock signals synchronous. Secondly, the FPGA has to exchange data with memory banks and peripheral devices. I/O Blocks (IOBs) are implemented on the chip for that purpose.

Figure 15 Block diagram of a Xilinx Virtex-2 FPGA. This chip is based on a regular replication of elementary building blocks that are the CLBs, BRAMs and mutlipliers. I/O Blocks are placed at the outskirts for handling the I/O

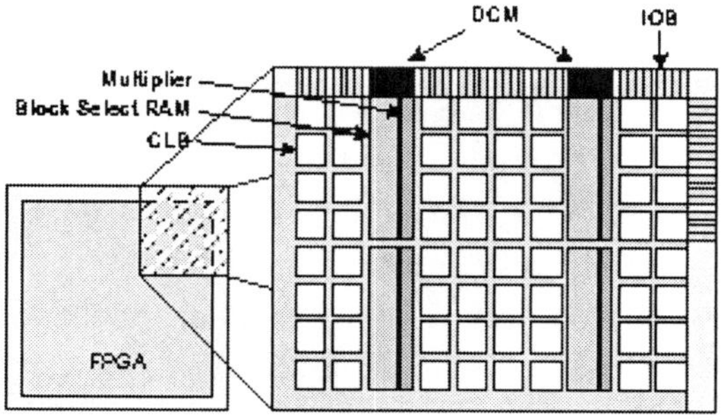

IOBs include the ability to drive signals and perform the required impedance adaptations. Since all IOBs have a similar capacity, a system architect can use them to best match the requirements of a given application. Indeed, there are no dedicated address or data busses. One can implement as many as needed and with the desired width; the only limiting factor is the number of IOBs or pins on the chip.

From the conceptual point of view, an FPGA can be considered as being a large collection of atomic elements that operates a clock frequency decided by the DCMs[11]. Every single element consumes and produces one result per clock cycle even if the production of the result consists in copying the result of the previous clock cycle. From this point of view, the application must be designed as a collection of processing pipelines. The VHDL language has been purposefully designed for supporting the keys building blocks of FPGAs (Pellerin 1997; Yalamanchili 1998). In VHDL, it is easy to specify signals, their width and the way operations happen synchronously with a given clock[12].

Specific resources like multipliers or BRAMs can be either synthesized by the appropriate development tools, or the programmer can select the option of manually deciding the use of a low-level component. In other words, the program can hold multiply instructions for which the synthesizer will decide which resource is best to use for this specific operation. On the other hand, the program can explicitly instantiate one of the multipliers available in the development libraries for the considered FPGA chip. For example, a 2-bits-by-2-bits multiplication can easily be implemented with the LUTs of the CLBs. Besides, such an operation would make poor usage of the multipliers.

On the Xilinx Virtex-2 FPGA family, the CLB is built around two Look Up Tables (LUT) and register circuitry. The LUTs can be used as RAM or registers, or perform some simple operation such as shifting (Figure 16). Since the CLB can perform simple arithmetic operations, it is also

Figure 16. Block diagram of a Configurable Logic Block (CLB)

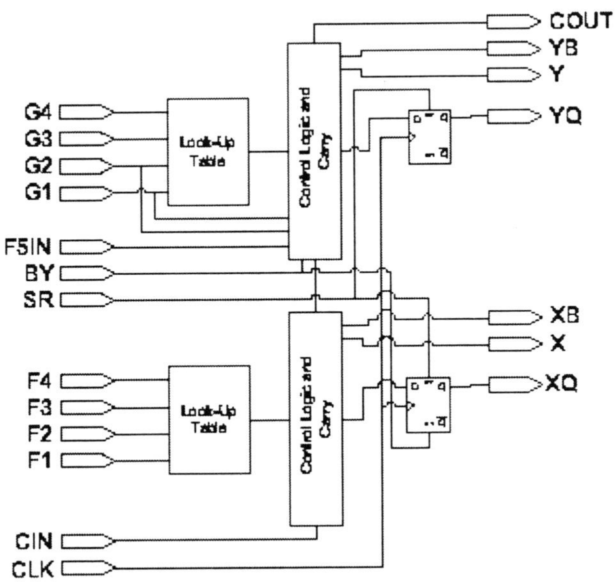

equipped with fast-Carry generation and propagation logic that spans across neighboring CLBs. This makes it possible to perform operations on data items wider than 4 bits.

The multipliers are capable of performing an 18-by-18-bits multiply at every clock cycle. The BRAM are built on dedicated resources. Their capacity is constant, but the width and number of atomic elements is configurable. BRAM are dual ported and can perform two read write operations during the same cycle. Moreover, the width of the data ports does not need to be the same, making the BRAM a handy device for performing data-width conversions or serializations.

For the implementation of a backprojection algorithm, the BRAM shall be used for holding the volume and the projection data. The logic and the multipliers shall be used for computing the projection points of the individual voxels and performing the accumulation onto the volume.

Nevertheless, the implementation of this computation based on equations (4) to (7) requires the use of operators like sine, cosine, the square root, and the inverse. There are no such operators on an FPGA, and it would be expensive in terms of real estate to try to build them from the underlying CLBs. There are several options for overcoming this difficulty. The most common approach is to use Look Up Tables (LUTs) to implement the desired function.

One should consider two cases. The first case appears where all the values are known in advance, such as the cosine of the projection angle as given in equations (6) and (7). In such cases, it is easier to take the index of projection to address the table holding the desired cosine value. The other case manifests itself when the input of the operator is not known in advance, such as the inverse in equation (4) and (5). In such situations, it is necessary to perform a true LUT operation. Such operations generally require a double access and an interpolation for obtaining the desired value. However, this mainly depends on the speed of variation of the function to implement, and the granularity of the LUT. With slowly varying functions and/or a fine granularity, the nearest neighbor approach may provide good enough results. In other cases, interpolation may be required. The compromise to make is to decide whether the program should consume more BRAM space or multipliers.

The second option is to revisit the way the coordinates of the projection points are computed. One can rewrite the equations (4) and (5) in the following way:

$$u(\alpha,\vec{r}) = (c_{00}x + c_{01}y + c_{02}z + c_{03})w(\alpha,\vec{r}) \quad (14)$$

$$v(\alpha,\vec{r}) = (c_{10}x + c_{11}y + c_{12}z + c_{13})w(\alpha,\vec{r}) \quad (15)$$

$$w(\alpha,\vec{r}) = \frac{1}{c_{20}x + c_{21}y + c_{22}z + c_{23}} \quad (16)$$

where

$$c_{ij} = c_{ij}(\alpha).c_{ij}=c_{ij}(\alpha) \quad (17)$$

Here, $\vec{r} = (x, y, z)$ denotes the voxel location, α is the trajectory parameter and u and v are the detector coordinates of voxel $\vec{r}$ at projection angle α. The coefficients $c_{ij}=c_{ij}(\alpha)$ that define the perspective transform from the detector into the volume are arbitrary functions of the projection angle α. In general. $w(\alpha,\vec{r})$ defines the distance weight function. The $c_{ij}(\alpha)$ can be thought of an other way to express equations (4) to (7).

The major advantage of this representation it that these formulas are capable of representing any trajectory, as well as variations in the scanner geometry of the C-arm[13]. This advantage naturally becomes a shortcoming when the trajectory of the source scanner system is perfect. In this case, some of the $c_{ij}(\alpha)$ are equal to zero, and hence the generalized approach would compute a number of values which are known to be zero as well. The case where the trajectory is perfect is one of the topics of the optimization section.

However, the important aspect for an FPGA implementation is that all needs for complex functions have been removed, except for the computation of the inverse. It makes it significantly easier to implement the backprojection. Moreover, this method allows maximizing the amount of BRAMs dedicated to volume and projection data. The prerequisite for having an efficient implementation on an FPGA is to have all of the $c_{ij}(\alpha)$ coefficients precomputed before handing projection data to the backprojection software on the FPGA[14].

Figure 17 shows a block diagram of an overly simplified implementation of the backprojection. Unlike processors, FPGAs are programmed through an inherently parallel paradigm, driven by a properly set clock (the clock signal has not been represented on Fig. 15; however all of the components need to receive it in order to keep the logic in sync). At every clock cycle, the "position generation" (PG) component sends new coordinates to the "coordinate computation" (CC) component. Once the CC has established the coordinates of the projection of point (x, y, z, q) on the detector, it issues the (u, v) coordinates to get the four surrounding pixels. Those pixels are sent to the "interpolation and accumulation" component that computes the final contribution of the considered projection to the voxel (x, y, z), taking the coefficients into account. This contribution is added to the volume data.

The $c_{ij}(\alpha)$ coefficients associated to a projection can be computed on-the-fly or just before the current projection is handed over to the backprojection. The VantageRT-FCN board from Mercury Computer Systems, Inc. is designed to handle this type of case (Figure 18). The board is designed around one Xilinx Virtex II and two PowerPC 7410 processors. The FPGA can process the projection data received on the LVDS links and the PPC processors can compute all the $c_{ij}(\alpha)$ coefficients for fast reconstruction. Extraordinary performance has been reported on other flavors of this board (Goddard 2002).

Beyond the ability to compute the coefficients for the backprojection, the PPCs can also be used

Figure 17. Block diagram of a simple implementation of the backprojection on an FPGA. All data items are carried along with the clock. This elementary set of components can be instanciated several times, until the real estate of the FPGA is saturated

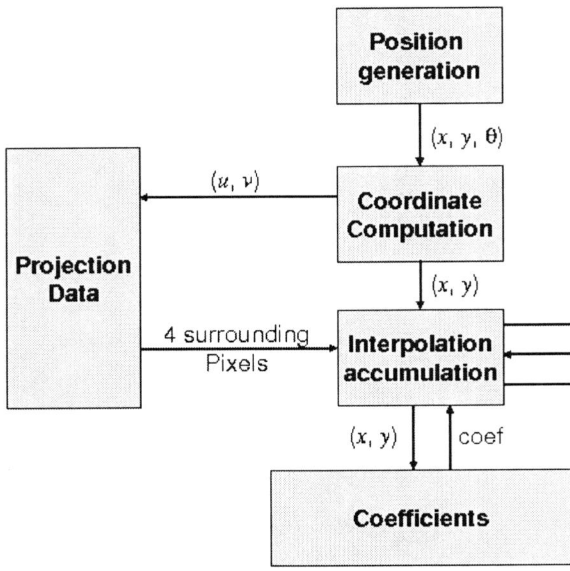

to perform the FFT-based filtering and all of the border and exceptional case processing.

4.1.4 GPGPU Platforms

GPUs were introduced in 1995 to perform graphical tasks such as volume rendering. GPUs are used through programming languages such as OpenGL and Direct-X. They have also been used for accelerating the reconstruction problem (Kole 2006, Müller 1999, Müller 2006, Xue 2006, Xu 2005). The general concept consists in describing the objects to render in the form of triangles whose vertex coordinates are known. The contents of this triangle are treated as a texture. In a given scene, there can be several objects, and depending on the angle from which they are observed, some may partially or totally hide the others. Therefore, the first task in the processing pipeline consists of mapping the 3D information into a 2D representation taking into account the relative position of the objects. This step is performed by the vertex shaders (Figure 20). After this step is completed, the information is represented as a collection of surfaces, each of those holding the information about the texture to use for rendering. These surfaces are passed to the pixel shaders (Figure 19) for final rendering of the 2D images.

The process of mapping a given texture to a coordinate-defined surface is done by the GPU. During the transformation, the value of individual pixels must be interpolated from the four neighboring pixels in the texture. This mechanism is implemented by dedicated interpolation hardware in the shaders.

The vertex shaders are located at the first stage of the pipeline to perform per-vertex transformations, and are hence connected to texture and vertex caches. The second stage of the pipeline consists of a collection of pixel shaders (aka fragment processors). They apply the same program to a collection of pixels in parallel.

Since it is likely that fragments hold more than one pixel, or that the image will not consist of single-pixel surfaces, the structure of a modern

Figure 18. Block diagram of the VantageRT-FCN board from Mercury Computer Systems. It is articulated around a fast interconnect fabric that the transfer of data simultaneously between the processing elements, the host, and peripheral devices

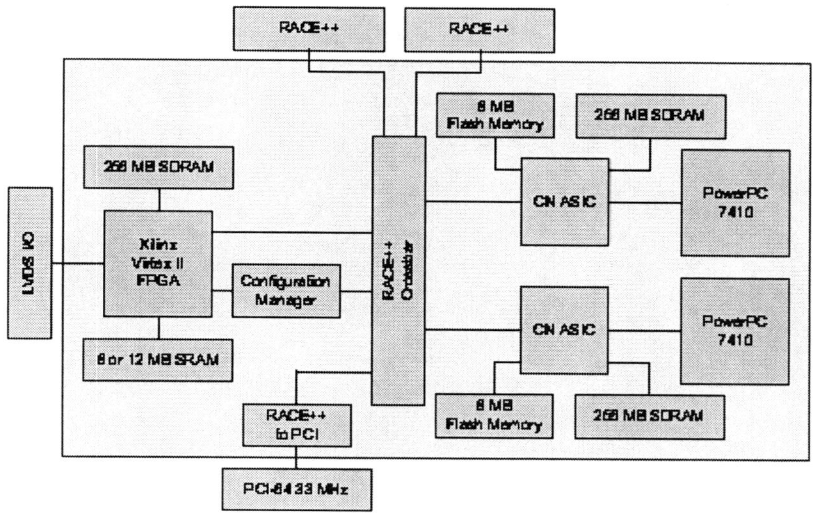

Figure 19. Block diagram of the pixel shader of the NVIDIA GPU. The processing core accesses the textures as indicated by the vertex shaders and computes the output for every pixel

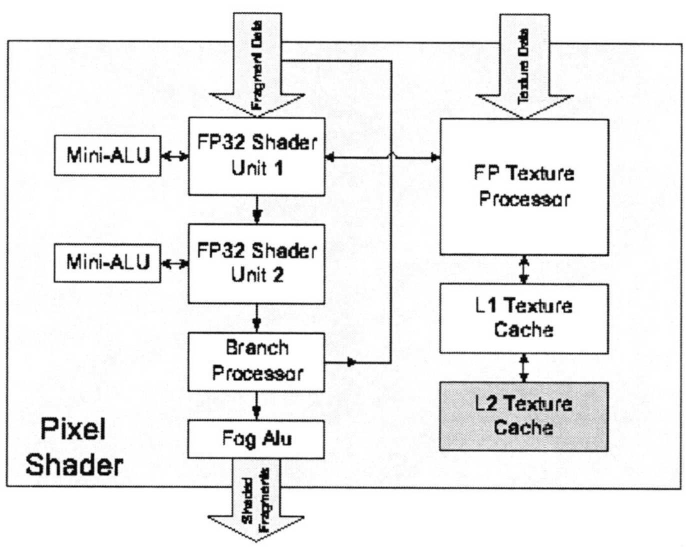

GPU has much more pixel shaders than vertex shaders.

Implementing the backprojection step on a modern GPU like an NVIDIA G71 (Figure 21) consists in loading the relevant part of each projection as texture data. The latest GPUs now have enough memory to hold both a 512^3 volume and 512 projections.

The basic step of the backprojection consists of taking a given slice in the volume, i.e. one xy

Figure 20. Block diagram of the vertex shader of the NVIDIA GPU

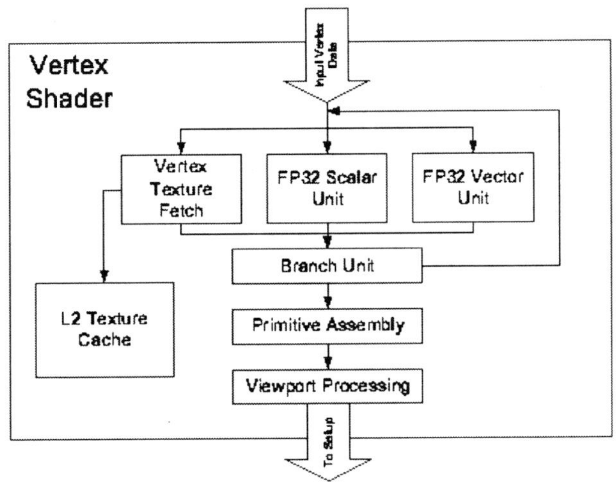

Figure 21. Block diagram of the NVIDIA G71 GPU. The vertex and pixel shaders are interconnected with a fast crossbar for dispatching the work

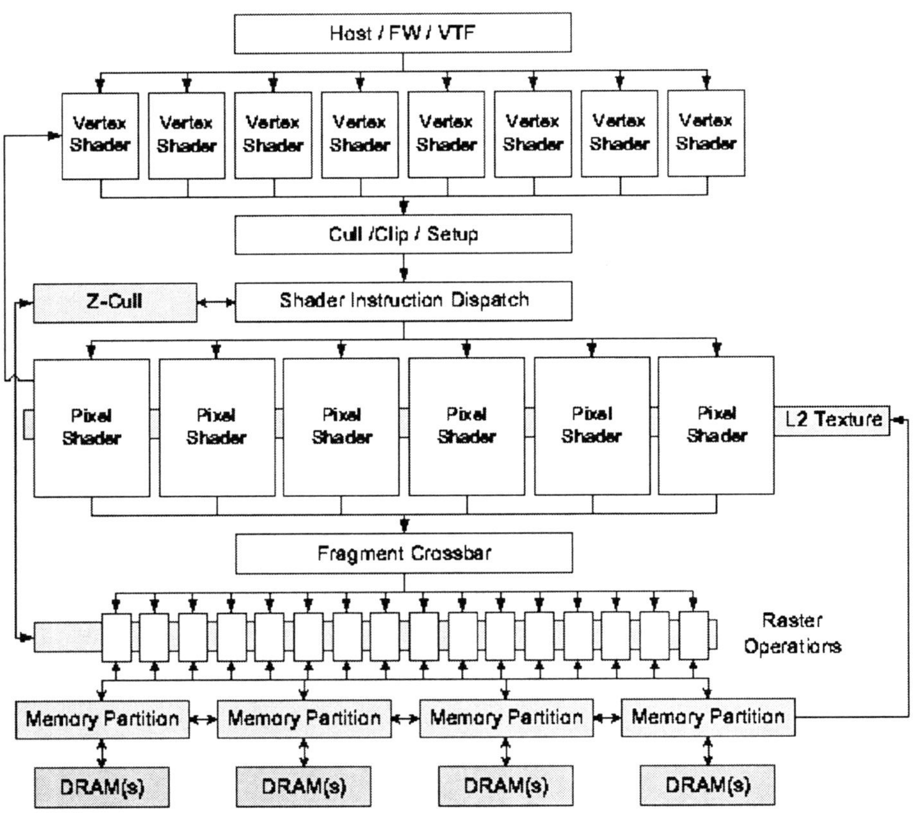

Figure 22. Block diagram of the Intel Quad Core architecture. It is actually built around two dual-core devices sharing the front side bus

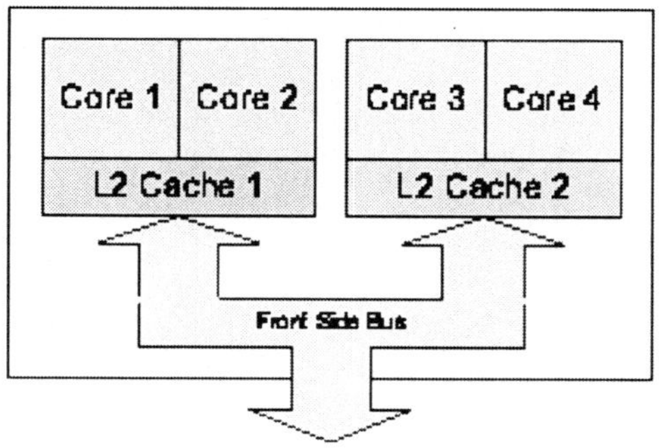

plane and to consider it as the render target. A given projection is then rendered onto this slice with the pixel shaders, the accumulation taking place through simple blending of the results of successive backprojection steps. Accounting for the $w(\alpha, \vec{r})$ coefficients is made through the definition of a mask that has the same size as the considered projection data and holds the coefficients to apply pixel by pixel.

4.1.5 Intel Multi Core Architecture

Intel has introduced processor with four cores (Figure 22). They are based on a duplication of the dual-core processors (Figure 8), and both dual cores share the same front side bus (FSB). The actual speed at which the processor and the FSB operate depends on the design of the motherboard. As in many SMP architectures, the true memory performance depends on the implementation of the Northbridge and its ability to handle multiple data transaction at the same time.

4.2 Optimization Techniques

The reconstruction challenges the designer with two major issues. The first is related to the size of the problem. There is indeed a lot of data to be processed in order to produce output slices. Without taking any precaution, the program ends up being strongly memory-bandwidth limited. The solution to this issue consists in trying to change the way the data is processed, and make best usage of the device's internal resources such as caches for processors or BRAMs for FPGAs. The second issue is related to the internal processing power of the device, and more specifically, the available parallelism. Modern processors have built-in SIMD features. They take the form of SSE units for Intel-based processors or AltiVec/VMX units for PowerPC-based processors. The SPEs on the CBE processor are SIMD only processors.

There are several ways to change the way of processing the data in order to achieve better performance (Knaup 2007), as described in the following sections.

4.2.1 Resampling to Ideal Geometry

The first method to make better use of the processor consists in simplifying the mathematical aspect of the problem. For C-arm based scanners, we know that we must take the imperfections of the C-arm into account and use special coefficients to compensate for the non-circularity of the trajectory of the source and detector (Ridell 2006). However, one can perform a resampling of the projection data in such a way that the projection looks as if it had been taken from a geometrically perfect scanner (Figure 23).

Once the transformation has been applied, it can be observed that the problem can be stated with the following equations:

$$u(\alpha, \vec{r}) = (c_{00}x + c_{01}y + c_{03})w(\alpha, \vec{r}) \tag{18}$$

$$v(\alpha, \vec{r}) = (c_{10}x + c_{11}y + c_{12}z + c_{13})w(\alpha, \vec{r}) \tag{19}$$

$$w(\alpha, \vec{r}) = \frac{1}{c_{20}x + c_{21}y + c_{23}} \tag{20}$$

Figure 23. Resampling the real detector to a detector that has an ideal trajectory and is alinged parallely to the z-axis

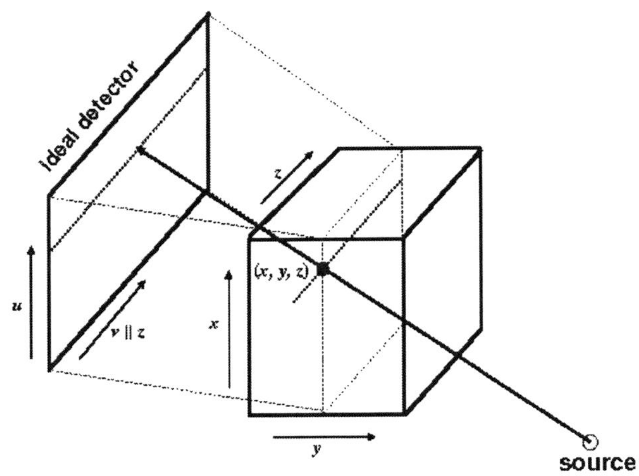

The comparison of those equations with equations (14) to (16) shows a significant simplification. Firstly, terms have been removed from the equation, so there will be an immediate gain in processing time. Secondly the $w(\alpha, \vec{r})$ term now does not depend on *z*. It is now possible to consider this term as a constant when progressing in the *z*-dimension.

The performance gain comes at the cost of an additional resampling step of the projection data. However, this resampling can be included in one of the preprocessing steps at minimal cost. Indeed, the preprocessing of the projection data involves simple operations for compensating for the variations in gain and offset for individual detector pixels. Those corrections are usually strongly memory-bandwidth bound. Adding a resampling at this stage will not change the memory bandwidth required and hence comes at no extra delay.

4.2.2 Oversampling Projection Data

It is also possible to simplify the code required to do the backprojection. Having a closer look at the code, it appears that it almost takes as many instructions to do the bilinear interpolation as to compute the coordinates of the projection point. In the general case, it is not possible to avoid this interpolation step without causing severe artifacts. On the other hand, it is possible to over-sample the projection data by bilinear interpolation of the original projection data in a pre-precessing step. During backprojection, it is sufficient to perform a nearest neighbour (NN) interpolation of the oversampled projection data (Figure 24). If the upsampling factor f_{ups} is high enough, this results in the same image quality as a bilinear interpolation on the original projection data (Kachelrieß 2007).

The performance gain requires an oversampling step, which can be implemented in conjunction with the resampling described above. However, implementing the oversampling of the projection data early in the processing pipeline also involves longer vectors of samples for the convolution. Depending on the relative speed of the filtering and backprojection steps, oversampling may accelerate or slow down the whole reconstruction, depending on the upsampling factor f_{ups}. A typical value is $f_{ups} = 1.5$.

Figure 24. Oversampling the projection data enables a nearest neighbor technique instead of using bilinear interpolation without loss in image quality

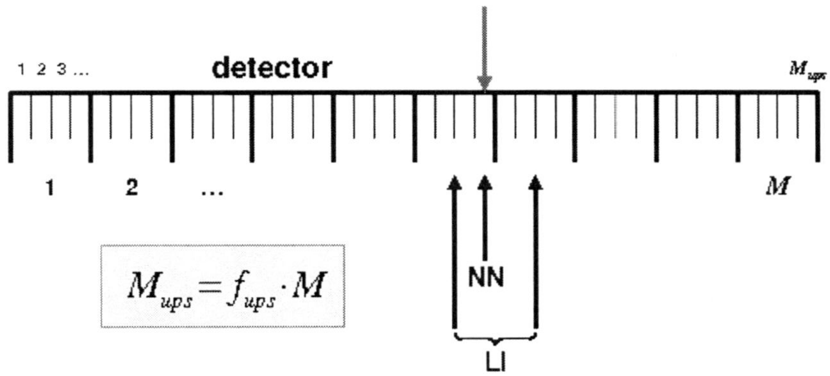

4.2.3 Using the SIMD Capability

Taking advantage of the SIMD units is not as trivial as it seems. The first idea is to try to process N voxels at the same time, i.e. perform a backprojection on four voxels from one projection. Looking at Figure 23, we see that, in the general case, this will be difficult to achieve: The pixels required for the four voxels are not on sequential positions in memory, and multiple loads are required for getting the relevant data into registers. However, in the special case of parallel geometry it is possible to process four slices at the same time (Figure 25). This exploits the fact that the coefficients are the same for all slices in this case.

4.2.4 Locality of Projection Data

In modern scanners, the number of projections taken around the object is rather large. Consequently, the difference in consecutive projection angles is rather small. When the sub-volume is small enough, the shadow of two neighboring sub-volumes overlap for a large part (Figure 26). This can be taken advantage of during the forward- and backprojection steps to reduce the amount of projection-data movement between the main memory and the cache, BRAMs or Local Store. Indeed, when the size of the sub-volume is small and shadows overlap for the major part, the amount of projection data needed for a collection of sub-volumes can be kept small enough to fit into fast memory. There are two consequences to this. Firstly, since the shadows overlap, one would repeatedly load the same projection data for neighboring sub-volumes, and this can be avoided. Secondly, the forward projection step requires walking through all the voxels along a given ray for computing the estimated projection. In order to avoid computing partial sums and recombining them, it is desirable to compute larger parts of the projection data with more sub-volumes.

4.3 Discussion

4.3.1 Results

The optimization methods mentioned in the previous sections have been used for implementing the reconstruction algorithm on the various platforms. The performance numbers are given in Table 1.

Table 1 needs comments. Firstly, the clock rates show a wide spectrum. The Virtex-2 Pro is an older generation of FPGA devices. However, recent FPGAs like the Virtex-5 do not come close to the 3 GHz of the multicore processors such as

Figure 25. Backprojectinging several slices at the same time enables the use of SIMD capabilities of the modern processor. In this figure, the data has been rebinned to parallel geometry

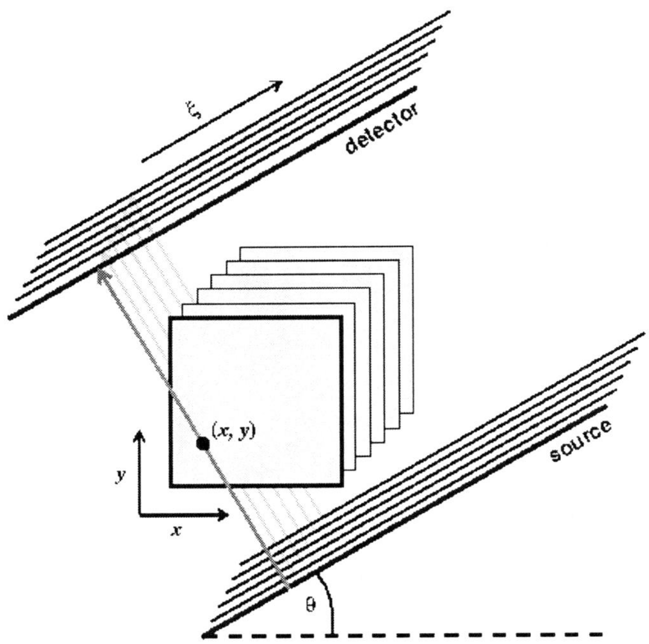

Figure 26. For different angles, one can hold a subset of the projections in such a way that several sub-volumes can be updated from those subsets, avoiding to repeatedly reload projection data

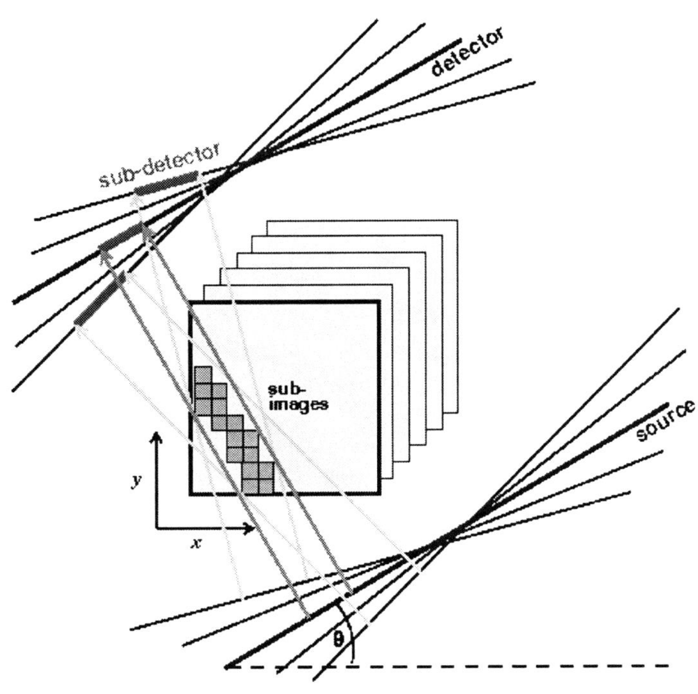

Table 1.

Architecture	Clock (GHz)	Fast Convolution (GC/s)	Backprojection (GU/s)
CBE (Mercury Computer Systems)	3.2	15	4.7
Playstation 3 (Sony)	3.2	11	3.5
Dual Quad Core 45 nm (Intel)	3.0	5.7	6.6
Virtex-2 Pro (Xilinx)	0.133	N/A	3.1
GPU G70 (NVIDIA)	1.35	N/A	7.5

the CBE processor. The major reason for this low-clock rate is the programmable interconnect. Between CLBs is an interconnect fabric, responsible for conveying data between a given CLB and the next one. The average transmission time between CLBs accounts for as much time as needed for a CLB to perform its task. Routing data between CLBs requires several levels of gates to come into play, lowering the capability for an FPGA to sustain higher clock rates. Therefore, the speed of the interconnect is unlikely to significantly change in the future.

Secondly, the CBE processor shows excellent results for the fast convolution, but only second order performance for the backprojection. Compared to a dual quad- core architecture from Intel that holds a similar number of cores, the CBE performs a lot better for the fast convolution but is significantly slower than the dual quad-core solution. There are several explanations for this. The CBE has an internal architecture designed for number crunching: the SPEs are SIMD only and scalar code cannot be easily dealt with. A Fast Fourier Transform (FFT), as needed for a fast convolution, exhibits the power hungriness that fits the CBE design. The Intel architecture is based on a replication of a powerful general-purpose core. Lacking the specialization for number crunching built into the CBE SPEs, the Intel solution cannot achieve the performance of the CBE. On the other hand, the backprojection keeps a significant part of code that cannot be easily vectorized without losing the flexibility required for solving arbitrary reconstruction problems. A general-purpose design handles the backprojection problem more efficiently.

Thirdly, the fast convolution has not been investigated for the FPGA and the GPU platforms. The FFT process cannot be easily dealt without floating-point capabilities. Even if attempts to implement FFTs on FPGAs have been made (Andraka 2006), the overall efficiency cannot compare with processors designed with the floating-point capability. The GPU is not a good target for the FFT, mainly because of structural reasons. A typical FFT performs a multistage "butterfly". It requires the capability to rapidly exchange the results of neighboring butterflies to implement the global FFT process. GPUs are designed at efficiently handling a collection of vertexes or pixels, all taken individually as needed for volume rendering. The exchange of data items between shaders is a delicate thing to do and make the implementation of FFTs a difficult problem.

4.3.2 Analysis

The goal of the optimization techniques described in the previous section is to enhance the utilization factor of the HPC platforms. Taking a closer look at the optimization problem, one can identify three categories of resources that require special attention:

1. processing power (e.g. the ALUs)
2. internal fast memory (e.g. the cache)
3. memory bandwidth.

Figure 27 plots the resource utilization on the different platforms when facing the optimized FDK backprojection algorithm for a problem consisting of 512 projections and a volume size of 512^3. The utilization factor is computed as being the ratio of the observed rates compared to the theoretical maximum for the given resource. The BW value indicates how much the memory subsystem is solicited by the task, while the Cache value indicates the effectiveness of the cache utilization; it is computed from the quantity of data that is maintained internally with respect to the total space available. Finally, the CPU value gives the percentage of the duty cycles the processor performs, which is computed in taking the number of Gflops sustained vs. the maximum processing power sustainable.

Figure 27 requires a number of comments. Firstly, for traditional processing elements like a multicore processor or a GPU, it seems rather difficult to achieve a high level of CPU utilization. The reason for this is that a thoroughly optimized backprojection algorithm only exhibits very few processing cycles and rather more load/store cycles, leaving a big part of the ALU core unemployed. Less sophisticated hardware such as FPGAs have more flexibility to accommodate a large variety of algorithms, and designers can make easily make good usage of their real estate.

Secondly, all Cache usage values are more than 70%. This level on this metric is rather difficult to achieve by a common approach for all platforms. The major reason resides in the drastic difference in the way fast memory is managed on the different devices. For the PC and the GPGPU, caches are automatically managed by the logic built into the silicone. It maintains the contents of the cache according to Least Recently Used (LRU) policies and proceeds to replacements according to the demands of the CPU. For the CBE and the FPGA, the internal memory resources need to be managed by hand. The moving of the data can be finely controlled on the CBE and the FPGA. In particular, manual data movement associated with double buffering allows for optimal performances: the backprojection problem is compute intensive enough to allow the loading of the data required for the next iteration, while the current iteration is in progress. This kind of optimization is difficult to achieve with caches.

Finally, the level of memory-bus-bandwidth utilization varies a lot from one platform to another. By design, the task for a GPU is to process every single pixel of an image according to simple rules. Doing so, it has to repeatedly access texture data. Therefore, the memory bandwidth has been the subject of a lot of attention to allow higher data rates. The CBE processor follows the same

Figure 27. Utilization factor of the key resources for the different devices

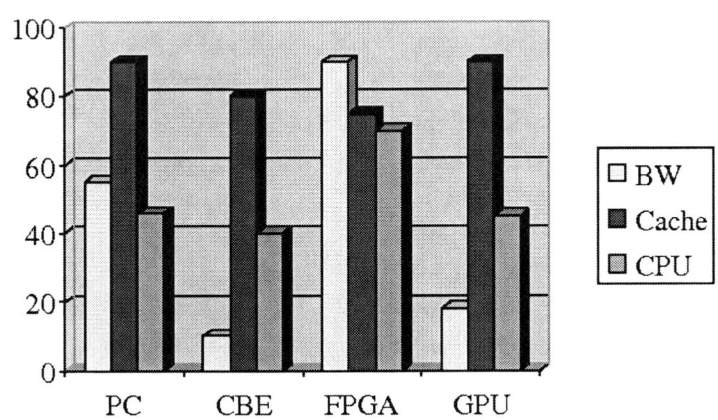

type of approaches: the SPEs don't have enough LS to allow working for a long time without requiring some data in main memory. Indeed, high-memory bandwidth is required to feed the 8 SPEs. The FPGA is a special case. All the logic to drive memory banks has to be built from the real estate on the chip. Indeed, using complex memory subsystems allowing for multiple data transactions at the same time certainly improve the memory bandwidth, but at the cost of a lot of real estate jeopardizing the ability to perform the intended backprojection task. Therefore, the memory subsystem has been kept in its simplest form allowing the fetch and store of the data at the appropriate speed, hence leading to a high factor of utilization.

4.4 A Glimpse Into the Future

4.4.1 Acceleration Hardware

There are significant changes taking place in the area of computing hardware designs. After a period where the easiest solution was to increase the clock frequency, designers are now gaining processing power in making denser packages. Those chips now use thinner technology, typically 45 nm. This has several advantages. Firstly, it is possible to implement more logic onto the same die surface. Secondly, the path between logic components is shorter, allowing for higher clock speed and less power consumption. Finally, it also allows drastic changes in the internal structure of the chips, allowing for a higher number of more complex functional units to be implemented on the same die.

Xilinx proposes the Virtex-4 and Virtex-5 chips in various configurations. The major change consists in adding the so called eXtreme DSP slices (Figure 28). Those small compute elements are in fact simple ALUs that can efficiently perform simple RISC-like instructions such as Multiply-Accumulate. Since the backprojection is based on the accumulating projection data on the volume data, these features are of highest interest for the backprojection. In addition to the changes in the internal structure, Xilinx proposes IP blocks for driving DDR2 memory banks at 667 MHz, significantly improving the capability for high-data transfer rates.

IBM announces the next generation of the CBE processor for 2010. It shall be built around

Figure 28. Block diagram of an eXtreme DSP slice from a Xilinx Virtex-4 FPGA. The actual operation performed by the slice can be decided through control bits, in a similar way an instruction is fed into an ALU

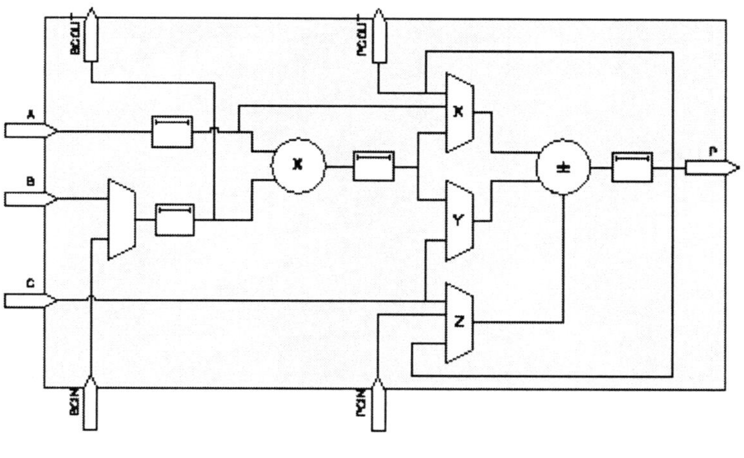

two PPEs and 32 SPEs, effectively proposing a CPU performance increase by a factor of four. RamBus proposes new memory architectures capable of reaching 1 TB/s. Without going to this extreme case, the future existence of a CBE-based architecture offering a bandwidth increase compatible with the performance increase sounds a reasonable guess.

It is possible to extrapolate the performance of these new devices from the utilization factor of the critical resources (i.e. CPU power, cache sizes and memory bandwidth) and the speedup ratio announced by the manufacturer. For the Xilinx Virtex-5, the clock rate can be set to 0.5 GHz, the real estate is growing by a factor of 6.5 and the DDR2 memory can now be clocked at 0.33 GHz effectively allowing 0.667 Gbps. Compared to the Virtex-2 Pro, the lowest increase ratio is related to the real estate[15]. For the CBE architecture, the utilization factor of the memory bandwidth is not the bottleneck. The performance increase shall be dictated by the increase in the number of SPEs.

Those performance numbers bring HPC platforms based on the FPGA of the CBE processor to reconstruct a volume of 512^3 voxels from 512 projections in less than 5s.

4.4.2 New Scanner Technology

In order to increase the spatial resolution of the reconstructed volume, the sampling of the projections must be improved. This is usually done by increasing the number of projections taken around the object as well as the resolution of the detector.

At constant sampling rate, the reconstruction time is a linear function of the number of projections. Similarly, the bandwidth required to transport the projection data is a function of the detector size. Spiral CT scanners have seen their detector sizes increase from 32 to 320 detector rows over the last five years. For a given number of projections per second, this represents a bandwidth increase by a factor of 10. A modern scanner takes about 1000 projections per rotation with each projection consisting in 320×1000 samples; it performs about three rotations per second. Assuming the samples are coded on 3 bytes, HPC platforms have to face a total bandwidth of 2.9 TB/s. Such data rates are challenging for the network and for the memory subsystem that receives the projection data.

The source and detector technologies are also evolving. The level of absorption of the X-rays is a function of the energy level and of the tissue. Taking the energy levels into consideration makes it possible to determine the atomic number of the exposed tissues. Some CT scanners intentionally use two sources with different energy levels (Alvarez 1976). Using this kind of technology to determine the atomic numbers of the exposed tissues requires two full reconstructions and the merging of their reconstructed volumes.

The X-ray radiation emitted by the source is polychromatic by nature. Using detectors based on Cadmium Zinc Telluride (CZT), that can separate photon beam into several energy bins, can achieve the same result as scanner with multiple energy levels managed by the sources. However, this information comes at the cost of a complete reconstruction per energy level. Indeed, taking full advantage of a detector with four energy bins also means four times more reconstruction efforts.

Table 2.

Architecture	Clock (GHz)	Fast Convolution (GC/s)	Backprojection (GU/s)
CBE (Mercury Computer Systems)	3.2	60	18.8
Virtex-2 Pro (Xilinx)	0.133	N/A	20.15

Finally, medical imaging requires higher resolution in the reconstructed volume. A typical example relates to the study of the calcium plaque in the coronary arteries. For evaluating the calcium level in these tiny blood vessels, the spatial resolution has to increase dramatically. The resolution increase leads to the reconstruction of more voxels for a constant physical volume size, typical 1024^3 instead of 512^3. This means an increase by a factor of eight in the backprojection effort.

4.4.3 New Applications

The ability to look inside the scanned object without opening it has a lot of new applications. In medical imaging, computer-aided intervention is a promising area. Real-time processing and display are the cornerstone for the success of these new applications. A typical example is pulmonary biopsies. The surgical act consists of inserting a needle into the body to reach the desired area before injecting fluid. Since the tissues are subject to deformations due to the insertion of the tool, is it desirable to obtain a view of the progress of the tool in real time. In this case, real time means introducing as little latency as possible and updating the view at least 10 times per second. Without applying any tricks, such applications require the reconstruction of the region of interest 10 times per second, while today's best platforms can perform only one reconstruction every 10 seconds.

Another area where real processing is required is related to luggage scanning. The objective of these scanners is to inspect the contents of bags without opening them. The bags are placed on a belt that moves at a constant speed through the source-detector system. Assuming the speed is 0.25m/s, the slices are 512^2 pixels large and the slice thickness is 1mm, such a scanner has to reconstruct 250 slices per second. In order to reach an image quality compatible with the application with a filtered backprojection algorithm, several hundreds of projections must be taken for a given volume. Extrapolating this problem to the reference case of 512^3 with 512 projections, the reconstruction needs to be performed in less than two seconds.

4.4.4 New Algorithms

The development of new algorithms is mainly driven by the need for improved image quality. Exact algorithms bring the computational artifacts to a very small level. Nevertheless, other sources of artifacts need to be corrected. The first source of annoying artifacts is due to the presence of metal inside the object, deflecting the X-rays from their ideal straight trajectory. Compensating for this phenomenon can be done in several ways, but the most common is to proceed in the volume space with an iterative approach. This method can be compared to the iterative reconstruction algorithms such as ART: every iteration consists of a forward projection and a backprojection step. Highly sophisticated artifact reduction algorithms require at least one iteration to reduce the metal artifacts to an acceptable level. Consequently the increase in the computational cost is at least a factor of two.

4.5 Compromises

Nevertheless, due to the sensitivity to price in markets where reconstruction is deployed, one has to consider how efficiently a given reconstruction algorithm can be implemented on a given HPC platform. Moreover, for maintenance-related cost reasons, scanner manufacturers prefer to reuse existing HPC platforms; HPC platforms that can serve more than one purpose are highly appreciated, even at the cost of inefficient processing.

4.5.1 Image Quality

The different implementations have been evaluated against the same data set and obtained clinical-quality reconstructed volumes for all of them. Figure 29 gives a typical example of the quality

Figure 29. Statistical image reconstruction can significantly improve image quality. Since statistical reconstruction is iterative, only HPIR solutions can provide the desired performance (Knaup 2006)

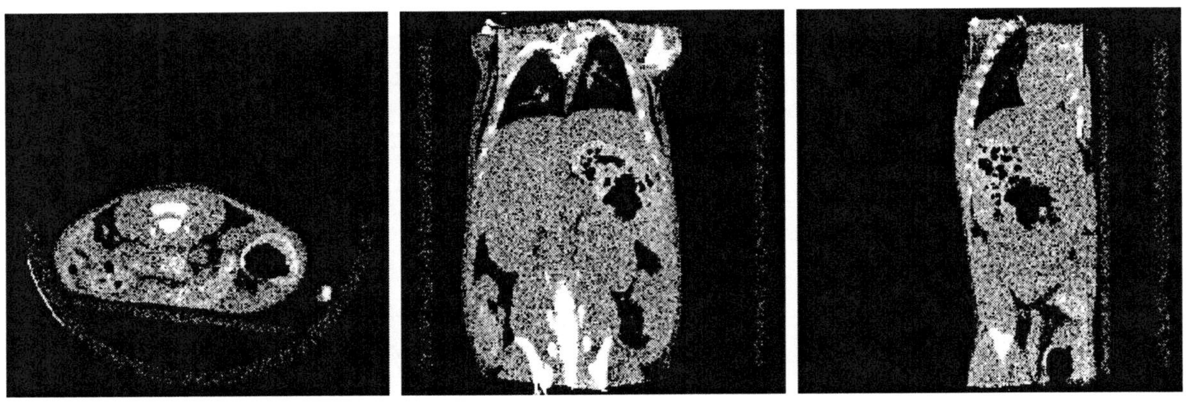

of those implementations. It depicts different views of the reconstruction of a mouse scanned with a micro-CT-scanner TomoScope 30s (VAMP GmbH, Erlangen, Germany).

However, there are slight differences to be observed between the different volumes and they can be taken care of at minimal processing expenses.

The FPGA version performs all of its computation in fixed point. Even if attempts to use floating point on FPGAs have been made (Andraka 2006), implementing the complete pipeline in floating-point math is questionable for real estate reasons, even on modern chips. It is preferable to use a fixed-point representation with the inherent limit imposed by the width of the multipliers embedded in the Virtex family chips. There is still the possibility to cascade multipliers to reach better accuracy, but the results turn out to be inefficient in terms of performance. The best way to overcome this kind of problem is to carefully design the computation pipeline to keep the relevant bits and to recondition the input data so that extreme values do not occur. However, some impact on the image quality can be observed.

The GPU-reconstructed volumes show the same kind of issues, but at a reduced level. This is mainly due to the fact that, however close to IEEE floating-point standards, the floating-point processing on an NVIDIA GPU still has some deviations with respect to the standard. It takes the form of incorrect handling of exceptional cases, such as Not A Number (NaN). One can use data-preconditioning techniques to avoid this kind of exception. It is rather easier than in the FPGA case, since the conditioning has to take care of only exceptional cases, while the accuracy of the implementation must be taken into account for the FPGA case.

The Cell implementation suffers to a low degree from inaccuracies related to the computations of estimates instead of real values for operators, like divide, square root and exponential. The estimates turn out to be accurate, up to the 6th digit after the floating point. Some special cases at low angles require more accuracy; Raphson-Newton kinds of algorithms can be employed to overcome this issue.

4.5.2 Complexity

There are different levels of complexity to be considered when one thinks of developing a reconstruction algorithm on a given platform. The first relates to the complexity of developing the algorithm, and acquiring adequate image quality. The second relates to the design of the system hosting the reconstruction part. Some implementations call for multi-chassis platforms with complex interconnects, while others need adequate cooling and power supplies. The third and final aspect relates to the engineering effort required to keep up with the latest technology to replace failing parts in the field, once the failing part has been end-of-lifed by the manufacturer.

The most obvious and stable implementation has been done on a PC. The Cell processor offers a multicomputer platform which is very comparable to multicomputers such as those developed by Mercury Computer Systems with RACEWay, RACE++ and RapidIO. They all can be programmed in a high level programming language.

Even though all GPU boards support OpenGL and DirectX, the level of efficiency for different GPU boards varies, even when they come from the same manufacturer. The internal features, such as the structure of the 2D-texture caches, are hidden to the developer for many reasonable reasons. The result is that performances are not predictable across GPU board generations. The coding of reconstruction algorithms are a lot more difficult on FPGAs, mainly because they don't offer floating-point operators, and that operators such as multiply, divide, sine and cosine must be coded as application-dependent LUTs.

GPUs are intended to be the graphical processor companion in every PC. Most of the modern PCs can accommodate the presence of a modern GPU for power supply and cooling. Consequently, all reconstruction hardware that fits in the same {cooling, power supply} envelope can be hosted in the same host PC. The CAB has been designed to fit into that envelope and can be hosted in any modern PC. FPGA-based boards are subject to the inspiration of the designer. FPGAs traditionally draw less power than high-clocked devices such as a GPU or the CBE processor, and are easier to cool. However, FPGA boards require special attention to ensure their power and cooling requirements are within the specifications of the host.

4.5.3 Life-Cycle Management

However much host processors have evolved in recent years, they all remain compatible with each other, usually even binary compatible. This means that a given executable instruction produced with a given version of tools for a given version of processors, is likely to work on many later processor versions without intervention. Therefore, PC-based implementations also offer the best solution for field repairs and upgrades, when the maintenance costs are considered. FPGAs and the Cell processor are designed to remain active for many years, and in fact, represent a valuable alternative for accelerating medical image reconstruction. GPUs represent the device family with the greatest variability in terms of architecture, structure, application programming interfaces and drivers.

5 CONCLUSION

High-Performance Computing has made tremendous progress over the last 10 years. There is now a large variety of devices and platforms that can be considered for solving the 3D reconstruction problems in a time that is compatible with the workflow in hospitals. However, the processing-power requirements of CT reconstruction applications are growing at a very fast rate. Depending on the final application, those requirements have been consistently growing three times faster than Moore's law over the last decade and are likely to continue that way for a non-predictable period.

There are numerous techniques that allow improving the performance of straight implementations. They belong either to the family of tricks that take advantage of the geometrical properties of the scanner or to the family using the knowledge of the internal structure of the device selected for accelerating the processing. The real art in engineering the reconstruction platform is the selection of the adequate combination of acceleration techniques.

Unfortunately, there are other considerations that need to be taken into account. Applications needing CT reconstruction are under high price pressure and require an intricate life cycle management of a complex platform. In a real life HPC platform for CT reconstruction, there will be devices responsible for the acquisition of the projections and devices in charge with the visualization. Because of the integer encoding of the samples, the former is usually implemented as an FPGA. GPUs are traditionally used for the latter. The FPGA and the GPU are likely to have some real estate or free cycles available for implementing a part of the reconstruction pipeline. As a consequence, there is a strong likelihood that the HPC platform architecture forces the consideration of using several different device types for the implementation of the complete reconstruction pipeline.

These potential combinations make the spectrum of possible HPC platforms for CT reconstruction extremely wide. Most of these combinations do not make the best utilization of all the involved acceleration devices. For the purpose of scalability, it is important that those components have a consistent utilization factor; for a slight increase of computing load, the whole architecture would have to be revisited in case one of the components gets saturated. This means that it may sometimes not be necessary to get to the highest possible performance: another component may already be the bottleneck and any further optimization on the considered device won't make the whole pipeline go faster.

The design of the ultimate reconstruction pipeline is based on the selection of the accelerating device and the knowledge of the acceleration techniques that can be efficiently used for those devices.

REFERENCES

Alvarez, R. E., & Macovski, A. (1976). Energy-Selective Reconstructions in X-Ray CT. *Physics in Medicine and Biology, 21*(5), 733–744. doi:10.1088/0031-9155/21/5/002

Andraka, R. (2006). Hybrid Floating Point Technique Yields 1.2 Gigasample Per Second 32 to 2048 point Floating Point FFT in a single FPGA (37K). *Proceedings of the 10th Annual High Performance Embedded Computing Workshop.*

Basu, S., & Bresler, Y. (2000). An O(N^2/log N) Filtered Backprojection Reconstruction Algorithm for Tomography. *IEEE Transactions on Medical Imaging, 9*, 1760–1773.

Beekman, F. J., & Kamphuis, C. (2001). Ordered Subset Reconstruction for X-Ray CT. *Physics in Medicine and Biology, 46*, 1835–1844. doi:10.1088/0031-9155/46/7/307

Bockenbach, O., Knaup, M., & Kachelriess, M. (2007). Real Time Adaptive Filtering for Computed Tomography Applications. *IEEE Medical Imaging Conference Proceedings 2007.*

Chen, G. H. (2003). From Tuy's Inversion Scheme to Katsevich's Inversion Scheme: Pulling a Rabbit out of the Hat. *Proceedings of the 7th Int. Meeting on Fully 3D Image Reconstruction, Saint Malo, France.*

Danielsson, P. E., & Ingerhed, M. (1998). Backprojection in O(N^2/log N) Time. *IEEE Nuclear Science Symposium Record, 2,* 1279-1283.

Feldkamp, L. A., Davis, L. C., & Kress, J. W. (1984). Practical Cone-Beam Algorithm. *Journal of the Optical Society of America, 1*, 612–619. doi:10.1364/JOSAA.1.000612

Flachs, B., Asano, S., Dhong, S. H., Hofstee, H. P., Gervais, G., Kim, R., et al. (2005). A Streaming Processing Unit for a Cell Processor. *IEEE International Solid-State Circuits Conference 2005.*

Goddard, I., & Trepanier, M. (2002). High-Speed Cone-Beam Reconstruction: An Embedded Systems Approach. *SPIE Medical Imaging Proceedings*, *4681*, 483–491.

Gordon, R. A. (1974). Tutorial on ART (Algebraic Reconstruction Techniques). *IEEE Transactions on Nuclear Science*, *NS-21*, 78–93.

Grangeat, P. (1987). *Analyse d'un système d'imagerie 3D par reconstruction à partir de radiographies X en géométrie conique.* Doctoral dissertation, Ecole Nationale Supérieure des Télécommunications, France.

Haykin, S. (2002). *Adaptive Filter Theory.* Prentice Hall Information and System Science Series, ISBN 0-130-90126-1, 4th Edition.

Herman, G. T. (1980). *Image Reconstruction from Projections: The Fundamentals of Computerized Tomography.* Computer Science and Applied Mathematics, Academic Press, New York, ISBN 0-123-42050-4.

Hofstee, H. P. (2005). Power Efficient Processor Architecture and the Cell Processor. *Proceedings of the 11th International Symposium on High-Performance Computer Architecture.*

Hounsfield, G. N. (1972). *A Method of and Apparatus for Examination of a Body by Radiation such as X or Gamma Radiation. Patent Specification 1283915.* London: The Patent Office.

Joseph, P. M. (1982). An Improved Algorithm for Reprojecting Rays through Pixel Images. *IEEE Transactions on Medical Imaging*, *2*(3), 192–196. doi:10.1109/TMI.1982.4307572

Kachelrieß, M., Knaup, M., & Bockenbach, O. (2007). Hyperfast Parallel-Beam and Cone-Beam Backprojection using the Cell General Purpose Hardware. *Medical Physics*, *34*, 1474–1486. doi:10.1118/1.2710328

Kachelrieß, M., Knaup, M., & Kalender, W. A. (2004). Extended parallel backprojection for standard 3D and phase-correlated 4D axial and spiral cone-beam CT with arbitrary pitch and 100% dose usage. *Medical Physics*, *31*(6), 1623–1641. doi:10.1118/1.1755569

Kachelrieß, M., Watzke, O., & Kalender, W. A. (2001). Generalized multi-dimensional adaptive filtering (MAF) for conventional and spiral single-slice, multi-slice and cone-beam CT. *Medical Physics*, *28*(4), 475–490. doi:10.1118/1.1358303

Kaczmarz, S. (1937). Angenäherte Auflösung von Systemen Linearer Gleichungen. *Bull. Acad. Polon. Sci. Lett. A*, *35*, 335–357.

Kak, A. C., & Slaney, M. (1988). *Principles of Computerized Tomographic Imaging.* Society of Industial and Applied Mathematics, Philadelphia, ISBN 0-898-71494-X.

Kalender, W. A. (2005). *Computed Tomography.* Wiley & Sons, ISBN 3-89578-216-5, 2nd Edition.

Katsevich, A. (2002). Analysis of an Exact Inversion Algorithm for Spiral Cone-Beam CT. *Physics in Medicine and Biology*, *47*, 2583–2597. doi:10.1088/0031-9155/47/15/302

Katsevich, A. (2003). A General Scheme for Constructing Inversion Algorithms for Cone Beam CT. *International Journal of Mathematics and Mathematical Sciences*, *21*, 1305–1321. doi:10.1155/S0161171203209315

Knaup, M., & Kachelriess, M. (2007). Acceleration techniques for 2D Parallel and 3D perspective Forward- and Backprojections. *Proceedings of the HPIR Workshop at the 9th Int. Meeting on Fully 3D Image Reconstruction, Lindau, Germany.*

Knaup, M., Kalender, W. A., & Kachelrieß, M. (2006). Statistical cone-beam CT image reconstruction using the Cell broadband engine. *IEEE Medical Imaging Conference Program, M11-422,* 2837-2840.

Kole, J. S., & Beekman, F. J. (2006). Evaluation of Accelerated Iterative X-Ray CT Image Reconstruction Using Floating Point Graphics Hardware. *Physics in Medicine and Biology*, *51*, 875–889. doi:10.1088/0031-9155/51/4/008

Leeser, M., Coric, S., Miller, E., Yu, H., & Trepanier, M. (2002). Parallel-Beam Backprojection: An FPGA Implementation Optimized for Medical Imaging. *Proceedings of the 10th Int. Symposium on FPGA, Monterey, CA.*

Müller, K., & Xu, F. (2006). Practical Considerations for GPU-Accelerated CT. *IEEE International Symposium on Biomedical Imaging 2006.*

Müller, K., Yagel, R., & Wheller, J. J. (1999). Fast Implementation of Algebraic Methods for Three-Dimensional Reconstruction from Cone-Beam Data. *IEEE Transactions on Medical Imaging*, *18*, 538–548. doi:10.1109/42.781018

Natterer, F. (1989). *The Mathematics of Computerized Tomography.* B.G. Teubner, Stuttgart, ISBN 0-898-71493-1.

Pellerin, D., & Taylor, D. (1997). *VHDL Made Easy.* Prentice Hall, ISBN 0-13-650763-8.

Pham, D., Asano, S., Bolliger, M., Day, M. N., Hofstee, H. P., Johns, C., et al. (2005). The Design and Implementation of a First-Generation Cell Processor. *Proceedings of the IEEE International Solid-State Circuits Conference 2005.*

Radon, J. (1986). On the Determination of Functions From Their Integral Values Along Certain Manifolds. *IEEE Transactions on Medical Imaging*, *MI-5*, 170–176. doi:10.1109/TMI.1986.4307775

Ramachandran, G. N., & Lakshminarayanan, A. V. (1971). Three-Dimensional Reconstruction from Radiographs and Electron Micrographs: Application of Convolution instead of Fourier Transforms. *Proceedings of the National Academy of Sciences of the United States of America*, *68*, 2236–2240. doi:10.1073/pnas.68.9.2236

Riddell, C., & Trousset, Y. (2006). Rectification for Cone-Beam Projection and Backprojection. *IEEE Transactions on Medical Imaging*, *25*, 950–962. doi:10.1109/TMI.2006.876169

Schaller, S., Flohr, T., & Steffen, P. (1998). An Efficient Fourier method in 3D reconstruction from cone-beam data. *IEEE Transactions on Medical Imaging*, *17*, 244–250. doi:10.1109/42.700736

Shepp, L. A., & Logan, B. F. (1974). The Fourier Reconstruction of a Head Section. *IEEE Transactions on Nuclear Science*, *NS-21*, 21–43.

Siddon, R. (1985). Fast calculation of the exact radiological path length for a three-dimensional CT array. *Medical Physics*, *12*, 252–255. doi:10.1118/1.595715

Trepanier, M., & Goddard, I. (2002). Adjunct Processors in Embedded Medical Imaging Systems. *SPIE Medical Imaging Proceedings*, *4681*, 416–424.

Turbell, H. (2001). *Cone Beam Reconstruction using filtered Backprojection.* Doctoral dissertation, University of Linköping, Sweden.

Tuy, H. K. (1983). An Inversion Formula for Cone-Beam Reconstruction. *SIAM Journal on Applied Mathematics*, *43*, 546–552. doi:10.1137/0143035

Xu, F., & Mueller, K. (2005). Accelerating Popular Tomographic Reconstruction Algorithms on Commodity PC Graphics Hardware. *IEEE Transactions on Nuclear Science*, *52*(3), 654–663. doi:10.1109/TNS.2005.851398

Xue, X., Cheryauka, A., & Tubbs, D. (2006). Acceleration of Fluoro-CT Reconstruction for a Mobile C-Arm on GPU and FPGA Hardware: A Simulation Study. *SPIE Medical Imaging Proceedings*, *6142*, 494–1501.

Yalamanchili, S. (1998). *VHDL Starter's Guide.* Prentice Hall, ISBN 0-13-519802-X.

Yu, R., Ning, R., & Chen, B. (2001). High-Speed Cone-Beam Reconstruction on PC. *SPIE Medical Imaging Proceedings*, *4322*, 964–973.

ENDNOTES

1 Although the optimization of the underlying mathematics is beyond the scope of this chapter, it is worth mentioning that there are methods to reduce the size of the problem. See, e.g. (Danielsson 1998, Basu 2000).

2 As a consequence, even one may consider storing the acquired data for a C-arm system before starting the reconstruction process; it can't be done for a CT gantry. Indeed, the quantity of data would require too large buffer space. Furthermore, it is desirable to be capable of processing at least a part of the data in real time or close to real time, in order to allow the operator to validate the scan protocol.

3 It is worth mentioning that although approximate algorithms do not solve the reconstruction problem in an exact way, the approximation is compatible with the scanner technology for which they are intended to be used, and that combination of scanner and algorithm is able to produce high-fidelity clinical image quality. Indeed, as the scanner technology evolves, some approximations introduce unacceptable artifacts and new algorithms need to be designed.

4 Due to the large size of the problem, inverting those equations is only possible using iterative matrix-inversion methods.

5 The original PI algorithm and the subsequent PI-Slant derivation show a different level of approximation in the filtering of the projection data. However, those approximations are related to the geometry of the problem, and the solution to this problem is beyond the scope of this chapter.

6 It is worth mentioning that the above equations do not account for the imperfections of the scanner. In real-life systems, the C-arm is not rigid enough to avoid changes in the relative position of the source with respect to the detector during the sweep round the object. In addition, the detector also tends to tilt along the *u*- and the *v*-axis. These distortions need to be included as specific terms in the above equations. The value of those terms varies on a per-projection basis and needs to be carefully calibrated in order to avoid reconstruction artifacts.

7 Even though a sophisticated program can influence the contents of the caches, the management of this fast-memory space is totally under the control of dedicated built-in logic. Furthermore, their structures vary between processors and an application that can take good advantage of a given cache may not experience the same advantages on another processor without rework. In some cases, the discrepancies can turn into performance losses due to cache trashing.

8 It is worth noting that a different optimization is required for the forward projection: in this step, the volume data remains constant.

9 The spatial and temporal locality of the memory-access pattern of the program in listing 1 is poorly adapted to the size of the caches. This example program ends up reading in, updating and writing back the whole volume for every single projection, resulting in high-data traffic on the memory bus. As a consequence, the backprojection problem becomes memory-bandwidth bound. This would not happen if the whole volume could fit into the internal caches of the processor.

10 The LS is organized as four banks of static RAM as opposed to core managed cache. Structuring the LS as four banks helps support the SIMD nature of the core as well as the instruction fetch mechanism.

11 DCMs can generate various clock frequencies, creating clock domains. The designer is responsible for creating the buffering facilities needed to accommodate the difference of speeds in two communicating-frequency domains.

12 The important notion to keep in mind is that there is no waiting inside an FPGA; there is always an operation in progress. It only depends on the control to decide weather a result is kept (latched), forwarded to the next stage or ignored. It is worth mentioning that VHDL allows for the definition of building blocks that can be individually instantiated depending on the requirements of the application and the real estate available in the selected FPGA chip. For example, after having implemented a backprojection algorithm, the amount of resources necessary for one instance can precisely be measured, and the effective number of instances decided on a chip-by-chip basis. The effective performance is then achieved by replicating the backprojection module.

13 These variations from the ideal trajectory are generally induced by gravity and produce deviations in the source to detector distance, as well as detector tilts along all possible angles.

14 Those coefficients usually require a floating-point representation, and FPGAs have poor floating-point computation capabilities. The most commonly used method is to convert the floating point $c_{ij}(\alpha)$ into a fixed-point representation that matches both the capabilities of the multipliers and the required accuracy. For example, an 18.7 fixed-point representation gives good results for typical FDK-based algorithms (Trepanier 2002, Leeser 2002).

15 This doesn't account for the presence of the new eXtreme DSP slices. These new components represent a significantly higher processing density than regular CLBs. However, it is difficult to predict how efficiently those DSP slices can be used without actually trying it. Therefore, the speedup that they could provide is ignored in this estimation.

Chapter 5
Compression of Surface Meshes

Frédéric Payan
Université de Nice - Sophia Antipolis, France

Marc Antonini
Université de Nice - Sophia Antipolis, France

1.1 ABSTRACT

The modelling of three-dimensional (3D) objects with triangular meshes represents a major interest for medical imagery. Indeed, visualization and handling of 3D representations of biological objects (like organs for instance) are very helpful for clinical diagnosis, telemedicine applications, or clinical research in general. Today, the increasing resolution of imaging equipments leads to densely sampled triangular meshes, but the resulting data are consequently huge. In this chapter, we present one specific lossy compression algorithm for such meshes that could be used in medical imagery. According to several state-of-the-art techniques, this scheme is based on wavelet filtering, and an original bit allocation process that optimizes the quantization of the data. This allocation process is the core of the algorithm, because it allows the users to always get the optimal trade-off between the quality of the compressed mesh and the compression ratio, whatever the user-given bitrate. By the end of the chapter, experimental results are discussed and compared with other approaches.

1.2 INTRODUCTION

The surface of a 3D object is most of times represented by a triangular mesh (see Figure 1). A triangular mesh is a set of triangles (defined by the 3D positions of three vertices in the space), and connected by their common edges. Generally, the triangular meshes are *irregular*, meaning that all the vertices do not have the same number of neighbours (each vertex of a *regular* mesh has 6 neighbours).

In medical imagery and numerous other domains, the resolution of 3D representations has to be high, in order to get the maximum of geometrical details. But designing such detailed surfaces leads to triangular meshes which can be defined today by several millions of vertices. Unfortunately, a raw representation of these

DOI: 10.4018/978-1-60566-280-0.ch005

Figure 1. 3D modelling of a tooth (on the left) defined by a triangular mesh (on the right)

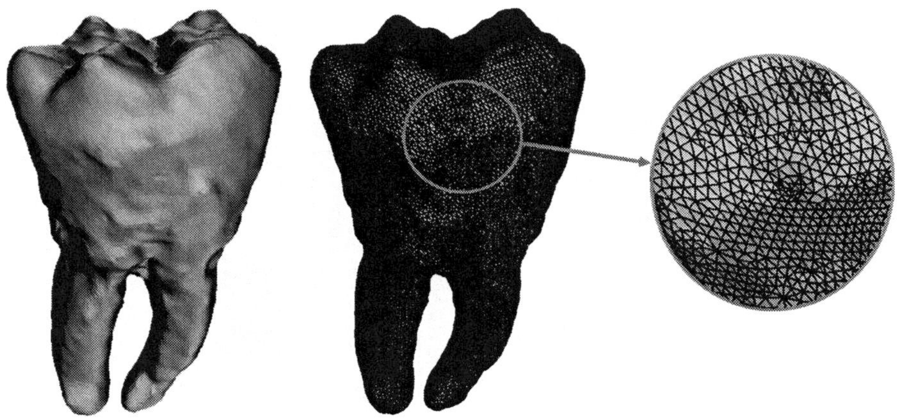

densely sampled meshes is huge, and it can be a major drawback for an efficient use of such data. For instance:

- archival or storage of a large quantity of similar data in a patient database is problematic (capacity of the servers);
- during clinical diagnosis or follow-up cares of patients, a remote access to database in particular with bandwidth-limited transmission systems, will be long and unpleasant for practitioners;
- real-time and bandwidth-limited constraints in general could restrict the applications in the domain of telemedicine.

In signal processing, compression is a relevant solution to allow a compact storage, an easy handling or a fast transmission in bandwidth-limited applications of large data. Two kinds of compression methods exist: the lossless and the lossy methods. With a lossless method, all original data can be recovered when the file is uncompressed. On the other hand, lossy compression reduces data by permanently eliminating certain information, especially irrelevant information. In this case, when the file is decompressed, the data may be different from the original, but close enough to be still useful. Lossy methods can produce a much smaller compressed file than any known lossless method, while still meeting the requirements of the application. Consequently, they always attempt to optimize the trade-off between bitrate (relative to the file size) and quality of compressed data (relative to the information loss).

When dealing with large data like densely sampled triangular meshes for instance, lossy methods are more relevant since it allows reaching higher compression ratios. However, in the domain of medical imagery, eliminating crucial geometrical details may be damaging, since it may lead, for instance, to false clinical diagnosis. Therefore the information loss must be absolutely well-controlled and also limited when compressing medical data.

One relevant way to overcome this crucial problem is to include an allocation process in the compression algorithm. The purpose of this process is generally to optimize lossy compression by minimizing the losses due to data quantization for one specific bitrate. But designing a fast and low-complex allocation process is not trivial. Therefore, in this chapter, we particularly explain how designing an allocation process for an efficient coding of large surface meshes.

The remainder of this chapter is organized as follows. Section 3 gives a short survey of the main methods of compression for 3D surface meshes. Section 4 introduces an overview of the proposed coder/decoder, the problem statement relative to the allocation process, and the major contributions of this work. In section 5 we detail the proposed bit allocation, and present a model-based algorithm in section 6. Then, we give some experimental results and discuss the advantages/disadvantages of this method in section 7. Finally, we conclude in section 8, and highlight the main future research directions in section 9.

1.3 SHORT SURVEY IN 3D SURFACE COMPRESSION

Connectivity-Guided Compression

The first approaches proposed for compressing surface meshes were connectivity-guided, in the sense that the connectivity were first encoded according to one deterministic path (following edges or triangles), while the positions of the vertices were predicted according to this path. Then the prediction errors were uniformly quantized (most of times at 12 bits). In this case, we generally talk about *mesh compression* (Alliez, 2003), and such approaches are generally viewed as lossless, in the sense that the connectivity is exactly the same before and after compression/decompression (even if quantization inescapably introduces geometrical deformations, since the original positions of vertices are defined by floating numbers; *i.e.*, 32 or 64 bits). One of the most popular methods is the *triangle mesh compression* developed by Touma (1998). The main advantage of those approaches is that connectivity is exactly preserved, which is relevant in certain application domains. Moreover, they reach good compression performances particularly with "small" meshes (in other words with few triangles), and above all when the meshes are fairly sampled. On the other hand, these methods are single-rate, and it consequently disables progressive processing.

Simplification-Based Compression

Another kind of approaches is based on surface simplification/refinement. In that case, the original mesh is simplified by subsequent decimations (of vertices, edges…) until a very coarse mesh is obtained. Conversely, during decoding, connectivity and geometry are reconstructed incrementally, from the coarse mesh until the whole original mesh. One of the most popular methods is the *progressive meshes* developed by Hoppe (1996). The main advantage of a progressive compression is that it provides access to intermediate states of the object during its reconstruction and/or its networked transmission. Finally, progressive compression can be lossless if the input mesh is reconstructed until its original resolution (with exactly the same connectivity), or lossy if the reconstruction is not complete (for instance if the user estimates that an intermediate resolution is sufficient for its visualization). Their main advantage is clearly the feature of progressive processing.

Geometry Compression

When dealing with surfaces designed by any kind of acquisition techniques (for instance, iso-surfaces extracted from volumes, geometry scanning), the associated meshes are most of times irregular, and above all, geometrically over-sampled. Therefore, currently, more and more works consider the original mesh to be just one instance of the surface geometry. In that case, we talk about *geometry compression* instead of *mesh compression* (Alliez, 2003). The *geometry compression* considers the geometry to be the most important component to represent a mesh. One relevant structure for such approaches is the *semi-regular mesh*, defined by a base mesh (a coarse approximation of a given surface) and several levels of refining details, added by successive regular subdivisions (see Figure 2). Semi-regular meshes are generally produced by a remeshing algorithm applied before compression (it transforms the irregular input mesh

Figure 2. Semi-regular mesh of the data MOLECULA

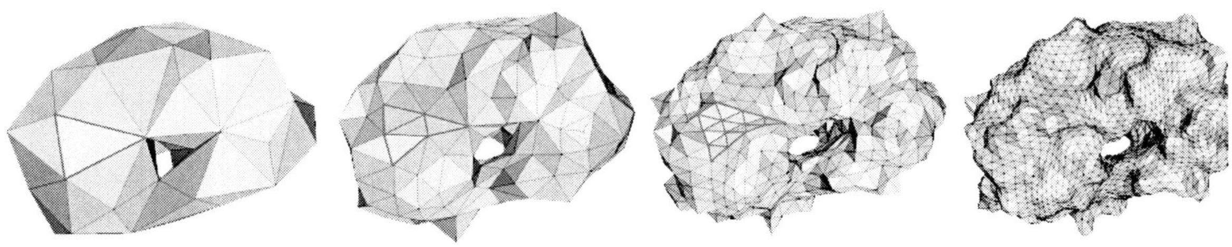

in a semi-regular one). Several methods exist, the most famous remeshers are certainly *MAPS* (Lee, 1998), *Normal Meshes* (Guskov, 2000), and *Trireme* (Guskov, 2007).

The first advantage of this structure is that the regular subdivision makes the connectivity information implicit, except the list of triangles of the base mesh. Another major advantage is the resulting "almost-regularity" of the sampling grid (see Figure 3) that leads to more efficient wavelet filtering.

Therefore wavelets are also exploited to perform efficient lossy compression of meshes (Khodakovsky, 2000, 2002, Payan, 2005). Based on multiresolution analysis, not only wavelet coders achieve better compression rates than methods based on uniform quantization, but also present scalability properties which make the progressive transmission, the adaptive displaying or the level of details control easier (like the progressive method based on simplification described before). In case of large meshes, geometry compression based on wavelet filtering is certainly one of the most relevant approaches, and this is why we propose in this chapter to develop and discuss such a method for large medical data.

1.4 BACKGROUND

Overview of a Wavelet-Based Coder

Figures 4 and 5 present an overall scheme of a wavelet-based coder/decoder for triangular meshes.

Figure 3. Irregular (on the left) versus semi-regular sampling (on the right)

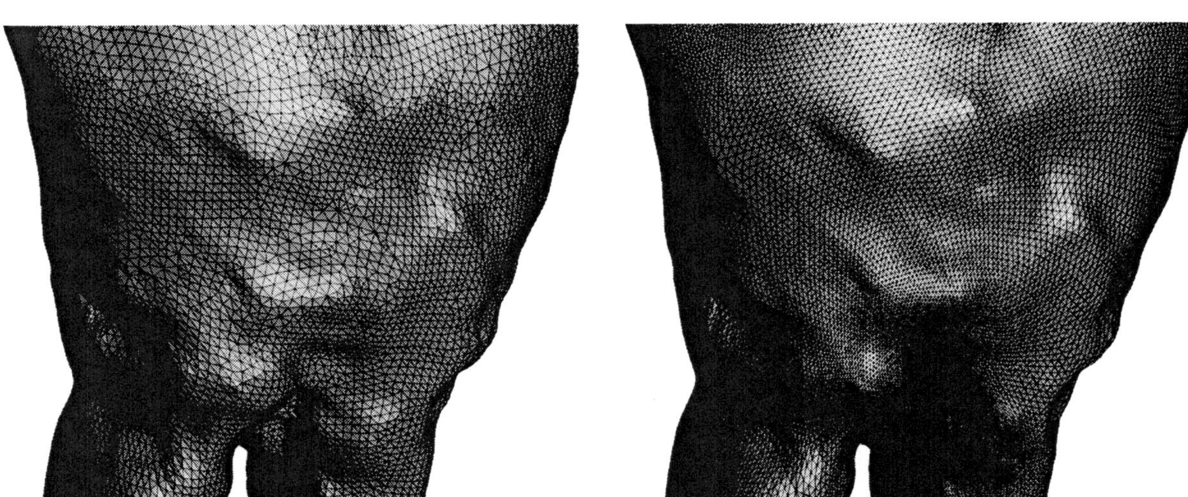

Figure 4. Proposed coder

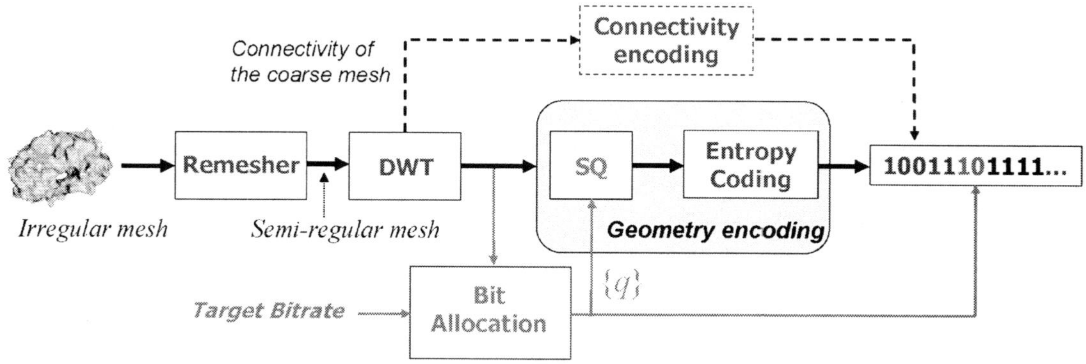

The principle of each stage is described hereinafter.

- **Remesher** - The remesher, if needed, provides a semi-regular mesh, from the irregular input one.
- **Multiresolution Analysis** - Wavelet filtering (Mallat, 1999) or **DWT** (Discrete Wavelet Transform) is then applied to obtain one low frequency (LF) signal (similar to the base mesh), and N subbands of 3D high frequency (HF) details (or *wavelet coefficients*): see Figure 6. During decoding, the associated inverse transform will have to be used to reconstruct the semi-regular meshes from the LF signal and the HF details.

Several wavelet filterings exist (Schröder, 1995, Khodakovsky, 2000, Khodakovsky, 2002, Bertram, 2002, Li, 2004). Here, we use the Butterfly-based wavelet transform (Khodakovsky, 2000, Khodakovsky, 2002), because it is one of the most efficient and has the advantage to be implemented in lifting scheme (Sweldens, 1998). The details are computed in a local frame (Zorin, 1997) induced by the tangent plane and the normal direction at the surface defined by the mesh of lower resolution. This involves the distinction between the so-called *tangential components* and *normal components* of detail vectors $d_{i,j}$: the *tangential components* are the coordinates $d^x_{i,j}$ and $d^y_{i,j}$ of detail vectors; the *normal components* are the coordinates $d^z_{i,j}$ of detail vectors (Khodakovsky, 2000).

- **Quantization (SQ)** - The *tangential* and *normal sets* are then encoded separately using scalar quantizers (Gersho, 1992) de-

Figure 5. Proposed decoder

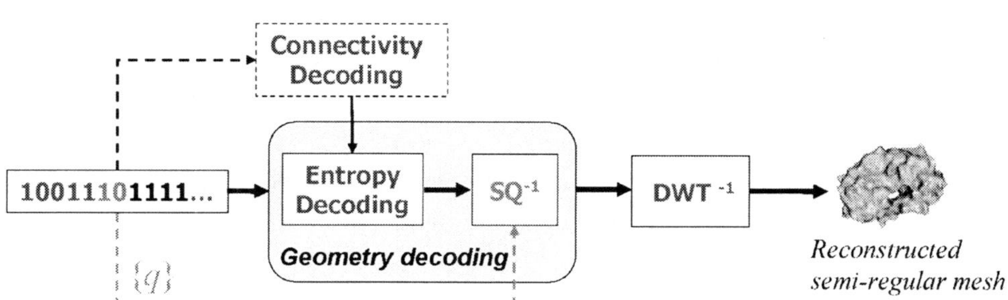

Figure 6. Multiresolution analysis of a semi-regular mesh

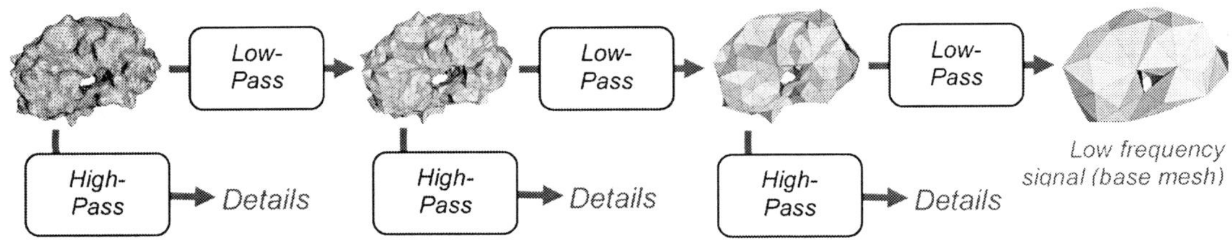

pending on the optimal quantization steps computed during the allocation process (detailed in the next section). When compressing semi-regular meshes with our compression scheme, the loss of geometrical details comes only from this stage. This is why the allocation is the key process.

- **Entropy coding -** An entropy coder is finally applied to transform the quantized data in binary file. In our case, we use a coder adapted to semi-regular meshes (Payan, 2003).
- **Connectivity coding -** In order to reconstruct the meshes after transmission, the list of triangles of the base mesh must be also encoded to be merged in the binary file. We use the method of Touma and Gotsman (1998).

Problem Statement and Contributions

The main problem with such an approach is relative to the multiresolution representation of the transformed data. Once transformed, the relevant information (from a coding point of view) is most of times concentrated in the LF signal, while having the fine and perhaps negligible details in the HF subbands. Therefore, we cannot use the same quantizer for all the subbands of a transformed data, the energy being not uniformly dispatched between them.

This is why we propose to include a bit allocation process in the compression algorithm. It will be the core of the coding scheme and consequently the main contribution of this chapter. Its goal will be the computation of the best quantizer for each subband, in order to obtain the best trade-off between rate (compressed file size) and quality of the reconstructed data (distortion).

1.5 BIT ALLOCATION PROCESS

General Purpose

The goal of the allocation process is to minimize the reconstruction error defined by the global distortion D_T relative to data quantization, with a constraint on the total bitrate R_T. As distortion criterion, we use the mean square error (MSE) $\sigma_\varepsilon^2\left(\{q\}\right)$ computed between the original and the quantized data. So, the allocation process can be modelled by the following problem P:

$$(P)\begin{cases} \text{minimize} & \sigma_\varepsilon^2\left(\{q\}\right) \\ \text{with constraint} & R_T\left(\{q\}\right) = R_{target} \end{cases}, \tag{1}$$

with R_{target} a target bitrate, given by users for instance, and $\{q\}$ the set of quantization steps that must be computed optimally. The principle is the following. The target bitrate is given, and then the reconstruction error is minimized for this specific bitrate. Once the allocation processed and the quantization steps computed, coding, transmission and decoding can be done progressively.

When developing this allocation process, one problem is how computing the MSE $\sigma_\varepsilon^2\left(\{q\}\right)$. The main problem is that the MSE $\sigma_\varepsilon^2\left(\{q\}\right)$ is relative to the geometry of the compressed mesh, *i.e.*, computed between the original semi-regular mesh and its reconstructed version in the *Euclidean* space. On the other hand, the losses due to quantization are relative to the subbands of wavelet coefficients, in the *transform* space. It means that, each time an estimation of the reconstructed MSE is required during the allocation process, we have to apply the synthesis filters of the wavelet transform on the quantized coefficients before its computation. This leads to a complex and time-consuming process, and consequently a slow compression algorithm. It should be more relevant to express the reconstructed MSE directly from the quantization errors of each coefficient subband, in order to reduce the algorithm complexity and to speed the process up.

MSE Across a Wavelet Coder

It has been shown that the MSE relative to the quantization of the mesh geometry encoded across a wavelet coder using a N-level decomposition is equivalent to a weighted sum of the MSE $\sigma_{\varepsilon_i}^2(q_i)$ introduced by the quantization of each wavelet coefficient subband i (Payan, 2006). Therefore, the MSE $\sigma_\varepsilon^2\left(\{q\}\right)$ between a semi-regular mesh and its reconstructed version can be written as

$$\sigma_\varepsilon^2\left(\{q\}\right) = \sum_{i=0}^{N} W_i \sigma_{\varepsilon_i}^2\left(q_i\right), \quad (2)$$

where $\sigma_{\varepsilon_i}^2$ and $\sigma_{\varepsilon_N}^2$ are respectively the MSE due to the quantization of the HF subband i ($\forall i \neq N$), and the MSE for the LF signal (*i.e.*, the base mesh).

The weights $\{W_i\}$ are due to the biorthogonality of wavelets (Usevitch, 1996, Payan, 2006), and are given by

$$\begin{cases} W_N = \dfrac{N_{s_N}}{N_s} \left(w_{lf}\right)^N \\ W_i = \dfrac{N_{s_i}}{N_s} \left(w_{lf}\right)^i w_{hf} \quad \forall\, i \neq N \end{cases}. \quad (3)$$

N_{s_i} and N_{s_N} are respectively the number of coefficients of a HF subband i, and the number of coefficients of the base mesh. For the lifted version of the butterfly-based wavelet transform (Khodakovsky, 2000), the weights w_{lf} and w_{hf} (Payan, 2006) are

$$\begin{cases} w_{lf} = \dfrac{169}{256} \simeq 0.66015625 \\ w_{hf} = \dfrac{1727}{2048} \simeq 0.843261715 \end{cases}. \quad (4)$$

For its unlifted version (Khodakovsky, 2002), w_{lf} is the same, but w_{hf} is equal to 1 (Payan, 2006).

Lagrangian Approach

The allocation problem P stated by (1) can be formulated by a lagrangian criterion

$$J_\lambda(\{q\}) = \sigma_\varepsilon^2\left(\{q\}\right) + \lambda\left(R_T - R_{target}\right), \quad (5)$$

with λ the lagrangian operator. Combining (2) and (5) gives

$$J_\lambda(\{q\}) = \sum_{i=0}^{N} W_i \sigma_{\varepsilon_i}^2(q_i) + \lambda\left(R_T - R_{target}\right). \quad (6)$$

Moreover, each subband of HF details is splitted in two scalar sets, the tangential and normal sets (see section "Background"). Consequently, the MSE $\sigma^2_{\varepsilon_i}$ of the ith i^{th} HF subband is the sum of the MSE $\sigma^2_{\varepsilon_{i,1}}$ and $\sigma^2_{\varepsilon_{i,2}}$ due to the quantization of the tangential and normal sets:

$$\sigma^2_{\varepsilon_i} = \sum_{j \in J_i} \sigma^2_{\varepsilon_{i,j}} \qquad \forall i \neq N, \tag{7}$$

where J_i is a set of indices defined by J_i={1,2}. On the other hand, the LF signal does not present specific properties, since it represents a coarse version of the input mesh. Therefore, the LF signal will be splitted in three scalar sets, and the MSE $\sigma^2_{\varepsilon_N}$ of the LF signal is the sum of the three MSE $\sigma^2_{\varepsilon_{N,j}}$ due to the quantization on each coordinate set:

$$\sigma^2_{\varepsilon_N} = \sum_{j \in J_N} \sigma^2_{\varepsilon_{N,j}}, \tag{8}$$

where J_N is a set of coordinate indices defined by J_N={1,2,3}. By using (7) and (8), the criterion (6) becomes:

$$J_\lambda(\{q\}) = \sum_{i=0}^{N} W_i \sum_{j \in J_i} \sigma^2_{\varepsilon_{i,j}}(q_{i,j}) + \lambda\left(R_T - R_{target}\right). \tag{9}$$

In parallel, the total bitrate can be formulated by

$$R_T = \sum_{i=0}^{N} \sum_{j \in J_i} a_{i,j} R_{i,j}(q_{i,j}) \tag{10}$$

where $R_{i,j}$ is the bitrate relative to the $(i,j)^{th}$ set. The coefficients $a_{i,j}$ depend on the subsampling associated to the multiresolution analysis, and correspond to the ratios between the size of the $(i,j)^{th}$ set and the total number of samples $3N_s$. Finally, the criterion becomes

$$J_\lambda(\{q\}) = \sum_{i=0}^{N} W_i \sum_{j \in J_i} \sigma^2_{\varepsilon_{i,j}}(q_{i,j}) + \lambda\left(\sum_{i=0}^{N} \sum_{j \in J_i} a_{i,j} R_{i,j}(q_{i,j}) - R_{target}\right). \tag{11}$$

Finally, the solutions of the allocation problem P (*i.e.*, the optimal quantization steps) are obtained by minimizing (11).

Optimal Solutions

The solutions of P can be obtained by solving the following system:

$$\begin{cases} \dfrac{\partial J_\lambda(\{q_{i,j}\})}{\partial q_{i,j}} = 0 \\ \dfrac{\partial J_\lambda(\{q_{i,j}\})}{\partial \lambda} = 0 \end{cases}, \tag{12}$$

which can be developed in

$$\begin{cases} \dfrac{\dfrac{\partial \sigma^2_{\varepsilon_{i,j}}(q_{i,j})}{\partial q_{i,j}}}{\dfrac{\partial R_{i,j}(q_{i,j})}{\partial q_{i,j}}} = -\lambda \dfrac{a_{i,j}}{W_i} \\ \sum_{i=0}^{N} \sum_{j \in J_i} a_{i,j} R_{i,j}(q_{i,j}) = R_{\text{target}} \end{cases}. \tag{13}$$

Finally, we have to solve this system of $(2N+4)$ equations with $(2N+4)$ unknowns (the set $\{q_{i,j}\}$ and λ). In order to obtain the optimal quantization steps analytically, the first equation of (13) requires to be inverted. Unfortunately, this stage is impossible due to the complexity of the equations. To overcome such a problem, an iterative algorithm depending on λ is generally proposed.

Overall Algorithm

The optimal solutions are computed thanks to the following overall algorithm:

Figure 7. Typical probability density function of tangential (on the left) and normal sets (on the right). The dash-dot lines represent the real density functions, and the solid lines represent the corresponding estimated GGD

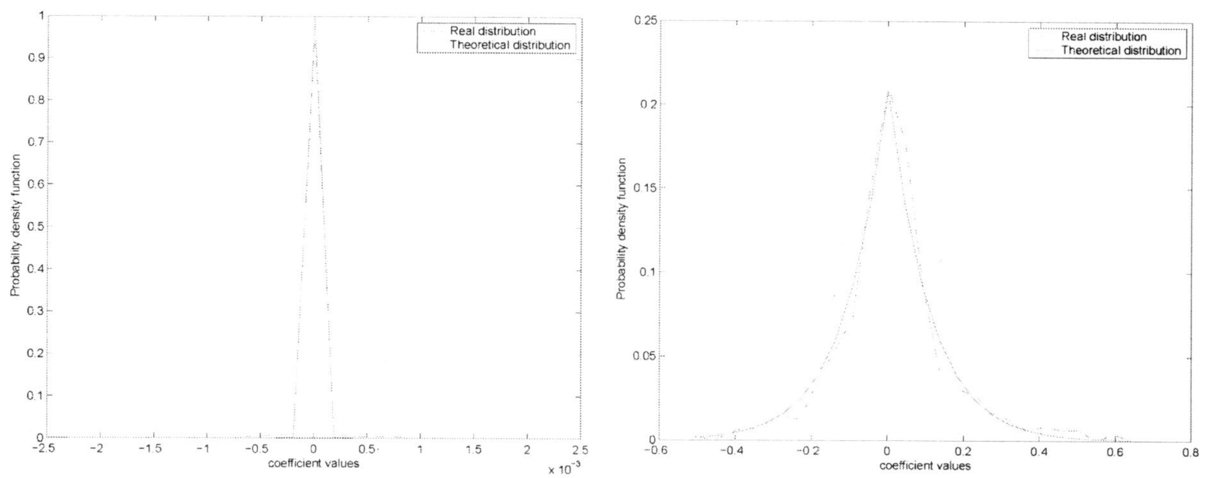

1. λ is given. For each set (i,j), compute $q_{i,j}$ verifying the first equation of (13);
2. while the second equation of (13) is not verified, calculate a new λ by dichotomy and return to step 1;
3. stop.

The computation of the quantization steps $\{q_{i,j}\}$ as solutions during Step 1 can be done according to different methods. In the following section, we propose to process this algorithm with an efficient analytical approach thanks to theoretical models for the bitrate and the MSE.

1.6 MODEL-BASED ALGORITHM

The only way to compute the bitrate and the MSE of the different subbands without real pre-quantization is to perform a model-based method. Therefore we introduce theoretical models for the distortion and the bitrate, depending on the probability density functions of each data set.

Wavelet Coefficient Distribution

Figure 7 shows typical probability density functions of the tangential and normal sets of wavelet coefficients (HF subbands).

We observe that distributions are zero-mean and all information is concentrated on few coefficients (small variances). It has been shown that these sets can be modelled by a *Generalized Gaussian Distribution* (GGD)

$$p_{\sigma,\alpha}(x) = a e^{-|bx|^{\alpha}}, \quad (14)$$

with $b = \frac{1}{\sigma}\sqrt{\frac{\Gamma(3/\alpha)}{\Gamma(1/\alpha)}}$ and $a = \frac{b\alpha}{2\Gamma(1/\alpha)}$. The parameter α is computed using the variance σ^2 and the fourth-order moment of each set. $\Gamma(.)$ stands for the Gamma function.

On the other hand, since the three subsets of the LF signal represent the geometry of the base mesh, they do not have any particular distribution and can not be modelled as the HF details. To overcome this problem, we use a differential technique, by modelling and encoding the differences between two LF components (instead of the components themselves). Indeed, these differences can be modelled by a GGD (Payan, 2005).

Theoretical Models for Distortion and Bitrate

When applying a uniform scalar quantization (with the center of the cells as decoding value), it can be shown (Parisot, 2003) that the MSE σ_{sq}^2 associated to a GGD can be rewritten as

$$\sigma_{sq}^2 = \sigma^2 D(\tilde{q}, \alpha), \tag{15}$$

with σ^2 the variance of the set, and $\tilde{q} = \frac{q}{\sigma}$. $D(\tilde{q}, \alpha)$ is given by

$$D(\tilde{q}, \alpha) = 1 + 2\sum_{m=1}^{+\infty} (m\tilde{q})^2 f_{0,m}(\tilde{q}, \alpha) - 4\sum_{m=1}^{+\infty} m\tilde{q} f_{1,m}(\tilde{q}, \alpha), \tag{16}$$

where functions $f_{n,m}$ are defined by

$$f_{n,m}(\tilde{q}, \alpha) = \int_{\frac{1}{2}\tilde{q}+(m-1)\tilde{q}}^{\frac{1}{2}\tilde{q}+m\tilde{q}} x^n p_{1,\alpha}(x)dx, \tag{17}$$

and by

$$f_{n,0}(\tilde{q}, \alpha) = \int_{-\frac{1}{2}\tilde{q}}^{\frac{1}{2}\tilde{q}} x^n p_{1,\alpha}(x)dx. \tag{18}$$

By the same way, the bitrate R associated to a GGD can be rewritten as

$$R(\tilde{q}, \alpha) = -f_{0,0}(\tilde{q}, \alpha)\log_2 f_{0,0}(\tilde{q}, \alpha) - 2\sum_{m=1}^{+\infty} f_{0,m}(\tilde{q}, \alpha)\log_2 f_{0,m}(\tilde{q}, \alpha). \tag{19}$$

According to these theoretical models for each component set, the system (13) becomes

$$\begin{cases} h_{\alpha_{i,j}}(\tilde{q}_{i,j}) = \dfrac{\frac{\partial D(\tilde{q}_{i,j}, \alpha_{i,j})}{\partial \tilde{q}_{i,j}}}{\frac{\partial R_{i,j}(\tilde{q}_{i,j}, \alpha_{i,j})}{\partial \tilde{q}_{i,j}}} = -\lambda \dfrac{a_{i,j}}{W_i \sigma_{i,j}^2} \\ \sum_{i=0}^{N} \sum_{j \in J_i} a_{i,j} R_{i,j}(\tilde{q}_{i,j}, \alpha_{i,j}) = R_{target} \end{cases}, \tag{20}$$

where $h_{\alpha_{i,j}}\left(\tilde{q}_{i,j}\right)$ is an analytic function detailed in Payan (2006).

Model-Based Algorithm

In order to speed the allocation process up, Parisot (2003) proposes to use some offline computed Look-Up Tables (LUT) to solve the system (20). Two parametric curves are exploited:

- $\left[ln(\tilde{q}); ln(-h_\alpha)\right]$: this LUT (Figure 8) allows to compute the quantization steps which verify the first equation of (20).
- $\left[R; ln(-h_\alpha)\right]$: this LUT (Figure 9) gives the bitrate R for a specific $h_\alpha\left(\tilde{q}_{i,j}\right)$, in order to verify the constraint on the target bitrate (second equation of (20)).

In that case, the algorithm given in the previous section becomes:

1. compute the variance $\sigma^2_{i,j}$ and the parameter $\alpha_{i,j}$ for each set (i,j);
2. a value of λ is given. For each set (i,j), compute $h_{\alpha_{i,j}}\left(\tilde{q}_{i,j}\right)$ thanks to the right-hand side of the first equation of (20). Then, use the second LUT to compute the corresponding bitrate $R_{i,j}$;
3. while the target is not reached, calculate a new λ by dichotomy and return to Step 2;
4. the optimal λ is known. For each set (i,j), use the first LUT to compute the optimal

Figure 8. First LUT used: $ln(-h_\alpha)$ according to $ln(\tilde{q})$, for different α

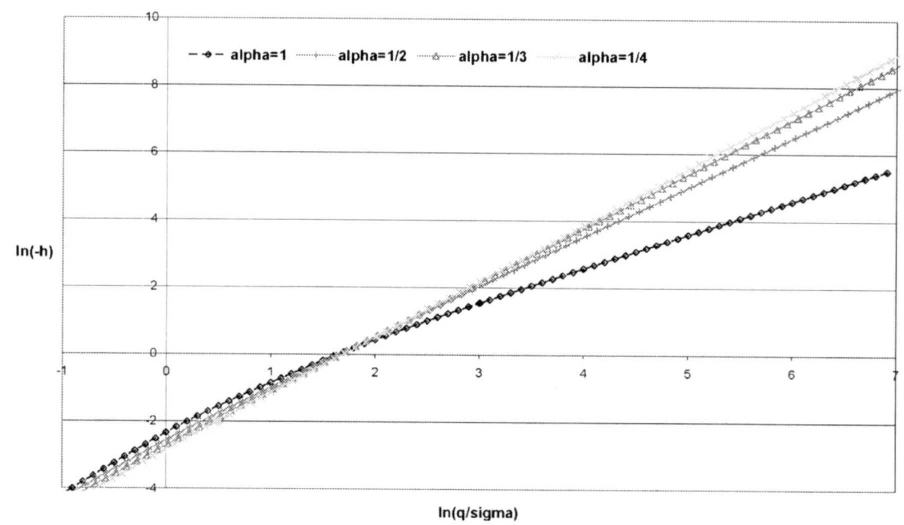

Figure 9. Second LUT used: $ln(-h_\alpha)$ according to R, for different α

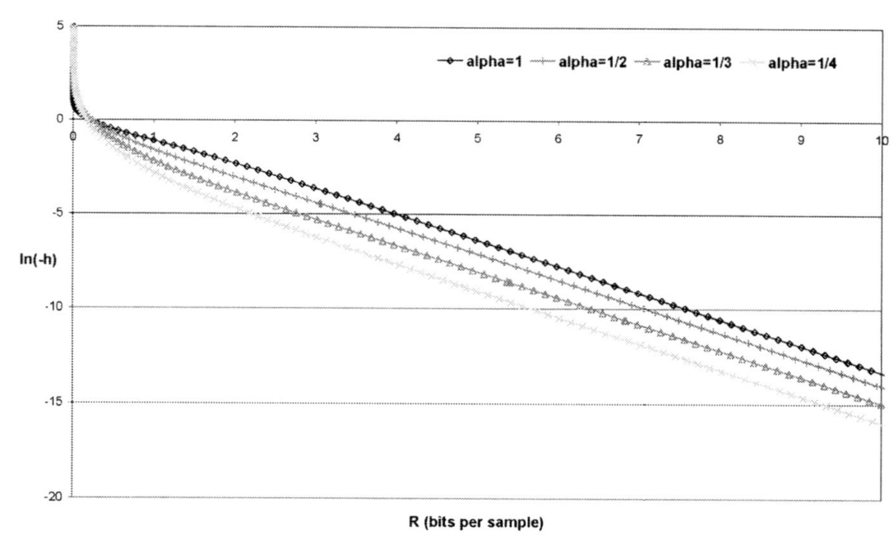

quantization step $q_{i,j}$ corresponding to the value of $h_{\alpha_{i,j}}\left(\tilde{q}_{i,j}\right)$ found in Step 2.

5. stop.

Complexity

Step 1 of the model-based algorithm permits the computation of the variance σ^2 and of the parameter α. The parameter α is computed from the variance and the fourth-order moment for each component set (Kasner, 1999). This step can be done in 4 operations per component. At step 2, after the computation of $ln(-h_\alpha)$ using λ, σ^2 and the second equation of (20), the set of $\{R_{i,j}\}$ is computed at low cost by addressing the second LUT. Step 3 consists in computing a simple weighted sum of the bitrates estimated at step 2 (2 arithmetic opera-

Table 1.

Data	Irregular mesh		Semi-regular mesh	
	# Vertices	# Faces	# Vertices	# Faces of the base mesh
Tooth	21,947	43,890	66,562	130 (5 resolution levels)
Skull	20,002	40,000	131,074	4 (8 resolution levels)
Molecula	10,028	20,056	54272	106 (5 resolution levels)
Tumour	3,422	1,713	4,802	150 (3 resolution levels)

tions per component set) to verify the constraint on the global bitrate. The computation of a new λ is done by a simple dichotomy. At step 4, the set of quantization steps $\{q_{i,j}\}$ is computed at low cost by addressing the first LUT.

The convergence of the algorithm is reached after few iterations (lower than 5). Finally, the step 1 represents the highest computational cost of this algorithm, with 4 operations per sample, hence a computational complexity of approximately 12 operations per semi-regular vertex. This involves a fast allocation process with a very low computational complexity, and negligible in time (in comparison with the whole algorithm).

1.7 EXPERIMENTATIONS AND DISCUSSIONS

In this section, we present experimental results obtained on several simulation cases. In order to discuss the efficiency and the relevance of the proposed approach, the tested data are more or less large. See Table 1 for data.

Comparison with the State-of-the-Art Geometry Coder

We first compare our geometry coder that includes the presented bit allocation process with the state-of-the-art geometry coder, *i.e.*, the method developed by Khodakovsky (2000) that uses a zerotree coder. This coder currently is the most efficient for semi-regular meshes. Moreover, to show that our method is relevant for any kind of lifting schemes and any kind of semi-regular meshes, we use semi-regular meshes obtained with the two remeshers *MAPS* (Lee, 1998) and *Normal Meshes* (Guskov, 2000). As wavelet transform, the lifted version of the butterfly-based wavelet transform and its unlifted version are used respectively with the MAPS meshes and the "Normal" ones.

Figures 10, 11, 12, and 13 show the resulting Peak Signal to Noise Ratio (PSNR) curves according to the bitrate per irregular vertex, for two MAPS meshes (Tooth and Tumour), and two "Normal" meshes (Molecula and Skull). The PSNR is given by

$$PSNR = 20 \log_{10}\left(\frac{\text{bb}}{d_S}\right),$$

where bb is the original bounding box diagonal and d_s is the surface-to-surface distance between the input irregular mesh and the reconstructed semi-regular one. d_s is computed with the software developed by Aspert (2002). We observe that the proposed coder always provides better or equal results than the state-of-the-art coder, for any bitrate, and whatever the number of vertices of the input meshes. We observe similar results for all the tested data.

In addition, Figure 14 gives some visual benefits relative to the use of the proposed coder. This figure shows the distribution of the reconstruction error on Tooth, quantized with the proposed coder (on the left) and with the Zerotree coder (on the

Figure 10. Bitrate-PSNR curve for TOOTH at its finest resolution

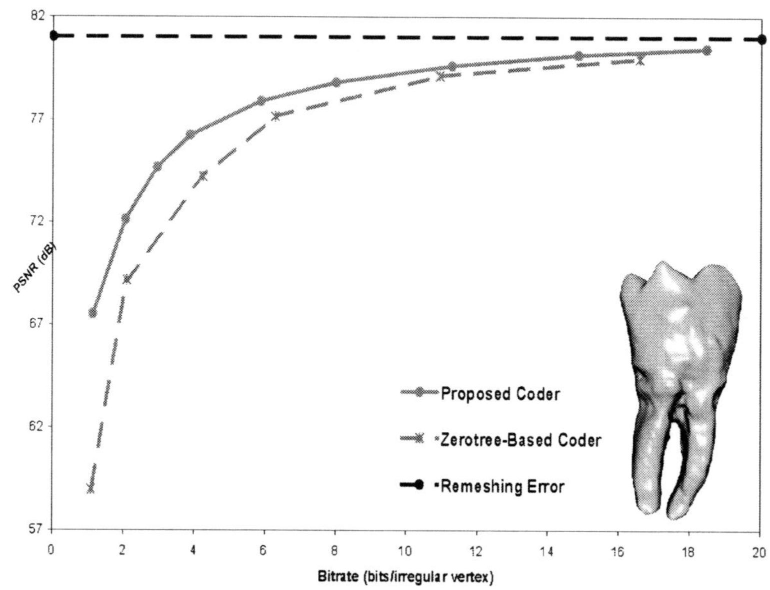

right) of Khodakovsky (2000). The colour corresponds to the magnitude of the distance point-surface normalized by the bounding box diagonal, between the input irregular mesh and the quantized one. One can argue that the zerotree coder leads to more local errors than the proposed algorithm.

To summarize, when compressing semi-regular meshes, the proposed bit allocation improves the quality of the compressed/uncompressed meshes, without increasing the complexity of the coding/decoding scheme.

Lossy vs. Lossless Compression In Medical Imaging

The previous section proves the interest of using an allocation process in lossy compression. Nevertheless, as previously stated, one major constraint for medical data is that eliminating

Figure 11. Bitrate-PSNR curve for TUMOUR at its finest resolution

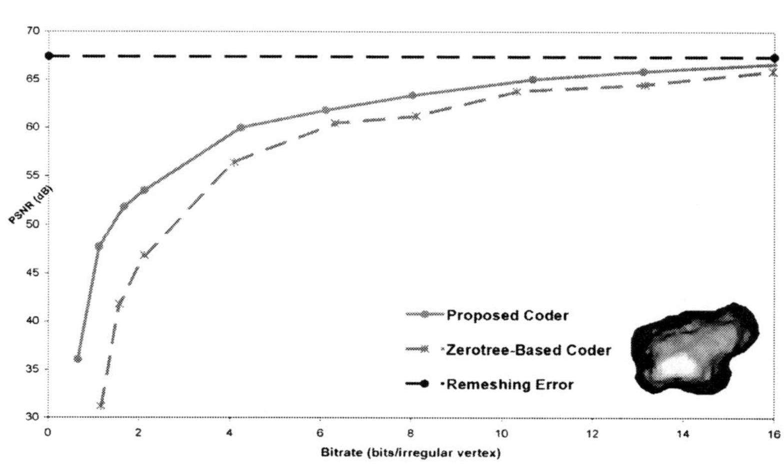

Figure 12. Bitrate-PSNR curve for Molecula *at its finest resolution*

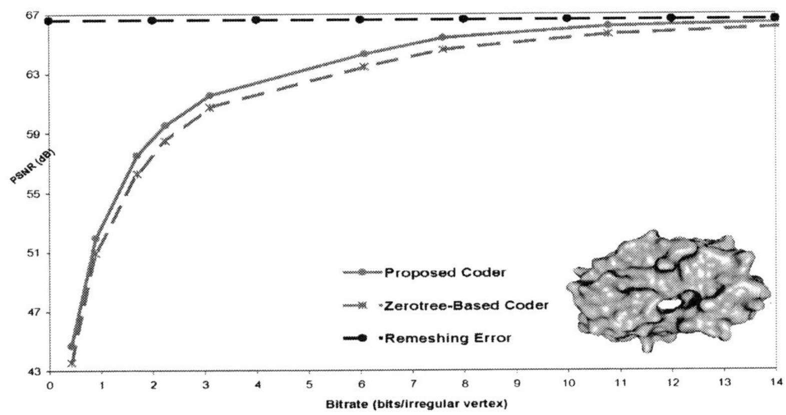

Figure 13. Bitrate-PSNR curve for Skull *at its finest resolution*

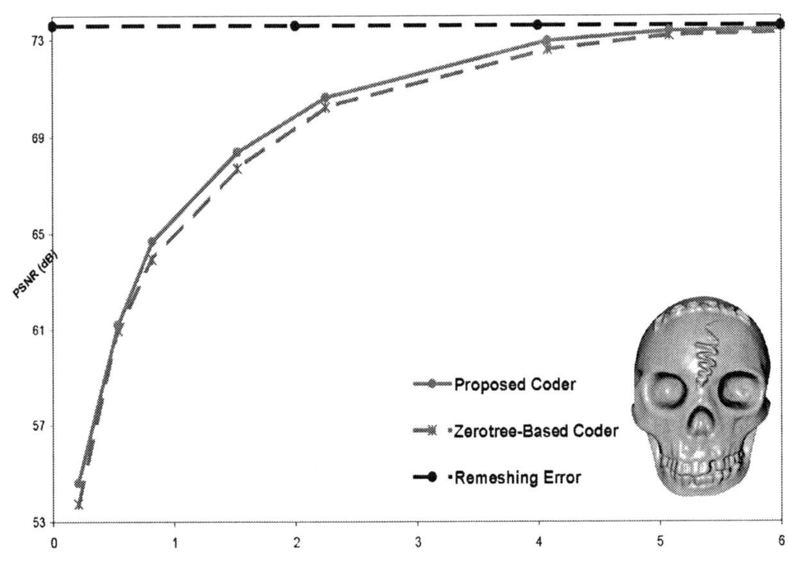

crucial geometrical details may be damaging since it may lead to false clinical diagnosis, for instance. So, lossy compression can not reach too high compression ratios. However, it is interesting to compare the visual quality of data compressed either with lossless methods or with our method.

Figure 15 compares renderings of Skull compressed with the lossless method *TG* of Touma (1998) and with our lossy method. On the left, the data are compressed with *TG* (21bits/irregular vertex). The three other ones are compressed with our method respectively at 4.4 bits/irregular vertex (middle left), at 2.2 bits/irregular vertex (middle right) and at 0.82 bits/irregular vertex (on the right). We can observe that, visually speaking, the differences between the mesh losslessly compressed and the mesh compressed with our method at 4.4 bits/irregular vertex are small, or even negligible. However, the compression ratio (difference of size between original data and compressed one) for the lossless *TG* is 8.7 while the compression ratio for the lossy approach is

Figure 14. Distribution of the geometric error on TOOTH compressed at 8 bits per irregular vertex (at its finest resolution) with the proposed coder on the left (78.8 dB), and with the zerotree coder on the right (77.8 dB)

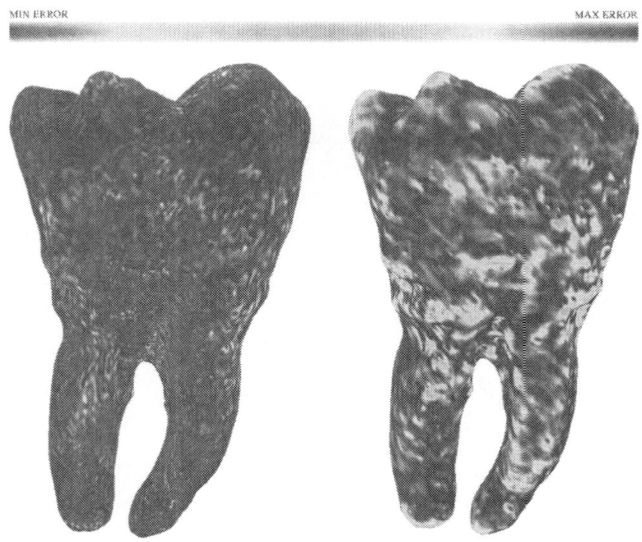

Figure 15. Rendering of different compressed versions of SKULL obtained with the lossless coder TG (on the left, 21bits/irregular vertex), and with the proposed coder at 4.4 bits/irregular vertex (middle left), at 2.2 bits/irregular vertex (middle right) and at 0.82 bits/irregular vertex (on the right)

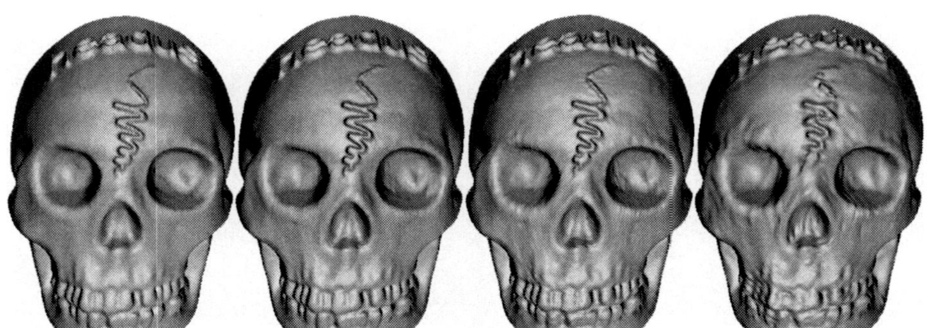

45. It means that our method reaches a compression ratio five times higher than the state-of-the-art lossless one. On the other hand, we observe that the deformations quickly become unacceptable when the compression ratio increases.

When dealing with other data, we obtain similar results. However, we observe that the gain in term of compression ratio between lossless and lossy compression tends to decrease with the number of vertices. With the model TUMOUR for instance, considered as a small mesh, it is not relevant to use our lossy compression. This is due to the fact that the semi-regular remeshers included in all the geometry compression algorithms as ours, are useful only with large and dense meshes.

To summarize, when considering lossy compression, at moderate bitrates for large meshes lossy methods tend to keep acceptable visual quality and preserve most of details, even fine (similar to lossless approaches) while reaching compression ratio higher than the state-of-the-art. So it is more relevant to use wavelet-based methods similar to the proposed one. On the other hand, in case of small meshes, lossless compression is more adapted.

In parallel, a lossy compression scheme based on wavelets and semi-regular meshes presents another feature which is relevant for bandwidth-limited transmission systems: the spatial scalability (or progressivity). Given the semi-regular meshes are multiresolution, it enables progressive coding, transmission, decoding, and displaying of the base mesh and then of the different levels of details, finer and finer. Even if the quality of the first intermediate versions during reconstruction may be insufficient for medical applications, this feature is still and all interesting since it is implicit at the semi-regular structure, without additional binary cost. Such a progressive displaying with successive levels of details is not possible with lossless connectivity-guided coders (like *TG*), since they are single-rate. On the other hand, note that simplification-based compression schemes (see Section "Short survey in 3D surface compression") also present the feature of scalability. However, since they do not reach compression ratios similar to the methods presented here, we do not further focus on such approaches.

1.8 CONCLUSION

We propose in this chapter a wavelet-based coder for 3D surfaces that could be used in medical imagery. The 3D surfaces being most of times defined by densely sampled and irregular triangular meshes, the proposed coder includes a pre-processing remeshing stage (if needed) that transforms the input data in semi-regular meshes before lossy compression. Even if lossy compression globally tends to eliminate geometrical information, experimental results demonstrate that including an efficient allocation process in a lossy compression scheme achieves good compression results for a very low computational cost. Moreover, after discussing the visual results of our compression scheme and the visual results of a frequently-used lossless coder, we conclude that, for large and dense meshes, a lossy compression scheme at medium bitrates achieves similar visual results for significantly higher compression performances.

1.9 FUTURE RESEARCH DIRECTIONS

There are two major lines of research for the future.

- Most of the meshes created by acquisition equipments today are irregular. So, the performances of a wavelet-based coder are highly dependent of the efficiency of the semi-regular remeshing algorithm used before compression. Some specific medical data may not be efficiently remeshed by the current techniques: in that case, our compression scheme would be inappropriate and lossless coders more relevant. Therefore a large experimentation has to be done with practitioners. In parallel, the semi-regular remeshing algorithms may be globally improved to be relevant with any kind of medical data.
- We have shown in this chapter that loss of geometrical details can be efficiently controlled by the allocation process on simulation cases. Now, the performances of our lossy compression have to be confirmed definitively by practitioners on study cases. One crucial information supplied by practitioners is the minimal threshold of visual quality for specific medical data. Once the threshold defined for each kind of medical data, tested, and validated for medical and biological applications, the proposed wavelet-based compression scheme could be incorporated into future acquisition systems.

ACKNOWLEDGMENT

Data are courtesy of CYBERWARE, HEADUS, the SCRIPPS research institute, the WASHINGTON University, the STANFORD University, the IMATI research institute, and the IRCAD research institute. We are particularly grateful to Igor Guskov, Aaron Lee, Andrei Khodakovsky, Shridar Lavu, Marco Attene, and Caroline Essert-Villard for providing us with these data and some results. We also particularly grateful to Aymen Kammoun for providing us the semi-regular versions of TOOTH, and TUMOUR.

REFERENCES

Alliez, P., & Gotsman, C. (2003). Recent advances in compression of 3D meshes. In *Symposium on Multiresolution in Geometric Modeling*.

Aspert, N., Santa-Cruz, D., & Ebrahimi, T. (2002). Mesh: Measuring errors between surfaces using the Hausdorff distance. In *International Conference on Multimedia & Expo*, (Vol. 1, pp. 705-708).

Bertram, M. (2004). Biorthogonal loop-subdivision wavelets. *Computing*, *72*(1-2), 29–39. doi:10.1007/s00607-003-0044-0

Guskov, I. (2007). Manifold-based approach to semi-regular remeshing. *Graphical Models*, *69*(1), 1–18. doi:10.1016/j.gmod.2006.05.001

Guskov, I., Vidimce, K., Sweldens, W., & Schröder, P. (2000). Normal Meshes. In *Computer Graphics Proceedings* (pp. 95-102).

Hoppe, H. (1996). Progressive Meshes. In *ACM SIGGRAPH Conference* (pp. 99-108).

Kasner, J., Marcellin, M., & Hunt, B. (1999). Universal trellis coded quantization. *IEEE Transactions on Image Processing*, *8*(12), 1677–1687. doi:10.1109/83.806615

Khodakovsky, A., & Guskov, I. (2002). Normal mesh compression . In *Geometric Modeling for Scientific Visualization*. Springer-Verlag.

Khodakovsky, A., Schröder, P., & Sweldens, W. (2000). Progressive Geometry Compression. In *Computer Graphics Proceedings, SIGGRAPH 2000* (pp. 271-278).

Lee, A., Sweldens, W., Schröder, P., Cowsar, P., & Dobkin, D. (1998). Multiresolution adaptive parameterization of surfaces . In *SIGGRAPH'98*. MAPS.

Li, D., Qin, K., & Sun, H. (2004). Unlifted loop subdivision wavelets. In *Pacific Graphics Conference on Computer Graphics and Applications* (pp. 25-33).

Mallat, S. (1999). *A Wavelet Tour of Signal Processing* (2nd ed.). Academic Press.

Parisot, C., Antonini, M., & Barlaud, M. (2003). *3D scan based wavelet transform and quality control for video coding*. EURASIP Journal on Applied Signal Processing.

Payan, F., & Antonini, M. (2003). 3D multiresolution context-based coding for geometry compression. In *IEEE International Conference in Image Processing (ICIP)*, Barcelona, Spain (pp. 785-788).

Payan, F., & Antonini, M. (2005). An efficient bit allocation for compressing normal meshes with an error-driven quantization. *Elsevier Computer Aided Geometric Design*, *22*, 466–486. doi:10.1016/j.cagd.2005.04.001

Payan, F., & Antonini, M. (2006). Mean Square Error Approximation for Wavelet-based Semiregular Mesh Compression. [TVCG]. *IEEE Transactions on Visualization and Computer Graphics*, *12*(4). doi:10.1109/TVCG.2006.73

Schröder, P., & Sweldens, W. (1995). Efficiently Representing Functions on the Sphere . In *SIGGRAPH'95* (pp. 161–172). Spherical Wavelets.

Sweldens, W. (1998). The lifting scheme: A construction of second generation wavelets. *SIAM Journal on Mathematical Analysis*, *29*(2), 511–546. doi:10.1137/S0036141095289051

Touma, C., & Gotsman, C. (1998). Triangle mesh compression. In *Graphics Interface'98* (pp. 26-34).

Usevitch, B. (1996). Optimal Bit Allocation for Biorthogonal Wavelet Coding. In *IEEE Data Compression Conference*.

Zorin, D., Schröder, P., & Sweldens, W. (1997). Interactive multiresolution mesh editing. In [Annual Conference Series]. *Computer Graphics*, *31*, 259–268.

ADDITIONAL READING

Alliez, P., & Gotsman, C. (2003). Recent advances in compression of 3D meshes. In *Symposium on Multiresolution in Geometric Modeling*.

Gersho, A., & Gray, R. (1992). *Vector Quantization and Signal Compression*. Norwell: Kluwer Academic Publishers.

Hoppe, H. (1996). Progressive Meshes. In *ACM SIGGRAPH Conference* (pp. 99-108).

Mallat, S. (1999). *A Wavelet Tour of Signal Processing* (2nd ed.). Academic Press.

Payan, F., & Antonini, M. (2005). An efficient bit allocation for compressing normal meshes with an error-driven quantization. *Elsevier Computer Aided Geometric Design*, *22*, 466–486. doi:10.1016/j.cagd.2005.04.001

Sweldens, W. (1998). The lifting scheme: A construction of second generation wavelets. *SIAM Journal on Mathematical Analysis*, *29*(2), 511–546. doi:10.1137/S0036141095289051

Touma, C., & Gotsman, C. (1998). Triangle mesh compression. In *Graphics Interface'98* (pp. 26-34).

Chapter 6
The Role of Self-Similarity for Computer Aided Detection Based on Mammogram Analysis

Filipe Soares
University of Beira Interior & Siemens S.A., Portugal

Mário M. Freire
University of Beira Interior, Portugal

Manuela Pereira
University of Beira Interior, Portugal

Filipe Janela
Siemens S.A., Portugal

João Seabra
Siemens S.A., Portugal

ABSTRACT

The improvement on Computer Aided Detection (CAD) systems has reached the point where it is offered extremely valuable information to the clinician, for the detection and classification of abnormalities at the earliest possible stage. This chapter covers the rapidly growing development of self-similarity models that can be applied to problems of fundamental significance, like the Breast Cancer detection through Digital Mammography. The main premise of this work was related to the fact that human tissue is characterized by a high degree of self-similarity, and that property has been found in medical images of breasts, through a qualitative appreciation of the existing self-similarity nature, by analyzing their fluctuations at different resolutions. There is no need to image pattern comparison in order to recognize the presence of cancer features. One just has to compare the self-similarity factor of the detected features that can be a new attribute for classification. In this chapter, the mostly used methods for self-similarity analysis and image segmentation are presented and explained. The self-similarity measure can be an excellent aid to evaluate cancer features, giving an indication to the radiologist diagnosis.

DOI: 10.4018/978-1-60566-280-0.ch006

INTRODUCTION

This chapter is mainly directed for professionals and students working in the area of medical applications and bioinformatics. The chapter covers the development of self-similarity models applied to breast cancer detection through digital mammography. The self-similarity formalism can consolidate the development of these CAD systems, helping the detection rate of techniques based on: contrast enhancement; edge detection, image segmentation, registration and subtraction; multiresolution analysis; statistics and neural networks.

The chapter starts with a clinical background of breast cancer and digital mammography. Afterwards, a comprehensive review of the mostly known self-similarity models is presented. Finally, the solutions for image segmentation of mammogram images are explained. The chapter ends with final remarks about the development of CAD systems based on self-similarity.

BACKGROUND

Breast cancer is one of the major causes for the increase of the mortality among women, especially in developed and under developed countries, and it can be curable if detected at early stages and given proper treatment. Mammography is currently the most effective screening technique capable of detecting the disease in an early stage. Together with breast physical examination, it has been shown to reduce breast cancer mortality by 18-30%. However, statistics show that 60-80% of biopsies, previously recommend for examination of the lesions, are performed on benign cases and approximately 25% of cancers are missed. Such numbers deserve our attention to the additional requirements of the diagnose process. Doctors are expected to find the least stressful and painful way to check the status of the disease. Regarding the unpleasantness of both mammogram and core biopsy exams, reducing the number of false positives becomes as equally important as reducing the number of false negatives.

The anatomy of the breast is the inevitable source of the highly textured structure of the mammograms. Due to its complexity, it provides a difficult input to analyze for radiologists, who are expected to distinguish very subtle abnormalities out of this mass of structural ambiguity. In addition, these abnormalities pointing for the disease are often immersed on a low contrast mammogram background, where the contrast between malignant and normal tissue may be present but below the threshold of human perception.

Mammographic early signs of breast cancer usually appear in the form of clusters of microcalcifications, in isolation or together with other readings, areas of high density breast tissue, called masses. The term mass arises from the characteristic well-defined mammographic appearance, and they tend to be brighter than their surroundings due to the high density within their boundaries.

In order to be able to characterize microcalcifications, radiologists generally rely on their shape and arrangement. Malignant calcifications are typically very numerous, clustered, small, dot-like or elongated, variable in size, shape and density. Benign calcifications are generally larger, more rounded, smaller in number, more diffusely distributed, and more homogeneous in size and shape. However, because of the small size of microcalcifications, the comparison and characterization of benign and malignant lesions represents a very complex problem even for an experienced radiologist (Salfity et al., 2001).

The nature of the two-dimensional mammography makes it very difficult to distinguish a cancer from overlying breast tissues. The mammographic features are generally hard to found because of their superimposition on the breast parenchymal textures and noise. Moreover, breast density is known to be the most affecting factor for mammographic accuracy (Pisano, et al., 2008).

These issues require dedicated methods that could, at the same time, extract relevant elements for cancer detection and obtain valuable information about these findings, in order to help the scrutiny.

The inter-subject variability increases the difficult task that the human decision maker faces, which emphasizes the need for reliable image processing tools to assist the process of detection and diagnosis. Radiologists will never see all the possible variations however long they practice or however many images they view (Kropinsky, 2003). According to studies, radiologists only investigate 87% of the mammogram area. In contrast, an automatic detection algorithm will not leave any area of the image unexamined (Nodine, 1994). Otherwise, the mammogram quality does not play such an important role in dianosis. In fact, the human eyes only perceives about ten tones of grey and as Julesz (1981) demonstrated it does not perceive variations statistics of superior orders of equal to the second.

A primary challenge of intelligent software in modern workstations is to assist the human expert in recognition and classification of disease by clever computer vision algorithms. The development of Computer Aided Detection (CAD) systems has reached the point where it is offered extremely valuable information to the clinician in the detection and classification of abnormalities, at the earliest possible stage. So far, they can only assist the medical staff in making a decision, but a CAD system performs about as well as a radiologist. However, the combination of both can perform better than either alone (Giordano et al., 1996; Amendolia et al., 2001; Blanks et al.,1998; Warren Burhenne, et al., 2000).

Traces of self-similar behaviors have been noticed in a vast number of natural processes (Oldershaw, 2002): rain fall patterns, seismic waves and biological signals are just a few examples of natural processes with a high degree of self-similarity. Stock market prices (Lo, 1991), fractal data and images (Le, 2003; Dryden, 2005; Dryden & Zempleni, 2004) or telecommunications traffic (Beran et al., 1992; Beran & Terrin, 1992; Cox, 1984; Hampel, 1987; Taqqu, 1985), are good examples of artificial processes with strong self-similar properties.

The degree of self-similarity of a signal, which can be extrapolated from the Hurst parameter (Hparam), is seen as an important statistic that provides means for describing the current and predicting the future behavior of the given signal. Hparam can be used in prediction mechanisms but also as an indicator of the trace characteristics. This property is particularly important considering that one can analyze any detect feature shape by the self-similarity point of view, and therefore obtain a new attribute for classification of the relevant elements found.

The presence of self-similarity issues has been discovered in a plethora of fields. Self-similar and fractal analysis of aging and health cycles in the field of medical sciences, as well as high frequency analysis of heart rate and brain waves, prove that a fast method of Hparam estimation might become a critical issue in the coming years, eventually being its immediate field of application. Growing applications of fractal image pattern coding techniques (Giordano et al., 1996; Mudigonda et al., 2000; Potlapalli & Luo, 1998; Kaplan L. M., 1999; Kaplan & Murenzi, 1997; Wen & Acharya, Self-Similar Texture Charcaterization Using Wigner-Ville Distribution, 1996; Wen & Acharya, Fractal Analysis of Self-Similar Textures Using a Fourier-Domain Maximum Likelihood Estimation Method, 1996; Pagano et al., 1996) and face / voice recognition methods, also require application of self-similarity detection procedures, though none is currently available.

The main advantage of the fractal and multifractal analyses (MFA) in signal processing, compared to classic signal processing, lie in the way of how the non-regularities are assumed. When irregularly shaped self-similar objects as typical tumor masses, are evaluated, described and classified from the fractal point of view, the

Figure 1. Screening mammograms from a 54-year old woman: mediolateral oblique (MLO) and craniocaudal (CC) views

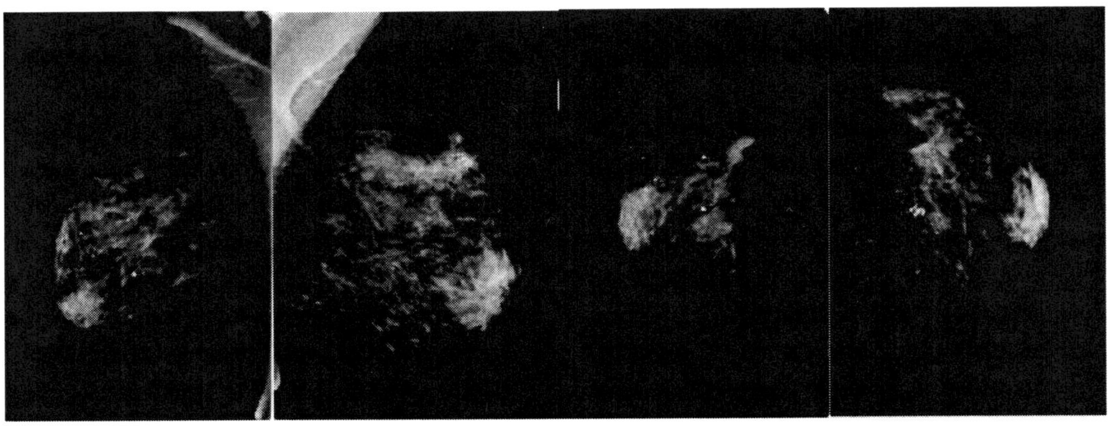

anomalies are then considered as structural deviations from global regularity of the background.

The classic signal processing usually deals with the smoothed version of the image in order to suppress the noise and extract irregularities, such as edges. The multifractal analysis tends to extract relevant information directly from the singularities and, by appropriate choice of multifractal parameters, different features may be recognized, extracted and even classified, both in geometric and probabilistic sense.

In X-ray mammography, CAD systems are mainly used in screening programs, where the large number of mammograms to be processed requires a large number of radiologists and the difficulty of their interpretation demand reliable assistance. In addition, the rapid development of digital mammography increases the utility of CAD in everyday image processing and fully automated detection methods. The self-similarity formalism can be supportive of this duty.

CLINICAL ASPECTS OF MAMMOGRAPHY

Too many factors characterize a mammogram: patient's age, type of parenchyma (fatty, glandular,

Figure 2. Different types of breast lesions. (Peters, 2007)

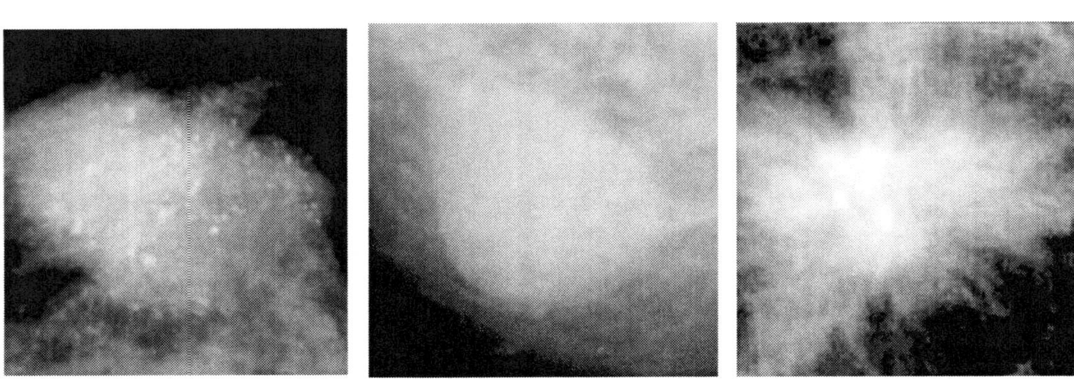

(a) clustered microcalcifications (b) dense kernel mass (c) spiculated mass fatty glandular), lesion location, etc. The numerical value of the features extracted has a proper valence only for the mammogram under examination. We think the mutual relations between different features are more useful for diagnosis than the absolute value of a single feature, and it is not that helpful to look for similarities between different mammograms.

It is preferable to examine the informative content of an under domain image if it is represented by a one-dimensional rather than by a two-dimensional signal, as it better highlights the features (texture, shape, periodicity).

Mammographic possible early signs of breast cancer are: masses (particularly with irregular margins); clusters of microcalcifications; and architectural distortions of breast structures. Figure 2 illustrates different types of breast lesions.

In order to be able to characterize a mass, radiologists generally rely on its contour and different kinds can be observed in mammograms (circumscribed, spiculated, microlobulated, with dense kernel). Usually circumscribed masses are related to benign lesions while speculated masses are related to malignant lesions.

Early detection through mammography in almost 50% of cases depends on the presence of particular microcalcifications in conjunction with other mammographic readings. Microcalcifications in isolation would account for about 30% of cancer detection. On screening studies, 90% of nonpalpable in situ ductal carcinomas and 70% of nonpalpable minimal carcinomas are visible on microcalcifications alone. Microcalcifications are found using high-resolution imaging techniques or direct radiological magnification, because they are the smallest structures identified on mammograms. Clinically, their size are from 0.1-1.0 mm, and the average diameter is about 0.3 mm. Small ones (ranging 0.1-0.2 mm) can hardly be seen on the mammogram due to their superimposition on the breast parenchymal textures and noise. Some parts of the background, such as dense tissue, may be brighter than the microcalcifications in the fatty part of the breast. The typical calcifications seen in the presence of breast cancer are clusters of tiny calcium based deposits having thin, linear, curvilinear, or branching shapes.

However, difficulties exist in interpreting some calcifications when they are tiny and clustered but do not conform to the recognized malignant characteristics, such as cluster shape, size and spatial distribution (Blanks et al., 1998; Warren Burhenne, et al., 2000; Giger, 1999; Boggis & Astley, 2000; Pisano, 2000; Li et al., 1997).

Whether or not they appear in independent clusters or associated with masses, the existence of microcalcifications in a mammogram is often a clear warning of abnormality. They can be visible long before any palpable lesion has developed and their early detection can indeed "make a difference" in the prognosis.

MAMMOGRAM ANALYSIS THROUGH SELF-SIMILARITY

Introduction

The property of self-similarity is present on many natural and artificial processes (Jones, 2004). The most usual records of observable quantities are in the form of time series and their fractal and multifractal properties have been extensively investigated. Description of such processes through mathematical models is difficult, mostly because of their apparent chaotic behavior. Nevertheless, their self-similarity degree, which can be extrapolated from a statistic known as the Hurst parameter (Hparam), can be used to classify them and anticipate their future status (Trovero, 2003).

Human tissue is characterized by a high degree of self-similarity (Mandelbrot, 1982). Self-similarity means that an object is composed of sub-units and sub-sub-units on multiple levels that resemble the structure of the whole object. Many natural phenomena exhibit self-similar or fractal property in which a structure is assumed as made of parts similar to the whole, exactly (monofractals) or statistically (random fractals). Random fractals have the same statistical properties for the entire data set and for sub-sections of the data set.

The self-similarity property has been found in mammograms, through a qualitative appreciation of the existing self-similarity nature, by analyzing their fluctuations at different resolutions.

The parameter characterizing such feature is called the fractal dimension, a non-integer value describing how the irregular structure of objects or phenomena is replicated in iterative way in enlarging scales. In an idealized model, the fractal dimension of a perfect fractal surface should remain constant over all ranges of scales. There are some restrictions of self-similar behaviour (beyond which a structure is no longer fractal), due to limitations in the compliance of medical images. For instance, the resolution limit of the image system sets a lower limit on the fractal scaling behaviour and an upper limit may be set by the size of the organ being examined.

The description of some of the mathematical concepts related to self-similarity and Hurst parameter estimation is presented here. Section B introduces basic concepts necessary to define the degree of self similarity. Four different Hurst parameter estimation methods are enunciated on sections C, D, and E.

Descriptions of all the Hurst parameter estimation methods are not included here, since it would increase significantly the size of this document without adding any novelty to the presented idea.

Please notice that, for the sake of clarity, some of the mathematical details are simplified. However, this simplification was carefully considered, so that it does not prejudice the general scientific precision.

Self-Similarity and the Hurst Parameter

The following description introduces the concept of self-similarity by defining the Hurst parameter of a given process.

Definition 1: Self-Similarity

Let (1) be a stochastic process defined for $t \geq 0$ and H in equations (3) and (5) be the Hurst parameter. The process is said to be self-similar with Hurst parameter H if equation (3) is satisfied under condition (4). In other terms, the statistical description of the process (1) does not change by scaling simultaneously its amplitude by a^{-H} and the time axis by a.

$$\{X(t)\}_{t\geq 0} \tag{1}$$

$$\overset{d}{=} \tag{2}$$

$$X(t) \overset{d}{=} a^{-H} X(at) \tag{3}$$

$$a>0 \tag{4}$$

$$H\geq 0 \tag{5}$$

Notice that (2) denotes equality in distribution. Equation (3) states that the distribution of $X(t)$ is equal to the distribution of $a^{-H}X(at)$.

Given this, the previous definition is equivalent to

Definition 2: Self-Similarity

A stochastic process (1), defined for $t \geq 0$ is self similar if the equations (6), (7) and (8) are satisfied under condition (4).

$$EX(t)=a^{-H}EX(at) \tag{6}$$

$$Var(X(t))=a^{-2H}Var(X(at)) \tag{7}$$

$$Corr(X(t),X(s))=a^{-2H}Corr(X(at),X(as)) \tag{8}$$

Definition 3: Short and Long Range dependence

If the Hurst parameter of a given stochastic process respects condition (9), then the process is said to exhibit short range dependence properties. If the Hurst parameter is bigger than 0,5 and smaller or equal than 1 (condition (10)), it is has long range dependence properties.

$$0 \le H < 0{,}5 \tag{9}$$

$$0{,}5 < H \le 1 \tag{10}$$

Definition 4: Degree of Self-Similarity

It can be said that the Hurst parameter is a measure of the length of short/long range dependence of a stochastic process. The degree of self-similarity increases as the value of the Hurst parameter increases. In this sense, the degree of self-similarity is the Hurst parameter itself.

Embedded Branching Process

The following mathematical explanation is partially based on (Jones, 2004).

Assuming that (1) is self-similar and belongs to the class of stochastic processes with stationary increments, let's suppose that the space dimension is always scaled by a fixed factor of *2*. This situation is depicted by expression (11).

$$\exists \mu \in R^{+} : X(t) \overset{d}{=} 2X(\mu . t) \tag{11}$$

$$2=\mu^{-H} \tag{12}$$

$$\Leftrightarrow H = -\log_{\mu} 2 \tag{13}$$

$$\Leftrightarrow H = -\frac{\log 2}{\log \mu} \tag{14}$$

If *X(t)* is self-similar, equations (11), (12), (13) and (14) are obvious and, thus, estimation of Hurst parameter confines itself to the estimation of the value of μ. This particular value is a measure of how much time the process spends until it double its probabilistic properties. To get this value, presume that ε is a fixed and positive real value (condition (14)). Expression (18) defines, for each *n*, a set of crossing points between *X(t)* and the parallel lines given by (16). Each crossing point is calculated through the intersection (if any) of the line segment that goes from *X(t-1)* to *X(t)* with one of the horizontal lines given by (16). The *inf* function assures that, from a series of followed crossings to the same line, only the initial moment *t* is added to the set T^n.

$$\varepsilon \in \mathrm{R} : \varepsilon > 0 \tag{15}$$

$$f(n)=\varepsilon . 2^{n} Z \tag{16}$$

$$T_{k+1}^{n} = \inf\left(t > T_{k}^{n} : X(t) \in \varepsilon . Z2^{n}, X(t) \neq X\left(T_{k}^{n}\right)\right) \tag{17}$$

$$T^{n} = \bigcup_{k} T_{k+1}^{n} \tag{18}$$

It is easy to see that, as *n* decreases, the cardinality of T^n increases (number of crossings increases because lines (16) become closer). Actually, given (19), condition (20) is always true (the number of crossings of level *n* always exceeds the double of the number of crossings for the level *n+1*).

$$R^{n}=\#(T^{n}) \tag{19}$$

$$2 \times R^{n+1} < R^{n} \tag{20}$$

Therefore, for each n, the ratio between R^n and R^{n+1} gives an estimate for μ (21). For well chosen values of ε and under condition (22), these values can be combined to get a more precise estimator using formula (23). In simple terms, the ergodic class is the class of sets with the same probabilistic properties.

$$\mu_n = \frac{R^n}{R^{n+1}} \tag{21}$$

$$\left(\forall n \in Z\right) \cap \left(R^{n+1} \neq 0\right) \cap \left(\left\{\#\left(T_k^n\right)\right\}_{k \in N} \in Ergodic\right) \tag{22}$$

$$\mu = \frac{R^1 \mu_0 + R^2 \mu_1 + \ldots + R^{n+1} \mu_n}{R^1 + R^2 + \ldots + R^{n+1}} \tag{23}$$

Until now, the number of crossings was calculated by constructing a tree structure. For each n, the crossings coincide with the nodes of the tree. Hence, the number of nodes was the cardinality of T^n. The original EBP estimator calculates the whole crossing tree structure for the given crossing level n at a time, resulting in the retrospective character of the estimation.

Variance Time

If (1) belongs to the class of stochastic processes with stationary increments, there is a Hurst parameter estimation method usually termed Variance Time (VT) method that is based on some properties of the logarithmic function.

$$Var(Y(t)) = m^{2-2H} Var(Y^{(m)}(t)) \tag{24}$$

Applying the logarithm function to both members of equation (24), we obtain equation (26), which is equivalent to equation (30). The deduction is described by transitions (27), (28) and (29). Note that, for simplicity, notation (25) is applied.

$$Y\left(t\right) \overset{n}{=} Y \tag{25}$$

$$\log(Var(Y)) = \log(m^{2-2H} Var(Y^{(m)})) \tag{26}$$

$$\Leftrightarrow \log\left(Var\left(Y\right)\right) = \log\left(m^{2-2H}\right) + \log\left(Var\left(Y^{(m)}\right)\right) \tag{27}$$

$$\Leftrightarrow \log\left(Var\left(Y\right)\right) = \left(2 - 2H\right)\log\left(m\right) + \log\left(Var\left(Y^{(m)}\right)\right) \tag{28}$$

$$\Leftrightarrow \frac{\log\left(Var\left(Y\right)\right) - \log\left(Var\left(Y^{(m)}\right)\right)}{\log\left(m\right)} = \left(2 - 2H\right) \tag{29}$$

$$\Leftrightarrow H = 1 - \frac{\beta}{2} : \beta = \frac{\log\left(Var\left(Y\right)\right) - \log\left(Var\left(Y^{(m)}\right)\right)}{\log\left(m\right)} \tag{30}$$

Estimation of the Hurst parameter is equivalent to the estimation of β, which is performed by taking a finite number of valid m values and by calculating, subsequently, the variance for Y and $Y^{(m)}$. Several values are obtained for β (one for each m) and a statistical function can be used to normalize them and retrieve a single value.

From the graphical point of view and as *Var(Y)* does not depend on m, the plot of $log(Var(Y^{(m)})$ versus $log(m)$ should be a straight line of slope $-\beta$. This fact is explained by equation (31). The method owns its name (Variance Time) to its graphical representation since the mentioned plot is usually called Variance/Time plot (VT plot).

$$\log\left(Var\left(Y^{(m)}\right)\right) = \log\left(Var\left(Y\right)\right) - \beta.\log\left(m\right) : \quad \beta = \frac{\log\left(Var\left(Y\right)\right) - \log\left(Var\left(Y^{(m)}\right)\right)}{\log\left(m\right)} \tag{31}$$

Detrended Fluctuation Analysis

It has been shown that any bounded time series can be mapped to a self-similar process by the process of integration (Beran, Statistics for Long-Memory Processes, 1994). However, another challenge faced by researchers applying this type of fractal analysis to physiologic data is that these time series are often highly non-stationary. A simplified and general definition characterizes a time series as stationary if the mean, standard deviation and higher moments, as well as the correlation functions are invariant under time translation. Signals that do not obey these conditions are nonstationary and thus the integration procedure will further exaggerate the nonstationarity of the original data.

To overcome this complication, a modified root mean square analysis of a random walk has been introduced, termed Detrended Fluctuation Analysis (DFA) (Peng et al., 1994; Goldberger et al., 2002). Advantages of DFA over conventional methods are that it permits the detection of intrinsic self-similarity embedded in a seemingly nonstationary time series, and also avoids the spurious detection of apparent self-similarity, which may be an artefact of extrinsic trends.

In the DFA Hurst parameter estimator, the original data sequence is first integrated by equation (32), where $X(i)$ is the actual sample of the data trace and $\hat{X}$ is the average value for the integrated series.

$$y(k) = \sum_{i=1}^{k} (X(i) - \hat{X}) \qquad (32)$$

As mentioned above, this calculation step maps the original time series to a self-similar process. Next we measure the vertical characteristic scale of the integrated time series. To do so, the integrated time series is divided into boxes of equal length, n. In each box, a least squares line is fit to the data (representing the trend in that box). The vertical coordinate of the approximation segments is designated by $y_n(k)$. In the final calculation step, the examined data trace is detrended by subtracting the local trend point $y_n(k)$ from the local original point $y(k)$ (deviation from its trend in each box) using the following formula (33). This represents the characteristic size of the fluctuations.

$$F(n) = \sqrt{\frac{1}{N}\sum_{k=1}^{N} (y(k) - y_n(k))^2} \qquad (33)$$

This computation process is repeated over all time scales (box sizes) to provide a relationship between $F(n)$ and the box size n. Typically, $F(n)$ will increase with box size n. A linear relationship on a double logarithm plot indicates the presence of scaling (self-similarity) – the fluctuations in small boxes are related to the fluctuations in larger boxes in a power-law fashion. The slope of the line relating $\log F(n)$ to $\log n$ determines the scaling exponent (Hurst parameter). This provides a measure of the regularity of the original time series.

The DFA algorithm is illustrated in Figure 3, applied in some cardiac interbeat signal. The solid black curve is the integrated time series, $y(k)$. The vertical dotted lines indicate boxes of size $n = 100$ beats. The solid straight line segments represent the trend estimated in each box by a linear least squares fit. $F(n)$, are plotted against the box size, n, in a double logarithmic plot. The red circle is the data point for $F(100)$, and the blue circle is the data point for $F(200)$. A straight-line graph indicates power-law scaling.

Multifractal Analysis as Image Segmentation Technique

When irregularly shaped self-similar objects are evaluated, described and classified from the fractal point of view, the anomalies are then considered as structural deviations from global regularity of the background.

In the Multifractal Analysis (MFA), conversely from the classical image analysis, edges are not

Figure 3. Illustration of the DFA algorithm to test for scale-invariance. (Peng, Havlin, Simons, Stanley, & Goldberger, 1994)

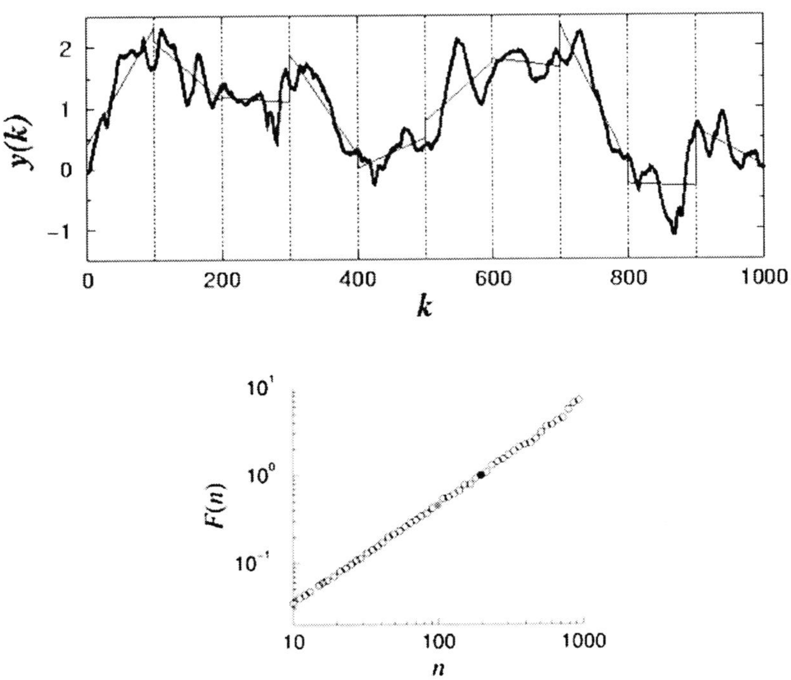

considered as points where sharp variations of the signal still exist after smoothing, but rather as points whose regularity differs from a background. More general, this approach is capable of describing image features both from local and global point of view. For instance, MFA permits the sharp distinction between edge points and isolated points. Although both types of points differ from background, edge points are locally connected, while isolated ones are not (Dathe et al., 2006; Kestener et al., 2001; Tarquis, et al., 2006). The multifractal analysis, as an emerging trend, is the basis of the method for extraction of small-sized isolated details in mammograms presented in this section.

Oppositely to the topological dimensions represented by a natural number of independent vectors, fractal elements are characterized by a fractal dimension, a real number, related to the degree of irregularity of the signal. One of the most popular methods for its calculation is the box-counting, due to its simplicity and fast computing procedure.

The method involves covering the observed structure with a grid of n-dimensional boxes (hyper-cubes) with a side length ε, and counting the number of non-empty boxes, $N(\varepsilon)$. Then, the log-log plot of $N(\varepsilon)$ and $1/\varepsilon$ is made. Now, one can change a side length progressively and count the corresponding number of non-empty boxes. From the slope of the fitted straight line (linear regression) to the plotted points of the diagram we derive the box-counting dimension D_B. Namely, as a limiting value, when $\varepsilon \longrightarrow 0$, the number of boxes $N(\varepsilon)$ is proportional to ε^{-D_B} as in equation (34) (Reljin & Reljin, 2002).

$$D_B = -\lim_{\varepsilon \to 0} \frac{\log N(\varepsilon)}{\log \varepsilon} \quad (34)$$

Artificially generated (deterministic) fractals exhibit hard fractal behaviour, by applying precise algorithms and rules. Conversely, natural objects and phenomena, do not exhibit so strict fractal behaviour even when they are classifiedas fractals. Natural objects have statistical self-similarity: by observing their structure in different scales a similar, but not exactly the same structure, is obtained. For instance, a magnified section of a coastline will resemble the whole in some way but not precisely. In this case we will consider multi-fractals rather than fractals. Multifractal parameters, used for describing such structures, can be applied to object classification (Uma et al., 1996), enabling a new approach for investigation of many phenomena.

Instead of one quantity or measure,μ, describing the phenomenon in all scales (as in case of fractals), a set of measures, $\sum \mu_i$ (a sort of weight factors) depicting statistically the same phenomenon in different scales, has to be used for characterizing such structures. Consequently, a theory of self-similarity is extended from fractals to multifractals.

Considering a 2D signal describing an object such as a grey scale image, the box-counting method is not appropriate since it gives only a relation between non-empty boxes and the box size, regardless of the signal level into the boxes.

In case of multifractals, the signal value (the measure μ_i) within the box is embedded into the process of signal characterization. At the first step, the quantity called the coarse *Hölder exponent* α is derived as in equation (35), where α quantifies the strength of the singularities of the measure, describing the pointwise singularity (local regularity) of the object, with the determined measure of the box $\mu(box)$ and size of the box ε. The limiting value of α is estimated as a slope of the linear regression line, taken from the plot corresponding points by bi-logarithmic diagram $\log\mu(box)$ against $\log \varepsilon$.

$$\alpha = \frac{\log \mu(box)}{\log \varepsilon} \tag{35}$$

Usually in the whole structure there are many boxes (or points) with the same parameter α. Once α has been derived, the frequency distribution of this parameter has to be established. For each value of α, one evaluates the number of boxes of size ε having the coarse *Hölder exponent* equal to α, $N_\varepsilon(\alpha)$. Since the total number of boxes of size ε is proportional to ε^{-D_E}, where D_E is the Euclidean dimension of the box, the probability of hitting the value of α is given by equation (36). Drawing the distribution of this probability would not be useful, since as $\varepsilon \longrightarrow 0$ this distribution no longer tends to a limit. Instead, it is more appropriate to consider the function given by equation (37). The limiting value of $f(\alpha)$ is estimated as a slope of the linear regression line (similar to α estimation), taken from the plot corresponding points by the respective bi-logarithmic diagram.

$$p_\varepsilon(\alpha) = \frac{N_\varepsilon(\alpha)}{\varepsilon^{-D_E}} \tag{36}$$

$$f_\varepsilon(\alpha) = \frac{-\log N_\varepsilon(\alpha)}{\log \varepsilon} \tag{37}$$

Such definition of $f(\alpha)$ means, that for each singularity α, the number of boxes increases for decreasing ε as $N_\varepsilon(\alpha) \sim \varepsilon^{-f(\alpha)}$. Then, $f(\alpha)$ may be seen as the fractal dimension of the set of points that corresponds to a singularity α, and a graph of $f(\alpha)$ plotted over subsets characterized by α is called the *multifractal* (MF) *spectrum* of the measure (also known as the *singularity spectrum* or the *Hausdorf dimension* of the distribution of α). $f(\alpha)$ is a continuous function of α. In many cases the graph of $f(\alpha)$ has the parabolic shape, having the maximum near α=1 (for 1D signals), or near α=2 (for 2D signals). The values of $f(\alpha)$ could be interpreted as a fractal dimension of the subset of boxes of size ε having coarse *Hölder exponenta* as $\varepsilon \longrightarrow 0$. Namely, when ε tends to 0, there is an increasing multitude of subsets, each characterized by its own α and a fractal dimension $f(\alpha)$. This is one of several reasons for the term multifractals (Uma et al., 1996).

In multifractal-based digital image processing, it is necessary to derive some kind of two-dimensional multi-fractal transform - a procedure enabling bi-directional mapping of pixel values from input image (original domain) to corresponding values of α and $f(\alpha)$ (transformed domain). By applying such procedure it is possible to extract details (pixels) belonging to particular image regions by the MF approach (Véhel, 1997).

The value α gives the local information of the point regularity: for fixed measure (grey level) each image pixel is characterized by its own value of α. For instance, image points having $\alpha \cong 2$ are the points where the measure is regular, i.e., where the probability of the change of the signal is small. Points with $\alpha \neq 2$denote he regions where "something happens", i.e. the non-regular zones exist.

The value of $f(\alpha)$ gives the global information of the signal (describes the global regularity of the observed structure (Barral & Seuret, 2007). For instance, points on the smooth contour belong to the point-set with $f(\alpha)$ close to 1, since this value corresponds to the Euclidean dimension of the line, while the points on the homogeneous region (surface) have $f(\alpha) \cong 2$, etc…

Regardless of a particular technique for deriving multifractal quantities α and $f(\alpha)$ (the box-counting is only one of the several possible methods for MF *spectrum* estimation, others can be found in (Tarquis et al., 2006; Barral & Seuret, 2007; Pesquet-Popescu & Vehel, 2002), all methods describe both local and global regularities of the process under investigation. Thereby, MFA may be used in a broad class of signal processing problems, as a robust method for describing or extracting some features hidden in large amount of data (Véhel, 1997; Pesquet-Popescu & Vehel, 2002).

The importance and the advantage of the fractal and multifractal analyses in signal processing, compared to classic signal processing, lie in the way of how the non-regularities are assumed. The classic approach usually deals with the smoothed version of the image in order to suppress the noise and extract irregularities, such as edges. The MFA tends to extract relevant information directly from the singularities.

Multifractal approach is already used in digital image processing, mainly for texture classification and segmentation (Pesquet-Popescu & Vehel, 2002; Reljin & Reljin, 2002). This approach exploits both local regularity of a given measure, described by the pointwise Hölder exponent α, and the global distribution of the regularity in a whole scene, described by multifractal spectrum $f(\alpha)$. By appropriate choice of a pair α and $f(\alpha)$, different features may be recognized, extracted and even classified, both in geometric and probabilistic sense.

In the research work by Soares et al. (2007) it was stated that the MFA can reveal details that can represent microcalcification regions. Technical details of MF image analysis are described, together with tests indicating that a suggested modified MFA scheme improves the accuracy of extraction of real microcalcifications mineral deposits as represented in Figure 4.

Wavelet Transform Modulus Maxima

To deriving and analyse the multifractal properties of experimental data, the wavelet transform modulus maxima (WTMM) (Muzy et al., 1991; Audit, 1999; Arneodo et al., 1995) technique can be used. The WTMM employs the wavelet transform, which is a very powerful tool for characterizing the scaling properties of multifractal measures (Budaev et al., 2006). The technique allows us to build an estimator that is based on the local maxima of the continuous wavelet transform. This method was proved very efficient to compute the *singularity spectrum* of multifractal signals.

Figure 4. Fragment of a mammogram with segmented microcalcifications. (Soares et al., 2007)

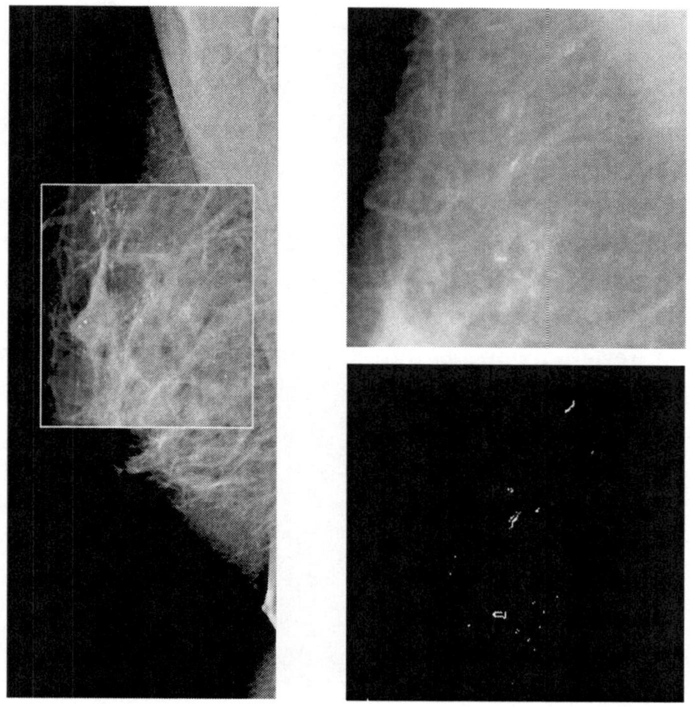

The basic idea is to describe the partition function over only the modulus maxima of the wavelet transform of the signal. We are going to decrease the redundancy of the continuous wavelet transform by just keeping the positions and the values of the wavelet transform at the local maxima.

A partition function $\tau(q)$ is found from a power-law dependence depicted by expression (38) where the structure function $Z(q,a)$ is the sum of the qth powers of the local maxima of the absolute modulus of the wavelet transform coefficients at scale a.

$$Z(q,a) \propto a^{\tau(q)} \tag{38}$$

When a function is continuously differentiable at a point there is no singularity present at that location. To precisely define what we mean by a local maxima of the wavelet transform modulus, let $Wf(x)$ be the wavelet transform of a function $f(x)$. We call a local extremum any point x_0 such that the derivative depicted by expression (39) has a zerocrossing at $x=x_0$, when x varies. We call a modulus maximum, any point x_0 such that (40) occur when x belongs to either a right or left neighbourhood of x_0, and (41) when x belongs to the other side of the neighbourhood of x_0. So, modulus maximum is a point whose absolute value is more than one of the neighbourhood and not less than the other neighborhood. These points, also called multiscale edge points, are points where the modulus is locally maximum with respect to its neighbours.

$$\frac{d(Wf(x))}{dx} \tag{39}$$

$$\left|Wf(x)\right| < \left|Wf(x_0)\right| \tag{40}$$

$$\left|Wf(x)\right| \le \left|Wf(x_0)\right| \tag{41}$$

A function is not singular in any neighbourhood where its wavelet transform has no modulus maxima at the finer scales (Jouck, 2004). We call maxima line, any connected curve in the scale space x along which all points are modulus maxima. At each scale, localized maxima in the modulus of the wavelet transform are identified, and these are then connected across scales to form maxima lines, essentially ridges identifying maxima across scale. There is always at least one maxima ridge line pointing toward any singularity. The singularities may be located and characterized (via α) using the maxima of the signal's wavelet coefficients: the so-called Wavelet Transform Modulus Maxima (WTMM). Measuring the slope of the logarithm of the WTMM associated with a singularity produces an estimate of α. The wavelet power spectrum can be averaged over time to produce a global wavelet spectrum analogous to the Fourier energy spectrum (Priest & Forbes, 2007).

The modulus maxima perform three useful tasks in the context of signal processing: i) the existence of local maxima marks the existence of a singularity (or discontinuity, or edge) in the signal. In this sense the wavelet transform is similar to well-known edge-detectors in image processing; ii) these maxima form paths which at fine scales locate the edge in the original function; iii) the modulus of these maxima can characterize the edge via its regularity, i.e. estimate the order of singularity which has led to the detected signal edge.

The Wavelet Transform Modulus Maxima 2D as Image Segmentation Technique

It was shown that WTMM can describe both local and global regularities of the process under investigation. Different features may be recognized, extracted and even classified, both in geometric and probabilistic sense.

An image is a positive function on R^2. The value of this function at each point specifies the brightness of the picture at that point. Digital images are sampled versions of such functions, where the value of the function is specified only at discrete locations on the image plane, known as pixels. One can derive a completely analogous theory for Fourier transform, filters, wavelet basis, etc in two variables. This leads to a theory of wavelets in two variables which are in general not separable, i.e., (x,y) cannot be written as a product $\psi 1(x)\psi 2(x)$. An easier approach is to construct tensor product wavelets which are separable. Separability gives separable scaling and wavelet functions so that the 2D transform is equivalent to two separate one dimensional transforms.

The wavelet decomposition of a 2D image f can be obtained by performing the filtering consecutively along horizontal and vertical directions (separable filter bank). by first applying the filtering in one dimension (e.g. row) and then the other (column) dimension, i.e., we use low pass (L) and high-pass (H) filters in both horizontal and vertical directions and get four filtered images at each level of the wavelet decomposition images:

1. LL: low pass filtering for rows and columns,
2. LH: low pass filtering for columns after high pass for rows,
3. HL: high pass filtering for columns after low pass for rows,
4. HH: high pass filtering for rows and columns.

The discrete wavelet is suitable for image compression because of its non-redundant information representation. This type of wavelets lacks of shift-invariant property and hence fails to perform some image processing such as feature extraction, edge detection, denoising and pattern recognition. To overcome this shortcoming, Mallat and Zhong (1992) proposed a *Dyadic Wavelet Transform* that possesses the shift-invariant property. Such wavelets can cope with those tasks and has been proved very useful when multiscale analysis is necessary.

At the foremost phase of the image processing algorithm using WTMM, we perform the 2D separable wavelet transform *Dyadic Wavelet Transform 2D* (DWT2)[1], implemented by first applying the filtering in one dimension and then the other, as aforementioned. For this 2D wavelet transform, the wavelet functions $\psi 1(x,y)$ and $\psi 2(x,y)$ are defined as equation (42) and (43), respectively. Let equation (44) and (45), ψ_s^1 and ψ_s^2 are referred to as the detail images, since they contain horizontal and vertical details of f at scale s. The transform of $f(x,y)$ at the scale s has two components defined by equation (46) and (47) where $*$ is the convolution operation. It is straight forward that the equations presented in (48) where ∇ is the gradient.

$$\psi^1(x,y) = \frac{\partial\theta(x,y)}{\partial x} \tag{42}$$

$$\psi^2(x,y) = \frac{\partial\theta(x,y)}{\partial y} \tag{43}$$

$$\psi_s^1(x,y) = \frac{1}{s^2}\psi^1(\frac{x}{s},\frac{y}{s}) \tag{44}$$

$$\psi_s^2(x,y) = \frac{1}{s^2}\psi^2(\frac{x}{s},\frac{y}{s}) \tag{45}$$

$$W_s^1 f(x,y) = f * \psi_s^1(x,y) \tag{46}$$

$$W_s^2 f(x,y) = f * \psi_s^2(x,y) \tag{47}$$

$$\begin{pmatrix} W_s^1 f(x,y) \\ W_s^2 f(x,y) \end{pmatrix} = s\begin{pmatrix} \frac{\partial}{dx}(f*\theta_s)(x,y) \\ \frac{\partial}{dy}(f*\theta_s)(x,y) \end{pmatrix} = s\nabla(f*\theta_s)(x,y) \tag{48}$$

The Canny algorithm defines (x_0,y_0) to belong to and edge if $\|\nabla f(x_0,y_0)\|$ is locally maximum at (x_0,y_0) in the direction of $\nabla f(x_0,y_0)$. The modulus of the gradient vector $\nabla(f*\theta_s)(x,y)$ is proportional to the wavelet transform modulus. Edges are often interpreted as one class of singularities, and thus are related to the local maxima of the wavelet transform modulus, defined as the local maxima of the gradient.

Remarking, the local maxima belong to curves in the (x,y) plane which are the edges of the image along each direction (locally maximum in the 1D neighbourhood that along each direction of the gradient vector). Hence, edge points can be located from the two components, (46) and (47), of the wavelet transform. The edge information of the image is given by the local extrema or the modulus maxima of the detail images.

In order to obey the second phase of the segmentation algorithm, the calculation of WTMM is depicted in the search of local maxima using the Canny edge detector. For each scale of the wavelet representation and for each pixel in the image, we check whether this pixel is a local modulus maximum along the gradient direction or not.

The third step of the procedure consists in the construction of the Maxima Chain (WTMM Chain). Singularities are tracked and chained to one another by similarity of wavelet modulus and position.

The forth step is the identification of the WTMM maxima (WTMMM) which is the local maxima along the WTMM chains.

In the fifth step the WTMMM are disposed along connected curves across the scales (maxima lines) forming a WT skeleton: i) If the value of wavelet power is similar to the wavelet power of the smaller scale ii) and if its position is close to the position of the smaller scale.

The computation of the partition function is then defined directly from the WTMMM that belong to the WT skeleton. The calculation of $\alpha, f(\alpha)$ is now possible as suggested in (Zhong & Mallat, 1992). Figure 5 shows that through the analysis of these multifractal parameters, it is possible to obtain microcalcifications (blue) or masses from

Figure 5. Extracted microcalcifications (black) from the background (grey), on a dense breast. (Kestener et al., 2001)

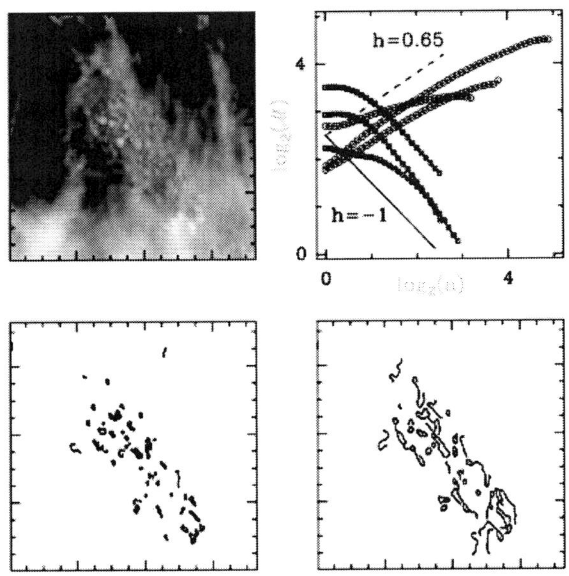

a defined background (red). Moreover, it is feasible to define the breast tissue by density.

CONCLUSION

Experience helps the radiologist to know what and where to look for when reading a mammogram: opacity near the mammary duct, the opacity shape, the tissue surrounding the opacity or nipple alterations in the surrounding area. However, with regard to microcalcifications, so important for precocious diagnosis, to measure or to confront the information in the interested areas would be little help. Indeed, it is very difficult to compare the distribution of the grey tones (texture), their value, the possible order or disorder of an area of the mammogram with another area of the same mammogram.

The self-similarity degree can be an excellent aid to compare and contrast the referred measures. There is no need to image pattern comparison in order to recognize the presence of cancer. One just has to compare the self-similarity factor of the detected features that can be a new attribute for classification. Actually, we noticed that in case of malignant masses, the self-similarity assumes very high values on the edge of the lesion. This can be an indicator for future research directions.

REFERENCES

Amendolia, S., Bisogni, M., Bottigli, U., Ceccopieri, A., Delogu, P., & Fantacci, M. (2001). The CALMA project: a CAD tool in breast radiography. *Nuclear Instruments and Methods, A460*, 107–112.

Arneodo, A., Bacry, E., & Muzy, J. (1995). The thermodynamics of fractals revisited with wavelets. *Physica A, 213*, 232–275. doi:10.1016/0378-4371(94)00163-N

Audit, B. (1999). *Analyse statistique des séquences d'ADN par l'intermédiaire de la transformée en ondelettes.* PhD dissertation, Université de Paris VI Pierre et Marie Curie.

Barral, J., & Seuret, S. (2007). *The singularity spectrum of levy processes in multifractal time.* Advances in Mathematics.

Beran, J. (1992). Statistical Methods for Data with Long-Range Dependence. *Statistical Science*, 7.

Beran, J. (1994). *Statistics for Long-Memory Processes.* New York: Chapman & Hal.

Beran, J., Sherman, R., Taqqu, M. S., & Willinger, W. (1992). *Variable-Bit-Rate Video Traffic and Long-Range Dependence.* IEEE Transactions on Networking.

Beran, J., & Terrin, N. (1992). *A Multivariate Central limit Theorem for Long-Memory Processes with Statistical Applications* [White paper].

Blanks, R., Wallis, M., & Moss, S. (1998). A Comparison of Cancer Detection Rates Achieved by Breast Cancer Screening Programmes by Number of Readers, for One and Two-View Mammography: Results from the UK National Health Breast Screening Programme. *J Med S, 5*, 195–201.

Boggis, C., & Astley, S. (2000). Computer-assisted mammographic imaging. *Breast Cancer Research, 2*, 392–395. doi:10.1186/bcr84

Budaev, V., Takamura, S., Ohno, N., & Masuzaki, S. (2006). Superdiffusion and multifractal statistics of edge plasma turbulence in fusion devices. *Nuclear Fusion, 46*, 181. doi:10.1088/0029-5515/46/4/S10

Cox, D. (1984). Long-range dependence: A review. *Statistics: An Appraisa.*

Dathe, A., Tarquis, A., & Perrier, E. (2006). Multifractal analysis of the pore and solid phases in binary twodimensional images of natural porous structures.

Dryden, L. (2005). *Statistical analysis on high-dimensional spheres and shape spaces.* Annals of Statistics.

Dryden, L., & Zempleni, A. (2004). Extreme shape analysis - Technical report. *Journal of the Royal Statistical Society, Series C, Applied Statistics.*

Giger, M. (1999). Computer-aided diagnosis. *RSNA Categorial Course in Breast Imaging*, 249-72.

Giordano, S., Pagano, M., Russo, F., & Sparano, D. (1996). *A Novel Multiscale Fractal Image Coding Algorithm based on SIMD Parallel Hardware.* Paper presented at Picture Coding Symposium PCS '96, Australia.

Goldberger, A., Amaral, L., Hausdorff, J., Ivanov, P., Peng, C., & Stanley, H. (2002). Fractal dynamics in physiology: Alterations with disease and aging. In *Proceedings of the National Academy of Sciences.*

Hampel, F. R. (1987). Data Analysis and Self-Similar Processes. In *Proceedings of 46th Session ISI.*

Jones, O. (2004). Analyzing self-similarity in network traffic via the crossing tree. In *Proceedings of Mathematics of Networks*. Ipswich, UK: BT Martlesham.

Jouck, P. (2004). *Application of the Wavelet Transform Modulus Maxima method to T-wave detection in cardiac.* Maastricht University.

Julesz, B. (1981). A theory of preattentive texture discrimination based on first-order statistics of textons. *Biological Cybernetics, 41*, 131–138. doi:10.1007/BF00335367

Kaplan, L., & Murenzi, R. (1997). Texture segmentation using multiscale Hurst features. *International Conference on Image Processing, 1997.* Santa Barbara, CA, USA.

Kaplan, L. M. (1999). Extended Fractal Analysis for Texture Classification and Segmentation. *IEEE Transactions on Image Processing*, *8*, 1572–1585. doi:10.1109/83.799885

Kestener, P., Lina, J., Saint-Jean, P., & Arneodo, A. (2001). Wavelet-based multifractal formalism to assist in diagnosis in digitized mammograms.

Kropinsky, E. (2003). The Future of Image Perception in Radiology. *Academic Radiology*, *10*(1).

Krupinskia, E., & Nodine, C. (1994). Gaze Duration Predicts the Locations of Missed Lesions in Mammography. In Gale, A. G., Astley, S. M., Dance, D. R., & Cairns, A. Y. (Eds.), *Digital Mammography* (pp. 399–405). Elsevier.

Le, H. (2003). Unrolling shape curves. *Journal of the London Mathematical Society*, *2*, 511–526. doi:10.1112/S0024610703004393

Li, H., Liu, K., Lo, S., Inc, O., & Jessup, M. (1997). Fractal Modeling and Segmentation for the Enhancement of Microcalcifications in Digital Mammograms. *IEEE Transactions on Medical Imaging*, *16*, 785–798. doi:10.1109/42.650875

Lo, A. W. (1991). Long-Term Memory in Stock Market Prices. *Econometrica*, *59*, 1279–1313. doi:10.2307/2938368

Mandelbrot, B. (1982). *The fractal geometry of nature*. WH Freeman.

Mudigonda, N., Rangayyan, R., & Desautels, J. (2000). Gradient and texture analysis for the classification of mammographic masses. *IEEE Transactions on Medical Imaging*, 1032–1043.

Muzy, J., Bacry, E., & Arneodo, A. (1991). Wavelets and multifractal formalism for singular signals: application to turbulence data. *Physical Review Letters*, *67*, 3515–3518. doi:10.1103/PhysRevLett.67.3515

Oldershaw, R. L. (2002). *Nature adores Self-Similarity*. Retrieved December 2008 from http://www3.amherst.edu/~rloldershaw/nature.html

Pagano, M., Giordano, S., Russo, F., & Sparano, D. (1996). Parallel Implementation of a Progressive Fractal Image Compression System. *IEEE International Workshop on Intelligent Signal Processing & Communication Systems ISPACS '96*.

Peng, C. K., Havlin, S., Simons, M., Stanley, H. E., & Goldberger, A. L. (1994). Mosaic organizatino of DNA nucleotides. *Physical Review E: Statistical Physics, Plasmas, Fluids, and Related Interdisciplinary Topics*, *49*, 49–54. doi:10.1103/PhysRevE.49.1685

Pesquet-Popescu, B., & Vehel, J. (2002). Stochastic fractal models for image processing.

Peters, G. (2007). Computer-aided detection for digital breast tomosynthesis.

Pisano, E. (2000). Current status of full-field digital mammography. *Academic Radiology*, *7*, 266–280. doi:10.1016/S1076-6332(00)80478-X

Pisano, E., Hendrick, R., Yaffe, M., Baum, J., Acharyya, S., & Cormack, J. (2008). Diagnostic accuracy of digital versus film mammography: exploratory analysis of selected population subgroups in DMIST. *Radiology*, *246*(2), 376. doi:10.1148/radiol.2461070200

Potlapalli, H., & Luo, R. (1998). Fractal-based classification of natural textures. *IEEE Transactions on Industrial Electronics*, *45*, 142–150. doi:10.1109/41.661315

Priest, E., & Forbes, T. (2007). The Bursty Nature Of Solar Flare X-Ray Emission. *The Astrophysical Journal*, 662-691Y700.

Reljin, I., & Reljin, B. (2002). Fractal geometry and multifractals in analyzing and processing medical data and images.

Salfity, M., Kaufmann, G., Granitto, P., & Ceccatto, H. (2001). *Automated detection and classification of clustered microcalcifications using morphological filtering and statistical techniques. IWDM2000*. Medical Physics Publishing.

Soares, F., & Andruszkiewicz, P. M., F., P, C., & Pereira, M. (2007). Self-Similarity Analysis Applied to 2D Breast Cancer Imaging. *The First International Workshop on High Performance Computing Applied to Medical Data and Bioinformatics (HPC-Bio 2007)*. IEEE.

Taqqu, M. S. (1985). A Bibliographical Guide to Self-Similar Processes and Long-Range Dependence. *Dependence in Probability and Statistic*, 137-165.

Tarquis, A., McInnes, K., Key, J., Saa, A., Garcia, M., & Diaz, M. (2006). Multiscaling analysis in a structured clay soil using 2D images.

Trovero, M. (2003). Long Range Dependence: a Light Tale for the Practitioner. In *Proceedings of Statistics students' seminar at UNC*.

Uma, K., Ramakrishnan, K., & Ananthakrishna, G. (1996). Image analysis using multifractals. *ICASSP*, *4*, 2188–2190.

Véhel, J. L. (1997). *Introduction to the multifractal analysis of images*. Fractal Image Encoding and Analysis.

Warren Burhenne, L., Wood, S., D'Orsi, C., Feig, S., Kopans, D., & O'Shaugnessy, K. (2000). The Potential Contribution of Computer Aided Detection to the Sensitivity of Screening Mammography. *Radiology*, *215*, 554–562.

Wen, C., & Acharya, R. (1996). Fractal Analysis of Self-Similar Textures Using a Fourier-Domain Maximum Likelihood Estimation Method. *International Conference on Image Processing*. Lausanne, Switzerland.

Wen, C., & Acharya, R. (1996). Self-Similar Texture Charcaterization Using Wigner-Ville Distribution. *International Conference on Image Processing*. Lausanne, Switzerland.

Zhong, S., & Mallat, S. (1992). Characterization of signals from multiscale edges. *IEEE Transactions on Pattern Analysis and Machine Intelligence*, *14*(7), 710–732. doi:10.1109/34.142909

ENDNOTE

1 *2D-Gaussian function* can be a good alternative.

Chapter 7
Volumetric Texture Analysis in Biomedical Imaging

Constantino Carlos Reyes-Aldasoro
The University of Sheffield, UK

Abhir Bhalerao
University of Warwick, UK

ABSTRACT

In recent years, the development of new and powerful image acquisition techniques has lead to a shift from purely qualitative observation of biomedical images towards more a quantitative examination of the data, which linked with statistical analysis and mathematical modeling has provided more interesting and solid results than the purely visual monitoring of an experiment. The resolution of the imaging equipment has increased considerably and the data provided in many cases is not just a simple image, but a three-dimensional volume. Texture provides interesting information that can characterize anatomical regions or cell populations whose intensities may not be different enough to discriminate between them. This chapter presents a tutorial on volumetric texture analysis. The chapter begins with different definitions of texture together with a literature review focused on the medical and biological applications of texture. A review of texture extraction techniques follows, with a special emphasis on the analysis of volumetric data and examples to visualize the techniques. By the end of the chapter, a review of advantages and disadvantages of all techniques is presented together with some important considerations regarding the classification of the measurement space.

INTRODUCTION

What is Texture?

Even when the concept of texture is intuitive, no single unifying definition has been given by the image analysis community. Most of the numerous definitions that are present in the literature have some common elements that emerge from the etymology of the word: texture comes from the Latin *textura*, the past participle of the verb *texere*, to weave (Webster, 2004). This implies that a texture will exhibit a certain structure created by common elements, repeated in a regular way, as in the threads that form a fabric. Three *ingredients* of texture were identified in (Hawkins, 1970):

DOI: 10.4018/978-1-60566-280-0.ch007

- some local 'order' is repeated over a region which is large in comparison to the order's size,
- the order consists of the non-random arrangement of elementary parts, and,
- the parts are roughly uniform entities having approximately the same dimensions everywhere within the textured region.

Yet these ingredients could still be found in the very different contexts, not just in imagery, such as food, painting, haptics or music. *Wikipedia* cites more than 10 contexts of tactile texture alone (http://en.wikipedia.org/wiki/Texture). In this work, we will limit ourselves to visual non-tactile textures, sometimes referred as *visual texture* or simply *image texture,* which is defined in (Tuceryan & Jain, 1998) as: *a function of the spatial variation in pixel intensities*. Although brief, this definition highlights a key characteristic of texture, that is, the spatial variation. Texture is therefore inherently *scale* dependent (Bouman & Liu, 1991; Hsu *et al.*, 1992; Sonka *et al.*, 1998). The texture of a brick wall will change completely if we get close enough to observe the texture of a single brick. Furthermore, the texture of an element (pixel or voxel) is implicitly related to its neighbors. It is not possible to describe the texture of a single element, as it will always depend on the neighbors to create the texture. This fact can be exploited through different methodologies that analyze neighboring elements, for example: Fourier domain methods, which extract frequency components according to the frequency of elements; a Markovian process in which the attention is restricted to the variations of a small neighborhood; a Fractal approach where the texture is seen as a series of self-similar shapes; a Wavelet analysis where the similarity to a prototypical pattern (the Mother wavelet) at different scales or shifts can describe distinctive characteristics; or a co-occurrence matrix where occurrence of the grey levels of neighboring elements is recorded for subsequent analysis.

Some authors have preferred to indicate properties of texture instead of attempting to provide a definition. For instance in (Gonzalez & Woods, 1992) texture analysis is related to its *Statistical* (smooth, coarse, grainy,...), *Structural* (arrangement of feature primitives sometimes called textons) and *Spectral* (global periodicity based on the Fourier spectrum) properties. Some of these properties are visually meaningful and are helpful to describe textures. In fact, studies have analyzed texture from a psycho-visual perspective (Ravishankar-Rao & Lohse, 1993; Tamura *et al.*, 1978) and have identified the properties such as: *Granular, marble-like, lace-like, random, random non-granular and somewhat repetitive, directional locally oriented, repetitive, coarse, contrast, directional, line-like, regular or rough*.

It is important to note that these *properties* are different from the *features* or *measurements* that can be extracted from the textured regions (although confusingly, some works refer to these properties as features of the data). When a methodology for texture analysis is applied, sub-band filtering for instance, a *measurement* is extracted from the original data and can be used to distinguish one texture from another one (Hand, 1981). A *measurement space* (it can also be called the *feature space* or *pattern representation* (Kittler, 1986)) is constructed when several measurements are obtained. Some of these measurements are selected to build the reduced set called a *feature space*. The process of choosing the most relevant measurements is known as *feature selection*, while the combination of certain measurements to create a new one is called *feature extraction* (Kittler, 1986).

Throughout this work we will refer to *Volumetric texture* as the texture that can be found in volumetric data ((Blot & Zwiggelaar, 2002) used the term *solid texture*). All the properties and ingredients that were previously mentioned about texture, or more specifically, visual, or 2D texture, can be applied to volumetric texture. Fig-

Figure 1. Three examples of volumetric data from where textures can be analyzed: (a) A sample of muscle from MRI, (b) A sample of bone from MRI, (c) The vasculature of a growing tumor from multiphoton microscopy. Unlike two dimensional textures, the characteristics of volumetric texture cannot always be observed from their 2D projection

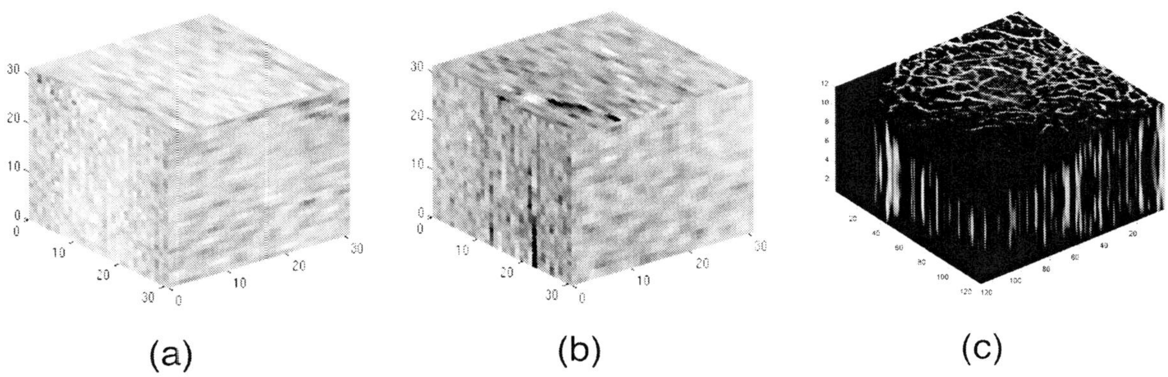

ure 1 shows three examples of volumetric data in which textured regions can be seen and analyzed.

Volumetric Texture

Volumetric Texture is different from 3D Texture, Volumetric Texturing or Texture Correlation. *3D Texture* (Chantler, 1995; Cula & Dana, 2004; Dana *et al.*, 1999; Leung & Malik, 1999; Lladó *et al.*, 2003) refers to the observed 2D texture of a 3D object that is being viewed from a particular angle and whose lighting conditions can alter the shadings that create the visual texture. This analysis is particularly important when the direction of view or lighting can vary from the training process to the classification of the images. Our volumetric study is considered as volume-based (or image-based for 2D); that is, we consider no change in the observation conditions. In Computer Graphics the rendering of repetitive geometries and reflectance into voxels is called *Volumetric Texturing* (Neyret, 1995). A different application of texture in Magnetic Resonance is the one described by the term *Texture Correlation* proposed in (Brian K. Bay, 1995) and now widely used (Brian K. Bay *et al.*, 1998; Gilchrist *et al.*, 2004; Porteneuve *et al.*, 2000), which refers to a method that measures the strain on trabecular bone under loading conditions by comparing loaded and unloaded digital images of the same specimen.

Throughout this work, we will consider that volumetric data, *VD*, will have dimensions for rows, columns and slices $N_r \times N_c \times N_s$ and is quantized to N_g levels. Let

$$L_r = \{1, 2, \ldots, r, \ldots, N_r\},$$

$$L_c = \{1, 2, \ldots, c, \ldots, N_c\} \text{ and}$$

$$L_s = \{1, 2, \ldots, s, \ldots, N_s\}$$

be the spatial domains of the data, (for an image L_r, L_c would be horizontal and vertical), *(r,c,s)* (rows, columns, slices) be a single point in the volumetric data, and $G = \{1, 2, \ldots, g, \ldots N_g\}$ the set of grey tones or grey levels in the case of grey scale and

$$G = \left[G_{red}, G_{green}, G_{blue}\right] =$$

$$\left[\{1, 2, \ldots, g_{red}, \ldots N_{g_{red}}\}, \{1, 2, \ldots, g_{green}, \ldots N_{g_{green}}\}, \{1, 2, \ldots, g_{blue}, \ldots N_{g_{blue}}\}\right]$$

for a color image where *G* corresponds to a triplet of values for red, green and blue channels.

The volumetric data *VD* can be represented then as a function that assigns a grey tone to each triplet of co-ordinates:

$$L_r \times L_c \times L_s; VD : L_r \times L_c \times L_s \rightarrow G \qquad (1)$$

An image then is a special case of volumetric data when $L_s=\{1\}$, that is (Haralick et al., 1973):

$$L_r \times L_c; I : L_r \times L_c \rightarrow G \qquad (2)$$

Literature Review

Texture analysis has been used with mixed success in medical and biological imaging: for detection of micro-calcification and lesions in breast imaging (James *et al.*, 2002; Sivaramakrishna *et al.*, 2002; Subramanian *et al.*, 2004), for knee segmentation (Kapur, 1999; Lorigo *et al.*, 1998) and knee cartilage segmentation (Reyes Aldasoro & Bhalerao, 2007), for the delineation of cerebellar volumes (Saeed & Puri, 2002), for quantifying contralateral differences in epilepsy subjects (Yu *et al.*, 2001; Yu *et al.*, 2002), to diagnose Alzheimer's disease (Sayeed *et al.*, 2002) and brain atrophy (Segovia-Martínez et al., 1999), to characterize spinal cord pathology in Multiple Sclerosis (Mathias *et al.*, 1999), to evaluate gliomas (Mahmoud-Ghoneim *et al.*, 2003), for the analysis of nuclear texture and its relationship to cancer (Jorgensen *et al.*, 1996; Mairinger *et al.*, 1999), to quantitate nuclear chromatin as an indication of malignant lesions (Beil *et al.*, 1995; Ercoli *et al.*, 2000; Rosito *et al.*, 2003), to evaluate invasive adenocarcinomas of the prostate gland (Mattfeldt *et al.*, 1993), to differentiate among types of normal leukocytes and chronic lymphocytic leukemia (Ushizima Sabino *et al.*, 2004), for the classification of plaque in intravascular ultrasound images (Pujol & Radeva, 2005), for the quantitative assessment of bladder cancer (Gschwendtner *et al.*, 1999), and for the detection of adenomas in gastrointestinal video as an aid for the endoscopist (Iakovidis *et al.*, 2006).

Volumetric texture has received much less attention than its spatial 2D counterpart which has seen the publication of numerous and differing approaches for texture analysis and feature extraction (Bigun, 1991; Bovik *et al.*, 1990; Cross & Jain, 1983; Haralick, 1979; Haralick et al., 1973; Tamura et al., 1978), and classification and segmentation (Bouman & Liu, 1991; Jain & Farrokhnia, 1991; Kadyrov *et al.*, 2002; Kervrann & Heitz, 1995; Unser, 1995; Weszka *et al.*, 1976). The considerable computational complexity that is introduced with the extra dimension is partly responsible for lack of research in volumetric texture. But also there are an important number of applications for 2D texture analysis, and yet, a growing number of problems where a study of volumetric texture is of interest.

In *Biology*, the introduction of confocal microscopy (Sheppard & Wilson, 1981; T. Wilson, 1989) has created a revolution since it is possible to obtain incredibly clear, thin optical sections and three-dimensional views from thick fluorescent specimens. The advent of multiphoton fluorescence microscopy has allowed 3D optical imaging *in vivo* of tissue at greater depth than confocal microscopy, with very precise geometric localization of the fluorophore and high spatial resolution (Masters & So, 2004). In *Medical Imaging*, the data provided by the scanners of several acquisition techniques such as Magnetic Resonance Imaging (MRI) (Kovalev *et al.*, 2001; Lerski *et al.*, 1993; Schad *et al.*, 1993), Ultrasound (Zhan & Shen, 2003) or Computed Tomography (CT) (Hoffman *et al.*, 2003; Segovia-Martínez *et al.*, 1999) deliver grey level data in three dimensions. Different textures in these data sets can allow the discrimination of anatomical structures. In *Food Science*, the visual texture of potatoes (Thybo *et al.*, 2003; Thybo *et al.*, 2004) and apples (Létal *et al.*, 2003) provided by MRI scanners has been used to analyze their varieties, freshness and proper cooking. In *Dentistry*, the texture of teeth, observed either by scanning electron microscopy or confocal microscopy, can reveal defects, its relation with attrition, erosion or caries-like processes (Tronstad, 1973) or even microwear, which can lead to infer aspects of diet in extinct primates (Merceron *et al.*, 2006; Scott *et al.*, 2006). The analysis of *crystallographic texture* - the organization of grains in polycrystalline materials - is of interest in relation to particular characteristics of ceramic materials such as for ferro- or piezoelectricity (Tai & Baba-Kishi, 2002). In *Stratigraphy*, also known as Seismic Facies Analysis (Carrillat *et al.*, 2002; Randen *et al.*, 2000), the volumetric texture of the patterns of seismic waves within sedimentary rock bodies can be used to locate potential hydrocarbon reservoirs.

Thus, the analysis of volumetric texture has many potential applications but most of the reported work, however, has employed solely 2D measures, usually co-occurrence matrices that are limited by computational cost. The most common technique to deal with volumetric data is to slice the volume in 2D cross-sections. The individual slices can be used in a 2D texture analysis (Blot & Zwiggelaar, 2002). A simple extension of the 2D slices is to use orthogonal 2D planes in the different axes, and then proceed with a 2D technique, using Gabor filters for instance (Zhan & Shen, 2003). However, high frequency oriented textures could easily be missed by these filter planes. In those cases it is important to conduct a volumetric analysis.

Objectives

This chapter will introduce six of the most important texture analysis methodologies, those that can be used to generate a volumetric Measurement Space. The methodologies presented are: *Spatial Domain techniques, Wavelets, Co-occurrence Matrix, Sub-band Filtering, Local Binary Patterns and Texture Spectra* and *The Trace Transform*. It is important to analyze different algorithms as one technique may capture the textural characteristics of one region but not another. While repetitive oriented patterns can be described by their energy patterns in the Fourier domain, Local Binary Patterns are fast to calculate and concentrate on small regions, Trace transforms are orientation independent, Wavelets can capture non-linear and non-intuitive patterns and in some other cases, simpler measurements like variance can capture different textures.

Each methodology will be presented with mathematical detail and examples. By the end of the chapter a summary will review the advantages and disadvantages of the techniques and their current applications and will give references to where the techniques have been used.

TEXTURE ANALYSIS: GENERATING A MEASUREMENT SPACE

In this section, a review of texture measurement extraction methods will be presented. A special emphasis will be placed on the use of these techniques in 3D. Some of the techniques have been widely used in 2D but not in 3D, and some others have already been extended. For visualization purposes, two data sets will be presented: an artificial set with two oriented patterns and one volumetric set of a human knee MRI set (Figure 2).

All the measurements extracted from the data, either 2D or 3D will form a multivariate space, regardless of the method used. The space will have as many dimensions or variables as measurements extracted. Of course, numerous measurements can be extracted from the data, but a higher number of measurements do not always imply a better space for classification purposes. In some cases, having more measurements can yield lower classification accuracy and in others a single measurement can provide the discrimination of a certain class. The set of all measurements extracted from the data will be called the *measurement space* and when a reduced set of relevant features is obtained, this will be called *feature*

Figure 2. Three-dimensional data sets with texture: (a) Artificial data set with two oriented patterns of [64×32×64] elements each, with different frequency and orientation, and (b) Magnetic Resonance of a human knee. Left: data in the spatial domain; right: data in the Fourier domain

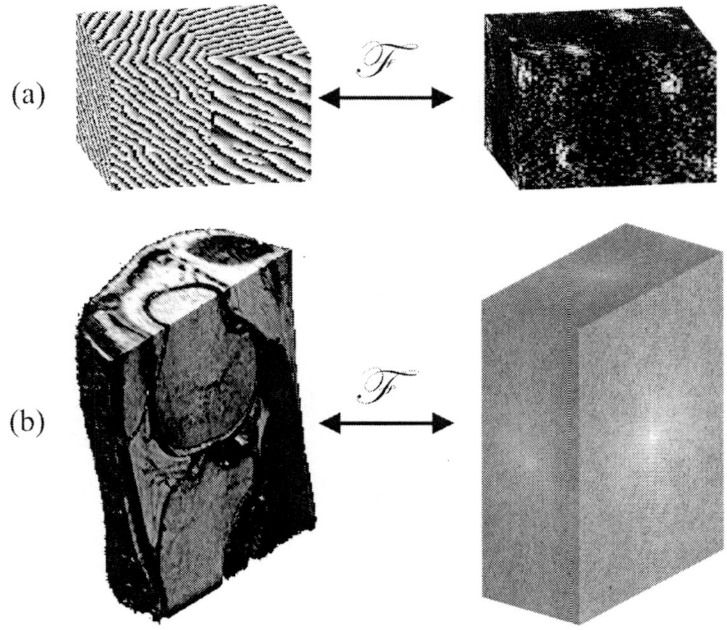

space (Hand, 1981). The selection of a proper set of measurements is a difficult task, which will not be covered here.

To obtain a measurement from a volumetric data set, it is necessary to perform a transformation of the data. A transformation can be understood as a modification of the data in any way, as simply as an arithmetic operation or as complicated as a translation to a different representation space. We will now describe different transformations that lead to measurement extraction techniques.

Spatial Domain Measurements

The spatial domain methods operate directly with the values of the pixels or voxels of the data:

$$V\tilde{D}(x) = T\left[VD\left(\mathcal{N}\right)\right], \quad \mathcal{N} \subset \left(L_r \times L_c \times L_d\right), \quad x \in \left(L_r^{\mathcal{N}} \times L_c^{\mathcal{N}} \times L_d^{\mathcal{N}}\right) \tag{3}$$

where T is an operator defined over a neighborhood N relative to the element x that belongs to the region $\left(L_r^{\mathcal{N}} \times L_c^{\mathcal{N}} \times L_d^{\mathcal{N}}\right)$. The result of any particular operator T^i will become one dimension of the multivariate measurement space S:

$$S^i = VD^i \tag{4}$$

and the measurement space will contain as many dimensions i as the operations performed on the data.

Single Element Mappings

The simplest spatial domain transformations arise when the neighborhood N is restricted to a single element x. T then becomes a mapping $T{:}G \longrightarrow G$ $T : G \to G$ on the intensity or grey level of the element: $\tilde{g} = T\left[g\right]$ and is sometimes called a *mapping function* (Gonzalez & Woods, 1992). Figure 3 shows two cases of these mappings; the

Figure 3. Mapping functions of the grey level. The horizontal axis represents the original value and the vertical axis the modified value: (a) Grey levels remain unchanged, (b) Thresholding between values g_l *and* g_h

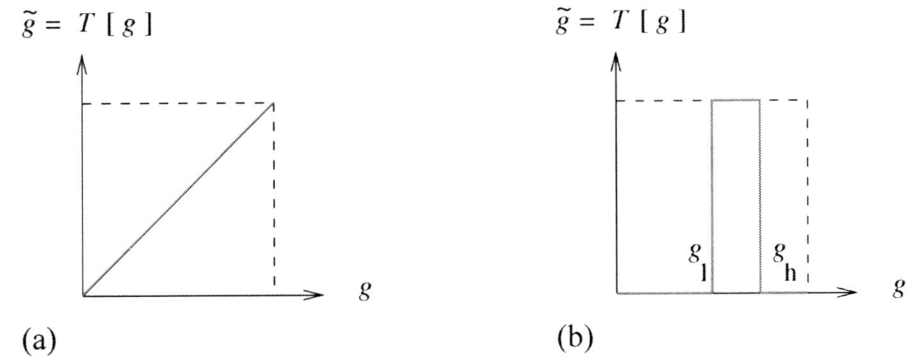

first involves no change of the grey level, while the second case thresholds the grey levels between certain arbitrary low and high values g_l, g_h.

This technique is simple and popular and is known as *grey level thresholding*, which can be based either on global (all the image or volume) or local information. In each scheme, single or multiple thresholds for the grey levels can be assigned. The philosophy is that pixels with a grey level below a threshold belong to one region and the remaining pixels to another region. The goal is to partition the image into regions, *object/ background*, or $object_a$ / $object_b$ / ... $background$. Thresholding methods rely on the assumption that the objects to segment are distinct in their grey levels and can use histogram information, thus ignoring spatial arrangement of pixels. Although in many cases good results can be obtained, in texture analysis there are several restrictions. First, since texture implies the variation of the intensities of neighboring elements, a single threshold can select only some elements of a single texture. In some cases like for MRI, the intensities of certain structures are often non-uniform, possibly due to inhomogeneities of the magnets, and therefore simple thresholding can wrongly divide a single structure into different regions. Another matter to consider is the noise intrinsic to the images that can lead to a misclassification. In many cases the optimal selection of the threshold is not a trivial matter.

The *histogram* (Winkler, 1995) of an image measures the relative occurrence of elements at certain grey levels. The histogram is defined as:

$$h(g) = \frac{\#\left\{x \in (L_r \times L_c \times L_d) : VD(x) = g\right\}}{\#\{L_r \times L_c \times L_d\}}, g \in G \tag{5}$$

where # denotes the number of elements in the set. This approach involves only the first-order measurements of a pixel (Coleman & Andrews, 1979) since the surrounding pixels (or voxels) are not considered to obtain higher order measurements. Figure 4 presents the two data sets and their corresponding histograms. The histogram of the human knee (b) is quite dense and although two local minima or valleys can be identified around the values of 300 and 900, using these thresholds may not be enough for segmenting the anatomical structures of the image. It can be observed that the lower grey levels, those below the threshold of 300 correspond mainly to background, which is highly noisy. The pixels with intensities between 301 and 900 roughly correspond to the region of muscle, but include parts of the skin,

Figure 4. Two images (one slice of the data sets) and their histograms: (a, b) Human Knee MRI, and (c, d) Oriented textures. It should be noticed how the MRI concentrates the intensities in certain grey levels while the oriented textures are spread (non-uniformly) over the whole range

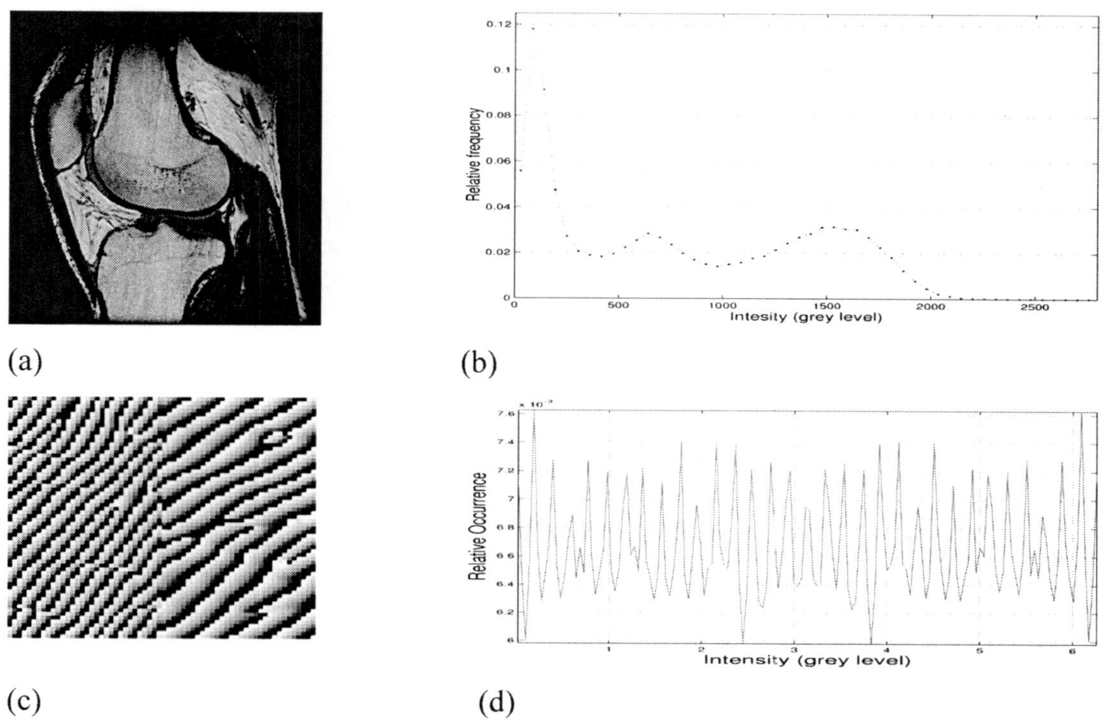

and the borders of other structures like bones and tissue. Many of the pixels in this grey level region correspond to transitions from one region to another. (The muscles of the thigh; Semimembranosus and Biceps Femoris in the hamstring region, do not appear as uniform as those in the calf; the Gastrocnemius, and Soleus.) The third class of pixels with intensities between 901-2787 roughly correspond to bones – femur, tibia and patella – and some tissue – Infrapatellar Fat Pad, and Suprapatellar Bursa. These tissues consist of fat and serous material, which have similar grey levels as the bones. The most important problem is that bone and tissue share the same range of grey levels in this MRI and using just thresholding it would not be possible to distinguish successfully between them. The histogram of the oriented textures (Figure 4 (d)) is not as dense and smooth as the one corresponding to the human knee and it spreads through the whole grey level region without showing any valleys or hills that could indicate that thresholding could help in separating the textures involved.

Figure 5 shows the result of thresholding over the data sets previously presented. The human knee was thresholded at the $g = 1500$ and the oriented data at $g = 5.9$. For the knee some structure of the leg is visible (like the Tibia and Fibula in the lower part) but this thresholding is far from useful. For the oriented data both regions contain pixels above the threshold.

Neighborhood Filters

When T comprises a neighborhood bigger than a single element, several important measurements can be used. When a convolution with kernels is performed, this can be considered as a filtering

Figure 5. Thresholding effect on 3D sets: (a) Oriented textures thresholded at g = 5.9, (b) Human knee thresholded at g = 1500. While the oriented textures have elements in the whole volume, the MRI is concentrated to the regions of bone and tissue

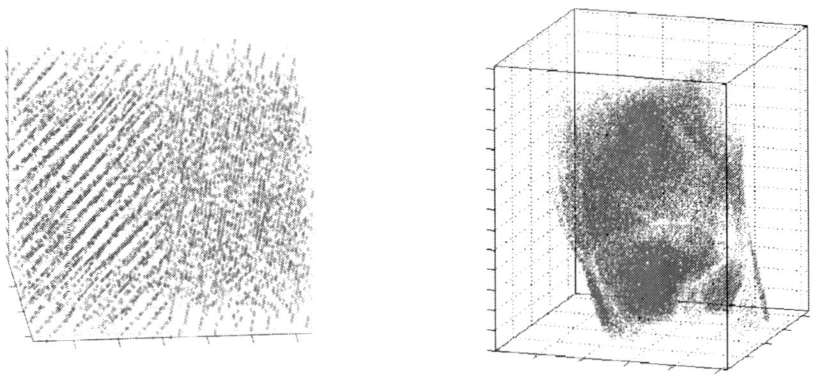

(a) (b)

operation, which is described below. If the relative position is not taken into account, the most common measurements that can be extracted are statistical moments. These moments can describe the distributions of the sample, that is the elements of the neighborhood, and in some cases these can help to distinguish different textures. Yet, since they do not take into account the particular position of any pixel, two very different textures could have the same distribution and therefore the same moments. Even with this limitation, some researchers use these measurements as descriptors for texture.

For a neighborhood related to the element $x = (r,c,s)$ a neighborhood can be seen as a subset N of the data with the domains $L_r^{\mathcal{N}} \times L_c^{\mathcal{N}} \times L_s^{\mathcal{N}}$ (of size $N_r^{\mathcal{N}}, N_c^{\mathcal{N}}, N_s^{\mathcal{N}}$) related to the data in the following relations:

$$L_r^{\mathcal{N}} \subset L_r \quad L_r^{\mathcal{N}} = \{r, r+1, \ldots, r+N_r^{\mathcal{N}}\}, \quad 1 \le r \le N_r - N_r^{\mathcal{N}}, \tag{6}$$

$$L_c^{\mathcal{N}} \subset L_c \quad L_c^{\mathcal{N}} = \{c, c+1, \ldots, c+N_c^{\mathcal{N}}\}, \quad 1 \le c \le N_c - N_c^{\mathcal{N}}, \tag{7}$$

$$L_s^{\mathcal{N}} \subset L_s \quad L_s^{\mathcal{N}} = \{s, s+1, \ldots, s+N_s^{\mathcal{N}}\}, \quad 1 \le s \le N_s - N_s^{\mathcal{N}}, \tag{8}$$

$$(r,c,s) \in (L_r^{\mathcal{N}} \times L_c^{\mathcal{N}} \times L_s^{\mathcal{N}})$$

The first four moments of the distribution; mean μ, standard deviation σ, skewness sk and kurtosis ku, are obtained by:

$$\mu_{VD} = \frac{1}{N_r^{\mathcal{N}} N_c^{\mathcal{N}} N_s^{\mathcal{N}}} \sum_{L_r^{\mathcal{N}} \times L_c^{\mathcal{N}} \times L_s^{\mathcal{N}}} VD\,(r,c,s) \tag{9}$$

$$\sigma_{VD} = +\sqrt{\frac{1}{N_r^{\mathcal{N}} N_c^{\mathcal{N}} N_s^{\mathcal{N}} - 1} \sum_{L_r^{\mathcal{N}} \times L_c^{\mathcal{N}} \times L_s^{\mathcal{N}}} \left(VD\,(r,c,s) - \mu_{VD}\right)^2} \tag{10}$$

$$sk_{VD} = \frac{1}{N_r^{\mathcal{N}} N_c^{\mathcal{N}} N_s^{\mathcal{N}} - 1} \sum_{L_r^{\mathcal{N}} \times L_c^{\mathcal{N}} \times L_s^{\mathcal{N}}} \left(\frac{VD\,(r,c,s) - \mu_{VD}}{\sigma}\right)^3 \tag{11}$$

$$ku_{VD} = \frac{1}{N_r^{\mathcal{N}} N_c^{\mathcal{N}} N_s^{\mathcal{N}} - 1} \sum_{L_r^{\mathcal{N}} \times L_c^{\mathcal{N}} \times L_s^{\mathcal{N}}} \left(\frac{VD\,(r,c,s) - \mu_{VD}}{\sigma}\right)^4 \tag{12}$$

Figure 6. Four moments for one slice of the examples: (a) Mean, (b) Standard Deviation, (c) Skewness, (d) Kurtosis

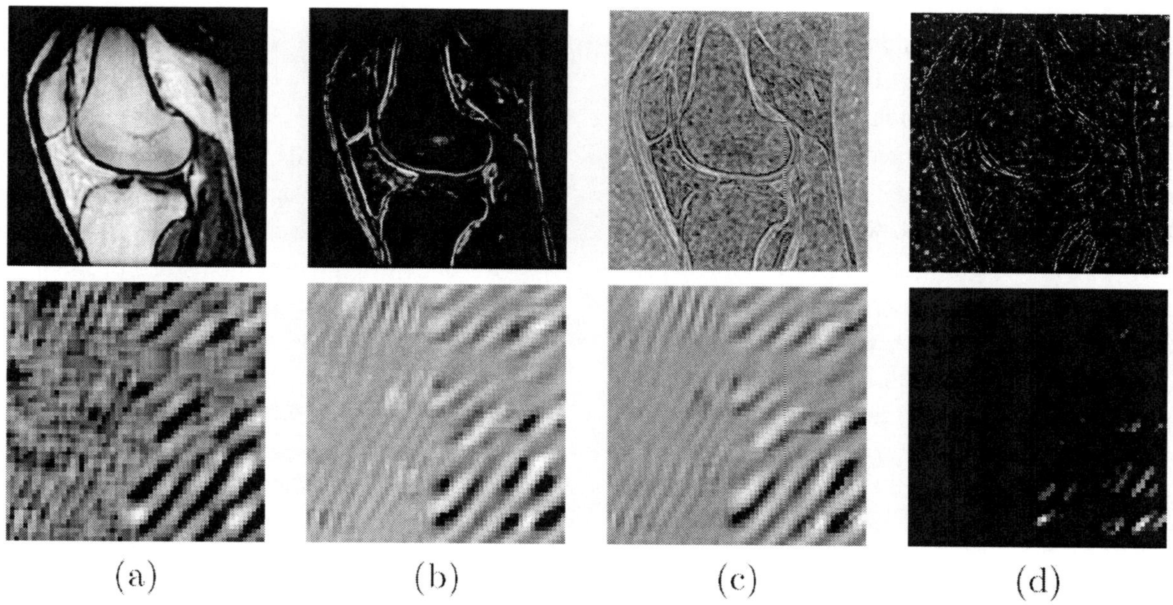

Figure 6 shows the results of calculating the four moments over a neighborhood of size 16×16 in a sliding window (overlapping) for the example data sets. It is important to mention that for higher moments the accuracy of the estimation will depend on the number of points. With only 256 points, the estimation is not very accurate.

For the knee data, it is interesting to observe that the higher values of the standard deviation correspond to the transition regions, roughly close to the edges of bones tissue and skin. The lower values correspond to more homogeneous regions, and account for more than 92% of the total elements.

While for the knee data, some of the results can be of interest, for the oriented textures the moments resemble a blurred version of the original image. From here we can observe that if these moments are of interest it will imply that a significant difference on the grey levels is present.

Convolutional Filters

The most important characteristic of the measurements that were presented in the previous section was that the relative position of the elements inside the neighborhood is not considered. In contrast to this, there are many methods in the literature that use a template to perform an operation among the elements inside a neighborhood. If the template is not isotropic then the relative position is taken into account. The template or filter is used as a sliding window over the data to extract the desired measurements. The operators respond differently to vertical, horizontal, or diagonal edges, corners, lines or isolated points.

The templates or filters will be arrays of different size: 2×2, 3×3, etc. To use these filters in 3D is just necessary to extend by one extra dimension and have filters of sizes: 2×2×2, 3×3×3, etc. The design and filtering effect will depend on the coefficients assigned to each element of the template: $z_1, z_2, z_3, \ldots$ that will interact with the voxels $x_1, x_2, x_3, \ldots$ of the data. If the coefficients of these filters are related to the values of the data through an equation $R=z_1x_1+z_2x_2+z_3x_3+\ldots$ this is considered as a *linear filter*. Other operations such as the *median, maximum, minimum, etc.* are possible. In those cases the filter is considered as a *non-linear filter*. The simplest case of these filters would be when all the elements z_i have equal values and the effect of the convolution is an averaging of neighboring elements. A very common set of filters is the one proposed in (Laws, 1980) that emerge from the combination of three basic vectors: [1 2 1] used for averaging, [-1 0 1] used for edges and [-1 2 -1] used for detecting spots. The outer product of two of these vectors can create many masks used for filtering.

These filters can easily be extended into 3D by using 3 vectors and have been used to analyze muscle fiber structures from confocal microscopic images (Lang *et al.*, 1991). The problem of Laws mask remains in the selection of the vectors; a great number of combinations can be generated in 3D and not all of them would be useful.

Differential filters are of particular importance for texture analysis. Applying a gradient operator ∇ to the data will result in a vector:

$$\nabla VD = \frac{\partial VD}{\partial r}\hat{r} + \frac{\partial VD}{\partial c}\hat{c} + \frac{\partial VD}{\partial s}\hat{s} \tag{13}$$

where $\left(\hat{r},\hat{c},\hat{s}\right)$ represent unitary vectors in the direction of each dimension. In practice the partial derivatives are obtained by the difference of elements, and while a simple template like $\begin{bmatrix}1 & -1\end{bmatrix}$, $\begin{bmatrix}1\\-1\end{bmatrix}$ would perform the difference of neighboring pixels in each direction, 3×3 operators like Sobel: $\begin{bmatrix}1 & 0 & -1\\2 & 0 & -2\\1 & 0 & -1\end{bmatrix}$, $\begin{bmatrix}1 & 2 & 1\\0 & 0 & 0\\-1 & -2 & -1\end{bmatrix}$ or Prewitt: $\begin{bmatrix}1 & 0 & -1\\1 & 0 & -1\\1 & 0 & -1\end{bmatrix}$, $\begin{bmatrix}1 & 1 & 1\\0 & 0 & 0\\-1 & -1 & -1\end{bmatrix}$, are commonly used. Roberts operator $\begin{bmatrix}1 & 0\\0 & -1\end{bmatrix}$, $\begin{bmatrix}0 & 1\\-1 & 0\end{bmatrix}$ is used to obtain differences in the diagonals. The differences between elements will visually sharpen the data; in contrast to the smoothing of the data created by averaging.

Other texture measurements use of the magnitude of the gradient (MG)

$$MG = \left(\left(\frac{\partial VD}{\partial r}\right)^2 + \left(\frac{\partial VD}{\partial c}\right)^2 + \left(\frac{\partial VD}{\partial s}\right)^2\right)^{\frac{1}{2}} \tag{14}$$

For example, the Zucker-Hummel filter (Zucker & Hummel, 1981):

$$\begin{bmatrix}\frac{1}{\sqrt{3}} & \frac{1}{\sqrt{2}} & \frac{1}{\sqrt{3}}\\ \frac{1}{\sqrt{2}} & 1 & \frac{1}{\sqrt{2}}\\ \frac{1}{\sqrt{3}} & \frac{1}{\sqrt{2}} & \frac{1}{\sqrt{3}}\end{bmatrix} \quad \begin{bmatrix}0 & 0 & 0\\0 & 0 & 0\\0 & 0 & 0\end{bmatrix} \quad \begin{bmatrix}\frac{-1}{\sqrt{3}} & \frac{-1}{\sqrt{2}} & \frac{-1}{\sqrt{3}}\\ \frac{-1}{\sqrt{2}} & -1 & \frac{-1}{\sqrt{2}}\\ \frac{-1}{\sqrt{3}} & \frac{-1}{\sqrt{2}} & \frac{-1}{\sqrt{3}}\end{bmatrix} \tag{15}$$

which has also been used as a gradient operator (Kovalev *et al.*, 2001; Kovalev *et al.*, 2003a; Kovalev *et al.*, 2003b; Segovia-Martínez *et al.*, 1999). Once the filter is convolved in each of the axis, either the magnitude or the orientation of the gradient at each voxel can be used to calculate three-dimensional histograms. If orientation is considered, the values are grouped into *bins* of solid angles. These histograms can be visualized with an extended Gaussian image (3D orientation indicatrix) (Kovalev *et al.*, 1999).

This filter is also used as a step of the 3D co-occurrence matrix proposed in (Kovalev et al., 1999; Kovalev & Petrou, 1996) and will be further discussed below.

Wavelets

Wavelet decomposition and Wavelet Packet are two common techniques used to extract measurements from textured data (Chang & Kuo, 1993; Fatemi-Ghomi, 1997; Fernández *et al.*, 2000; Laine & Fan, 1993; Rajpoot, 2002; Unser, 1995) since they provide a tractable way of decomposing images (or volumes) into different frequency components sub-bands at different scales.

Wavelet analysis is based on mathematical functions, the *Wavelets*, which present certain advantages over Fourier domain analysis when discontinuities appear in the data, since the *analyzing* or *mother* Wavelet ψ is a localized function limited in space (or time) and does not assume a function that stretches infinitely as do the sinusoidals of the Fourier domain analysis. The Wavelets or *small waves* should decay to zero at $\pm\infty$ (in practice they decay very fast) so in order to cover the space of interest (which can be the real line R) they need to be shifted along R. This could be done with integral shifts:

$$\psi(r-k), k \in Z, \tag{16}$$

where Z=[...,-1,0,1,...] is the set of integers. To consider different frequencies, the Wavelet needs to be dilated, one way of doing it is with a binary dilation in integral powers of 2:

$$\Psi(2^l r-k),\ k,l \in Z. \tag{17}$$

The signal $\Psi(2^l r-k)$ is obtained from the mother Wavelet $\psi(r)$ by a binary dilation 2^l and a dyadic translation $k/2^l$. The function $\Psi_{k,l}$ is defined as:

$$\Psi_{k,l}(r)=\Psi(2^l r-k),\ k,l \in Z. \tag{18}$$

The scaled and translated Wavelets need to be orthogonal to each other in the same way that sine and cosine are orthogonal, i.e.:

$$\langle \psi_{k,l}(r), \psi_{m,n}(r) \rangle = 0, \quad \text{for} \quad (k,l) \neq (m,n) \quad k,l,m,n \in \mathbb{Z} \tag{19}$$

Next, for the basis to be orthonormal, the functions need to have unit length. If ψ has unit length, then all of the functions $\Psi_{k,l}$ will also have unit length:

$$\| \Psi_{k,l}(r) \|_2 = 1. \tag{20}$$

Then, any function f can be written as:

$$f(r) = \sum_{k,l=-\infty} c_{k,l} \psi_{k,l}(r), \tag{21}$$

where $c_{k,l}$ are called the *Wavelet coefficients*, analogous to the notion of the Fourier coefficients and are given by the inner product of the function and the Wavelet:

$$c_{k,l} = \langle f, \psi_{k,l}(r) \rangle = \int_{-\infty}^{\infty} f(r)\, \psi_{k,l}^{*}(r) dr. \tag{22}$$

The Wavelet transform of a function $f(r)$ is defined as (Chui, 1992):

$$\Psi(a,b) = \frac{1}{\sqrt{|a|}} \int_{-\infty}^{\infty} f(r)\, \psi^{*}\left(\frac{r-b}{a}\right) dr. \tag{23}$$

The Wavelets must satisfy certain conditions, of which perhaps the most important one is the *admissibility condition*, which states that:

$$\int_{-\infty}^{\infty} \frac{|\psi_{\omega}(\rho)|^2}{|\omega|} d\rho < \infty, \tag{24}$$

where $\Psi_{\omega}(\rho)$ is the Fourier transform of the mother Wavelet $\psi(r)$. This condition implies that the function has zero mean:

$$\int_{\infty}^{\infty} \psi(r) dr = 0, \tag{25}$$

and that the Fourier transform of the Wavelet ψ vanishes at zero frequency. This condition prevents a Gabor filter from being a Wavelet since it is possible that a Gabor filter will have a value different from zero at the origin of the Fourier domain.

From a signal processing point of view, it may be useful to think of the coefficients and the Wavelets as filters, in other words, we are dealing with band pass filters, not low pass filters. To cover the low pass regions, a *scaling function* (Mallat, 1989) is used. This function does not satisfy the previous admissibility condition (and therefore it is not a Wavelet) but covers the low pass regions. In fact, this function should integrate to 1. So, by a combination of a Wavelet and a scaling function it is possible to split the spectrum of a signal into a low pass region and a high pass region. This combination of filters is sometimes called a *quadrature mirror filter pair* (Graps, 1995). The decomposition can continue by splitting the low pass region into another low pass and a band pass. This process is represented in Figure 7. To prevent the dimensions of the decomposition expanding at every step, a down-sampling (subsampling) step is performed in order to keep the dimensions constant. In many cases the down-sampling presents no degradation of the signals but it may not always be the case. If the down-sampling step is eliminated, the decomposition will provide an over-complete representation called *Wavelet Frames* (Unser, 1995).

It is important to remember that $e^{jx} = \cos(x)+j\sin(x)$ is the only function necessary to generate the orthogonal space in Fourier analysis. While through the use of Wavelets, it is possible to extract information that can be obscured by the sinusoidals. There is a large number of Wavelets to choose from: *Haar, Daubechies, Symlets, Coiflets, Biorthogonal, Meyer, etc.*, and some of them have variations according to the moments of the function. The nature of the data and the application can determine which family to use, but even with this knowledge, it is not always clear how to select a particular family of Wavelets.

The decomposition is normally performed only in the low pass region, but any other section can also be decomposed. When the high pass region (or band pass) is decomposed, an *adaptive Wavelet decomposition* or *Wavelet packet* is used. Figure 8 shows a schematic representation of a Wavelet packet.

The previous description of the Wavelet decomposition was based on a 1D function $f(r)$. When dealing with more than one dimension, the extension is usually performed by separable Wavelets and scaling functions applied in each dimension. In 2D, 4 options are obtained in one level of decomposition: **LL, LH, HL, HH**, that

Figure 7. (a) Wavelet decomposition by successively splitting the spectrum. (b) Schematic representation of the decomposition. In both cases the spectrum is subdivided first into low-pass and high pass, then the low-pass is subdivided into low-pass and high-pass successively until a desired level is reached

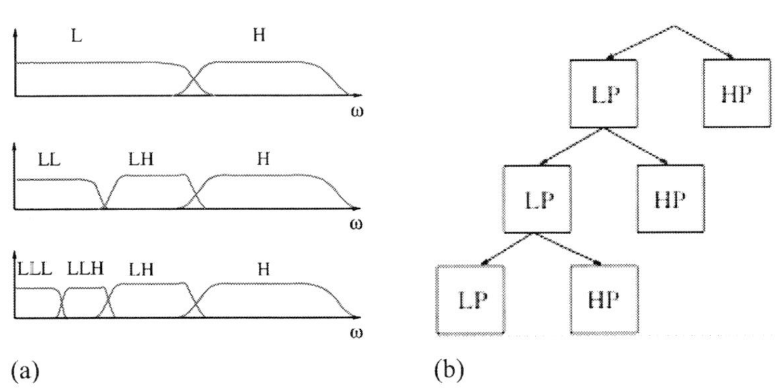

Figure 8. Wavelet packet decomposition. Both high pass and low pass are further split until a desired level of decomposition is reached

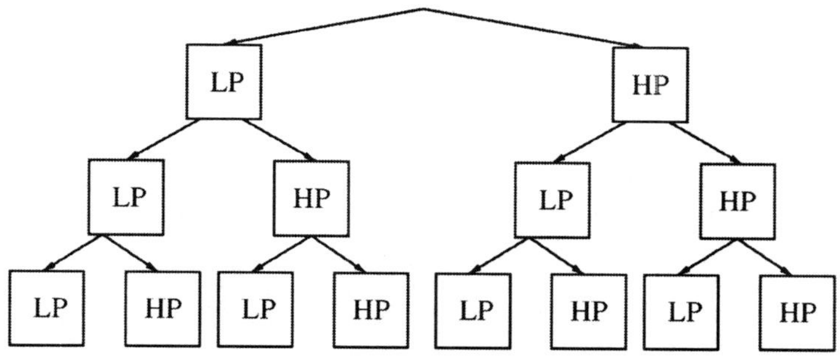

is low pass in both dimensions (LL), one low pass and one high pass in opposite dimensions (LH, HL) and high pass in both dimensions (HH). Figure 9 represents schematically a 3D separable Wavelet decomposition, eight different combinations of the filters (**LLL, LLH, LHL, LHH, HLL, HLH, HHL, HHH**) can be achieved in the first level of a 3D decomposition.

Figure 10 presents the first two levels of a 2D Wavelet decomposition (*Coiflet 1* used) of one slice of the human knee MRI.

Joint Statistics: The Co-Occurrence Matrix

The co-occurrence matrix defines the joint occurrences of grey tones (or ranges of tones) and is constructed by analyzing the grey levels of neighboring pixels. The co-occurrence matrix is a widely used technique over 2D images and some extensions to three dimensions have been proposed. We begin with a description of 2D co-occurrence.

2D Co-Occurrence

Let the original image I with dimensions for rows and columns $N_r \times N_c$ be quantized to N_g grey levels. The co-occurrence matrix will be a symmetric $N_g \times N_g$ matrix that will describe the number of co-occurrences of grey levels in a certain orientation and a certain element distance. The distance can be understood as a *chess-board* distance (D_8) (Gonzalez & Woods, 1992). The un-normalized co-occurrence matrix entry $\mathrm{CM}(g_1, g_2, D_8, \theta)$ records the number of times that grey levels g_1 and g_2 jointly occur at a neighboring distance D_8, in the orientation θ. For example, if $L_c=\{1,2,\ldots,N_c\}$ and $L_r=\{1,2,\ldots,N_r\}$ are the horizontal and vertical co-ordinates of an image I, and $G=\{1,\ldots,g_1,\ldots,g_2,\ldots,N_g\}$ the set of quantized grey levels, then the values of the un-normalized co-occurrence matrix $\mathrm{CM}(g_1,g_2)$ within a distance $D_8=1$ and $\theta = \frac{3\pi}{4}$ is given by:

Figure 9. A schematic representation of a 3D Wavelet decomposition

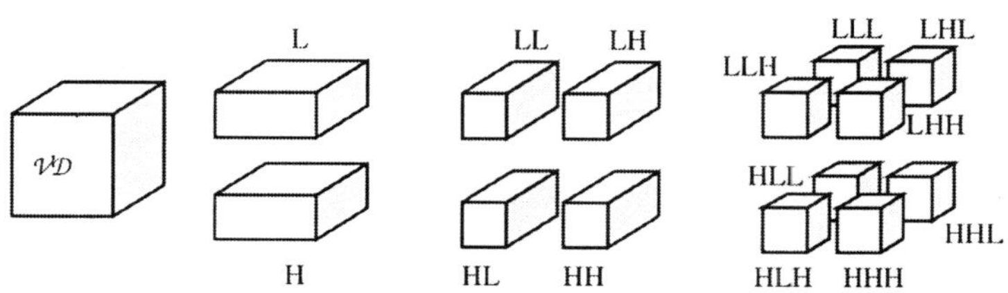

Figure 10. Two levels of a 2D Wavelet decomposition of one slice of the human knee MRI, (a) Level 1, (b) Level 2. In some cases, the four images of second level are placed in the upper-left quadrant of Level 1. In this case, they are presented separately to appreciate the filtering effect of the wavelets

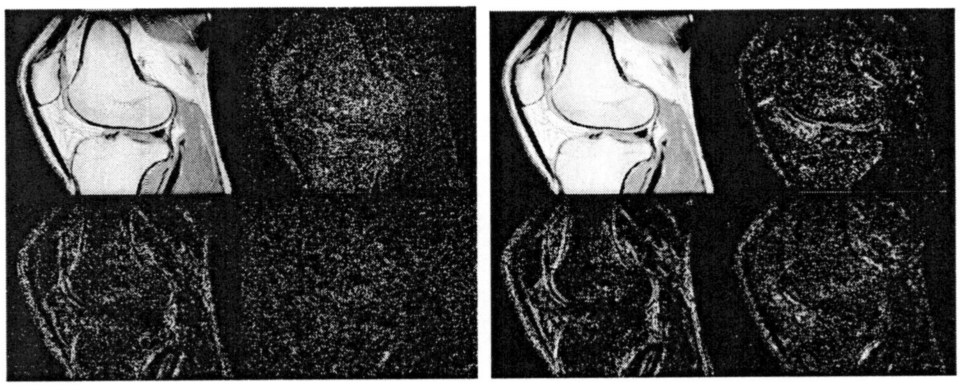

(a) (b)

$$CM(g_1, g_2, 1, 135^o) = \#\{((r_1, c_1), (r_2, c_2)) \in (L_r \times L_c) \times (L_r \times L_c) \mid ((r_1 - r_2 = 1, c_1 - c_2 = 1), I(r_1, c_1) = g_1, I(r_2, c_2) = g_2\}, \quad (26)$$

where # denotes the number of elements in the set. In other words, the matrix will be formed counting the number of times that two pixels with values g_1,g_2 appear contiguous in the direction down and to the right (south-east). In this way, a co-occurrence matrix is able to measure local grey level dependence: textural coarseness and directionality. For example, in coarse images, the grey level of the pixels change slightly with distance, while for fine textures the levels change rapidly. From this matrix, different features such as: *entropy, uniformity, maximum probability, contrast, correlation, difference moment, inverse difference moment, correlation* can be calculated (Haralick et al., 1973). It is assumed that all the texture information is contained in this matrix.

As an example to illustrate the properties of the co-occurrence matrix, 4 training regions, namely, *background, muscle, bone, tissue*, were selected from the MRI. Figure 11 shows the training samples location in the original image. For every texture, the co-occurrence matrix was calculated for 4 different orientations $\theta = \{0, \frac{\pi}{4}, \frac{\pi}{2}, \frac{3\pi}{4}\}$ and three distances D_8={1,2,3}. The results are presented in the Figure 12, Figure 13, Figure 14, Figure 15. Here are some brief observations about the co-occurrence matrices and their distributions:

- **Background**. The distribution of the co-occurrence matrix suggests a highly noisy nature with a skew towards the darker regions. There is a certain tendency to be more uniform in the horizontal direction (θ = 0) at a distance of D_8=1 which is the only matrix that is significantly different from the rest of the set.
- **Muscle**. The co-occurrence matrix is highly concentrated in the central region, the middle grey levels, and there is a lower spread compared with the background. A vertical structure can be observed, this in turn gives a certain vertical and horizontal (θ=0,π/2) uniformity, only at distance D_8=1.
- **Bone**. The nature of the bone is highly noisy as it can be observed from the matrices, but compared with the background,

Figure 11. Human knee MRI and four selected regions. These regions have different intensity levels and different textures that will be analyzed with co-occurrence matrices

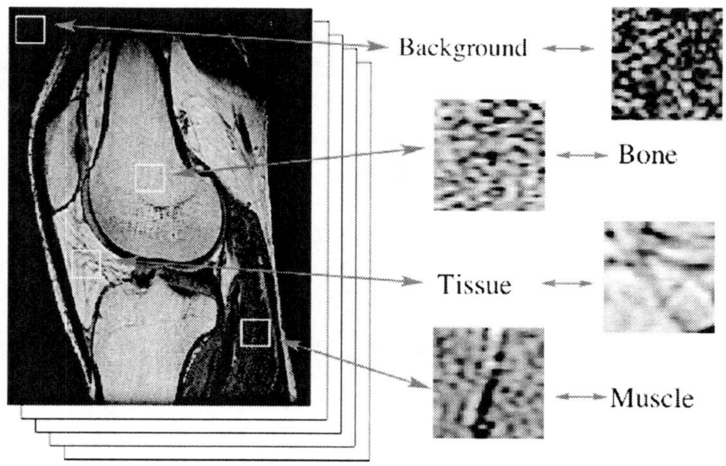

Figure 12. A sample of background, its histogram and co-occurrence matrices. The matrices describe a fairly uniform texture concentrated on the low intensity regions

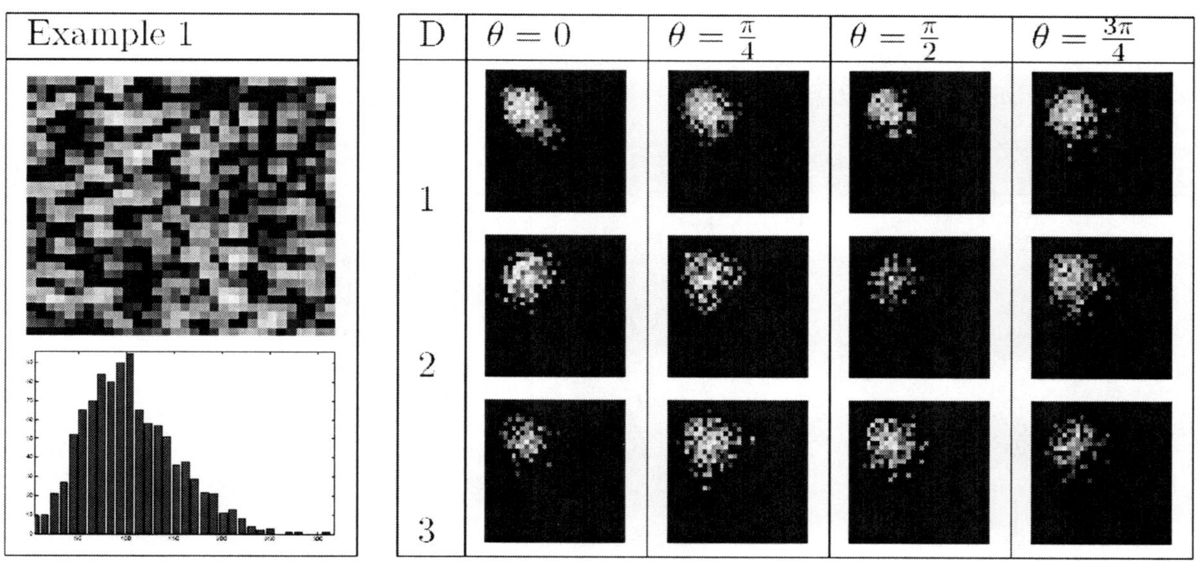

there is no skew towards dark or bright. As in the case of the muscle there is certain horizontal uniformity, but not vertical.

- **Tissue**. The distribution is skewed towards the brighter levels. The tissue presents several major structures with a 135° orientation, this makes the $\theta=\pi/4$ matrix to be more dispersed than the other orientations for distance $D_8=1$. As the distance increases the matrices spread towards a noisy configuration.

When observing the matrices, it is important to note which textures are invariant to distance or angle. Some useful characteristics of the co-occurrence matrix are presented in Table 1.

Figure 13. A sample of muscle, its histogram and co-occurrence matrices. The matrices describe a texture concentrated on the middle levels

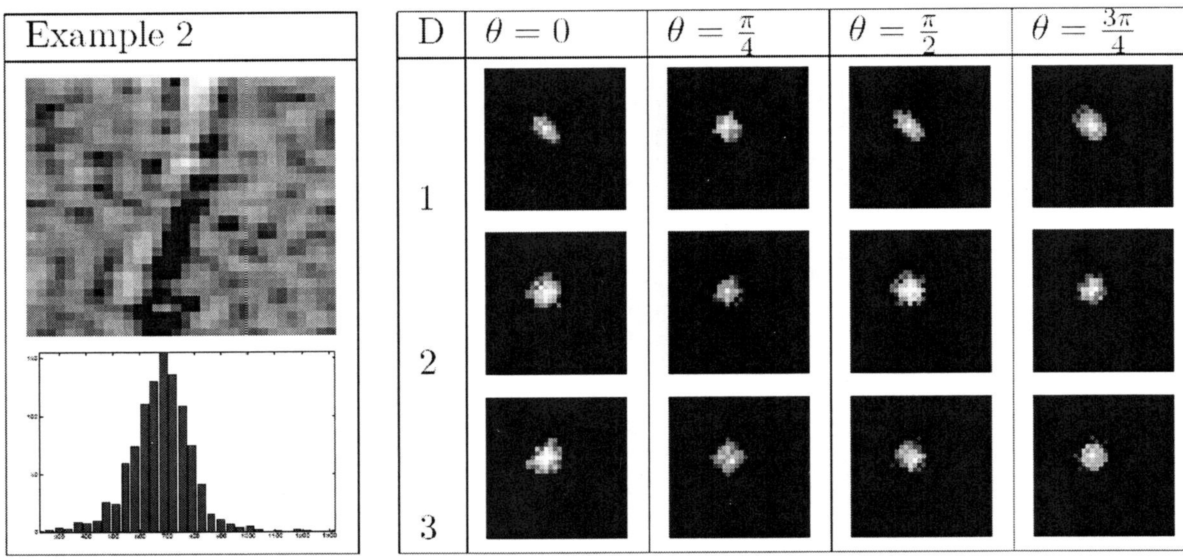

Figure 14. A sample of bone, its histogram and co-occurrence matrices. With the exception of the first matrix, the texture co-occurrences are rather uniform and spread. This suggests that bone has a strong component of orientation at ($\theta = 0$)

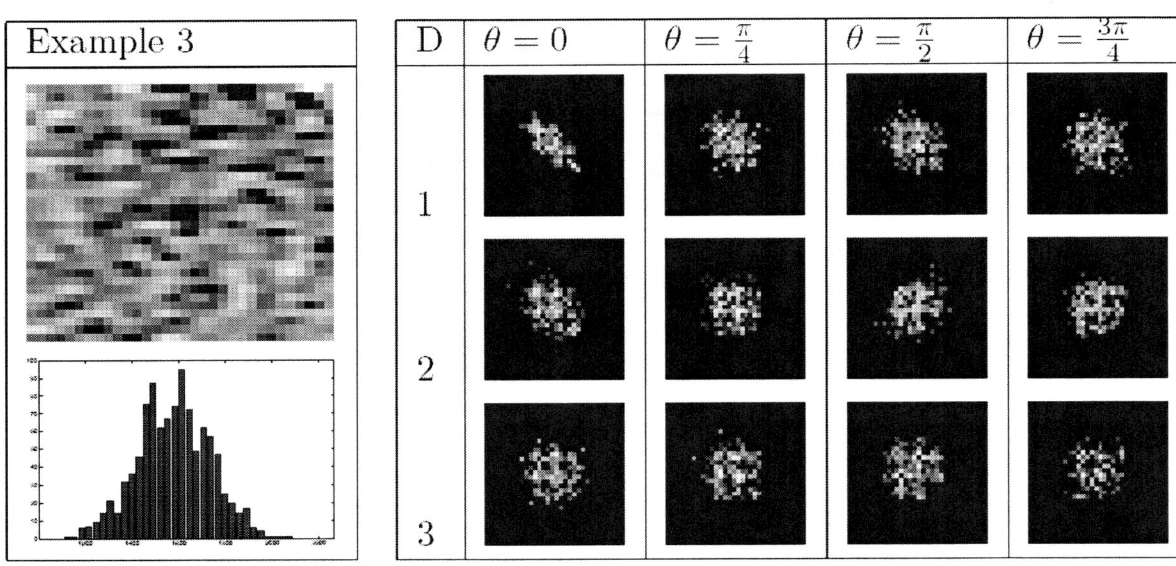

Some of the features determine the presence of a certain degree of organization, but others measure the complexity of the grey level transitions, and therefore are more difficult to identify. The textural features as defined in (Haralick et al., 1973) and (Haralick, 1979) are presented in Table 2 and Table 3. There are slight differences in the features presented in both texts, notice for instance that Contrast and Correlation are sometimes equivalently displayed as:

Figure 15. A sample of tissue, its histogram and co-occurrence matrices. The matrices indicate a highly concentrated texture towards the higher levels

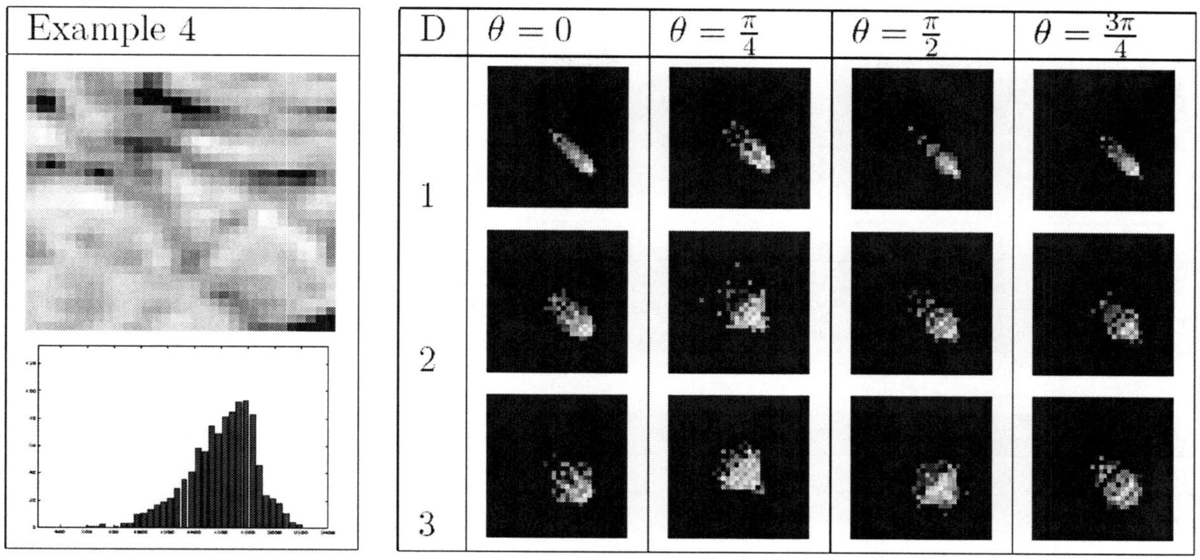

$$\varphi_2 = \sum_{g_1=1}^{N_g} \sum_{g_2=1}^{N_g} \left|g_1 - g_2\right|^k \left(cm(g_1, g_2)\right),$$

$$\varphi_3 = \sum_{g_1=1}^{N_g} \sum_{g_2=1}^{N_g} \frac{(g_1 - \mu)(g_2 - \mu)cm(g_1, g_2)}{\sigma^2}$$

Any single matrix feature or combination can be used to represent the local regional properties but it can be difficult to predict which combination will help discriminate regions without some experimentation.

The major disadvantage of the co-occurrence matrix is that its dimensions will depend on the number of grey levels. In many cases, the grey levels are quantized to reduce the computational cost and information is inevitably lost. Otherwise, the computational burden is huge. To keep computation tractable, the grey levels are quantized, D_8 is restricted to a small neighborhood and a limited number of angles θ are chosen. An important implication of quantizing the grey levels is that the sparsity of the co-occurrence matrix is reduced.

The images are normally processed by blocks of a certain size 4×4, 8×8, 16×16, etc., and they have an overlap which allows for rapid computation of the matrix (Alparonte *et al.*, 1990; Clausi & Jernigan, 1998). Even with these restrictions, the number of features can be very high and a selection method is required. If 4 angles are selected, with 15 textural features, the space will be of 60 features for every distance D_8; if D_8={1,2,3}, the feature space will have 180 dimensions. Figure 16 presents 60 features calculated on one slice of the MRI.

3D Co-Occurrence

When the co-occurrence of volumetric data sets *VD* is to be analyzed, the un-normalized co-occurrence matrix will become a five dimensional matrix:

$$CM(g_1, g_2, D_8, \theta, d), \tag{27}$$

where *d* will represent the slice separation of the voxels. Alternatively, two directions: θ, ϕ could be used. The computational complexity of this technique will grow considerably with this extension; the co-occurrence matrix could also be a very sparse matrix. The sparsity of the matrix could imply that quantizing could improve the

Table 1. Graphical characteristics of the co-occurrence matrix

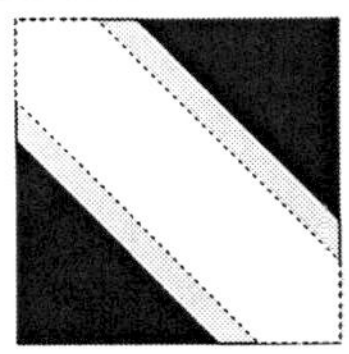	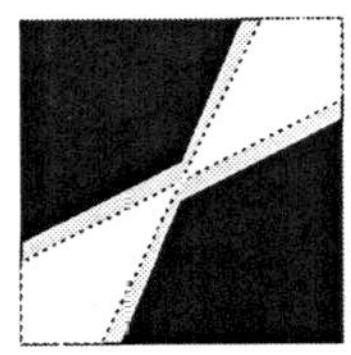	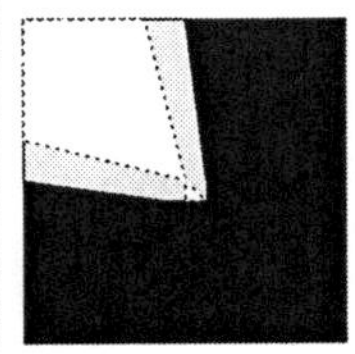	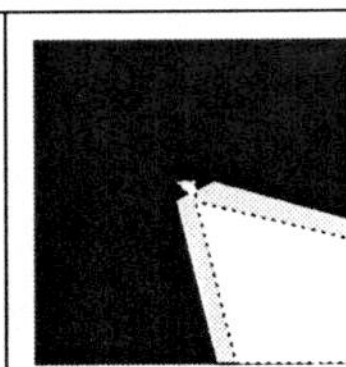	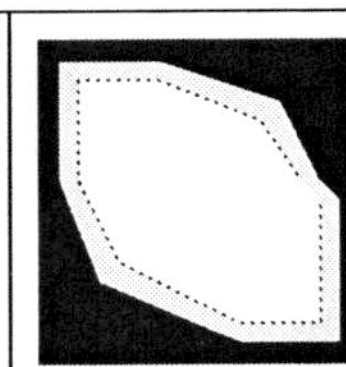	
(a)	(b)	(c)	(d)	(e)	(f)

	When the co-occurrence matrix is displayed as a grey-level intensity image, dark represents low occurrence, i.e. no transitions simultaneous occurrence of those intensity levels and bright represents high occurrence of those transitions. The main diagonal if formed by the occurrences of the transitions when $g_1 = g_2$.
(a)	High values in the main diagonal imply uniformity in the image. That is, most transitions occur between similar levels of grey for g_1 and g_2.
(b)	High values outside the main diagonal imply abrupt changes in the grey level, from very dark to very bright.
(c)	High values in the upper part imply a darker image.
(d)	High values in the lower part imply a brighter image.
(e)	High values in the lower central region part imply an image whose transitions occur mainly between similar grey levels and whose histogram is roughly of Gaussian shape.
(f)	In a noise image, the transitions between different grey levels should be balanced and it should be invariant to D_g and θ. The reverse, a balanced matrix, does not imply a noisy image.

complexity, or special techniques of sparse matrix could also be used (Clausi & Jernigan, 1998).

Early use of co-occurrence matrices with 3D data was reported by in (Ip & Lam, 1994) where data was partitioned, the co-occurrence matrix calculated, and three features for each partition were selected and then classified the data into homogeneous regions. The homogeneity is based on the features of the sub-partitions.

A generalized multidimensional co-occurrence matrix was presented in (Kovalev & Petrou, 1996). The authors propose *M*-dimensional matrices, which measure the occurrence of *attributes* or *relations* of the elements of the data; grey level is one attribute but others (such as magnitude of a local gradient) are possible. Rather than using the matrices themselves, features are extracted and used in several applications: to discriminate between normal brains and brains with pathologies, to detect defects on textures, and to recognize shapes.

Another variation of the co-occurrence matrix is reported in (Kovalev et al., 2001) where the matrix will include both grey level intensity and gradient magnitude:

$$CM(g_1,g_2,MG_1,MG_2,D_g,\theta,d). \qquad (28)$$

This matrix is called by the authors IIGGAD (Two Intensities, Two Gradients, Angle, Distance) who also consider reduced versions of the form: IID, GGD, GAD. The traditional co-occurrence matrix will be a particular case of the IIGGAD matrix. This matrix was used in the discrimination of brain data sets of patients with mild cognitive disturbance. This technique was also used to segment brain lesions but the method is not straightforward. First, a representative descriptor of the lesion is required. For this, a VOI that contains the lesion is required, which leads to a training set manually determined. Then, a mapping function is used to determine the probability of a voxel being in the lesion or not, based on

Table 2. Textural features of the co-occurrence matrix (Haralick, 1979; Haralick et al., 1973):

Angular Second Moment (Uniformity)	$\varphi_1 = \sum_{g_1=1}^{N_g} \sum_{g_2=1}^{N_g} \{cm(g_1, g_2)\}^2$
Element Difference Moment (Constrast)	$\varphi_2 = \sum_{n=0}^{N_g-1} n^2 \left\{ \begin{array}{c} \sum_{g_1=1}^{N_g} \sum_{g_2=1}^{N_g} \{cm(g_1, g_2)\}^2 \\ \lvert g_1 - g_2 \rvert = n \end{array} \right\}$
Correlation	$\varphi_3 = \dfrac{\sum_{g_1=1}^{N_g} \sum_{g_2=1}^{N_g} (g_1 g_2) cm(g_1, g_2) - \mu_x \mu_y}{\sigma_x \sigma_y}$
Sum of Squares (Variance)	$\varphi_4 = \sum_{g_1=1}^{N_g} \sum_{g_2=1}^{N_g} (g_1 - \mu)^2 \, cm(g_1, g_2)$
Inverse Difference Moment	$\varphi_5 = \sum_{g_1=1}^{N_g} \sum_{g_2=1}^{N_g} \dfrac{cm(g_1, g_2)}{1 + \lvert g_1 - g_2 \rvert^k}$
Sum Average	$\varphi_6 = \sum_{g_1=2}^{2N_g} g_1 p_{x+y}(g_1)$
Sum Variance	$\varphi_7 = \sum_{g_1=2}^{2N_g} (g_1 - \varphi_8)^2 p_{x+y}(g_1)$
Sum Entropy	$\varphi_8 = -\sum_{g_1=2}^{2N_g} p_{x+y}(g_1) \log\{p_{x+y}(g_1)\}$
Entropy	$\varphi_9 = -\sum_{g_1=1}^{N_g} \sum_{g_2=1}^{N_g} cm(g_1, g_2) \log\{cm(g_1, g_2)\}$
Difference Variance	$\varphi_{10} = Var\{p_{x-y}(g_3)\}$
Difference Entropy	$\varphi_{11} = -\sum_{g_1=0}^{N_g-1} p_{x-y}(g_1) \log\{p_{x-y}(g_1)\}$
Information Measures of Correlation	$\varphi_{12} = -\dfrac{HXY - HXY1}{\max\{HX, HY\}}$ $\varphi_{13} = (1 - e^{-2(HXY2 - HXY)})^{\frac{1}{2}}$
Maximal Correlation Coefficient	$\varphi_{14} = (\text{Sec. Larg. Eigenvalue of } Q)^{\frac{1}{2}}$
Maximum Pr *obability*	$\varphi_{15} = \max\{cm(g_1, g_2)\}$

the distances between the current VOI and the representative VOI of the lesion. Again this step needs tuning. The segmentation is carried out with a sliding-window analyzing the data for each VOI. Post-processing with knowledge of the WM area is required to discard false positives. The method segments the lesions of the WM but there is no clinical validation of the results.

Table 3. Notation used for the co-occurrence matrix and its features (Haralick, 1979; Haralick et al., 1973):

$cm(g_1, g_2) = \dfrac{CM(g_1, g_2)}{\sum CM}$	$(g_1, g_2)th$ entry in a normalized matrix
N_g	Number of gray levels of the quantized image
$p_x(g_1) = \sum_{g_2=1}^{N_g} cm(g_1, g_2)$	$g_1 th$ entry in the marginal probability matrix by summing the rows
$p_y(g_2) = \sum_{g_1=1}^{N_g} cm(g_1, g_2)$	$g_2 th$ entry in the marginal probability matrix by summing the columns
$p_{x+y}(g_3) = \sum_{g_1=1}^{N_g} \sum_{\substack{g_2=1 \\ g_1+g_2=g_3}}^{N_g} cm(g_1, g_2)$	$g_3 = 2, 3, \ldots, 2N_g$
$p_{x-y}(g_3) = \sum_{g_1=1}^{N_g} \sum_{\substack{g_2=1 \\ \|g_1+g_2=g_3\|}}^{N_g} cm(g_1, g_2)$	$g_3 = 0, 1, \ldots, N_g - 1$
$HXY = -\sum_{g_1=1}^{N_g} \sum_{g_2=1}^{N_g} cm(g_1, g_2) \log\{cm(g_1, g_2)\}$	Entropy of $cm(g_1, g_2)$
$HX = -\sum_{g_1=1}^{N_g} p_x(g_1) \log\{p_x(g_1)\}$	Entropy of $p_x(g_1)$
$HY = -\sum_{g_1=1}^{N_g} p_y(g_2) \log\{p_y(g_2)\}$	Entropy of $p_y(g_2)$
$HXY1 = -\sum_{g_1=1}^{N_g} \sum_{g_2=1}^{N_g} cm(g_1, g_2) \log\{p_x(g_1) p_y(g_2)\}$	
$HXY2 = -\sum_{g_1=1}^{N_g} \sum_{g_2=1}^{N_g} p_x(g_1) p_y(g_2) \log\{p_x(g_1) p_y(g_2)\}$	
$Q(g_1, g_2) = \sum_{g_3} \dfrac{cm(g_1, g_3)\, cm(g_2, g_3)}{p_x(g_1)\, p_y(g_2)}$	

In summary, co-occurrence matrices can be extended without much trouble to 3D and are a good way of characterizing textural properties of the data. The segmentation or classification with these matrices presents several disadvantages: first, the computational complexity of calculating the matrix is considerable for even small ranges of grey levels (even with fast methods (Alparonte et al., 1990; Clausi & Jernigan, 1998)). In many cases the range is quantized to fewer levels with possible loss of information. Second, the parameters on which the matrix depends: distance, orientation and number of bins in the 3D cases can yield a huge number of possible different matrices. If this dimensionality issue was not problematic enough, because there are a large number of features that can be extracted from the matrix, choosing the appropriate features will depend on the data and the specific analysis to be performed.

Figure 16. Features of the co-occurrence matrix for 4 different angles and distance $D_8=1$

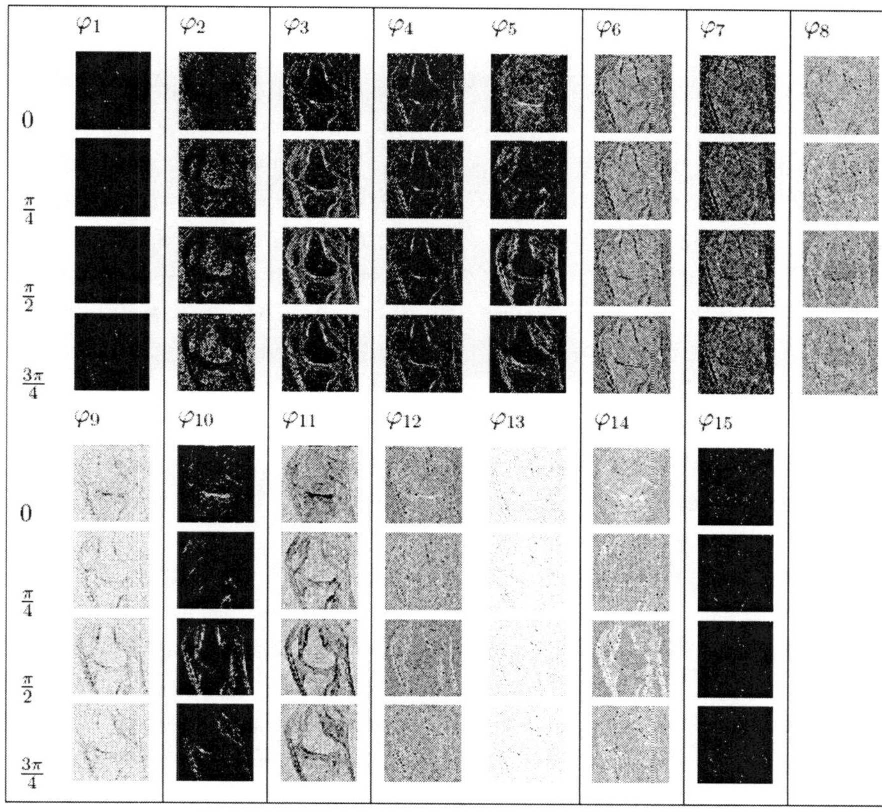

Sub-Band Filtering

In this section we will discuss some filters that can be applied to textured data. In the context of images or volumes, these filters can be understood as a technique that will modify the spectral content of the data. As mentioned before, textures can vary in their spectral distribution in the frequency domain, and therefore a set of sub-band filters can help in their discrimination.

The spatial and frequency domains are related through the use of the Fourier transform, such that a filter F in the spatial domain (that is the mask or template) will be used through a convolution with the data:

$$\tilde{VD} = F * VD \qquad (29)$$

where $\tilde{VD}$ is the filtered data. From the convolution theorem (Gonzalez & Woods, 1992) the same effect can be obtained in the frequency domain:

$$\tilde{VD}_\omega = F_\omega VD_\omega \qquad (30)$$

where the $\tilde{VD}_\omega = \mathcal{F}[\tilde{VD}]$, $VD_\omega = \mathcal{F}[VD]$, and $F_\omega = \mathcal{F}[F]$ are the corresponding Fourier transforms. The filters in the Fourier domain are named after the frequencies that are to be allowed to pass through them: *low pass, band pass* and *high pass* filters. Figure 17 shows the filter impulse response and the resulting filtered human knee for low pass, high pass and band pass filters.

The filters just presented have a very simple formulation and combinations through different frequencies will form a *filter bank*, which is an array of band pass filters that span the whole frequency domain spectrum. The idea behind the filter bank is to select and isolate individual frequency components. Besides the frequency, in 2D and 3D there is another important element of the filters, the *orientation*. The filters previously presented vary only in their frequency but remain isotropic with respect to the orientation of the filter; these filters are considered *ring* filters for the shape of the magnitude in the frequency domain. In contrast, the *wedge* filters will span the whole frequencies but only in certain orientations. Figure 18 presents some examples of these filters. Of course, the filters can be combined to concentrate only on a certain frequency and a certain orientation, so called *sub-band filtering*. Many varieties of sub-band filtering schemes exist; perhaps the most common is *Gabor filters*, described in the next section.

It is important to bear in mind that the classification process goes beyond the filtering stage as in some cases the results of filters have to be modified before obtaining a proper measurement to be used in a classifier. According to (Randen & Husøy, 1999) the classification process consists of the following steps: *filtering, non-linearity, smoothing, normalizing non-linearity* and *classification*. The first step corresponds to the output of the filters, then, a local energy function (LEF) is obtained with the non-linearity and the smoothing. The normalizing is an optional step before feeding everything to a classifier. Figure 19 demonstrates some of these steps. In this section we will concentrate on the filter responses and for all of them and use the magnitude as the non-linearity. The smoothing step is quite an important part of the classification as it may influence considerably the results.

Sub-Band Filtering with Gabor Filters

This multichannel filtering approach to texture is inspired by the human visual system that can segment textures preattentively (Malik & Perona, 1990). Experiments on psychophysical and neurophysiological data have led us to believe that the human visual system performs some local spatial-frequency analysis on the retinal image by a bank of tuned band pass filters (Dunn *et al.*,

Figure 17. Frequency filtering of the Human knee MR: Top Row (a) Low pass filter, (b) High pass filter, (c) Band pass filter. Bottom Row (d,e,f) Corresponding filtered images

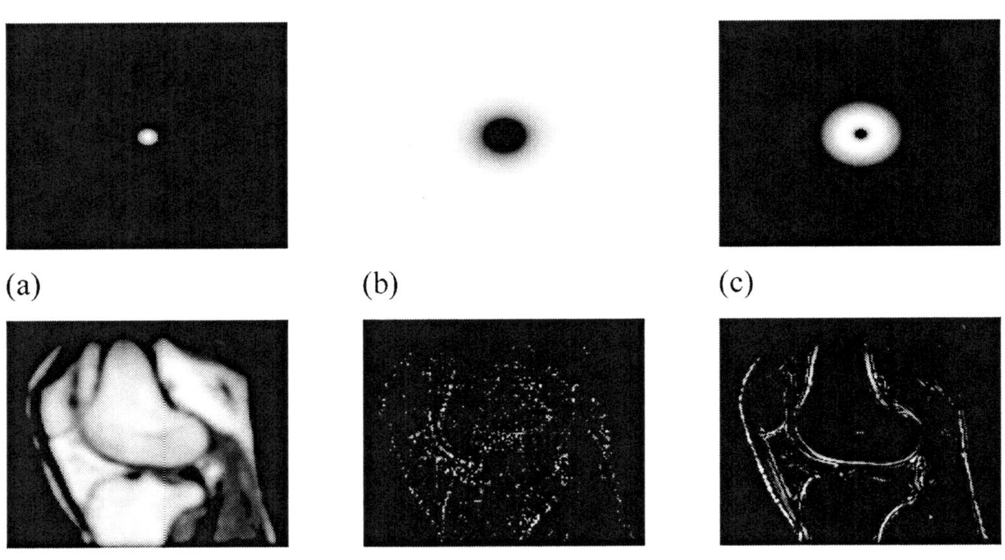

Figure 18. Different frequency filters: (a) Ring filter, (b) Wedge filter (c) Lognormal filter (Westin et al., 1997)

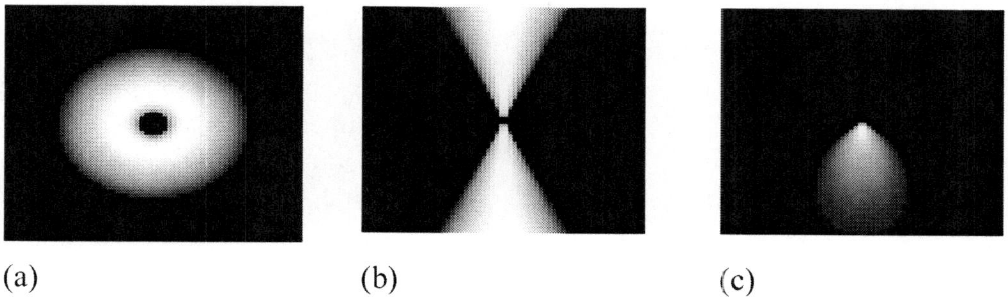

1994). In the context of communication systems, presented the concept of local frequency was presented in (Gabor, 1946), which has been used in computer vision by many researchers in the form of a multichannel filter bank (Bovik et al., 1990; Jain & Farrokhnia, 1991; Knutsson & Granlund, 1983). One of the advantages of this approach is the use of simple statistics of grey values of the filtered images as features or measurements of the textures.

The Gabor filter is presented in (Jain & Farrokhnia, 1991) as an even-symmetric function whose impulse response is the product of a Gaussian function $\mathcal{G}_a$ of parameters (μ,σ^2) and a modulating cosine. In 3D, the function is:

$$F^{\mathcal{G}} = \exp\left\{-\frac{1}{2}\left(\frac{r^2}{\sigma_r^2} + \frac{c^2}{\sigma_c^2} + \frac{s^2}{\sigma_s^2}\right)\right\}\cos\left(2\pi(r\rho_0 + c\kappa_0 + s\varsigma_0)\right), \quad (31)$$

where $\rho_0,\kappa_0,\varsigma_0$ are the frequencies corresponding to the center of the filter, and $\sigma_r^2,\sigma_c^2,\sigma_s^2$ are the constants that define the Gaussian envelope. The Fourier transform of the previous equation:

Figure 19. A filtering measurement extraction process

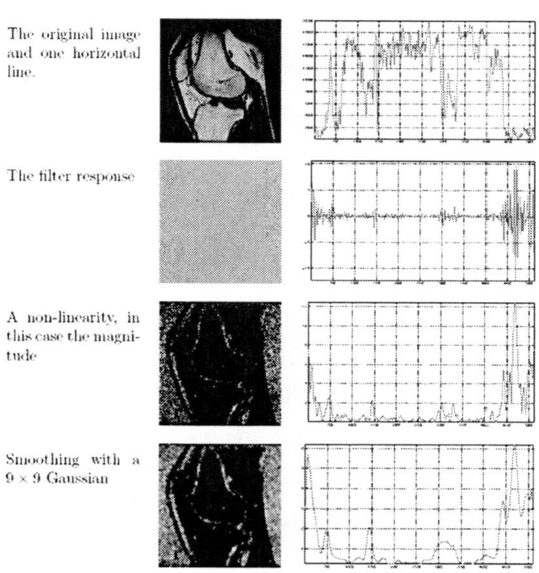

$$F_{\omega}^{\mathcal{G}} = A\exp\left\{-\frac{1}{2}\left[\frac{(\rho-\rho_0)^2}{\sigma_\rho^2}+\frac{(\kappa-\kappa_0)^2}{\sigma_\kappa^2}+\frac{(\varsigma-\varsigma_0)^2}{\sigma_\varsigma^2}\right]\right\}$$
$$A\exp\left\{-\frac{1}{2}\left[\frac{(\rho+\rho_0)^2}{\sigma_\rho^2}+\frac{(\kappa+\kappa_0)^2}{\sigma_\kappa^2}+\frac{(\varsigma+\varsigma_0)^2}{\sigma_\varsigma^2}\right]\right\} \quad (32)$$

where $\sigma_\rho = \frac{1}{2\pi\sigma_r}, \sigma_\kappa = \frac{1}{2\pi\sigma_c}, \sigma_\varsigma = \frac{1}{2\pi\sigma_s}$, and $A=2\pi\sigma_r\sigma_c\sigma_s$. The filter has two real-valued lobes, of Gaussian shape that have been shifted by $\pm(\rho_0,\kappa_0,\varsigma_0)$ frequency units along the frequency axes $\pm(\rho,\kappa,\varsigma)$ and rotated by an angle (θ,ϕ) with respect to the positive ρ axis. Figure 20 (a,b) presents a 2D filter in the spatial and Fourier domains.

The filter-bank is typically arranged in a *rosette* (Figure 20(c)) with several radial frequencies and orientations. The rosette is designed to cover the 2D frequency plane by overlapping filters whose centers lie in concentric circles with respect to the origin. The orientation and bandwidths are designed such that filters with the same radial frequency will overlap at the 50% of their amplitudes. In (Jain & Farrokhnia, 1991) it is recommended to use four orientations $\theta = \{0, \frac{\pi}{4}, \frac{\pi}{2}, \frac{3\pi}{4}\}$, and radial frequencies at octaves. The use of Gabor filters for the extraction of texture measurements has been widely used in 2D (Bigun & du-Buf, 1994; Bovik et al., 1990; Dunn & Higgins, 1995; Dunn et al., 1994; Jain & Farrokhnia, 1991; Randen & Husøy, 1999; Weldon *et al.*, 1996).

As an example, the example oriented pattern data was filtered with a 3D Gabor filter bank. Figure 21 (a) shows the envelope of the filter in the Fourier domain, this filter was multiplied with the data in the Fourier domain and one slice of the result in the spatial domain is presented in Figure 21 (c). The presence of two classes appears clearly. By thresholding at the midpoint between the grey levels of the filtered data, two classes can be roughly segmented (Figure 21 (d,e)).

The use of Gabor filters in 3D is not as common as in 2D. In (Zhan & Shen, 2003) the complete set of 3D Gabor features is approximated with two banks of 2D filters located at the orthogonal coronal and axial planes. In their application of Ultrasound prostate images, they claim that this approximation is sufficient to characterize the texture of the prostate. This approach is clearly limited since it is only analyzing 2 planes of a whole 3D volume. If the texture were of high frequencies that do not lie in either plane, then the characterization would fail.

In some cases, 1D Gabor filters have been used over data of more than one dimension (Kumar *et al.*, 2000; Randen *et al.*, 2003). The essence of the Gabor filter remains, in the sense

Figure 20. 2D even symmetric Gabor filters in: (a) Spatial domain, (b) Fourier domain. (c) A filter bank arranged in a rosette, 5 frequencies, 4 orientations

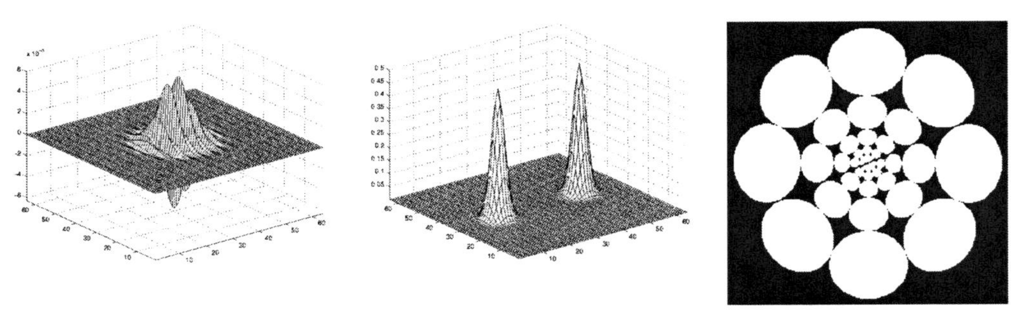

(a) (b) (c)

that a cosine modulates a Gaussian function, but the filters change notoriously. Consider the following comparison between 1D and 2D filters presented in Figure 22. The 2D filter is localized in frequency while the 1D filter spans through the Fourier domain in one dimension allowing a range of radial frequencies and orientations to be covered by the filter.

Sub-Band Filtering with Second Orientation Pyramid

A set of operations that subdivide the frequency domain of an image into smaller regions by the use of two operators *quadrature* and *center-surround* was proposed in (Wilson & Spann, 1988). By the combination of these operations, it is possible to construct different tessellations of the space, one of which is the Second Order Pyramid (SOP) (Figure 23). In this work, a band-limited filter based on truncated Gaussians (Figure 24) has been used to approximate the Finite Prolate Spheroidal Sequences (FPSS) used by Wilson and Spann. The filters are real, band-limited functions which cover the Fourier half-plane. Since the Fourier transform is symmetric, it is possible to use only half-plane or half-volume and still keep the fre-

Figure 21. (a) An even symmetric 3D Gabor in the Fourier domain, (b) One slice of the Oriented pattern data and (c) its filtered version with the filter from (a). (c,d) Two classes obtained from thresholding the filtered data

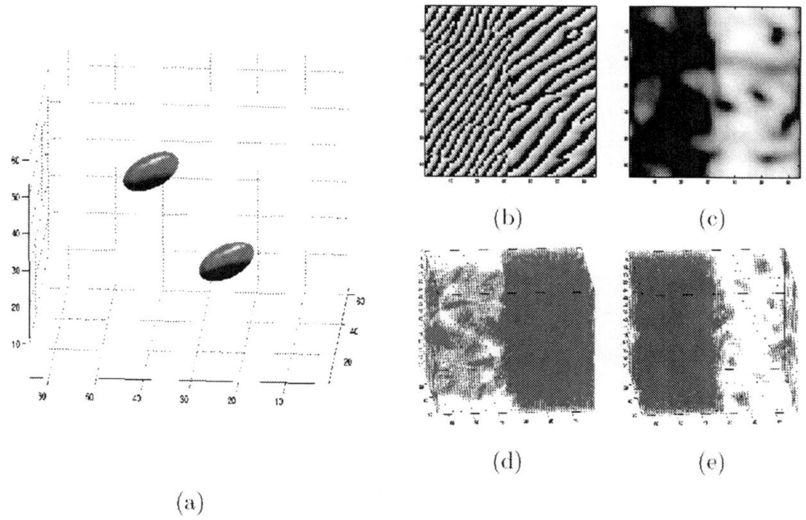

Figure 22. Comparison of 2D and 1D Gabor filters. An even symmetric 2D Gabor in: (a) spatial domain, and (b) Fourier domain. A 1D Gabor filter in: (c) spatial domain, and (d) Fourier domain

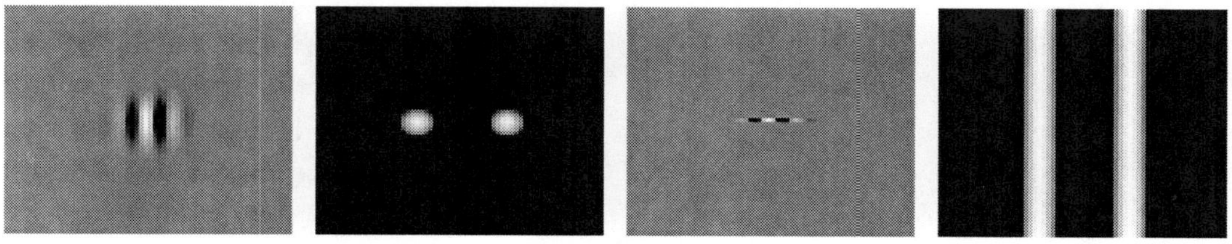

(a) (b) (c) (d)

Figure 23. 2D and 3D Second Orientation Pyramid (SOP) tessellation. Solid lines indicate the filters added at the present order while dotted lines indicate filters added in higher orders, as the central region is sub-divided. (a) 2D order 1, (b) 2D order 2, (c) 2D order 3, and (d) 3D order 1

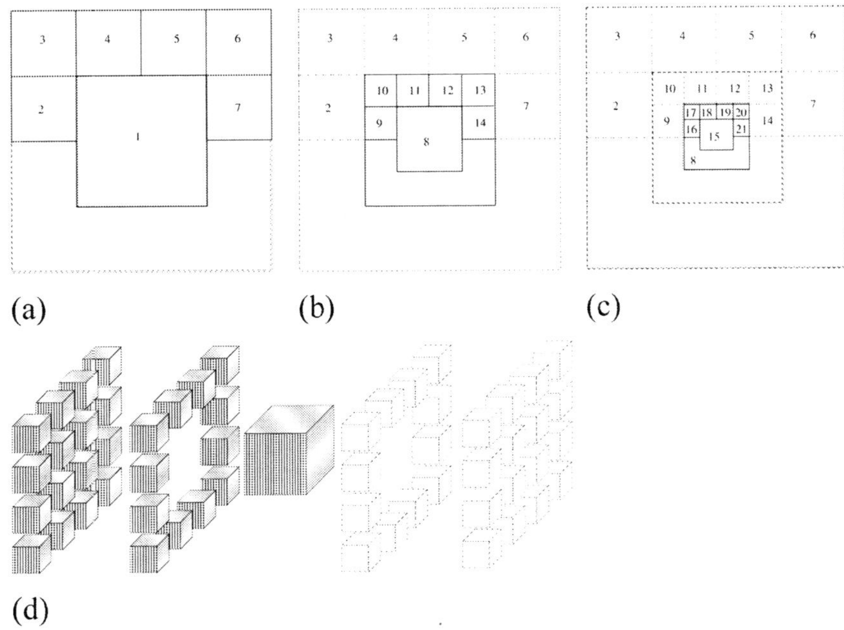

quency information. A description of the sub-band filtering with SOP process follows.

Any given volume VD whose centered Fourier transform is $VD_\omega = \mathscr{F}[VD]$ can be subdivided into a set of i regions $L_r^i \times L_c^i \times L_s^i$:

$$L_r^i = \{r, r+1, \ldots, r+N_r^i\}, 1 \le r \le N_r - N_r^i,$$

$$L_c^i = \{c, c+1, \ldots, c+N_c^i\}, 1 \le c \le N_c - N_c^i,$$

$$L_s^i = \{s, s+1, \ldots, s+N_s^i\}, 1 \le s \le N_s - N_s^i,$$

that follow the conditions:

$$\begin{aligned} &L_r^i \subset L_r, \sum_i N_r^i = N_r, \\ &L_c^i \subset L_c, \sum_i N_c^i = N_c, \\ &L_s^i \subset L_s, \sum_i N_s^i = N_s, \\ &(L_r^i \times L_c^i \times L_s^i) \cap (L_r^j \times L_c^j \times L_s^j) = \{\phi\}, \quad i \ne j. \end{aligned} \tag{33}$$

In 2D, the SOP tessellation involves a set of 7 filters, one for the low pass region and six for the high pass (Figure 23 (a)). In 3D, the tessellation will consist of 28 filters for the high pass region and one for the low pass (Figure 23 (d)). The i-th filter F_ω^i in the Fourier domain ($F_\omega^i = \mathscr{F}[F^i]$) is related to the i-th subdivision of the frequency domain as:

$$L_r \times L_c \times L_s; F_\omega^i : \begin{cases} L_r^i \times L_c^i \times L_s^i & \to \mathscr{G}_a(\mu^i, \Sigma^i) \\ (L_r^i \times L_c^i \times L_s^i)^c & \to 0 \end{cases} \quad \forall i \in SOP \tag{34}$$

where a $\mathscr{G}_a$ describes a Gaussian function, with parameters μ^i, the center of the region i, and $\sum^i$ is the co-variance matrix that will provide a cut-off of 0.5 at the limit of the band (for 2D Figure 24). In 3D, the filters will again be formed by truncated 3D Gaussians in an octave-wise tessellation that resembles a regular Oct-tree configuration. In the case of MRI data, these filters can be ap-

Figure 24. Band-limited 2D Gaussian filter (a) Frequency domain F^i_ω, (b) Magnitude of spatial domain $|F^i|$

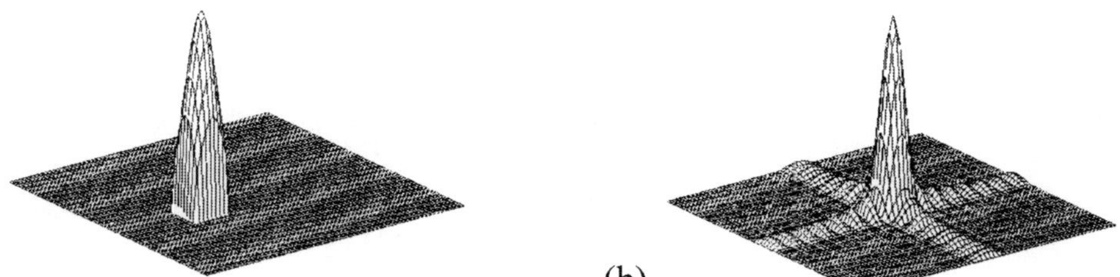

(a) (b)

plied directly to the K-space. (The image that is presented as an MRI is actually the inverse Fourier transform of signals detected in the MRI process, thus the K-space looks like the Fourier transform of the image that is being filtered.)

The measurement space S in its frequency and spatial domains will be defined as:

$$S^i_\omega(\rho,\kappa,\varsigma) = F^i_\omega(\rho,\kappa,\varsigma)\,VD^i_\omega(\rho,\kappa,\varsigma)$$
$$\forall(\rho,\kappa,\varsigma) \in (L_r \times L_c \times L_s),$$

$$S^i = \left|\mathcal{F}^{-1}[S^i_\omega]\right| \qquad (35)$$

The same scheme used for the first order of the SOP can be applied to subsequent orders of the decomposition. At every step, one of the filters will contain the low pass (i.e. the center) of the region analyzed, VD_w for the first order, and the six (2D) or 28 (3D) remaining will subdivide the high pass bands of the surround of the region.

For simplicity we detail only the co-ordinate systems in 2D:

$$\textbf{Centre}: F^1: \quad L^1_r = \{\frac{N_r}{4}+1,\ldots,\frac{3N_r}{4}\}, L^1_c = \{\frac{N_c}{4}+1,\ldots,\frac{3N_c}{4}\}, \qquad (36)$$

$$\textbf{Surround}: F^{2-7}: \quad L^{3,4,5,6}_r = \{1,\ldots,\frac{N_r}{4}\}, L^{2,7}_r = \{\frac{N_r}{4}+1,\ldots,\frac{N_r}{2}\},$$
$$L^{2,3}_c = \{1,\ldots,\frac{N_c}{4}\}, L^4_c = \{\frac{N_c}{4}+1,\ldots,\frac{N_c}{2}\},$$
$$L^5_c = \{\frac{N_c}{2}+1,\ldots,\frac{3N_c}{4}\}, L^{6,7}_c = \{\frac{3N_c}{4}+1,\ldots,N_c\}.$$

For a pyramid of order 2, the region to be subdivided will be the central region (of order 1) described by $(L^1_r(1) \times L^1_c(1))$ which will become $(L_r(2)\times L_c(2))$ with dimensions

$$N_r(2) = \frac{N_r(1)}{2}, \quad N_c(2) = \frac{N_c(1)}{2},$$

(or in general $N_{r,c}(o+1) = \frac{N_{r,c}(o)}{2}$, for any order o). It is assumed that $N_r(1)=2^a$, $N_c(1)=2^b$, $N_d(1)=2^c$ so that the results of the divisions are always integer values. The horizontal and vertical frequency domains are expressed by:

$$L_r(2) = \{\frac{N_r(1)}{4}+1,\ldots,\frac{3N_r(1)}{4}\},$$
$$L_c(2) = \{\frac{N_c(1)}{4}+1,\ldots,\frac{3N_c(1)}{4}\}$$

and the next filters can be calculated recursively: $L^8_r(1) = L^1_r(2)$, $L^8_c(1) = L^1_c(2)$, $L^9_r(1) = L^2_r(2)$, etc. To visualize the SOP on a textured image, an example is presented in Figure 25.

Figure 26 shows a slice from a different MRI set and the measurement space S for the first two orders of the SOP: S^{2-14}. The effect of the filtering becomes clear now, as some regions (corresponding to a particular texture) are highlighted by some filters and blocked by others. S^8 is a low pass filter and keeps a blurred resemblance to the original image. The background is highlighted in

Figure 25. A graphical example of the sub-band filtering. The top row corresponds to the spatial domain and the bottom row to the Fourier domain. A textured image is filtered with a sub-band filter with a particular frequency and orientation by a product in the Fourier domain, which is equivalent to a convolution in the spatial domain. The filtered image becomes one measurement of the space **S**, *S^2 in this case*

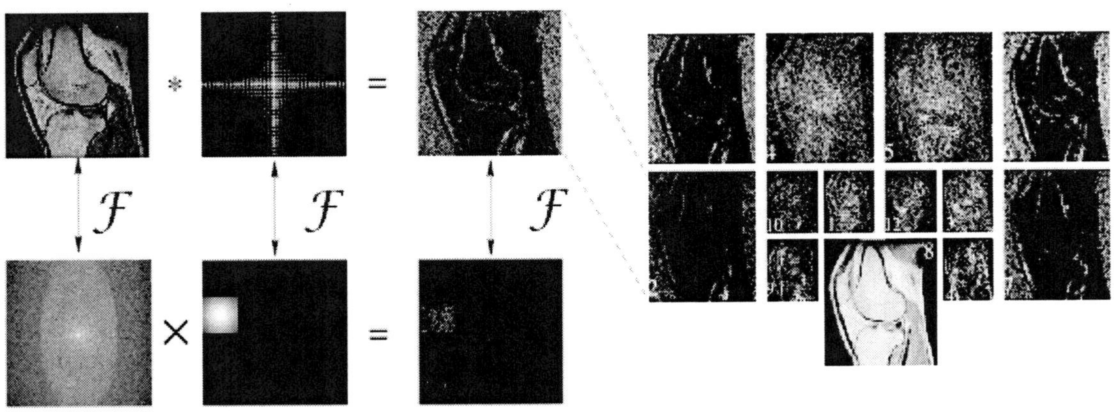

the high frequency filters, as should be expected of a noisy nature.

It should be mentioned that the previous analysis focuses on the magnitude of the inverse Fourier transform. The phase information (Boashash, 1992; Chung *et al.*, 2002; Knutsson *et al.*, 1994) has not been thoroughly studied, partly because of the problem of unwrapping in the presence of noise, but it deserves more attention in the future. The phase unwrapping in the presence of noise is a difficult problem since the errors that are introduced by noise accumulate as the phase is unwrapped. If the K-space is available, it should be used and this problem would be avoided since the K-space is real.

Local Binary Patterns and Texture Spectra

Two similar methods that try to explore the relations between neighboring pixels have been proposed in (He & Wang, 1991; Wang & He, 1990) and (Ojala *et al.*, 1996). These methods concentrate on the relative intensity relations between the pixels in a small neighborhood and not in their absolute intensity values or the spatial relationship of the whole data. The underlying assumption is that texture is not properly described by the Fourier spectrum (Wang & He, 1990) or traditional low pass / band pass / high pass filters.

To overcome the problem of characterizing texture, Wang and He proposed a texture filter based on the relationship of the pixels of a 3×3 neighborhood. A *Texture Unit* (*TU*) is first calculated by differentiating the grey level of a central pixel x_0 with the grey level of its 8 neighbors x_i. The difference is measured as 0 if the neighbor x_i has a lower grey level, 1 if they are equal and 2 if the neighbor has a bigger grey level. It is possible to quantize *G* by introducing a small positive value Δ. Thus the *TU* is defined as:

$$TU = \begin{bmatrix} E_1 & E_8 & E_7 \\ E_2 & & E_6 \\ E_3 & E_4 & E_5 \end{bmatrix} = \{E_1, \ldots, E_8\}, \quad E_i = \begin{cases} 0 & \text{if} \quad g_i \le (g_0 - \Delta) \\ 1 & \text{if} \quad (g_0 - \Delta) \le g_i \le (g_0 + \Delta) \\ 2 & \text{if} \quad g_i \ge (g_0 + \Delta) \end{cases} \tag{37}$$

After the *TU* has been obtained, a *texture unit number* (N_{TU}) is obtained by weighting each element of the *TU* vector:

$$N_{TU} = \sum_{i=1}^{8} E_i \times 3^{i-1}, \quad N_{TU} \in \{0, 1, \ldots, 6560\} \tag{38}$$

Figure 26. (a) One slice of a human knee MRI and (b) Measurements 2 to 14 of the textured image. (Note how different textures are highlighted by different measurements. In each set, the measurement S^i is placed in the position corresponding to the filter F^i_ω in the frequency domain).

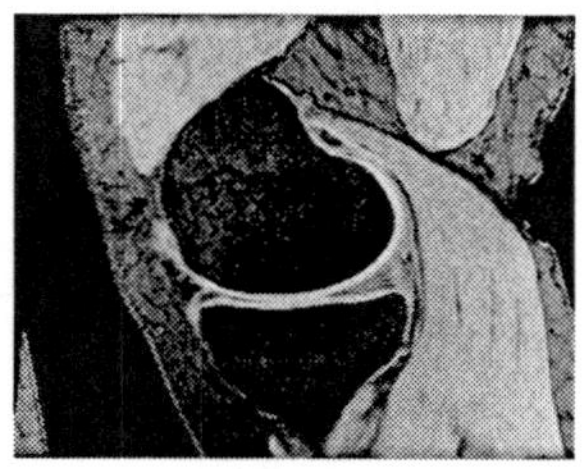

(a)

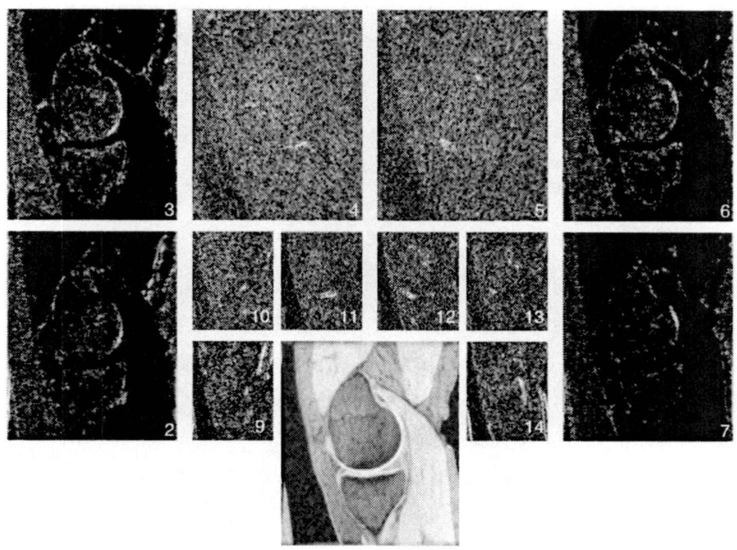

(b)

The sum of all N_{TU} elements for a given image will span from 0 to 6560 () and it is called the *texture spectrum*, which is a histogram of the filtered image. Since there is no unique way of labeling and ordering the texture units, the results of a texture spectrum are difficult to compare. For example, two slices of our example data were processed with the following configuration: $\begin{bmatrix} 1 & 27 & 243 \\ 3 & & 729 \\ 9 & 81 & 2187 \end{bmatrix}$ with Δ=0. Figure 27 shows the spectra and the filtered images.

The first observation of the texture spectrum comes from the filtered images. The oriented data seem to be filtered by an edge detection filter, the human knee also shows this characteristic around the edges of the bones and the skin. He and Wang claim that the filtering effect of the texture spectrum *enhances subjectively the textural perception*. This may well be an edge enhancement, which for certain textures could be an advantage; as an example they cite lithological units in a geological study. However, not every texture would benefit from this filtering. Another serious disadvantage is that this filtering is presented as a pre-processing step for a co-occurrence analysis. Co-occurrence by itself can provide many features, if this Texture spectrum filter is added as a pre-processing step, a huge amount of combinations

Figure 27. The Texture Spectrum and its corresponding filtered image of (a,b). Oriented data, (c,d) Human knee MRI

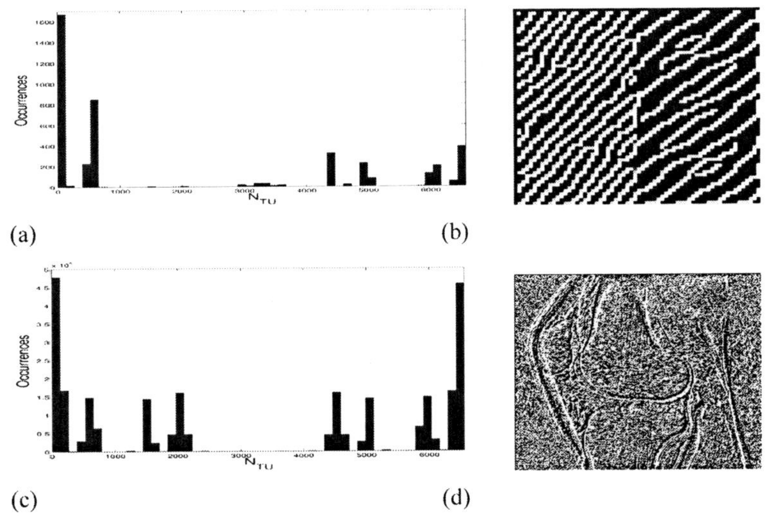

are possible, just the labeling to obtain the N_{TU} could alter significantly the results. Figure 28 shows the result of using a different order for the N_{TU}.

To the best of the authors' knowledge, this technique has not been extended to 3D yet. To do so, a neighborhood of size 3×3×3 should be used as a *TU*, and then N_{TU} of 3^{26}=2.5×10^{12} combinations would result. The texture spectrum would not be very dense with that many possible texture units. In our opinion, this would not be a good method in 3D.

A variation of the previous algorithm, called *Local Binary Pattern* (LBP) is presented in (Ojala et al., 1996). The pixel difference is limited to two options: $g_i \geq g_0, g_i < g_0$ and instead of 3^8=6561 there are only 2^8=256 possible texture units, which simplifies considerably the spectrum. If this method were to be extended into 3D the texture units would drop to 2^{26}=67,108,864, perhaps still too large. Two main advantages of texture spectrum and LBP is that there is no need to quantize the feature space and there is some immunity to low frequency artifacts such as those created by inhomogeneities of the MRI process. In the same paper, another measure is presented; the grey level difference method (DIFFX DIFFY) where a histogram of the absolute grey-level differences between neighboring pixels is computed in vertical and horizontal directions. This measure is a variation of a co-occurrence matrix but instead of registering the pairs of grey levels, the method registers the absolute differences. The distance is restricted to 1 and the directions are restricted to 2. They report that the results of this method are better than other texture measures, such as Laws masks or Gaussian Markov Random Fields.

In a more recent paper (Ojala *et al.*, 2001) another variation to the LBP considered the sign of the difference of the grey-level differences histograms. Under the new scheme, LBP is a particular case of the new operator called p_8. This operator is considered as a probability distribution of grey levels, where $p(g_0,g_1)$ denotes the co-occurrence probabilities, they use $p(g_0,g_1-g_0)$ as a joint distribution. Then, a strong assumption is made on the independence of the distribution, which they manipulate such that $p(g_0,g_1-g_0)=p(g_0)p(g_1-g_0)$. The authors present an error graph, which does not fall to zero, yet they consider this average error to be small and therefore independence to be a reasonable assumption. This comparison was

Figure 28. Filtered versions of the oriented data with different labelings (a,b) Filtered data, (c,d) arrangements of E_i

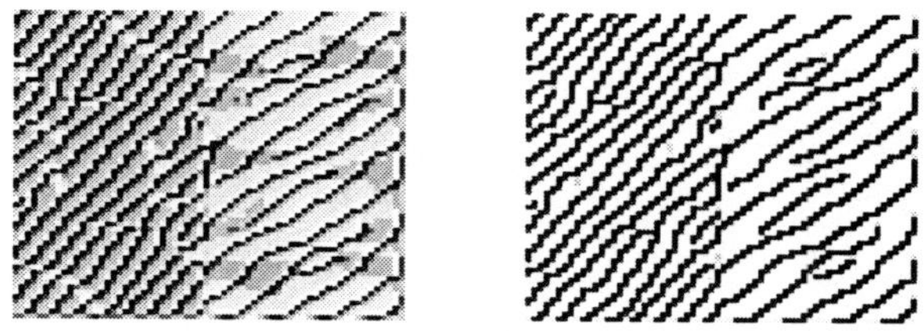

(a) (b)

$$\begin{bmatrix} 3 & 9 & 27 \\ 1 & & 81 \\ 2187 & 729 & 243 \end{bmatrix} \qquad \begin{bmatrix} 2187 & 81 & 9 \\ 729 & & 3 \\ 243 & 27 & 1 \end{bmatrix}$$

(c) (d)

made for only 16 grey levels, it would be very interesting to report for 256 or 4096 grey levels.

Besides the texture measurement extraction with the signed grey-level differences, a discrimination process is presented. The authors present their segmentation results on the images arranged in (Randen & Husøy, 1999) which allows comparison of their method, but they do not present a comparison for the measurements separated from their segmentation method, which could influence considerably. This method quantizes the difference space to reduce the dimensionality, then uses a sampling disk to obtain a sample histogram, uses a small number of bins, lower than their own reliability criterion, and also uses a local adjustment of the grey scales for certain images.

The Trace Transform

The *Trace Transform* (Kadyrov & Petrou, 2001; Petrou & Kadyrov, 2004) is a generalized version of the Radon transform and has seen recent applications in texture classification (Kadyrov *et al.*, 2002). As some other transforms, the Trace transform measures image characteristics in a space that is non-intuitive. One of the main advantages of the Trace transform is its invariance to affine transformations, that is, translation, rotation and scaling.

The basis of the transformation is to scan an image with a series of lines or traces defined by two parameters: an orientation ϕ and a radius p, relative to an origin O shown in Figure 29. The Trace transform calculates a functional T_r over the line t defined by (ϕ, p); with the functional, the variable t is eliminated. If an integral is used as the functional, a Radon transform is calculated, but one is not restricted to the integral as the functional. Some of the functionals proposed in (Kadyrov et al., 2002) are shown in Table 4, but many other options are possible. The Trace transform results in a 2D function of the variables (ϕ, p). As an example, Figure 30 show the Trace transform of one slice of the oriented data with three different functionals.

With the use of two more functionals over each of the variables, a single number called the *triple feature* can be obtained: $\Phi[P[T_r[I]]]$. These features are called the *diametrical* functional P, and the *circus* functional Φ. Again there are many options for each of the functionals, (Table 4). The combinations of different functionals can easily lead to thousand of features. The relevance of the features has to be evaluated in a training phase and then a set of weighted features can be used to form a similarity measure between images. In (Kadyrov et al., 2002) it is reported that the Trace transform is much more powerful than the co-

Figure 29. The Trace transform parameters. A trace (t) that scans the image will have a certain angle (ϕ) and a distance (p) from the origin of the image

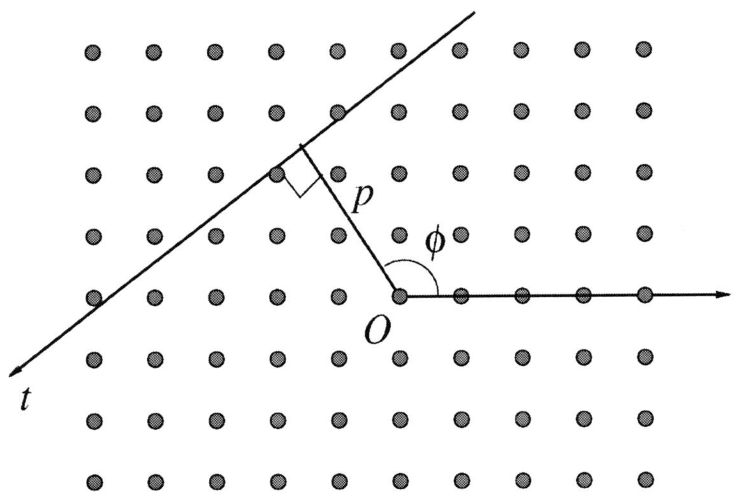

Table 4. Some functionals for Trace $\mathbf{T}_r$*, diametrical* **P** *and circus* **Φ**

	T_r	P	Φ
1	$\sum_{i=0}^{N} t_i$	$\max(t_i)$	$\sum_{i=0}^{N-1} \lvert t_{i+1} - t_i \rvert^2$
2	$\sum_{i=0}^{N} it_i$	$\min(t_i)$	$\sum_{i=0}^{N-1} \lvert t_{i+1} - t_i \rvert$
3	$\sqrt{\sum_{i=0}^{N} t_i^2}$	$\sqrt{\sum_{i=0}^{N} t_i^2}$	$\sqrt{\sum_{i=0}^{N} t_i^2}$
4	$\max(t_i)$	$\sum_{i=0}^{N} it_i \Big/ \sum_{i=0}^{N} t_i$	$\sum_{i=0}^{N} t_i$
5	$\sum_{i=0}^{N-1} \lvert t_{i+1} - t_i \rvert$	$\sum_{i=0}^{N} it_i$	$\max(t_i)$
6	$\sum_{i=0}^{N-1} \lvert t_{i+1} - t_i \rvert^2$	$\frac{1}{N}\sum_{i=0}^{N} (t_i - t)^2$	$\max(t_i) - \min(t_i)$
7	$\sum_{i=0}^{N-2} \lvert t_{i-2} + t_{i-1} - t_{i+1} - t_{i+2} \rvert$	c so that $\sum_{i=0}^{c} t_i = \sum_{i=c}^{N} t_i$	i so that $t_i = \max(t_i)$

Figure 30. Three examples of the Trace transform of the Oriented Pattern: (a) Functional 1, (b) Functional 4 and (c) Functional 5. The transformations do not present an intuitive image but important metrics can be extracted with different functions

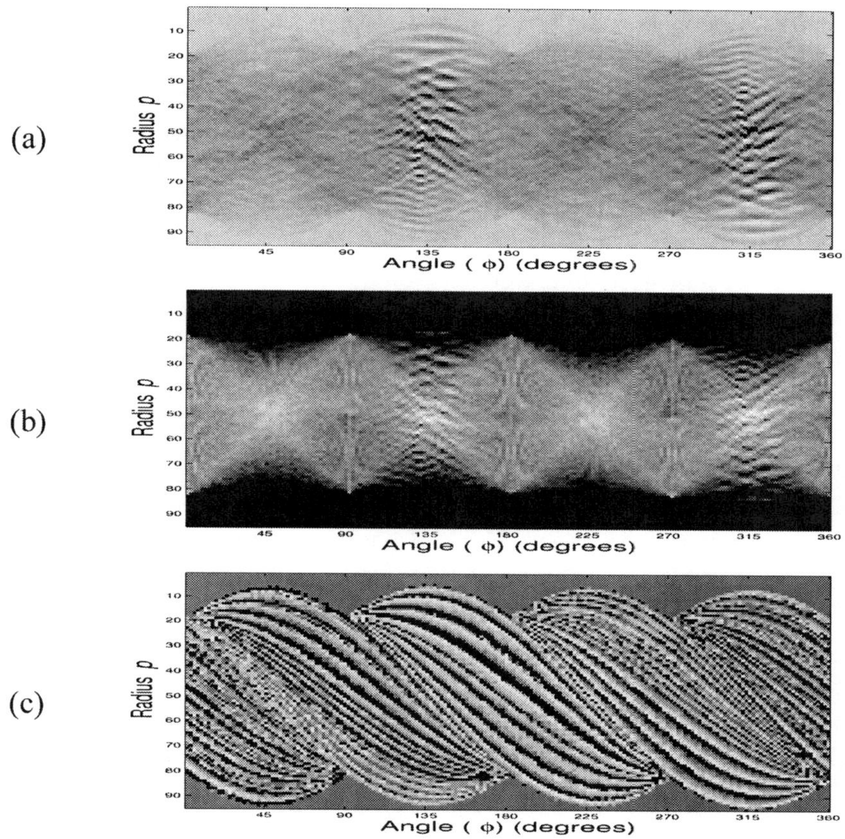

occurrence matrix to distinguish between pairs of Brodatz textures.

In order to extend this method into 3D, the trace along the data will be defined by three parameters, (ϕ, p) and another angle of orientation, say θ, so the Trace transform would produce a 3D set. This can be reduced again by a series of functionals into a single value without complications, but the computational complexity is increased considerably.

Summary

Texture is not a properly defined concept and textured images or volumes can vary widely. This has led to a great number of texture measurement extraction methods. We have concentrated on techniques that can be used in 3D and thus only those techniques for 3D measurement extraction were presented in this chapter.

Spatial domain methods such as local mean and standard deviation can be used for their simplicity, and for some applications this can be good enough to extract textural differences between regions. Also, these methods can be used as a pre-processing step for other extraction techniques. **Neighborhood filters** have been used in burn diagnosis to distinguish healthy skin from burn wounds (Acha *et al.*, 2003). Their textural measurements were a set of parameters; mean, standard deviation, and skewness, of the color components of their images. Their feature selection invariably selected the mean values of lightness, hue, and chromaticity, so perhaps the discrimination power resides in the amplitude levels more than the texture of the images. 3D medical data was studied in a model-based analysis where a spatial relationship, measuring distance and orientation, between bone and cartilage is modeled from a set of manually segmented images and is later used in model-based segmentation (Kapur, 1999). Segmentation of the bone in MRI using active contours is presented in (Lorigo *et al.*, 1998). Both used local variance as a measure of texture.

Convolution filters have been applied to analyze the transition between grey matter (GM) and white matter (WM) in brain MRIs (Bernasconi *et al.*, 2001). A blurred transition between GM and WM, (lower magnitude values) could be linked to Focal cortical dysplasia (FCD), a neuronal disorder. Bernasconi proposed a ratio map of GM thickness multiplied by the relative intensity of voxel values with respect to a histogram-based threshold that divides GM and WM and then divide this product by the grey level intensity gradient. Their results enhance the visual detection of lesions. In seismic applications Randen used the gradient to detect two attributes of texture: dip and azimuth (Randen et al., 2000). Instead of the magnitude, they were interested in the direction, which in turn poses the problem of unwrapping in presence of noise - a non-trivial problem. They first obtain the gradient of the data and then calculate a local covariance matrix whose eigenvalues are said to describe dip and azimuth. These measures are said to be adequate for seismic data where parallel planes run along the data, but when other seismic objects are present, like faults, other processing is required.

Three-dimensional histograms obtained from the Zucker-Hummel filter and the metrics that can be extracted from them - anisotropy coefficient, integral anisotropy measure or local mean curvature - can reveal important characteristics of the original data, like the anisotropy, which can be linked to different brain conditions. The measure of anisotropy in brains has shown that there is some indication of higher degree of anisotropy in brains with brain atrophy than in normal brains (Segovia-Martínez et al., 1999).

Wavelets are a popular and powerful technique for measurement generation. By the use of separable functions a 3D volume can be easily decomposed. A disadvantage of Wavelet techniques is that there is not an easy way to select the best Wavelet family, which can lead to many different options and therefore a great number of measurements. When classification is performed, having a larger number of measurements does not imply a better classification result, nor does it ease the computational complexity. The main problem in Wavelet analysis is determining the decomposition level that yields the best results (Pichler *et al.*, 1996). He also reports that since the channel parameters cannot be freely selected, the Wavelet transform is sub-optimal for feature extraction purposes. Texture with Wavelets has been analyzed in (Unser, 1995) concluding that Wavelet transform is an attractive tool for characterizing textures due to its properties of multiresolution and orthogonality; it is also mentioned that having more than one level led to better results than a single resolution analysis. Wavelets in 2D and 3D have been used for the study of temporal lobe epilepsy (TLE) and concluded that the extracted features are linearly separable and the energy features derived from the 2D Wavelet transform provide higher separability compared with 3D Wavelet decomposition of the hippocampus (Jafari-Khouzani *et al.*, 2004). The endoscopic images of the colonic mucosal surface have been analyzed with color wavelet features in (Karkanis *et al.*, 2003), for the detection of abnormal colonic regions corresponding to adenomatous polyps with a reported high performance.

Although easy to implement, **co-occurrence matrices** are outperformed by filtering techniques, the computational complexity is high and can have prohibitive costs when extended to 3D. Another strong drawback of co-occurrence is that the range of grey levels can increase the computational complexity of the technique. In most cases, the number of grey levels is quantized to a small number, this can be done either directly on the data or in the measurements that are extracted, but inevitably they result in a loss of information. When the range of grey levels exceeds the typical 0-255 that is used in images, this issue is even more critical. Some of the extensions proposed for 3D have been used as global techniques, that is, that the features are obtained from a whole region of interest. Generalized multidimensional co-occurrence matrices have been used in several publications: to measure texture anisotropy (Kovalev & Petrou, 1996), for the analysis of MRI brain data sets (Kovalev et al., 2001), to detect age and gender effects in structural brain asymmetry (Kovalev et al., 2003a), and the detection of schizophrenic patients (Kovalev et al., 2003b). In (Kovalev et al., 2003b) Kovalev, Petrou and Suckling use the magnitude of the gradient calculated with the Zucker-Hummel filter over the data. The authors use 3D co-occurrence to discriminate between schizophrenic patients and controls. The data of T1-MRIs are filtered spatially and then the co-occurrence matrix will be a function of

$$CM(MG_1, MG_2, D_8, \theta, d), \quad (39)$$

where MG is the magnitude of the gradient at a certain voxel. This method requires an empirical threshold to discard gradient vectors with magnitudes lower than 75 units (from a range 0-600) as a noise removal of the data. The authors reported that not all the slices of the brain were suitable for discrimination between schizophrenics and normal control subjects. It is the most inferior part of the brain, in particular the tissue close to the sulci, which gives the slices whose features provide discrimination between the populations.

Brain asymmetry in 3D MRI with co-occurrence matrices was also studied in (Kovalev et al., 2001). Gradients as well as intensities are included in the matrix, which is then used to analyze the brain asymmetry. It was found that male brains are more asymmetric than females and that changes of asymmetry with age are less prominent. The results reported correspond closely to other techniques and they propose the use of texture-based methods for digital morphometry in neuroscience.

3D co-occurrence matrices have been reported in MRI data for evaluation of gliomas (Mahmoud-Ghoneim *et al.*, 2003). An experienced neuroradiologist selected homogeneous volumes of interest (VOI) corresponding to a particular tissue: WM, active tumor, necrosis, edema, etc. Co-occurrence matrices were obtained from these VOIs and their parameters were used in a pair-wise discrimination between the classes. The results were compared against 2D co-occurrence matrices, which were outperformed by the 3D approach. Herlidou has used a similar methodology for the evaluation of osteoporosis (Herlidou *et al.*, 2004), diseased skeletal muscle (Herlidou *et al.*, 1999) and intracranial tumors (Herlidou-Même *et al.*, 2001). Regions of interest (ROI) were manually selected from the data and then measurements were extracted with different techniques with the objective of discriminating between the classes of the ROIs. As with other techniques, the partitioning of the data presents a problem: if the region or volume of interest (VOI/ROI) selected is too small, it will not capture the structure of a texture, if it is too big, it will not be good for segmentation.

The extraction of textural measurements with **Gabor filters** is a powerful and versatile method that has been widely used. While the *rosette* configuration is good for many textures in some cases will not be able to distinguish some textures. Also, the origin of the filters in the Fourier domain has to be set to zero to avoid that the filters react to regions with constant intensity (Jain & Farrokhnia, 1991). Another disadvantage of the Gabor filters is their non-orthogonality due to their overlapping nature that leads to redundant features in different channels (Li, 1998). Other cases of 3D Gabor filters have been reported where Wavelets and Gabor filters are combined for segmentation of 3D seismic sections and filters were applied to clinical ultrasound volumes of carotid (Fernández et al., 2000). For the design of a filter bank in 3D the radial frequencies are also taken in octaves and the orientation of azimuth and elevation can be both restricted to 4 angles: $(\theta, \phi) = \{0, \frac{\pi}{4}, \frac{\pi}{2}, \frac{3\pi}{4}\}$ which yield a total of 13 orientations. Pichler compared Wavelets and Gabor filters and overall Gabor filtering had better results than Wavelets but with a higher computational effort (Pichler *et al.*, 1996). In another comparison of Wavelets and Gabor filters (Chang & Kuo, 1993) it is mentioned that Wavelets are more natural and effective for textures with dominant middle frequency channels and Gabor is suitable for images with energy in the low frequency region.

A technique that escapes the problem of the range of grey levels is the **Texture Spectrum** and **Local Binary Pattern** (LBP) (Harwood *et al.*, 1993; Ojala et al., 1996) by taking the sign of the difference between grey level values of neighboring pixels and weighting the orientation by a power of 2. LBP has been used in combination with Wavelets and co-occurrence matrices for the detection of adenomas in gastrointestinal video as an aid for the endoscopist (Iakovidis *et al.*, 2006) with good results but LBP underperforms against filter banks and co-occurrence in (Pujol & Radeva, 2005) while trying to classify plaque in intravascular ultrasound images. Both LBP and signed grey level differences provide good segmentation results in 2D but the extension to 3D will imply having a very large number of combinations. The possibility of different labelings of the elements in a neighborhood can lead to many different measurements.

The **Trace transform** provides a way of characterizing textures with invariance to rotation, translation and scaling, that enables this relatively new technique to discriminate between pairs of texture with success over co-occurrence matrices. The trace transform has been applied for face recognition based on the textural Triple features of faces (Srisuk *et al.*, 2003). The three dimensional structure of protein structures has been analyzed by the trace transform, which provided good results when applied to single domain chains but not for multidomain (Daras *et al.*, 2006). The detection of Alzheimer's disease (AD) applied to position emission tomography (PET) images of the brain has also seen applications of this algorithm (Sayeed et al., 2002). Accuracies of more that 90% in specificity and sensitivity were obtained discriminating between patients with AD and healthy controls.

Final Considerations

In the previous sections, processing of the textured data produced a series of measurements, either the results of filters, features of the co-occurrence matrix or Wavelets, that belong to a *Measurement Space (Hand, 1981)*, which is then used as the input data of a classifier. Classification, that is, assigning every element of the data, or the measurements extracted from the data, into one of several possible classes is in itself a broad area of research, which is outside the scope of this chapter. However, for the particular case of texture analysis there are four important aspects that can affect the classification results and will be briefly mentioned here.

First, not all the measurements dimensions will contribute to the discrimination of the different textures that compose the original data, therefore it is important to evaluate the discrimination power of the measurements and perform *feature selection or extraction*. The feature selection and extraction problem selects a subset of features that will reduce the complexity and improve the performance of the classification with mathematical tools (Kittler, 1986). In feature selection, a set of the original measurements is discarded and the ones that are selected, which will be the most useful ones, will constitute the *Feature Space*. In contrast, the combination of a series of measurements in a linear or non-linear mapping to a new reduced dimensionality is called feature extraction. Perhaps the most common feature extraction method is the *Principal Components Analysis* (PCA) where the new features are uncorrelated and these are the projections into new axes that maximize the variances of the data. As well as making each feature linearly independent, PCA allows the ranking of features according to the size of the variance in each principal axis from which a 'subspace' of features can be presented to a classifier. However, while this eigenspace method is very effective in many cases, it requires the computation of all the features for given data. If the classes are known, an algorithm for feature selection through the use of a novel *Bhattacharyya Space* provides a good way of selecting the most discriminant features of a measurement space (Reyes Aldasoro & Bhalerao, 2006). This algorithm can also be used for detecting which pairs of classes would be particularly hard to discriminate over all the space and in some cases, the individual use of one point of the space can be also of interest. When the number of classes is not known, other methods like the *Two-point correlation function* or the *distance histogram* (Fatemi-Ghomi, 1997) could be used.

Second, it is important to observe that if one measurement is several orders of magnitude greater than others, the former will dominate the result. It may help thus to *normalize* or scale the measurements in order for the measurements to be comparable. This whitening of the distributions presents another problem that is exemplified in Figure 31. By scaling the measurements, the elements can change their distribution and different structures can appear.

Third, the choice of a *local energy function* (LEF) can influence considerably the classification process. The simplest, and perhaps most common way to use a LEF is to smooth the space with a convolution of a kernel, either Gaussian or uniform. Another way of averaging the values of neighbors is through the construction of a pyramid (Burt & Adelson, 1983) or tree (Samet, 1984). These methods have the advantage of reducing the dimensions of the space at higher levels. Yet another averaging can be performed with an anisotropic operator, namely butterfly filters (Schroeter & Bigun, 1995). This option can be used to improve the classification, especially

Figure 31. The scaling of the measurements can yield different structures. In the first case, the data could be separated into two clusters that appear above an below of a imaginary diagonal while on the second case, the clusters appear to be on the left and right

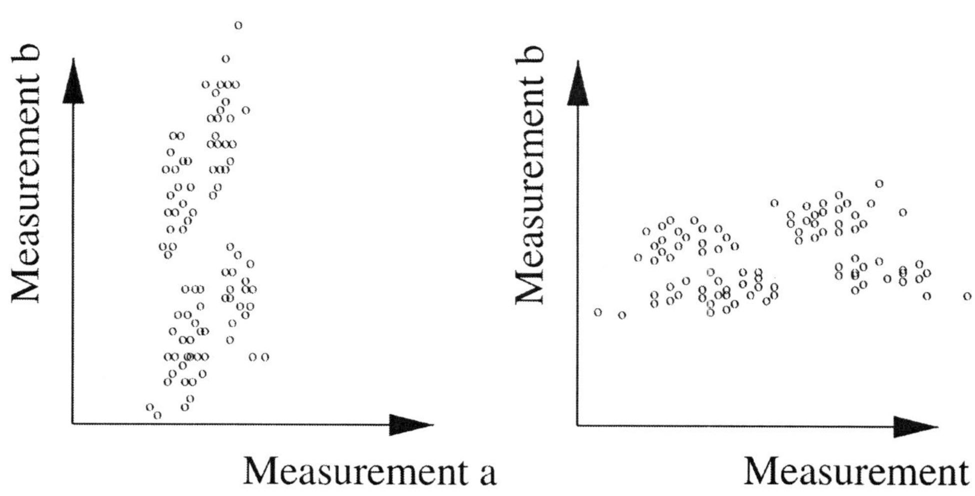

near the borders between textures. Previous research shows that a Gaussian smoothing (Bovik et al., 1990; Jain & Farrokhnia, 1991; Randen & Husøy, 1994, 1999) is better than uniform, yet the issue of the size of the smoothing filter is quite important.

Finally, since texture is scale-dependent a multiresolution classification may provide a lower misclassification than a single resolution classifier. Multiresolution will consist of three main stages: the process of *climbing* the levels or stages of a pyramid or tree, a decision or analysis at the highest level is performed, and the process of *descending* from the highest level down to the original resolution. The basic idea of the method is to reduce number of elements of the data, by climbing a tree, in order to reduce the uncertainty at the expense of spatial resolution (Schroeter & Bigun, 1995). This climbing stage represents the decrease in dimensions of the data by means of averaging a set of neighbors on one level (which are called *children* elements or nodes) up to a *parent* element on the upper level. The decrease of elements should decrease the uncertainty in the elements values since they are tending to a mean. In contrast, the spatial position increases its uncertainty at every stage (Wilson & Spann, 1988). Interaction of the neighbors can reduce the uncertainty in spatial position that is inherited from the parent node. This process is known as spatial restoration and boundary refining, which is repeated at every stage until the bottom of the tree or pyramid is reached. A comparison between *volumetric pyramidal butterfly filters*, which outperform a *Markov Random Field* approach is presented in (Reyes Aldasoro, 2004).

CONCLUSION

Texture analysis presents an attractive route to analyze medical or biological images as different tissues or cell populations, which would present similar intensity characteristics, can be differentiated by their textures. As the resolution of the imaging equipment (CCD cameras, laser scanners of multiphoton microscopes or Magnetic Resonance imaging) continues to increase, texture will play an important role in the discrimination and analysis of biomedical imaging. Furthermore, the use of the volumetric data provided by the scanners as a volume and not just as slices can reveal important information that is normally lost when data is analyzed only in 2D.

The fundamental ideas of several texture analysis techniques have been presented in this chapter, together with some examples and applications, such that a reader will be able to select an adequate technique to generate a measurement space that will capture some characteristics of the data being considered.

FUTURE RESEARCH DIRECTIONS

There are three important lines of research for the future:

1) Algorithms should be compared in performance and computational complexity. For 2D, the images proposed in (Randen & Husøy, 1999) have become a benchmark against which many authors test their extraction techniques and classifiers. There is not such a reliable and interesting database in 3D and, as such, the algorithms presented tend to be optimized for a particular data set. It is also important to consider the measurement extraction separate from classification, feature selection and intermediate steps like the local energy function, otherwise a bad measurement may be obscured by a sophisticated classifier.
2) Volumetric texture analysis deals with large datasets, for a typical $256 \times 256 \times 256$ voxel MRI, the measurement space is correspondingly large. In the future, the use of High Performance Clusters will be necessary if

images with more resolution are to be analyzed. The evolution of volumetric texture analysis should grow hand in hand with parallel-distributed algorithms; otherwise, the analysis will remain restricted to small areas, volumes whose intensities have been quantized to limit computational complexity.

3) As algorithms are tested, and more importantly, validated for medical and biological applications, these could be incorporated into acquisition equipment and in this way, volumetric texture analysis would be able to provide important information about lesions or abnormalities without needing off-line analysis, which may take several weeks after the data has been acquired.

REFERENCES

Acha, B., Serrano, C., Acha, J. I., & Roa, L. M. (2003). CAD tool for burn diagnosis. In Taylor, C., & Noble, A. (Eds.), *Proceedings of information processing in medical imaging* (pp. 282–293). Ambleside, UK.

Alparonte, L., Argenti, F., & Benelli, G. (1990). Fast calculation of co-occurrence matrix parameters for image segmentation. *Electronics Letters*, *26*(1), 23–24. doi:10.1049/el:19900015

Bay, B. K. (1995). Texture correlation. A method for the measurement of detailed strain distributions within trabecular bone. *Journal of Orthopaedic Research*, *13*(2), 258–267. doi:10.1002/jor.1100130214

Bay, B. K., Smith, T. S., Fyhrie, D. P., Martin, R. B., Reimann, D. A., & Saad, M. (1998). Three-dimensional texture correlation measurement of strain in trabecular bone. In *Orthopaedic research society, transactions of the 44th annual meeting* (p. 109). New Orleans, Louisiana.

Beil, M., Irinopoulou, T., Vassy, J., & Rigaut, J. P. (1995). Chromatin texture analysis in three-dimensional images from confocal scanning laser microscopy. *Analytical and Quantitative Cytology and Histology*, *17*(5), 323–331.

Bernasconi, A., Antel, S. B., Collins, D. L., Bernasconi, N., Olivier, A., & Dubeau, F. (2001). Texture analysis and morphological processing of MRI assist detection of focal cortical dysplasia in extra-temporal partial epilepsy. *Annals of Neurology*, *49*(6), 770–775. doi:10.1002/ana.1013

Bigun, J. (1991). Multidimensional orientation estimation with applications to texture analysis and optical flow. *IEEE Transactions on Pattern Analysis and Machine Intelligence*, *13*(8), 775–790. doi:10.1109/34.85668

Bigun, J., & du-Buf, J. M. H. (1994). N-folded symmetries by complex moments in Gabor space and their application to unsupervised texture segmentation. *IEEE Transactions on Pattern Analysis and Machine Intelligence*, *16*(1), 80–87. doi:10.1109/34.273714

Blot, L., & Zwiggelaar, R. (2002). Synthesis and analysis of solid texture: Application in medical imaging. In *Texture 2002: The 2nd international workshop on texture analysis and synthesis* (pp. 9-14). Copenhagen.

Boashash, B. (1992). Estimating and interpreting the instantaneous frequency of a signal; part i: Fundamentals, part ii: Algorithms. *Proceedings of the IEEE*, *80*(4), 519–569.

Bouman, C., & Liu, B. (1991). Multiple resolution segmentation of textured images. *IEEE Transactions on Pattern Analysis and Machine Intelligence*, *13*(2), 99–113. doi:10.1109/34.67641

Bovik, A. C., Clark, M., & Geisler, W. S. (1990). Multichannel texture analysis using localized spatial filters. *IEEE Transactions on Pattern Analysis and Machine Intelligence*, *12*(1), 55–73. doi:10.1109/34.41384

Burt, P. J., & Adelson, E. H. (1983). The Laplacian pyramid as a compact image code. *IEEE Transactions on Communications, 31*(4), 532–540. doi:10.1109/TCOM.1983.1095851

Carrillat, A., Randen, T., Sönneland, L., & Elvebakk, G. (2002). Seismic stratigraphic mapping of carbonate mounds using 3D texture attributes. In *Extended abstracts, annual meeting, European association of geoscientists and engineers*. Florence, Italy.

Chang, T., & Kuo, C. C. J. (1993). Texture analysis and classification with tree-structured wavelet transform. *IEEE Transactions on Image Processing, 2*(4), 429–441. doi:10.1109/83.242353

Chantler, M. J. (1995). Why illuminant direction is fundamental to texture analysis. *IEEE Proceedings in Vision. Image and Signal Processing, 142*(4), 199–206. doi:10.1049/ip-vis:19952065

Chui, C. K. (1992). *An introduction to wavelets*. Boston: Academic Press Inc.

Chung, A. C. S., Noble, J. A., & Summers, P. (2002). Fusing magnitude and phase information for vascular segmentation in phase contrast MR angiography. *Medical Image Analysis Journal, 6*(2), 109–128. doi:10.1016/S1361-8415(02)00057-9

Clausi, D. A., & Jernigan, M. E. (1998). A fast method to determine co-occurrence texture features. *IEEE Transactions on Geoscience and Remote Sensing, 36*(1), 298–300. doi:10.1109/36.655338

Coleman, G. B., & Andrews, H. C. (1979). Image segmentation by clustering. *Proceedings of the IEEE, 67*(5), 773–785. doi:10.1109/PROC.1979.11327

Cross, G. R., & Jain, A. K. (1983). Markov random field texture models. *IEEE Transactions on Pattern Analysis and Machine Intelligence, 5*(1), 25–39. doi:10.1109/TPAMI.1983.4767341

Cula, O. G., & Dana, K. J. (2004). 3D texture recognition using bidirectional feature histograms. *International Journal of Computer Vision, 59*(1), 33–60. doi:10.1023/B:VISI.0000020670.05764.55

Dana, K. J., van-Ginneken, B., Nayar, S. K., & Koenderink, J. J. (1999). Reflectance and texture of real-world surfaces. *ACM Transactions on Graphics, 18*(1), 1–34. doi:10.1145/300776.300778

Daras, P., Zarpalas, D., Axenopoulos, A., Tzovaras, D., & Strintzis, M. G. (2006). Three-dimensional shape-structure comparison method for protein classification. *IEEE/ACM Transactions on Computational Biology and Bioinformatics, 3*(3), 193–207. doi:10.1109/TCBB.2006.43

Dunn, D., & Higgins, W. E. (1995). Optimal Gabor filters for texture segmentation. *IEEE Transactions on Image Processing, 4*(7), 947–964. doi:10.1109/83.392336

Dunn, D., Higgins, W. E., & Wakeley, J. (1994). Texture segmentation using 2-D Gabor elementary functions. *IEEE Transactions on Pattern Analysis and Machine Intelligence, 16*(2), 130–149. doi:10.1109/34.273736

Ercoli, A., Battaglia, A., Raspaglio, G., Fattorossi, A., Alimonti, A., & Petrucci, F. (2000). Activity of cisplatin and ici 182,780 on estrogen receptor negative ovarian cancer cells: Cell cycle and cell replication rate perturbation, chromatin texture alteration and apoptosis induction. *International Journal of Cancer, 85*(1), 98–103. doi:10.1002/(SICI)1097-0215(20000101)85:1<98::AID-IJC18>3.0.CO;2-A

Fatemi-Ghomi, N. (1997). *Performance measures for wavelet-based segmentation algorithms*. Centre for Vision, Speech and Signal Processing, University of Surrey.

Fernández, M., Mavilio, A., & Tejera, M. (2000). Texture segmentation of a 3D seismic section with wavelet transform and Gabor filters. In *International conference on pattern recognition, ICPR 00* (Vol. 3, pp. 358-361). Barcelona.

Gabor, D. (1946). Theory of communication. *Journal of the IEE, 93*(26), 429–457.

Gilchrist, C. L., Xia, J. Q., Setton, L. A., & Hsu, E. W. (2004). High-resolution determination of soft tissue deformations using MRI and first-order texture correlation. *IEEE Transactions on Medical Imaging, 23*(5), 546–553. doi:10.1109/TMI.2004.825616

Gonzalez, R. C., & Woods, R. E. (1992). *Digital image processing*. Reading, MA: Addison Wesley.

Graps, A. (1995). An introduction to wavelets. *IEEE Computational Science & Engineering, 2*(2), 50–61. doi:10.1109/99.388960

Gschwendtner, A., Hoffmann-Weltin, Y., Mikuz, G., & Mairinger, T. (1999). Quantitative assessment of bladder cancer by nuclear texture analysis using automated high resolution image cytometry. *Modern Pathology, 12*(8), 806–813.

Hand, D. J. (1981). *Discrimination and classification*. Chichester: Wiley.

Haralick, R. M. (1979). Statistical and structural approaches to texture. *Proceedings of the IEEE, 67*(5), 786–804. doi:10.1109/PROC.1979.11328

Haralick, R. M., Shanmugam, K., & Dinstein, I. h. (1973). Textural features for image classification. *IEEE Transactions on Systems, Man, and Cybernetics, 3*(6), 610–621. doi:10.1109/TSMC.1973.4309314

Harwood, D., Ojala, T., Petrou, P., Kelman, S., & Davis, S. (1993). *Texture classification by center-symmetric auto-correlation, using kullback discrimination of distributions*. College Park, Maryland: Computer Vision Laboratory, Center for Automation Research, University of Maryland.

Hawkins, J. K. (1970). Textural properties for pattern recognition. In Lipkin, B., & Rosenfeld, A. (Eds.), *Picture processing and psychopictorics* (pp. 347–370). New York.

He, D. C., & Wang, L. (1991). Textural filters based on the texture spectrum. *Pattern Recognition, 24*(12), 1187–1195. doi:10.1016/0031-3203(91)90144-T

Herlidou, S., Grebve, R., Grados, F., Leuyer, N., Fardellone, P., & Meyer, M. E. (2004). Influence of age and osteoporosis on calcaneus trabecular bone structure: A preliminary in vivo MRI study by quantitative texture analysis. *Magnetic Resonance Imaging, 22*(2), 237–243. doi:10.1016/j.mri.2003.07.007

Herlidou, S., Rolland, Y., Bansard, J. Y., Le-Rumeur, E., & Certaines, J. D. (1999). Comparison of automated and visual texture analysis in MRI: Characterization of normal and diseased skeletal muscle. *Magnetic Resonance Imaging, 17*(9), 1393–1397. doi:10.1016/S0730-725X(99)00066-1

Herlidou-Même, S., Constans, J. M., Carsin, B., Olivie, D., Eliat, P. A., & Nadal Desbarats, L. (2001). MRI texture analysis on texture text objects, normal brain and intracranial tumors. *Magnetic Resonance Imaging, 21*(9), 989–993. doi:10.1016/S0730-725X(03)00212-1

Hoffman, E. A., Reinhardt, J. M., Sonka, M., Simon, B. A., Guo, J., & Saba, O. (2003). Characterization of the interstitial lung diseases via density-based and texture-based analysis of computed tomography images of lung structure and function. *Academic Radiology, 10*(10), 1104–1118. doi:10.1016/S1076-6332(03)00330-1

Hsu, T. I., Calway, A., & Wilson, R. (1992). *Analysis of structured texture using the multiresolution Fourier transform*. Department of Computer Science, University of Warwick.

Iakovidis, D. K., Maroulis, D. E., & Karkanis, S. A. (2006). An intelligent system for automatic detection of gastrointestinal adenomas in video endoscopy. *Computers in Biology and Medicine*, *36*(10), 1084–1103. doi:10.1016/j.compbiomed.2005.09.008

Ip, H. H. S., & Lam, S. W. C. (1994). Using an octree-based rag in hyper-irregular pyramid segmentation of texture volume. In *Proceedings of the IAPR workshop on machine vision applications* (pp. 259-262). Kawasaki, Japan.

Jafari-Khouzani, K., Soltanian-Zadeh, H., Elisevich, K., & Patel, S. (2004). Comparison of 2D and 3D wavelet features for TLE lateralization. In A. A. Amir & M. Armando (Eds.), *Proceedings of SPIE vol. 5369, medical imaging 2004: Physiology, function, and structure from medical images* (pp. 593-601). San Diego, CA, USA.

Jain, A. K., & Farrokhnia, F. (1991). Unsupervised texture segmentation using Gabor filters. *Pattern Recognition*, *24*(12), 1167–1186. doi:10.1016/0031-3203(91)90143-S

James, D., Clymer, B. D., & Schmalbrock, P. (2002). Texture detection of simulated microcalcification susceptibility effects in magnetic resonance imaging of the breasts. *Journal of Magnetic Resonance Imaging*, *13*(6), 876–881. doi:10.1002/jmri.1125

Jorgensen, T., Yogesan, K., Tveter, K. J., Skjorten, F., & Danielsen, H. E. (1996). Nuclear texture analysis: A new prognostic tool in metastatic prostate cancer. *Cytometry*, *24*(3), 277–283. doi:10.1002/(SICI)1097-0320(19960701)24:3<277::AID-CYTO11>3.0.CO;2-N

Kadyrov, A., & Petrou, M. (2001). The trace transform and its applications. *IEEE Transactions on Pattern Analysis and Machine Intelligence*, *23*(8), 811–828. doi:10.1109/34.946986

Kadyrov, A., Talepbour, A., & Petrou, M. (2002). Texture classification with thousand of features. In *British machine vision conference* (pp. 656–665). Cardiff, UK: BMVC.

Kapur, T. (1999). *Model-based three dimensional medical image segmentation*. AI Lab, Massachusetts Institute of Technology.

Karkanis, S. A., Iakovidis, D. K., Maroulis, D. E., Karras, D. A., & Tzivras, M. (2003). Computer-aided tumor detection in endoscopic video using color wavelet features. *IEEE Transactions on Information Technology in Biomedicine*, *7*(3), 141–152. doi:10.1109/TITB.2003.813794

Kervrann, C., & Heitz, F. (1995). A Markov random field model-based approach to unsupervised texture segmentation using local and global spatial statistics. *IEEE Transactions on Image Processing*, *4*(6), 856–862. doi:10.1109/83.388090

Kittler, J. (1986). Feature selection and extraction. In Fu, Y. (Ed.), *Handbook of pattern recognition and image processing* (pp. 59–83). New York: Academic Press.

Knutsson, H., & Granlund, G. H. (1983). Texture analysis using two-dimensional quadrature filters. In *IEEE computer society workshop on computer architecture for pattern analysis and image database management - capaidm* (pp. 206-213). Pasadena.

Knutsson, H., Westin, C. F., & Granlund, G. H. (1994). Local multiscale frequency and bandwidth estimation. In *Proceedings of the IEEE international conference on image processing* (pp. 36-40). Austin, Texas: IEEE.

Kovalev, V. A., Kruggel, F., Gertz, H.-J., & von Cramon, D. Y. (2001). Three-dimensional texture analysis of MRI brain datasets. *IEEE Transactions on Medical Imaging*, *20*(5), 424–433. doi:10.1109/42.925295

Kovalev, V. A., Kruggel, F., & von Cramon, D. Y. (2003a). Gender and age effects in structural brain asymmetry as measured by MRI texture analysis. *NeuroImage, 19*(3), 895–905. doi:10.1016/S1053-8119(03)00140-X

Kovalev, V. A., & Petrou, M. (1996). Multidimensional co-occurrence matrices for object recognition and matching. *Graphical Models and Image Processing, 58*(3), 187–197. doi:10.1006/gmip.1996.0016

Kovalev, V. A., Petrou, M., & Bondar, Y. S. (1999). Texture anisotropy in 3D images. *IEEE Transactions on Image Processing, 8*(3), 346–360. doi:10.1109/83.748890

Kovalev, V. A., Petrou, M., & Suckling, J. (2003b). Detection of structural differences between the brains of schizophrenic patients and controls. *Psychiatry Research: Neuroimaging, 124*(3), 177–189. doi:10.1016/S0925-4927(03)00070-2

Kumar, P. K., Yegnanarayana, B., & Das, S. (2000). 1-d Gabor for edge detection in texture images. In *International conference on communications, computers and devices (ICCCD 2000)* (pp. 425-428). IIT Kharagpur, INDIA.

Laine, A., & Fan, J. (1993). Texture classification by wavelet packet signatures. *IEEE Transactions on Pattern Analysis and Machine Intelligence, 15*(11), 1186–1191. doi:10.1109/34.244679

Lang, Z., Scarberry, R. E., Zhang, Z., Shao, W., & Sun, X. (1991). A texture-based direct 3D segmentation system for confocal scanning fluorescence microscopic images. In *Twenty-third southeastern symposium on system theory* (pp. 472-476). Columbia, SC.

Laws, K. (1980). *Textured image segmentation.* University of Southern California.

Lerski, R. A., Straughan, K., Schad, L. R., Boyce, D., Bluml, S., & Zuna, I. (1993). MR image texture analysis - an approach to tissue characterization. *Magnetic Resonance Imaging, 11*(6), 873–887. doi:10.1016/0730-725X(93)90205-R

Létal, J., Jirák, D., Šuderlová, L., & Hájek, M. (2003). MRI 'texture' analysis of MR images of apples during ripening and storage. *Lebensmittel-Wissenschaft und-Technologie, 36*(7), 719-727.

Leung, T. K., & Malik, J. (1999). Recognizing surfaces using three-dimensional textons. In *ICCV (2)* (pp. 1010-1017). Corfu, Greece.

Li, C.-T. (1998). *Unsupervised texture segmentation using multiresolution Markov random fields.* Coventry: Department of Computer Science, University of Warwick.

Lladó, X., Oliver, A., Petrou, M., Freixenet, J., & Mart, J. (2003). Simultaneous surface texture classification and illumination tilt angle prediction. In *British machine vision conference* (pp. 789–798). Norwich, UK: BMVC.

Lorigo, L. M., Faugeras, O. D., Grimson, W. E. L., Keriven, R., & Kikinis, R. (1998). Segmentation of bone in clinical knee MRI using texture-based geodesic active contours. In *Medical image computing and computer-assisted interventions* (pp. 1195–1204). Cambridge, USA: MICCAI.

Mahmoud-Ghoneim, D., Grégoire, T., Constans, J. M., & Certaines, J. D. d. (2003). Three dimensional texture analysis in MRI: A preliminary evaluation in gliomas. *Magnetic Resonance Imaging, 21*(9), 983–987. doi:10.1016/S0730-725X(03)00201-7

Mairinger, T., Mikuz, G., & Gschwendtner, A. (1999). Are nuclear texture features a suitable tool for predicting non-organ-confined prostate cancer? *The Journal of Urology, 162*(1), 258–262. doi:10.1097/00005392-199907000-00078

Malik, J., & Perona, P. (1990). Preattentive texture discrimination with early vision mechanisms. *Journal of the Optical Society of America. A, Optics and Image Science*, *7*(5), 923–932. doi:10.1364/JOSAA.7.000923

Mallat, S. G. (1989). A theory for multiresolution signal decomposition: The wavelet representation. *IEEE Transactions on Pattern Analysis and Machine Intelligence*, *11*(7), 674–693. doi:10.1109/34.192463

Masters, B. R., & So, P. T. C. (2004). Antecedents of two-photon excitation laser scanning microscopy, microscopy research and technique. *Microscopy Research and Technique*, *63*, 3–11. doi:10.1002/jemt.10418

Mathias, J. M., Tofts, P. S., & Losseff, N. A. (1999). Texture analysis of spinal cord pathology in multiple sclerosis. *Magnetic Resonance in Medicine*, *42*(5), 929–935. doi:10.1002/(SICI)1522-2594(199911)42:5<929::AID-MRM13>3.0.CO;2-2

Mattfeldt, T., Vogel, U., & Gottfried, H. W. (1993). Three-dimensional spatial texture of adenocarcinoma of the prostate by a combination of stereology and digital image analysis. *Verhandlungen der Deutschen Gesellschaft fur Pathologie*, *77*, 73–77.

Merceron, G., Taylor, S., Scott, R., Chaimanee, Y., & Jaeger, J. J. (2006). Dietary characterization of the hominoid khoratpithecus (Miocene of Thailand): Evidence from dental topographic and microwear texture analyses. *Naturwissenschaften*, *93*(7), 329–333. doi:10.1007/s00114-006-0107-0

Neyret, F. (1995). *A general and multiscale model for volumetric textures.* Paper presented at the Graphics Interface, Canadian Human-Computer Communications Society, Québec, Canada.

Ojala, T., Pietikinen, M., & Harwood, D. (1996). A comparative study of texture measures with classification based on feature distributions. *Pattern Recognition*, *29*(1), 51–59. doi:10.1016/0031-3203(95)00067-4

Ojala, T., Valkealahti, K., Oja, R., & Pietikinen, M. (2001). Texture discrimination with multidimensional distributions of signed gray level differences. *Pattern Recognition*, *34*(3), 727–739. doi:10.1016/S0031-3203(00)00010-8

Petrou, M., & Kadyrov, A. (2004). Affine invariant features from the trace transform. *IEEE Transactions on Pattern Analysis and Machine Intelligence*, *26*(1), 30–44. doi:10.1109/TPAMI.2004.1261077

Pichler, O., Teuner, A., & Hosticka, B. J. (1996). A comparison of texture feature extraction using adaptive Gabor filtering, pyramidal and tree structured wavelet transforms. *Pattern Recognition*, *29*(5), 733–742. doi:10.1016/0031-3203(95)00127-1

Porteneuve, C., Korb, J.-P., Petit, D., & Zanni, H. (2000). Structure-texture correlation in ultra high performance concrete: A nuclear magnetic resonance study. In *Franco-Italian conference on magnetic resonance*. France: La Londe Les Maures.

Pujol, O., & Radeva, P. (2005). On the assessment of texture feature descriptors in intravascular ultrasound images: A boosting approach to a feasible plaque classification. *Studies in Health Technology and Informatics*, *113*, 276–299.

Rajpoot, N. M. (2002). Texture classification using discriminant wavelet packet subbands. In *Proceedings 45th IEEE Midwest symposium on circuits and systems (MWSCAS 2002)*. Tulsa, OK, USA.

Randen, T., & Husøy, J. H. (1994). Texture segmentation with optimal linear prediction error filters. *Piksel'n*, *11*(3), 25–28.

Randen, T., & Husøy, J. H. (1999). Filtering for texture classification: A comparative study. *IEEE Transactions on Pattern Analysis and Machine Intelligence*, *21*(4), 291–310. doi:10.1109/34.761261

Randen, T., Monsen, E., Abrahamsen, A., Hansen, J. O., Shlaf, J., & Sønneland, L. (2000). Three-dimensional texture attributes for seismic data analysis. In *Ann. Int. Mtg., soc. Expl. Geophys., exp. Abstr.* Calgary, Canada.

Randen, T., Sønneland, L., Carrillat, A., Valen, S., Skov, T., Pedersen, S. I., et al. (2003). Preconditioning for optimal 3D stratigraphical and structural inversion. In *65th EAGE conference & exhibition*. Stavanger.

Ravishankar-Rao, A., & Lohse, G. L. (1993). Towards a texture naming system: Identifying relevant dimensions of texture. In *Proceedings of the 4th conference on visualization* (pp. 220-227). San Jose, California.

Reyes Aldasoro, C. C. (2004). *Multiresolution volumetric texture segmentation*. Coventry: The University of Warwick.

Reyes Aldasoro, C. C., & Bhalerao, A. (2006). The Bhattacharyya space for feature selection and its application to texture segmentation. *Pattern Recognition*, *39*(5), 812–826. doi:10.1016/j.patcog.2005.12.003

Reyes Aldasoro, C. C., & Bhalerao, A. (2007). Volumetric texture segmentation by discriminant feature selection and multiresolution classification. *IEEE Transactions on Medical Imaging*, *26*(1), 1–14. doi:10.1109/TMI.2006.884637

Rosito, M. A., Moreira, L. F., da Silva, V. D., Damin, D. C., & Prolla, J. C. (2003). Nuclear chromatin texture in rectal cancer. Relationship to tumor stage. *Analytical and Quantitative Cytology and Histology*, *25*(1), 25–30.

Saeed, N., & Puri, B. K. (2002). Cerebellum segmentation employing texture properties and knowledge based image processing: Applied to normal adult controls and patients. *Magnetic Resonance Imaging*, *20*(5), 425–429. doi:10.1016/S0730-725X(02)00508-8

Samet, H. (1984). The quadtree and related hierarchical data structures. *Computing Surveys*, *16*(2), 187–260. doi:10.1145/356924.356930

Sayeed, A., Petrou, M., Spyrou, N., Kadyrov, A., & Spinks, T. (2002). Diagnostic features of Alzheimer's disease extracted from PET sinograms. *Physics in Medicine and Biology*, *47*(1), 137–148. doi:10.1088/0031-9155/47/1/310

Schad, L. R., Bluml, S., & Zuna, I. (1993). MR tissue characterization of intracranial tumors by means of texture analysis. *Magnetic Resonance Imaging*, *11*(6), 889–896. doi:10.1016/0730-725X(93)90206-S

Schroeter, P., & Bigun, J. (1995). Hierarchical image segmentation by multi-dimensional clustering and orientation-adaptive boundary refinement. *Pattern Recognition*, *28*(5), 695–709. doi:10.1016/0031-3203(94)00133-7

Scott, R. S., Ungar, P. S., Bergstrom, T. S., Brown, C. A., Childs, B. E., & Teaford, M. F. (2006). Dental microwear texture analysis: Technical considerations. *Journal of Human Evolution*, *51*(4), 339–349. doi:10.1016/j.jhevol.2006.04.006

Segovia-Martínez, M., Petrou, M., Kovalev, V. A., & Perner, P. (1999). Quantifying level of brain atrophy using texture anisotropy in ct data. In *Medical imaging understanding and analysis* (pp. 173-176). Oxford, UK.

Sheppard, C. J., & Wilson, T. (1981). The theory of the direct-view confocal microscope. *Journal of Microscopy*, *124*(Pt 2), 107–117.

Sivaramakrishna, R., Powell, K. A., Lieber, M. L., Chilcote, W. A., & Shekhar, R. (2002). Texture analysis of lesions in breast ultrasound images. *Computerized Medical Imaging and Graphics*, *26*(5), 303–307. doi:10.1016/S0895-6111(02)00027-7

Sonka, M., Hlavac, V., & Boyle, R. (1998). *Image processing, analysis and machine vision*. Pacific Grove, USA: PWS.

Srisuk, S., Ratanarangsank, K., Kurutach, W., & Waraklang, S. (2003). Face recognition using a new texture representation of face images. In *Proceedings of electrical engineering conference* (pp. 1097-1102). Cha-am, Thailand.

Subramanian, K. R., Brockway, J. P., & Carruthers, W. B. (2004). Interactive detection and visualization of breast lesions from dynamic contrast enhanced MRI volumes. *Computerized Medical Imaging and Graphics*, *28*(8), 435–444. doi:10.1016/j.compmedimag.2004.07.004

Tai, C. W., & Baba-Kishi, K. Z. (2002). Microtexture studies of pst and pzt ceramics and pzt thin film by electron backscatter diffraction patterns. *Textures and Microstructures*, *35*(2), 71–86. doi:10.1080/07303300210000000191

Tamura, H., Mori, S., & Yamawaki, T. (1978). Texture features corresponding to visual perception. *IEEE Transactions on Systems, Man, and Cybernetics*, *8*(6), 460–473. doi:10.1109/TSMC.1978.4309999

Thybo, A. K., Andersen, H. J., Karlsson, A. H., Dønstrup, S., & Stødkilde-Jorgensen, H. S. (2003). Low-field NMR relaxation and NMR-imaging as tools in different determination of dry matter content in potatoes. *Lebensmittel-Wissenschaft und-Technologie, 36*(3), 315-322.

Thybo, A. K., Szczypiński, P. M., Karlsson, A. H., Dønstrup, S., Stødkilde-Jorgensen, H. S., & Andersen, H. J. (2004). Prediction of sensory texture quality attributes of cooked potatoes by NMR-imaging (MRI) of raw potatoes in combination with different image analysis methods. *Journal of Food Engineering*, *61*, 91–100. doi:10.1016/S0260-8774(03)00190-0

Tronstad, L. (1973). Scanning electron microscopy of attrited dentinal surfaces and subjacent dentin in human teeth. *Scandinavian Journal of Dental Research*, *81*(2), 112–122.

Tuceryan, M., & Jain, A. K. (1998). Texture analysis. In Chen, C. H., Pau, L. F., & Wang, P. S. P. (Eds.), *Handbook of pattern recognition and computer vision* (pp. 207–248). World Scientific Publishing.

Unser, M. (1995). Texture classification and segmentation using wavelet frames. *IEEE Transactions on Image Processing*, *4*(11), 1549–1560. doi:10.1109/83.469936

Ushizima Sabino, D. M., Da Fontoura Costa, L., Gil Rizzati, E., & Zago, M. A. (2004). A texture approach to leukocyte recognition. *Real-time imaging, 10*, 205-216.

Wang, L., & He, D. C. (1990). Texture classification using texture spectrum. *Pattern Recognition*, *23*(8), 905–910. doi:10.1016/0031-3203(90)90135-8

Webster, M. (2004). *Merriam-Webster's collegiate dictionary*. USA: NY.

Weldon, T. P., Higgins, W. E., & Dunn, D. F. (1996). Efficient Gabor filter design for texture segmentation. *Pattern Recognition*, *29*(12), 2005–2015. doi:10.1016/S0031-3203(96)00047-7

Westin, C. F., Abhir, B., Knutsson, H., & Kikinis, R. (1997). Using local 3D structure for segmentation of bone from computer tomography images. In *Proceedings of IEEE computer society conference on computer vision and pattern recognition*. San Juan, Puerto Rico: IEEE.

Weszka, J. S., Dyer, C. R., & Rosenfeld, A. (1976). A comparative study of texture measures for terrain classification. *IEEE Transactions on Systems, Man, and Cybernetics*, *6*(4), 269–285.

Wilson, R. G., & Spann, M. (1988). Finite prolate spheroidal sequences and their applications: Image feature description and segmentation. *IEEE Transactions on Pattern Analysis and Machine Intelligence*, *10*(2), 193–203. doi:10.1109/34.3882

Wilson, T. (1989). Three-dimensional imaging in confocal systems. *Journal of Microscopy*, *153*(Pt 2), 161–169.

Winkler, G. (1995). *Image analysis, random fields and dynamic Monte Carlo methods*. Berlin, Germany: Springer.

Yu, O., Mauss, Y., Namer, I. J., & Chambron, J. (2001). Existence of contralateral abnormalities revealed by texture analysis in unilateral intractable hippocampal epilepsy. *Magnetic Resonance Imaging*, *19*(10), 1305–1310. doi:10.1016/S0730-725X(01)00464-7

Yu, O., Roch, C., Namer, I. J., Chambron, J., & Mauss, Y. (2002). Detection of late epilepsy by the texture analysis of MR brain images in the lithium-pilocarpine rat model. *Magnetic Resonance Imaging*, *20*(10), 771–775. doi:10.1016/S0730-725X(02)00621-5

Zhan, Y., & Shen, D. (2003). Automated segmentation of 3D US prostate images using statistical texture-based matching method. In *Medical image computing and computer-assisted intervention* (pp. 688–696). Canada: MICCAI. doi:10.1007/978-3-540-39899-8_84

Zucker, S. W., & Hummel, R. A. (1981). A three-dimensional edge operator. *IEEE Transactions on Pattern Analysis and Machine Intelligence*, *3*(3), 324–331. doi:10.1109/TPAMI.1981.4767105

ADDITIONAL READING

Blot, L., & Zwiggelaar, R. (2002). Synthesis and analysis of solid texture: Application in medical imaging. In *Texture 2002: The 2nd international workshop on texture analysis and synthesis* (pp. 9-14). Copenhagen.

Haralick, R. M. (1979). Statistical and structural approaches to texture. *Proceedings of the IEEE*, *67*(5), 786–804. doi:10.1109/PROC.1979.11328

Jain, A. K., & Farrokhnia, F. (1991). Unsupervised texture segmentation using Gabor filters. *Pattern Recognition*, *24*(12), 1167–1186. doi:10.1016/0031-3203(91)90143-S

Kittler, J. (1986). Feature selection and extraction. In Fu, Y. (Ed.), *Handbook of pattern recognition and image processing* (pp. 59–83). New York: Academic Press.

Lerski, R. A., Straughan, K., Schad, L. R., Boyce, D., Bluml, S., & Zuna, I. (1993). MR image texture analysis - an approach to tissue characterization. *Magnetic Resonance Imaging*, *11*(6), 873–887. doi:10.1016/0730-725X(93)90205-R

Mallat, S. G. (1989). A theory for multiresolution signal decomposition: The wavelet representation. *IEEE Transactions on Pattern Analysis and Machine Intelligence*, *11*(7), 674–693. doi:10.1109/34.192463

Petrou, M., & Garcia-Sevilla, P. (2006). *Image processing: Dealing with texture*. Chichester, UK: John Wiley & Sons. doi:10.1002/047003534X

Randen, T., & Husøy, J. H. (1999). Filtering for texture classification: A comparative study. *IEEE Transactions on Pattern Analysis and Machine Intelligence*, *21*(4), 291–310. doi:10.1109/34.761261

Reyes Aldasoro, C. C., & Bhalerao, A. (2007). Volumetric texture segmentation by discriminant feature selection and multiresolution classification. *IEEE Transactions on Medical Imaging*, *26*(1), 1–14. doi:10.1109/TMI.2006.884637

Sonka, M., Hlavac, V., & Boyle, R. (1998). *Image processing, analysis and machine vision*. Pacific Grove, USA: PWS.

Tuceryan, M., & Jain, A. K. (1998). Texture analysis. In Chen, C. H., Pau, L. F., & Wang, P. S. P. (Eds.), *Handbook of pattern recognition and computer vision* (pp. 207–248). World Scientific Publishing.

Unser, M. (1995). Texture classification and segmentation using wavelet frames. *IEEE Transactions on Image Processing*, *4*(11), 1549–1560. doi:10.1109/83.469936

Chapter 8
Analysis of Doppler Embolic Signals

Ana Leiria
Universidade do Algarve, Portugal

M. M. M. Moura
Universidade do Algarve, Portugal

ABSTRACT

A broad view on the analysis of Doppler embolic signals is presented, uniting physics, engineering and computing, and clinical aspects. The overview of the field discusses the physiological significance of emboli and Doppler ultrasound with particular attention given to Transcranial Doppler; an outline of high-performance computing is presented, disambiguating the terminology and concepts used thereafter. The presentation of the major diagnostic approaches to Doppler embolic signals focuses on the most significant methods and techniques used to detect and classify embolic events including the clinical relevancy. Coverage of estimators such as time-frequency, time-scale, and displacement-frequency is included. The discussion of current approaches targets areas of identified need for improvement. A brief historical perspective of high-performance computing of Doppler blood flow signals and particularly Doppler embolic signals is accompanied by the reasoning behind the technological trends and approaches. The final remarks include, as a conclusion, a summary of the contribution and as future trends, some pathways hinting to where new developments might be expected.

INTRODUCTION

Increasing technological developments, together with the emergence of new diseases, prompted the association of engineering and medicine areas. The work developed in the intersection of these areas led to methods of higher accuracy in diagnosis, and encourages research towards new challenges. The developments that have occurred in Doppler ultrasound instrumentation are examples of the successful application of engineering in medical vascular diagnosis. Clinical Doppler instrumentation and the corresponding mathematical models became particularly relevant tools, allowing the use of non-surgical methods in the measurement of blood flow characteristics.

DOI: 10.4018/978-1-60566-280-0.ch008

The study of blood flow includes, among other goals, the detection, and characterization of emboli in the cerebral circulation. In particular, Transcranial Doppler (TCD) ultrasound instrumentation allows for the assessment of blood flow information from intracranial arteries, namely from middle cerebral arteries (MCA), where cerebral embolic events can be observed. The assessment of blood flow and embolic events is especially relevant because cardiovascular diseases are the major cause of mortality worldwide (Gatzoulis & Iakovidis, 2007). Ischemic stroke, predominantly due to cerebral embolism (Zuilen, Gijn, & Ackerstaff, 1998), is one of the most important disorders, highly contributing to these statistics. The accurate detection and classification of emboli in the blood circulation of the brain might help the prevention of such strokes.

Nowadays, many clinical and hospital units are equipped with TCD instrumentation. These devices enable emboli detection, but still present some difficulties in identifying micro-emboli. The understanding of Transcranial Doppler, also pursued in this chapter, is relevant to the articulation between medical physics and biomedical signal processing and the potential contribution to the clinical diagnosis. The significance and implications of the equipment employed allows critically examining the estimation results and deciding upon the clinical relevancy. These issues will be presented in the background section.

It should be noted that the correct characterization of blood flow and cerebral emboli by TCD instrumentation depends on the precision obtained by the spectral estimation process. Most TCD equipments use conventional spectral estimation methods based on the application of Short Time Fourier Transform (STFT) and STFT presents well identified limitations that lead to inaccurate quantitative measurements, especially when small embolus detection is required. Several published studies have reported improvement in blood flow spectral estimation with methods other than the STFT. An overview of these methods will be presented in this chapter. Most of these studies, aiming several arteries, made use of simulated Doppler ultrasound signals to test the alternative spectral estimators. Although the simulation of ultrasound signals is out of the scope of this work, the entire setup to study the alternatives frequently leads to the adoption of high-performance computing strategies. An overview of the field and the presentation of taxonomy are addressed in the background section.

Embolic signals (ES) are very complex and demand optimized methods and methodologies. Detection and classification of embolic events in the blood flow have been addressed using time-domain processing (TD), time-frequency (TF) processing, and time-scale processing. The study and development of alternative estimators can help the choice of the best approach to process embolic signals. A strong emphasis will be given to the current approaches to the analysis of embolic signals targeting clinical diagnosis.

Although techniques allowing ultrasonic emboli detection and characterization have been reported in the literature, these reports are scarce and do not convey a unique approach. The field of analysis of Doppler embolic signals has been, since its inception, strongly dependant of the computational power required to sustain its development. While other areas of Doppler blood flow somehow strived, only recently have the researchers been able to gather the signal processing methods and the computational power to overcome the challenges. A perspective of high-performance computing will give the reader a broad idea of the field in order to be able to select and /or adopt a solution to support further studies.

To conclude, final remarks are drawn and future trends identified, focusing not only on embolic signals analysis but also on telemedicine and the use of grid technologies to provide for the computational power necessary to support medical decisions.

This chapter aims to present an integrated view to the Analysis of Doppler Embolic Signals using High-Performance Computing, addressing foundation issues such as physiological aspects of emboli, Transcranial Doppler ultrasound, estimation methods, clinically relevant metrics, and some supporting high-performance cluster and grid technologies.

BACKGROUND

High-Performance Cluster and Grid Computing

High-performance computing aims to deliver the computational power and resources necessary to address issues with performance requirements that would require expensive resources or would otherwise be unavailable. The performance requirements vary with the particular application concerned and thus the requirements being evaluated. When the quality of the system being assessed is associated with time, the systems are designated real-time systems. In a hard real-time system, it is a failure not to comply with a deadline or not to be able to sustain the required rate of production of results; these occurrences in a soft real-time system would not be qualified as failure but as loss of quality.

In the context of the analysis of Doppler embolic signals the use of high-performance computing may be required in order to enable the deliverance of the required computing power in clinical or research settings. In a clinical setting, it is often required the timely presentation of the clinically relevant indicators. In the context of research, the investigation of methods and techniques require that significant amounts of data are repeatedly computed and results evaluated. The former case might be a hard real-time system and the latter a soft real-time system. In any case, the use of high-performance computing is driven by the requirements of the application, and, like so many other areas, a continuous increase is felt.

The first approaches to high-performance computing consisted in trying to harness the computational power of several processing elements. Later, this kind of solution involved parallel computing where multiprocessor or multicomputer systems were used. These systems would deliver the required computational power, greater than the one that could be achieved by a single machine or at a lower cost.

Nowadays, performance requirements are more elaborate and the solutions may involve the use of distributed systems, where several systems cooperate in order to achieve some goals. Stressing that the underlying motivation to high-performance computing is the harvesting and sharing of resources, it should be noted that these resources are not restricted to devices and peripherals but may extend to computational power, storage capacity or sharing the software infrastructure.

The terminology used in high-performance computing systems is not a closed issue. Distinctions are made as time passes and technology evolves, as illustrated by Dongarra, Sterling, Simon & Strohmaier (2005). Sometimes, the name translates more than the architecture of the system, conveying the hierarchy of decision or the sharing policy.

In mid 1990's, the distinction of parallel and distributed systems was based on whether a direct coupling between CPUs existed. This implied that in a parallel system all CPUs were in the same box or frame and anything else with more than one CPU was a distributed system. Tanenbaum (2001) proposes the designation of multiprocessor system for a computer system with two or more CPU's that fully share a common RAM and multicomputers (or cluster of computers) for tightly-coupled CPUs that do not share memory. Parallel systems are under the same administrative domain and the composing elements are tightly-coupled.

Cluster computing is the term used for a parallel system where tightly-coupled CPU's from multiple computers are brought together, under a common administration sharing its resources. The popularity of clusters is largely due to high-performance, high-availability, and high-throughput processing characteristics obtainable from commodity-off-the-shelf computers (Yeo, Buyya, Pourreza, Eskicioglu, Graham, & Sommers, 2006).

One of the advantages of cluster computing is to make available, at low cost, the computational power to address in manageable time some categories of problems. Clusters can be built from identical or different computers, with one or more processors. Parallelism and data movement (communication) may be obtained explicitly, by including directives or parallelisation-specific instructions in the application code, or implicitly by making use of libraries or compilers that produce the corresponding code to a target system. For instance, deploying parallel application on a cluster may rely on the Message Passing Interface (MPI) standard or the Parallel Virtual Machine (PVM™) framework for communication support or rely on the OpenMP™ standard for explicit parallelism (Oliveira & du Buf, 2003); an implicit parallel application may be obtained using a High Performance Fortran compiler, or using a tailored library (Latt & Chopard, 2003).

A distributed system may be defined as a collection of independent computers that, to its users, appear as a single coherent system (Tanenbaum & Van Steen, 2002) or as one in which components, located at networked computers, communicate and coordinate their actions only by passing messages (Coulouris, Dollimore, & Kindberg, 2001). The models to unite independent computers or systems into a distributed system vary. In any case, computers under different administration and that do not share a common clock are brought together to achieve a high-performance goal.

In a distributed system, it is common to distinguish three layers. The top layer is the application level, at the intermediate level the middleware provides the communication and resource sharing services and the lower level is the communication layer, usually the Internet. Ideally a distributed system should be transparent, secure and scalable, allow for heterogeneity of its components and for the security of the system and data, handle failures or faults and manage the concurrency of its components. Independently of the model used (master-slave, client-server with or without mobile computing, or peer-to-peer), it can be noted an increasing presence of distributed applications over Internet, such as electronic banking or audio and video sharing.

Progressive advances in device miniaturization and power consumption have favoured, increasingly, the use of small and portable computing devices in everyday life. These devices may range from laptop computers to devices embedded in appliances thus including personal digital assistants (PDAs), mobile phones, digital cameras or wearable devices (such as smart watches). The pervasiveness of these portable computing devices allied with wireless communication facilitated the integration of these devices with distributed systems, not only to network remote sensors but also as mobile computing platforms.

Taking advantage of the consolidation of Internet technologies, grid computing appears as a particular kind of distributed computing. The concept of the grid is to foster the development of large scientific applications combining different resources that cover many disciplines and organizations, complementing the existing solutions (Foster, Kesselman, & Tuecke, 2001). Separate systems (massively parallel systems, clusters of computers or portable and mobile devices) are the building blocks of a grid. In such a grid the resources shared are physical (hardware), informational (data), capabilities (software) and frameworks (grid middleware) (Blanquer, Hernández, Mas, & Segrelles, 2004). A key concept in grid computing is a virtual organization. An organization is represented by a set of resources and services made accessible through an interface, subject to protocols that define the sequence of interactions among the resources and services in order to implement a policy. This policy defines the rules that specify the admissible patterns of use of types of resources and/or services (Foster, Kesselman, & Tuecke, 2001).

A grid integrates and coordinates resources and users that live within different control domains, being built from multi-purpose protocols and interfaces that address fundamental issues as authentication, authorization, resource discovery and resource access. It allows the constituent resources to be used in a coordinated fashion to deliver various qualities of service such as response time, security and/or co-allocation of multiple resource types to meet complex user demands (Foster, 2002). With this in mind, grid environments are inherently large, heterogeneous, dynamic and unreliable. Grid applications are equally complex, heterogeneous and highly dynamic in their behaviours and interactions (Parashair & Browne, 2005).

The use of high-performance computing in health related applications ranges from wearable devices for home monitoring to grid applications to enable a diagnose in reasonable time or to plan a surgery.

Physiological Significance of Emboli

Emboli are particles, gas bubbles or fat substances that travel through circulation. Most emboli are derived from thrombus and are called thromboemboli. Other emboli are originated by bone or haematopoietic medulla fragments, atheromatous detritus from atherosclerotic plaques, little fat drops, tumour fragments, and organism's foreign bodies and air or nitrogen bubbles (Hudorović, 2006).

Several cardiovascular disorders are usually associated to embolic occurrence. There are evidences of the significance of accurately detect and characterize embolic events; for example, the identification of risk of stroke in asymptomatic patients, the therapeutic decision in symptomatic patients, the identification of the type of stroke or the identification of the source of emboli (Azarpazhooh & Chambers, 2006), (Hudorović, 2006), (Sloan, et al., 2004).

Hemorrhagic stroke is the most common kind of stroke. It occurs due to the rupture of vascular lesions (blood involves the cerebral tissue around the injury). Ischemic strokes, on the other hand, are derived by an obstruction (arteriosclerosis, embolus, thrombus, haemorrhage, or vasospasms) of the bigger arteries from the cerebral circulation (Hademenos, 1997).

Embolism is classified according to the place of occlusion or the nature of the embolic material as pulmonary, systemic, infusion, gaseous or fat. Pulmonary emboli can obstruct smaller branches of the pulmonary arteries and are frequent cause of death; systemic emboli often result in infarction, and, a small embolus obstructing the MCA can lead to death in a few days or hours; infusion emboli, caused by amniotic liquid, occur with parturition or immediately after, and frequently lead to the death of the mother; gaseous emboli are air or gas bubbles that obstruct the vascular flow due to lesions in the tissues (barotraumas), and eventually, can lead to problems on the cerebral vessels resulting on coma or death; fat emboli are small drops of fat that are not usually lethal, although fat micro-aggregates might lead to pulmonary or cerebral occlusion (Hademenos, 1997).

Embolic diagnosis requirements are not limited to the detection and quantification of emboli. It is necessary to be capable of distinguishing artefacts (patient movements, tissue vibration, etc) from real circulating emboli, determining the nature of emboli (gaseous, particulate or fat), differentiating between different types of solid emboli, and evaluating micro-emboli size.

Doppler Ultrasound TCD

Since the 40s, when the first work on ultrasound medical diagnosis was published (Hagen-Ansert, 2006), ultrasound has been increasingly used for medical diagnosis purposes. Ultrasound devices provide a non-surgical way for observing the interior of the human body. The amount of publications in reference literature on this subject reveals the attention that has been drawn to this technology across the years.

Ultrasound is a sound wave with frequencies above the human audible range of frequencies, i.e., above 20 kHz. Diagnostic ultrasound devices emit ultrasound waves to the human body, and collect and analyse the echoes returned by the structures reached by the wave.

Dispersion, reflection, and absorption are the main causes of ultrasound attenuation. Higher transmitted frequencies of the waves produce more attenuation, decrease the penetration capability, but improve the skill of imaging near structures with increased resolution. The choice of the transmitting frequency depends on the depth willing to be reached and the resolution to be sought.

The Doppler Effect is a physical principle observed from the relative movement between a source of waves and an observer. If the source and the observer are moving close to each other, the relative frequency perceived by the observer is higher than the emitted frequency. Otherwise, if the observer and the source are moving away from each other, the frequency measured by the observer is lower than the emitted frequency. The signal representing the difference between the emitted and the received signals is called the Doppler signal (Evans & McDicken, 2000).

Doppler ultrasound, in particular, is mostly applied in medicine for analysing the blood flow behaviour and finding possible disease patterns. Examples of Doppler systems are Continuous Wave Doppler (CW), Pulse Wave Doppler (PW), Multigate Doppler system, Duplex scanning, that combines PW or CW with B-Mode scanning systems, and Colour Flow Imaging, that combines a Multigate Doppler system with B-scanning system (Hoskins, Thrush, Martin, & Whittingham, 2003). These systems make use of the Doppler Effect: phase information from the echoes returned by moving structures in the body can be extracted, and used to produce images, blood velocity spectra and estimates of several hemodynamic quantities.

On Doppler ultrasound systems, an ultrasound beam is emitted using a transmitting transducer towards the target to be analysed; then the ultrasound waves echoed by the moving targets will be caught by a receiving transducer and compared with the emitted waves to compute the Doppler signal.

In what concerns diagnosis, one should consider the combination of two Doppler Effects: the source (transducer) as a static subject and the target (blood cells) are considered as moving structures, and the opposite effect, this is, the source (blood cells) are considered moving and the target (transducer) is assumed static.

Doppler signals can be represented by the Doppler equation,

$$f_d = f_t - f_r = 2f_t \frac{v \cos(\theta)}{c} \qquad (1)$$

where f_d, f_t and f_r are respectively the Doppler frequency, the transmitted and received frequencies, v is the velocity of the target, θ the angle between the ultrasound beam and the direction of the moving target and c is the velocity of the sound on the medium.

The values of f_t, θ and c are known. Therefore, the target velocity can be found if the Doppler frequency is also known,

$$v = \frac{c\, f_d}{2f_t \cos(\theta)} \qquad (2)$$

When a wave is transmitted at a known frequency in direction to a specific vessel, the targets (mainly red blood cells) reflect the wave, originating several echoes. Comparing those echoes with the transmitted frequency according to (1), the velocity of the targets can be found from (2).

For medical applications the transmission frequency is usually in the range of 2 to 10 MHz, depending on the depth demanded and the sort of tissues that the ultrasound will cross (Evans & McDicken, 2000).

Two main classes of Doppler ultrasound equipments can be considered, according to the instrument's operating method: Continuous Wave and Pulsed Wave Doppler.

Pulsed Wave Doppler devices use a single transducer working on two periods, for sending and receiving the echoes. In particular, TCD Pulsed Wave instrumentation allows the insonation of the basal portions of the major cerebral arteries.

Doppler ultrasound analysis of cerebral arteries located under the skull, present some technical difficulties. The bony skull greatly attenuates ultrasound beams. In addition, cerebral blood vessels are small and tightly packed together, making the identification of a vessel or its location difficult. In fact, the vessels cannot be directly visualised and their locations and identification must be deducted from the Doppler signals (Zuilen, Gijn, & Ackerstaff, 1998).

Although ordinary medical ultrasound Doppler diagnosis applications use frequency values between 5 and 8 MHz, TCD instrumentation operates around 2 MHz to enable the penetration of the skull; however, even such frequencies cannot adequately penetrate most bones.

For most purposes, the only part of the skull that provides a suitable ultrasonic "window" is the thinnest portion of the squamous part of the temporal bone, just in front of the ear. This transtemporal window is usually used to insonate the vessels of the circle of Willis (see Figure 1).

The quality of the Doppler signal varies with the thickness of the bone which depends on the age, gender, and ethnic group of the patient. The transtemporal window can be localised quite anteriorly (close to the vertical portion of the zygomatic bone) or, more frequently, posteriorly (close to the pinna of the ear). The vessels that can be examined through this window include the terminal portion of the internal carotid artery, its bifurcation into the middle and the anterior cerebral arteries, and the posterior cerebral artery. Sometimes the communicating arteries (either

Figure 1. Temporal bone structure

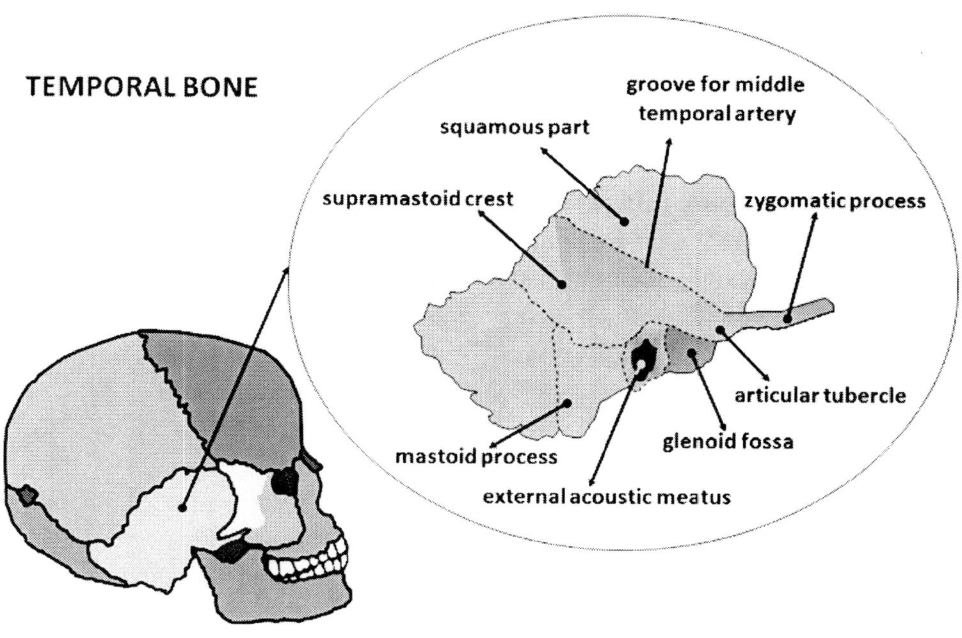

anterior or posterior) can also be sampled, but they are more dependent upon the hemodynamic variability of the circle of Willis.

CURRENT DIAGNOSTIC APPROACHES TO TCD EMBOLIC ANALYSIS

First studies on emboli detection were reported in the decade of 1960. **Emboli** are often identified as high intensity transient signals, and their detection, through TCD, depends on the power returned from emboli being higher than the one returned from the background blood flow. The effective power of the embolic signals cannot be accurately measured, as the attenuation by the tissues between the transducer and the embolus is not known. The estimated power of the background signal, which suffers similar attenuation, is typically used as a basis of comparison (Evans D. H., 1999).

Embolic signals are usually described as amplitude modulated sine waves, sometimes also containing frequency modulation. Emboli duration frequently varies between 2 and 100ms and their powers range from 3dB to more than 60dB above the power of the background signal. Embolic events are also characterized by a random occurrence within the cardiac cycle. Within the proper dynamic range of the bidirectional instrumentation, the signal should be unidirectional within the Doppler spectrum. Depending on the equipment used and on the velocity of the emboli, the embolic signals can be identified as a snap, a chirp or a moan on an audible output (Ackerstaff, et al., 1995), (Evans D. H., 1999), (Hudorović, 2006).

Detection of embolic events can be thought as a statistical process, on which an occurrence with a small size and power has less probability of being detected. Also, emboli have higher probability of being detected during the diastolic phase of the cardiac cycle. Velocities are higher in systole, and thus, emboli can only be seen for a shorter period. Furthermore, the higher amount of blood in the artery during systole might increase the risk of confusing the power of emboli with the power of background blood (Leiria, 2005).

The "gold standard" for embolic detection remains the human observer (Azarpazhooh & Chambers, 2006). However, people are vulnerable to factors like fatigue and distraction that might lead to mistakes. On the other hand, automatic detection systems are not simple. These systems must include features such as the determination of ratio between the power backscattered by the embolus and the power of the remaining signal; the detection threshold (measured in decibels) chosen to classify an event as being or not an emboli; the position in the cardiac cycle at which the event occurs; the size of the sample volume. The performance of these automatic systems is affected by the spectral estimation method used and time and frequency resolutions achieved; the dynamic range of the instrumentation (in decibels); the transmitted ultrasound frequency (in megahertz); the filter settings in kilohertz (high pass filters should suppress low frequencies from arterial wall oscillations); and the recording time (Ringelstein B. E., et al., 1998), (Ringelstein & Droste, 1999).

The pursuit of automatic systems for emboli detection and characterization that can substitute the current "gold standard" with improved performance and new capabilities has been a recurrent subject in literature. These systems have been provided with alternative spectral (and time) estimators, with intelligent classification methods and with alternative device configuration.

Spectral Representation of Doppler Signals

Correct characterization of cerebral emboli depends on the performance of signal processing techniques involved. Different methodologies have been used and there is no consensus as to

Figure 2. Excerpt of an MCA TCD signal represented in time (left) and time-frequency (right) domains

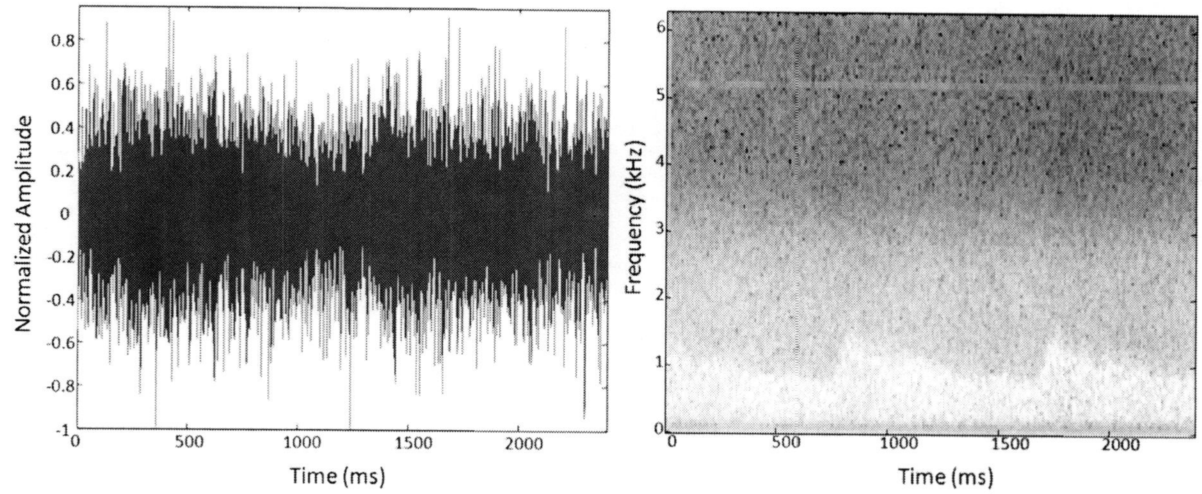

whether time domain or TF domain processing should be used. Excerpts of MCA signals obtained with TCD and the corresponding time-frequency representations are depicted in Figures 2, 3 and 4, without and with emboli.

Time-domain processing was reported as the most accurate method for extracting the relevant parameters for embolic characterization (Cowe, Gittins, Naylor, & Evans, 2005), but signals represented in the TF domain are easier to manipulate and enable a more friendly display (Leiria, Moura, Ruano, & Evans, 2005). A presentation of the most commonly used estimators, namely STFT, time-frequency distributions of the Cohen's class, parametric methods, wavelets and the displacement-frequency method follows.

Figure 3. Excerpt of an MCA TCD signal with a particulate embolus represented in time (left) and time-frequency (right) domains

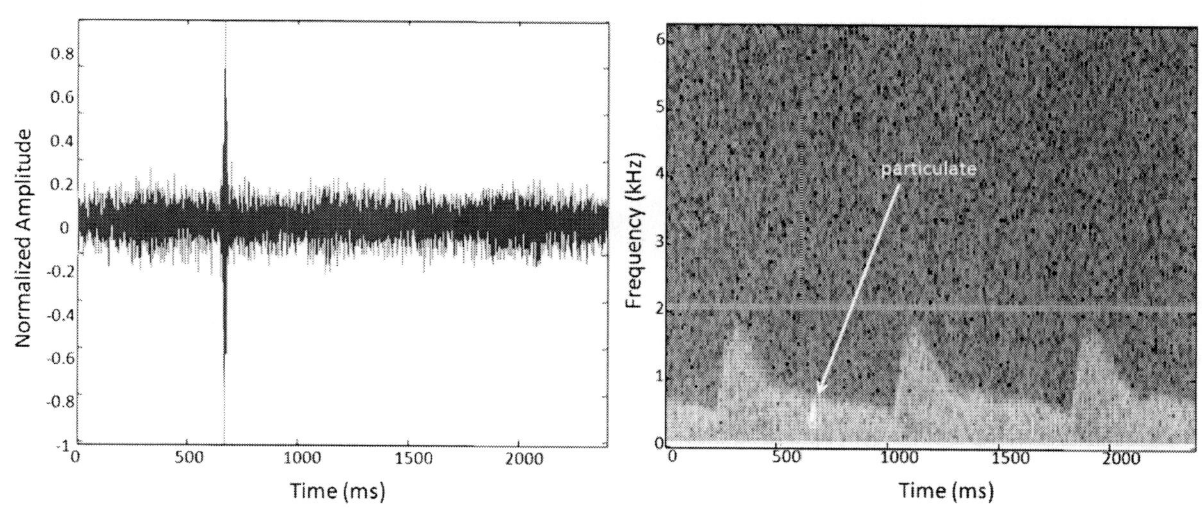

Figure 4. Excerpt of an MCA TCD signal, with two gaseous emboli with an artefact in between, represented in time (left) and time-frequency (right) domains

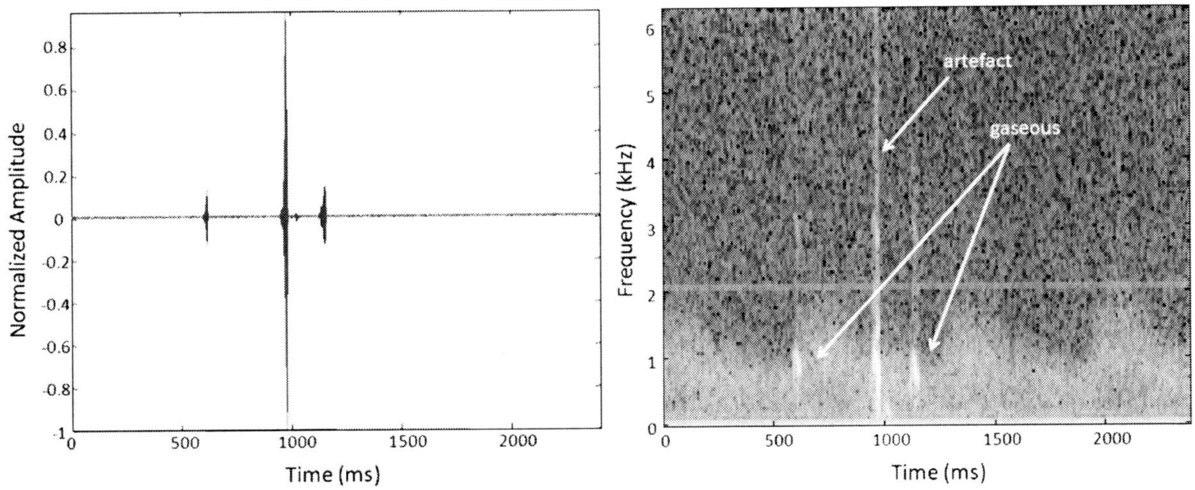

Time-Frequency Estimators

The classical approach is the spectral estimation based on Fourier Transform (Aydin & Markus, 2000). Fourier analysis is an important tool for determining the frequencies in a signal. The main limitation is its inadequacy to deal with most non-stationary signals, as it is not able to distinguish the times at which each frequency occurs. The need for studying general non-stationary signals led to the development of TF estimators capable of describing the density of energy of the signals in time and frequency simultaneously. TF spectra convey the complete information: which frequencies are present in the signal and when do they occur (Cohen, 1989).

The classical approach to TF spectrum estimation is the STFT. It can be computed by taking successive Fourier Transforms over short time sections of the signal, becoming, in the discrete formulation:

$$TF_{STFT} = \left| \sum_{\tau=0}^{N} x(\tau) w(\tau + n) e^{\frac{-j2k\pi\tau}{N}} \right|^2 \qquad (3)$$

where n and k are respectively the discrete time and frequency indices, $x(n)$ is the time domain Doppler signal, $w(n)$ a symmetric sliding window function centred on n, and N is the number of points of the window. The time lag is represented by τ.

The choice of $w(n)$ length remains an issue. It should be large enough to diminish the spectral leakage introduced by windowing the signal, and short enough to deal with the very short durations of some embolic events. Other open issues are the window function that shapes $w(n)$ and the percentage of overlap between windows. The International Consensus Group on Microembolus Detection advises the usage of windows between 5 and 10ms and at least 50% of overlap (Ringelstein B. E., et al., 1998). A more recent study suggests that the length of windows should be between 8.9 and 17.9ms, the overlap between 55% and 97%, also advising for the use of Hamming, Hanning or Bartlet windows (Aydin & Markus, 2000). It should be noted that these choices depend on the particularities of the study, namely on the specifications of the signals being address, the settings of the acquisition system, and the measures being performed.

TF distributions are among the most popular alternatives to STFT. The Cohen's class TF distributions are characterised by a kernel function $\phi(\xi,\tau)$, and can be obtained by:

$$TDF(t,\omega) = \int_{-\infty}^{+\infty}\int_{-\infty}^{+\infty} R_x(t,\tau)\Psi(t-\mu,\tau)e^{-j\tau\omega}d\mu d\tau \quad (4)$$

where the instantaneous autocorrelation function of $x(t)$ is defined by

$$R_x(\mu,\tau) = x\left(\mu + \frac{\tau}{2}\right)x^*\left(\mu - \frac{\tau}{2}\right) \quad (5)$$

and the autocorrelation domain kernel is given by:

$$\Psi(t,\tau) = \int_{-\infty}^{+\infty} \varphi(\xi,\tau)e^{-j\xi t}d\xi \quad (6)$$

being ξ the frequency lag.

Examples of commonly used kernels functions are $\phi(\xi,\tau) = 1$ that characterizes the Wigner distribution, or $\varphi(\xi,\tau) = e^{-\xi^2\tau^2/\sigma}$ (σ is a scaling factor) that characterizes the Choi-Williams distribution (CWD) (Cohen, 1989), (Choi & Williams, 1989).

The use of alternative TF estimation methods has been widely reported. Just to mention some in the context of embolic signals analysis: the Wigner analysis (Smith J. L., Evans, Fan, Thrush, & Naylor, 1997), Bessel, Cone-kernel distribution (Roy, Abraham, Montresor, & Saumet, 2000) and Choi-Williams Distribution (Leiria, 2005), Modified Group Delay Function based on STFT (Xu & Wang, 2006), or the Hilbert-Huang Transform (Hao & Zhang, 2007).

Another approach to TF estimators is based on parametric methods. These estimators have been reported to improve the performance achieved by conventional methods, namely on what concerns to embolic analysis. Unlike the conventional methods, parametric methods do not assume that the non-available data, or the data points that fall outside of the window, are null. They operate on a model of the signal rather than directly on the signal.

Among the parametric estimators, Autoregressive (AR) method has been preferred mainly due to the computational efficiency. AR models the current value of a process $x(n)$ as a linear sum of previous values of the same process and current estimation error $e(n)$.

$$x(n) = \sum_{l=1}^{p} a(l)x(n-l) + e(n) \quad (7)$$

In the above equation, $a(l)$ stand for the parameters of the model and p for the order of the model.

The Modified Covariance spectral estimator is an AR parametric method that estimates the parameters of the model from the solution of the covariance matrix

$$\begin{bmatrix} c_{xx}[1,1] & c_{xx}[1,2] & \cdots & c_{xx}[1,p] \\ c_{xx}[2,1] & c_{xx}[2,2] & \cdots & c_{xx}[2,p] \\ \vdots & \vdots & \ddots & \vdots \\ c_{xx}[p,1] & c_{xx}[p,2] & \cdots & c_{xx}[p,p] \end{bmatrix} \begin{bmatrix} \hat{a}[1] \\ \hat{a}[2] \\ \vdots \\ \hat{a}[p] \end{bmatrix} = -\begin{bmatrix} c_{xx}[1,0] \\ c_{xx}[2,0] \\ \vdots \\ c_{xx}[p,0] \end{bmatrix} \quad (8)$$

where

$$c_{xx}[i,j] = \frac{1}{2(N-p)}\left(\sum_{n=p}^{N-1} x^*[n-i]x[n-j] + \sum_{n=p}^{N-1-p} x[n+i]x^*[n+j]\right) \quad (9)$$

The power spectrum can be computed from

$$P_{AR}(k) = \frac{\hat{\sigma}^2}{\left|1 + \hat{a}[1]e^{-j2k\pi} + \cdots + \hat{a}[p]e^{-j2k\pi p}\right|} \quad (10)$$

where the white noise variance estimate is given by

$$\hat{\sigma} = c_{xx}\left[0,0\right] + \sum_{l=1}^{p} \hat{a}\left[l\right] c_{xx}\left[0,k\right] \quad (11)$$

Parametric methods, as conventional methods, are prepared to deal with stationary signals. To obtain proper TF spectra, an algorithm similar to the one used for STFT must be adopted. It should be noted that the same issues concerning the type, size and overlap of the window apply. The TF version of the AR Modified Covariance, the Short Time Modified Covariance (STMC), is recurrently applied to estimate Doppler blood flow spectra.

The choice of the model order is an issue to be addressed. Although $p = 2$ has been used (Guetbi, Kouame, Ouahabi, & Remenieras, 1997), (Girault, Kouamé, Ouahabi, & Patat, 2000), values of $p \geq 4$ have been advised (Leiria, 2005).

Spectral analysis based on parametric modelling has been further addressed in other studies (Kouamé, Girault, Ouahabi, & Patat, 1999) (Girault, Kouamé, Ouahabi, & Patat, 2000) (Kouamé, Biard, Girault, & Bleuzen, 2006).

Wavelets

The Wavelet Transform (WT) has been described as an extension of the Fourier transform that works on a multi-scale basis instead of on a single scale (time or frequency) (Güler & Übeyli, 2006). Therefore WT represents variable time and frequency resolutions over the entire TF plane, enabling the analysis of non-stationary signals.

This TF multi-resolution is achieved by decomposing the signal on a set of functions. These functions are obtained from translation and dilation operations applied to a single prototype function $\psi(t)$, the mother wavelet function. Translation will shift $\psi(t)$ along the time axis while dilation or scaling will compress or stretch it. The adequate choice of $\psi(t)$ and of the shifting and scaling parameters will enable approximations of the signal $x(t)$.

The Continuous Wavelet Transform (CWT) of a signal $x(t)$ is defined by

$$CWT\left(\tau, s\right) = \frac{1}{\sqrt{|s|}} \int x\left(t\right) \psi^{*}\left(\frac{t-\tau}{s}\right) dt \quad (12)$$

where t and s are the time and scale parameters, $x(t)$ the time domain signal, and $\psi^*(t)$ the complex conjugate of the wavelet function. Factor $1/\sqrt{|s|}$ ensures energy preservation.

The relationship between scale (s) and frequency (f) is given by $s=f_0/f$, for f_0 being the central frequency of the Fourier Transform of the wavelet (Matos, Leiria, & Ruano, 2000).

Continuous, in the context of the WT, implies that the scaling and translation parameters change continuously, what results in a significant effort and amount of data (Güler & Übeyli, 2006).

The decomposition of the wavelet series can be obtained by sampling the time and scale parameters of the CWT. Like so, the scale parameter is sampled at a logarithmic scale and the time parameter is sampled according to s:

$$\begin{aligned} s &= s_0^j \\ \tau &= k s_0^j \tau_0 \qquad j,k \in Z \end{aligned} \quad (13)$$

The Discrete Wavelet Transform (DWT) can be obtained by the output of the filter bank that describes this decomposition (see Figure 5).

In Figure 5, $h[n]$ and $g[n]$ are half-band low-pass and high-pass filters respectively, and $\downarrow 2$ represents a down-sampling by 2.

The wavelet function $\psi(t)$ can be obtained from the scaling function $\phi(t)$:

$$\psi\left(t\right) = \sum_{n} g_n \varphi\left(2t + n\right) \quad (14)$$

Figure 5. DWT filter bank

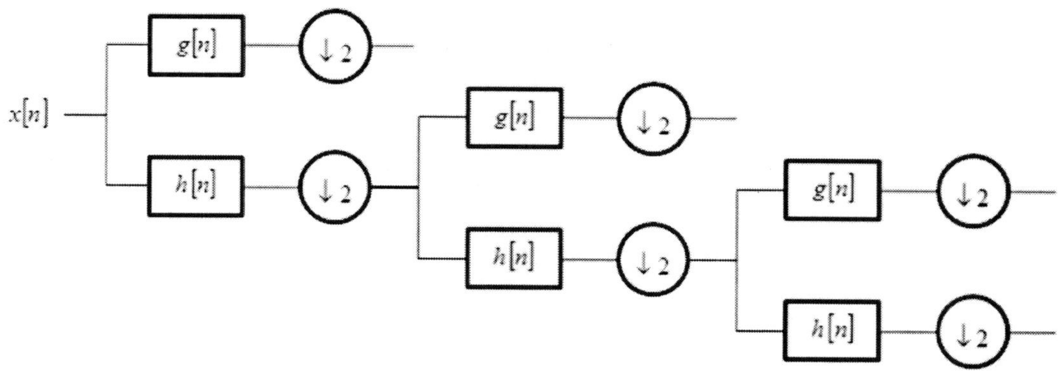

and the filter impulse responses are given by:

$$\Psi\left(t\right)=\sum_{n}h_{n}\varphi\left(2t+n\right) \tag{15}$$

The DWT can be computed from:

$$\begin{aligned} c_k^j &= \sum_n c_k^{j-1} h_{2n-k} \\ d_k^j &= \sum_n c_k^{j-1} g_{2n-k} \qquad j=1,\ldots,J; k\in Z \end{aligned} \tag{16}$$

being c_n^j and d_n^j are the output of the transform and c_n^0 is the signal to analyse, $x[n]$. The filter bank of Figure 5 is implemented by the set of equations defining the DWT.

Wavelet Packets Algorithm (WPA) is another approach to WT, a generalisation of the DWT where, instead of iterating only the lower branch of the filter bank, as shown on Figure 5, the upper branch is also iterated, as shown on Figure 6.

The issue in the application of wavelets is the choice of the wavelet function to be used. A study using different sets of signals indicates that a suitable wavelet for a particular application should be determined experimentally but filters length should be chosen to be higher than 4 (Aydin N., 2006). Among the most commonly used are the Daubechies wavelet of order 8 (Aydin, Marvasti, & Markus, 2004) (Marvasti, Gillies, Marvasti, & Markus, 2004) and the Morlet wavelet (Aydin, Padayachee, & Markus, 1999), (Girault, Kouamé, Ouahabi, & Patat, 2000), (Guetbi, Kouame, Ouahabi, & Remenieras, 1997).

Displacement-Frequency

In the time-domain signal, each bin contains information about all the blood cells in the sample volume at a given time (Leiria, Ruano, & Evans, 2007). Considering that the time signal must be sampled at least twice the maximum frequency observed anywhere in the signal, during some parts of the cardiac cycle, all the relevant information must be contained in just some of the bins, and during other in several bins. The time bins in which new information occurs, assuming that the maximum velocity is relatively static between relevant bins, can be found from:

$$n\left(s\right)=n\left(s-1\right)+\frac{s_{vl}}{v\left(s-1\right)} \qquad s=1,\ldots,M \tag{17}$$

where M is the number of relevant time instants in the time domain signal, s the time bin, s_{vl} is the sample volume length along the axis of the vessel and $v(s)$ the highest component of velocity along the vessel at time $n(s)$. The time resolution required depends on the quantity $\gamma_{\min}$ defined by:

Figure 6. WPA filter bank

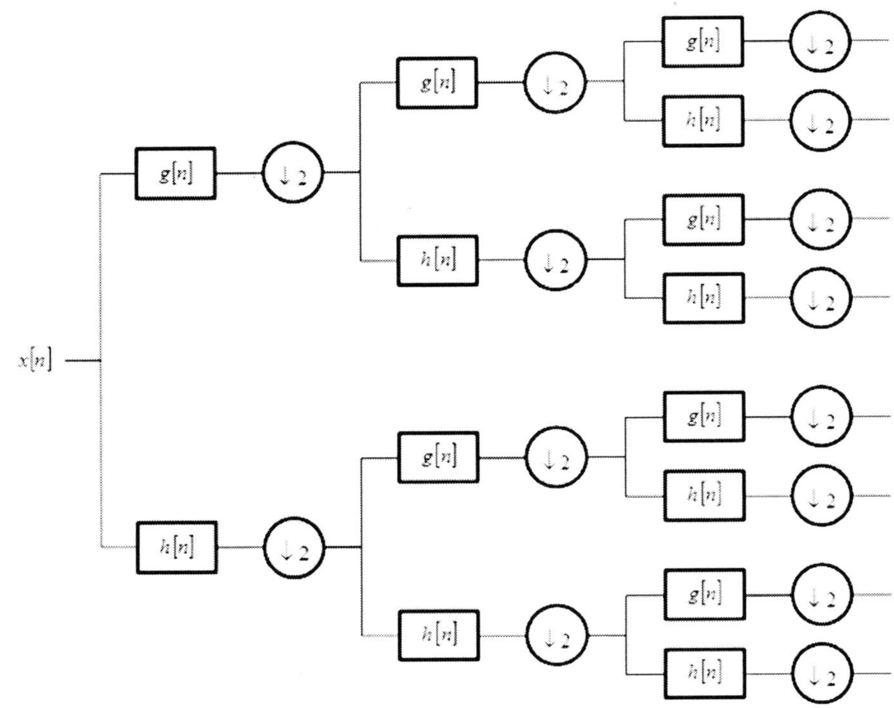

$$\gamma_{\min} = \min\left[n\left(s\right) - n\left(s-1\right)\right] \quad s = 1,\ldots,M \tag{18}$$

The amount of redundant information in the resulting TF representation depends on the bandwidth of the signal (Leiria, 2005).

DF representation is a non-linear function of the time-axis and a linear function of the maximum axial space traversed by the blood cells in a pathway parallel to the ultrasound beam within the sample volume. It can be computed resourcing to any TF representation method. For example, considering the STFT estimation, the corresponding DF becomes:

$$DF_{STFT}\left(s,k\right) = \left|\sum_{\tau=0}^{N-1} x\left(\tau\right) w\left(\tau + n\left(s\right)\right) e^{-\frac{j2k\pi\tau}{N}}\right|^2 \tag{19}$$

The characteristics of DF encouraged its usage for embolic analysis. The highest velocities of blood occur during systole, resulting in a shorter record of the emboli. Thus, when signals are represented in time or TF domain, the probability of missing an embolic event or underestimating its duration is higher when it is travelling during systole (Leiria, Moura, Ruano, & Evans, 2005).

Preliminary studies, with encouraging results, on the spectral analysis of embolic signals resourcing to DF estimation were already published (Leiria, 2005), (Leiria, Moura, Ruano, & Evans, 2005).

The performance of DF is related with the TF representation method chosen, the size and type of the window used, and the displacement resolution given by s_{vl}. The choice of these parameters remains an issue but preliminary studies suggest the use of Hanning windows of 20ms and s_{vl} to be half the size of the sample volume length of the probe (Leiria, Moura, Ruano, & Evans, 2005), (Leiria, 2005).

Clinically Relevant Metrics

Important characteristics of the source of the signals can be directly extracted from their spectra. Spectral parameters usually considered for Doppler blood flow evaluation are maximum and mean frequencies, bandwidth and power variation over time.

According to the Doppler Equation (2), spectral maximum and mean frequencies are proportional to respectively maximum and mean velocities in the signal.

For each time instant (or displacement index), the mean frequency is given by the average of the frequencies weighted by the corresponding spectral intensity. For TF, this is computed from:

$$f_m\left(n\right) = \frac{\sum_{k=0}^{N.1} f\left(n,k\right) TF\left(n,k\right)}{\sum_{k=0}^{N.1} TF\left(n,k\right)} \tag{20}$$

Similar representation can be derived using the DF methodology.

There are several possible approaches for extracting the maximum frequency envelope from clinical data (Evans & McDicken, 2000). The Modified Geometric Method is one of the most used. According to this method, for each time point, the maximum frequency corresponds to the frequency point registering the maximum vertical distance between two lines: the one representing the integrated Doppler power, and, the slope of the curve joining the extremities. Only frequencies above a predetermined threshold should be considered, to exclude the lower frequency interval where noise cannot be assumed to be white Gaussian.

Recall that, according to (17), the maximum frequency estimation is required to implement DF.

The bandwidth is proportional to the flow turbulence observed in the sample volume. The root mean square bandwidth waveform corresponds to the standard deviation of the density function obtained by normalizing the area of the spectral density to unity:

$$b\left(n\right) = \sqrt{\frac{\sum_{k=0}^{N-1} \left[f_m\left(n\right) - f\left(n,k\right)\right]^2 TF\left(n,k\right)}{\sum_{k=0}^{N-1} TF\left(n,k\right)}} \tag{21}$$

The nature and the quantity of scatterers in the sample volume can be accessed from the power variation over time (or displacement). For the TF representation it is given by:

$$p\left(n\right) = \frac{1}{NE_N} \sum_{k=0}^{N-1} \left|TF\left(n,k\right)\right|^2 \tag{22}$$

where E_N is the power density of the window. The DF bandwidth and power variation can be computed similarly (Leiria, Moura, Ruano, & Evans, 2005).

Embolic analysis mostly relies on the observation of the increased power in the Doppler signal during the passage of emboli through the sample volume. Other features, like the duration or the velocities associated to such occurrences, or the sample length over which it can be detected can also be analysed to distinguish embolic events from artefacts or to characterise emboli (Smith J., Evans, Bell, & Naylor, 1998), (Evans D. H., 2003). These characteristics can be extracted from the time domain signal or from its spectrum. Figure 7 depicts a normal (without embolic events) time-frequency spectrum of MCA TCD signal with the mean velocity and normalized power curves superimposed.

A proper observation of those properties is deeply related with many other factors. Some of those factors can be mathematically manipulated, as the choice or tuning of the signal processing

Figure 7. Mean velocity and normalized power superimposed on the time-frequency spectrum

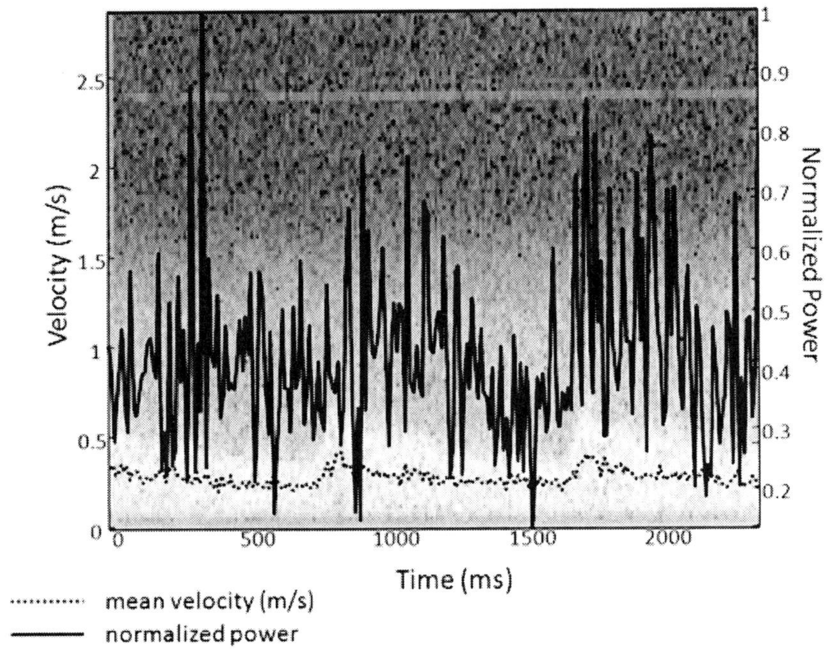

techniques, but others depend on the conditions under which the Doppler signal was recorded.

Embolic signals usually backscatter more power than blood. The power returned by gaseous emboli is even higher than that returned by approximately equally sized solid emboli (Evans D. H., 2003). Figure 8 and Figure 9 depict the time-frequency spectrum of MCA TCD signals, with mean velocity and normalized power curves, upon the occurrence of gaseous and particulate emboli, respectively. Note that in Figure 8 between the two gaseous emboli there is an artefact.

There is still no consensus on the best way to compute the backscattered power ratio. The power of embolic signals can be estimated from the peak intensity measurement or from averaged intensity over a period and frequency frame. The power of the background signal can be computed from the mean intensity of the embolus location for different cardiac cycles; from the frames subsequent to emboli; or from the whole sweep. In spite of these alternative approaches, the Measured Embolic Power (MEP) is used to access the relationship between powers of emboli and blood. It can be computed from

$$MEP = 10\log_{10}\left(\frac{P_E + P_B}{P_B}\right) \tag{23}$$

where P_E is the power backscattered by the embolus and P_B the power backscattered by blood.

The number of samples in the signal with increased power due to emboli can be accessed from the sample volume length (SVL). For time and TF domain representation, SVL is computed from:

$$SVL = D_E v_E \tag{24}$$

where D_E is the time duration of increased power (observed in the signal) and v_E the estimated mean velocity of the embolus.

In DF domain, SVL is given by

Figure 8. Mean velocity and normalized power superimposed on the time-frequency spectrum with gaseous emboli

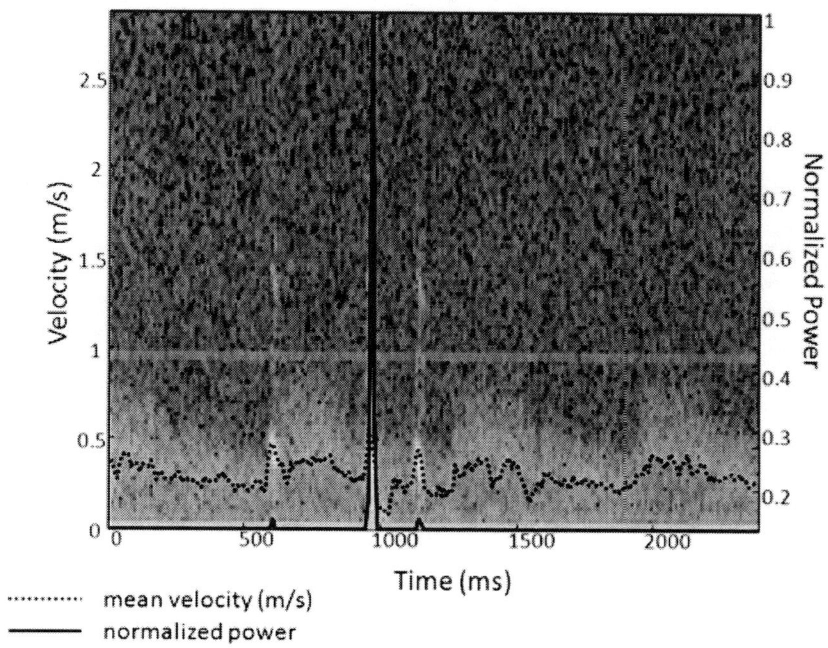

$$SVL = \frac{Lv_E}{v_M} \quad (25)$$

where L is the displacement with increased power (observed in the signal) and v_M is the highest maximum velocity in the signal. This is a simplified expression based on the unrealistic assumption that velocity does not change during the period of observation.

For spectral analysis v_E can be found using (2) and (20), and for the time domain, the embolic frequency is given by the evaluation of (2) considering

$$f_E = \frac{N_{hc}}{2D_E} \quad (26)$$

where N_{hc} is the number of complete half cycles in the time signal during the record of emboli.

Current Approaches

One of the recurring issues in literature concerns the best way to observe the features of TCD embolic signals.

The TF domain representation of blood flow Doppler signals has been widely used in the analysis the behaviour of the blood stream and its relationship with eventual disorders on the circulatory system. However, spectral analysis of emboli and spectral analysis of background blood have different requirements, and depend on distinct relevant parameters. Usually, analysis of blood flow requires accurate estimation of mean frequency and bandwidth, while embolic analysis requires accurate estimation of maximum and mean frequencies and power variation over time.

The application of Cohen's class distributions to embolic signals has been repeatedly questioned due to the trade-off required between time and frequency resolutions (Zhang, Zhang, & Zhang,

Figure 9. Mean velocity and normalized power superimposed on the time-frequency spectrum with a particulate embolus

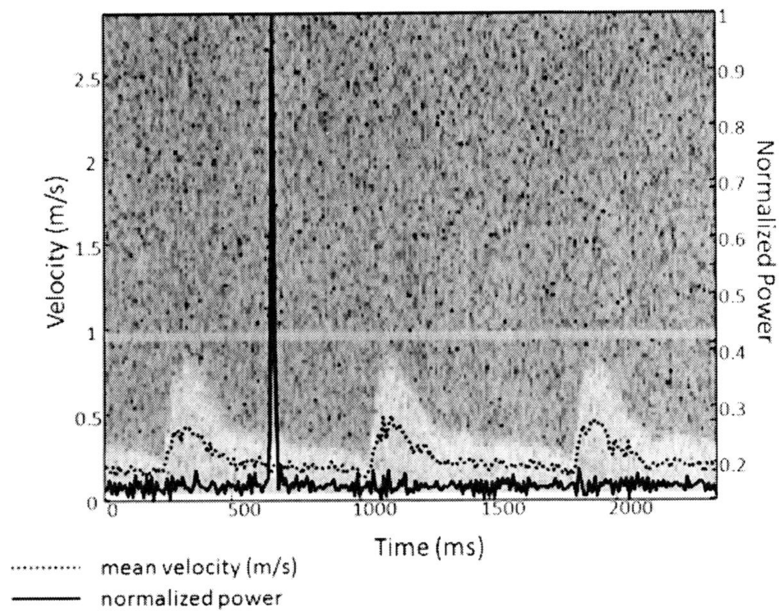

2005), (Xu & Wang, 2007), (Hao & Zhang, 2007), (Chen & Wang, 2008).

Among these methods, STFT is still very used, and has been reported as presenting better results when compared to other Cohen's class distributions (Leiria, 2005), (Roy, Abraham, Montresor, & Saumet, 2000). The only exception is the performance achieved with Wigner distribution that was reported to achieve a performance similar to the time-domain approach in the detection and characterization of embolic events (Smith J., Evans, Bell, & Naylor, 1998).

Figure 10, shows the comparison between the performance of time-domain (TD in the figure), STFT and displacement–frequency STFT (DF in the figure) while distinguishing particulate from gaseous emboli (Leiria, 2005). Notice that although DF does not achieve the same performance of TD, it increases the performance of STFT while diminishing the computational burden. Used together with other spectral estimators, namely the Wigner distribution, the overall performance of DF would probably be improved.

Standard applications of AR methods and WT, although considered very promising, did not provide significant improvements. Nevertheless, it was reported that while the STFT would allow to detect embolic signals with MEP of 20dB and higher, the WT would allow the detection of 9dB and the AR of 6dB (Guetbi, Kouame, Ouahabi, & Remenieras, 1997). Considering both a positive predicted value (PPV) and a negative predicted value (NPV) not higher than 10% it was possible to obtain a threshold for MEP detection of 12dB, 10dB and 4dB for respectively STFT, WT and AR (Girault, Kouamé, Ouahabi, & Patat, 2000).

The results obtained with the above mentioned methods rely, in addition to the settings of the signals acquisition system, on the choice of parameters or functions. Considering the nonstationary nature of the signals, these choices may translate into different performances, according to the part of the signal being analyzed. The amount of possible combination of alternatives strongly limits the optimal tuning of the methods. The optimization of these choices resourcing to, for

Figure 10. Comparison of the performance of time-domain, STFT and displacement-frequency STFT approaches

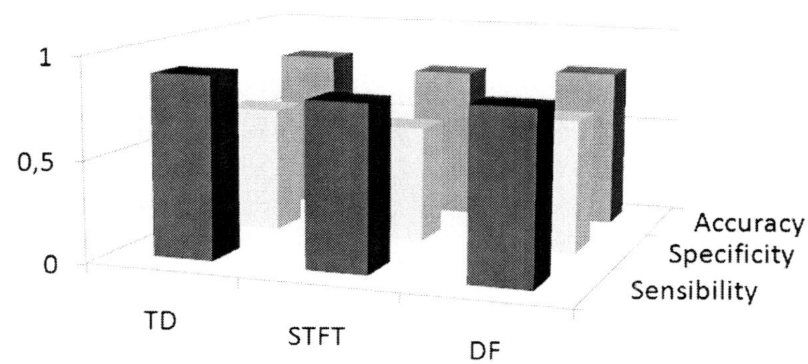

example, multi-objective evolutionary strategies, could lead to fairly good conclusions. Adaptive methods, also being considered in literature, can provide more interesting results (Chen & Wang, 2008). Several authors also claim that time-domain processing can lead to a better signal characterization (Müller, Pan, Walter, & Klaus, 1998), (Smith J., Evans, Bell, & Naylor, 1998), (Cowe, Gittins, Naylor, & Evans, 2005).

Regardless the domain considered to observe the features of the signals, intelligent systems for classifying the emboli are also being addressed; examples are fuzzy systems and neural networks (Teixeira, Ruano, & Ruano, 2004) (Kouamé, Biard, Girault, & Bleuzen, 2006) (Güler & Übeyli, 2006).

New approaches to the configuration of TCD devices, regarding the improvement of embolic analysis were also reported. These approaches include: the usage of two channels, one for the normal forward display and measurements of the blood flow signal, and the other containing the attenuated signal appropriate for the analysis of emboli (Smith J. L., Evans, Fan, Thrush, & Naylor, 1997); the multigated or multidepth technique, which consists of tracing the embolus at two or more depths in the same artery (Devuyst, et al., 2001), (Smith, Evans, & Naylor, 1997); or a variant of the multigated technique, where one of the sample volumes is placed outside the vessel and any event producing increase of power in both channels is considered an artefact was also considered (Georgiadis, Uhlmann, Lindner, & Zierz, 2000).

The results obtained in the analysis of Doppler embolic signals have proven that it is possible to detect values of MEP in the order of 4dB and SVL in the order of 0,01mm (Smith J., Evans, Bell, & Naylor, 1998), (Leiria, 2005). The thresholds for MEP and SVL used for distinguishing between different kind of embolic events depend on the method used, but reference values are MEP=30dB and SVL=12.8mm with Wigner analysis (Smith J. L., Evans, Bell, & Naylor, 1998). Values above 90% for sensibility, specificity and accuracy are currently achievable in ordinary conditions.

Although the different interpretation of the comparative performance of the methods, it is clear that current systems and methods are becoming more reliable (Evans D. H., 2003).

HIGH-PERFORMANCE IMPLEMENTATIONS

The analysis of Doppler embolic signals may be done in a clinical or research setting and accordingly, the processing load and requirements will vary. High-performance implementations will be required whenever the commonly available computers and applications are unable to meet the required performance.

For instance, in a clinical setting offline or real-time processing of Doppler embolic signals may occur. For offline processing of data, a reasonable amount of time can be tolerated. If needed be, dedicated equipment will be devoted to the task, eventually making use of more than one processing unit. Real-time processing will require that the data acquisition and processing should proceed at an adequate rate. The requirements of real-time processing of Doppler embolic signals will take into consideration the sampling frequency and the processing required thus producing a sustainable output rate.

Since the time when the current practice was to record the Doppler raw data for offline processing (Aydin, Padayachee, & Markus, 1999) and the clinical significance of circulating emboli was still an open issue (Markus H., 2000), the requirements in a clinical setting of the analysis of Doppler embolic signals have evolved. At that time, future work aimed to be able to monitor the blood stream as the signals were being collected (i.e. in real time), to be able to distinguish the nature of emboli and, be able to have a battery-powered portable device that would allow to extend the monitoring time up to 8 or 12 hours.

Before the attention was drawn to the clinical significance of Doppler embolic signals, the real-time estimation of Doppler blood flow signals was being investigated aiming the early detection of cardiovascular abnormalities. The estimation of the Doppler spectrum from simulated signals was addressed using different processing elements such as T8 transputers™ (INMOS, Limited, n.d.), the TMS320™ C40 (Texas Instruments, 1991) and the ADSP2016x (Analog Devices SHARC®) (Alex Parallel Computers, Inc., 1996) digital signal processors, using field-programmable gate arrays from Xilink (Xilink, 1995) or general-purpose computer with one or two processors; real-time implementations of the several TF spectral estimators (STFT, STMC, CWD and Bessel time-frequency distribution) were achieved on the processing of common carotid artery and aortic valve ((Leiria, Madeira, & Ruano, ICSPAT'99, 1999; Madeira, Tokhi, & Ruano, 1997) (Madeira, et al., 1999) (Madeira, Tokhi, & Ruano, 2000)). These works considered not only the computational performance of the implementations but also the produced results in consequence of the processing parameters used.

The statistical quality of the results, targeting the optimization of processing parameters for the analysis and detection of Doppler embolic signals was initially addressed by Aydin & Markus (2000), being noted that the performance of the estimator was enhanced by the use of overlapped running windows, with the consequent increase of the computational burden as more data elements must be computed.

The change from offline processing to real-time processing of Doppler embolic signals was done gradually (Mess, Willigers, Ledoux, Ackerstaff, & Hoeks, 2002) (Mackinnon, Aaslid, & Markus, 2004) (Marvasti, Gillies, Marvasti, & Markus, 2004).

In a research setting it is desirable and necessary to test multiple alternatives. In this context, testing implies offline processing of Doppler embolic signals, the estimation of the relevant metrics and the evaluating of the statistical performance of the estimation. It should be noted that the load requirements for the evaluation of performance varies. Results may be compared to previous human classification or, when using a simulation based system, to the waveforms used to generate the simulated signals. In either case, the computational burden is in orders of magnitude higher than the one required when online detection and/or classification of emboli is addressed.

Thus, when in a research context testing alternative approaches is ordinary and repeatedly done, it may be justifiable to make the effort to make use of high-performance solutions and, to the highest possible extent, to automate the procedures.

Such a scenario is described in (Leiria, Moura, Solano, Ruano, & Evans, 2004), illustrating the need for high-performance systems to support research. In order to evaluate the most suitable estimators and the optimal processing parameters for the detection and classification of Doppler embolic signals present in the middle cerebral artery blood flow, signals were simulated, estimated and the quality of the estimation evaluated. Three sets of 100 MCA blood flow signal simulations at different signal-to-noise ratios were generated. STFT, STMC and CWD estimators were used with variable sets of parameters, totalling 4180 different ways to estimate the spectral content of the 300 signals. Assuming that each cardiac cycle has the average duration of 800 ms, and real-time implementations are used, each alternative would require 240 s. Continuing this line of reasoning, using a single machine the time needed just to complete the estimation of the 1 254 000 signal-study cases would be $t = 0.8s \times 300 \times 4\ 180 = 1\ 003\ 200s$ = 11d 14h 40m, simulation and evaluation steps not included. The simulation was done in a single step and the signals generated were used thereafter. The necessary steps to evaluate the quality of the estimation were programmed in Matlab® (Mathworks Inc., 2002). In this case, a **cluster** with eight machines running Debian® GNU®/Linux® was used to diminish the total time.

One of the possible solutions to high-performance computing supporting research would be the use of cluster computing. Not going into too much technical detail due to the inevitable writing/reading gap, some approaches will be described.

The first decision that is presented to a prospective user of cluster computing might be either to buy one or to build one. Both have their cost, moneywise or time wise. If the choice is not buying, next decision is to build a Linux® cluster (Sloan J. D., 2004) (Wanous, 2008) or simply to use one. It should be noted that to deploy an efficient parallel solution, the application may need to be redone. Considering that minimal or no changes are to be made to the application, a simple approach might be a SSI (Single System Image) cluster. Ideally **SSI** clusters will automatically distribute the load and are easily manageable. Main choices are openMosix©, openSSI or Kerrighed® (Lottiaux, Gallard, Vallee, Morin, & Boissinot, 2005).

For cases of higher computational demand, grid computing might be useful. The suggested entry point is the integration of the cluster in the grid.

At the time of writing, the computational power available in commodity computers is enough for detect and classify Doppler embolic signals using time-frequency or time-scale distributions. However, high-performance implementations are still necessary to support more elaborate approaches to such as time domain analysis (Chung, L., Degg, & Evans, 2005) (Mess, Willigers, Ledoux, Ackerstaff, & Hoeks, 2002).

CONCLUDING REMARKS

The objective of this chapter was to present an integrated view of Analysis of Doppler Embolic Signals using High-Performance Computing.

A background section presents the basic aspects of the physics of ultrasound, Doppler Effect, the physiological significance of emboli, and of the Transcranial Doppler instrumentation. The fundamental issues that will constrain the analysis of embolic signals are addressed in an historical perspective of the development of the field. A key aspect that is highlighted is the estimation of the blood flow carrying the emboli. Also in the background section, an overview of high-performance computing and taxonomy is presented.

From the early goals of detection of emboli to the current practice of real-time monitoring of basal circulation, the estimators have gone through tremendous change. The survey includes the main domains of signal representation: time, time-frequency, time-scale and displacement-frequency. Each of the estimators is addressed and the mathematical formulation presented.

Relevant spectral parameters are identified and the mathematical formulation to determine the clinically relevant metrics is clearly presented. The choice of settings required for each of the estimators and the most relevant reports of its use are included. The discussion of results and current approaches draws the attention to the multiplicity of approaches and the lack of a consensus on what is expected from embolic signal analysis as newer and more complex systems are being created.

The use of high-performance computing in clinical and research environment is addressed, illustrating the difference of requirements in each case. The use of high-performance computing on the estimation of Doppler blood flow signals is addressed, noting on the capacity of current commodity computers to be used on the real-time analysis of Doppler embolic systems. Considering the creation of a research scenario where multiple tries are to be conducted, various alternatives are identified discussing the major opportunities and obstacles.

The steep road that the Analysis of Doppler Embolic Signals has been following lately hardens the identification of future trends, because the dreamt future is a step away.

It is expected that future advances will result from synergies from all involved, medical doctors, biomedical, electronic, and/or computer engineers and, last but not least, the patients themselves.

Future Trends

Developments registered in the computer industry have fuelled the demand for further services and facilities. Industries such as banking or entertainment have diversified their offer and increased their presence near the targeted public. This narrowing of distance was the effect of the increased availability of communication systems–either through landlines, fibre optic cable or wireless–and the commodity of computer systems and applications.

Likewise medical and clinical care services were prompted to extend their reach (Krishnan, 2004). Telemedicine added to the performance and security requirements of the computer industry, as dedicated computational and data centres started to emerge. For some time, cluster computing was able to provide the high-performance support necessary to acquire data, process it, analyze it and classify the huge amounts of data that were being fed to the computation systems.

Beyond the manipulation of data, information management became the next goal. Image registration, medical decision support systems, and portable, mobile and wearable devices servicing medical goals exhausted the computational power installed opening the way to grid-enabled solutions and grid applications (Blanquer, Hernández, Mas, & Segrelles, 2004) (Erberich, Silverstein, Chervenak, Schuler, Nelson, & Kesselman, 2007) (Frank, Stotzka, Jejkal, Hartmann, Sutter, & Gemmeke, 2007) (Gutierrez, Lage, Lee, & Zhou, 2007) (Ni, Youn, Kim, Han, & Liu, 2007).

Towards more precise estimation of ES, it is expected that adaptive methods together with intelligent classification systems will have a profounder influence on the actual techniques employed. Amongst the adaptive methods, the displacement-frequency methodology, allied with other techniques namely time-domain ones, inspires confidence on the results obtainable.

Future developments, such as the reduction of the sample volume length of the probes, will further the achievements of signal processing towards the improvement of Health by contributing to diminish the impact of cardiovascular incidents.

REFERENCES

Ackerstaff, R. G., Babikian, V. L., Georgiadis, D., Russell, D., Siebler, M., & Spencer, M. P. (1995). Basic identification criteria of Doppler microembolic signals. Consensus Committee of the Ninth International Cerebral Hemodynamic Symposium. *Stroke*, *26*(6), 1123.

Alex Parallel Computers, Inc. (1996). *Sharc1000 user's manual.*

Aydin, N., & Markus, H. S. (2000). Optimization of processing parameters for the analysis and detection of embolic signals. *European Journal of Ultrasound, 12*(1), 69–79. doi:10.1016/S0929-8266(00)00104-X

Aydin, N., Padayachee, S., & Markus, H. S. (1999). The use of the wavelet transform to describe embolic signals. *Ultrasound in Medicine & Biology, 25*(6), 953–958. doi:10.1016/S0301-5629(99)00052-6

Azarpazhooh, M. R., & Chambers, B. R. (2006). Clinical Application of Transcranial Doppler Monitoring for Embolic Signals. *Journal of Clinical Neuroscience, 6*(8), 799–810. doi:10.1016/j.jocn.2005.12.026

Blanquer, I., Hernández, V., Mas, F., & Segrelles, D. (2004). A Middleware Grid for Storing, Retrieving and Processing DICOM Medical Images. *Working Notes of the Workshop on Distributed Databases and Processing in Medical Image Computing (DIDAMIC).* Rennes, France.

Cardoso, J., Ruano, M. G., & Fish, P. (1996). Non-Stationary Broadening Reduction in Pulsed Doppler Spectrum Measurements Using Time-Frequency Estimators. *IEEE Transactions on Bio-Medical Engineering, 43*(12), 1176–1186. doi:10.1109/10.544341

Chen, Y., & Wang, Y. (2008). Doppler Embolic Signal Detection Using the Adaptive Wavelet Packet Basis and Neurofuzzy Classification. *Pattern Recognition Letters, 29*(10), 1589–1595. doi:10.1016/j.patrec.2008.03.015

Choi, H.-I., & Williams, W. J. (1989). Improved Time-Frequency of Multicomponent Signals using Exponential Kernels. *IEEE Transactions on Acoustics, Speech, and Signal Processing, 37*(6), 862–871. doi:10.1109/ASSP.1989.28057

Chung, E., L., F., Degg, C., & Evans, D. H. (2005). Detection of Doppler embolic signals: Psychoacoustic considerations. *Ultrasound in Medicine & Biology, 31*(9), 1177–1184. doi:10.1016/j.ultrasmedbio.2005.05.001

Cohen, L. (1989). Time-Frequency Distributions – A Review. *Proceedings of the IEEE, 77*(7), 941–981. doi:10.1109/5.30749

Coulouris, G., Dollimore, J., & Kindberg, T. (2001). *Distributed Systems: Concepts and Design* (3rd ed.). Addison Wesley, Pearson Education.

Cowe, J., & Evans, D. H. (2006). Automatic Detection of Emboli in the TCD RF Signal Using Principal Component Analysis. *Ultrasound in Medicine & Biology, 3*(12), 1853–1867. doi:10.1016/j.ultrasmedbio.2006.06.019

Cowe, J., Gittins, J., Naylor, A., & Evans, D. (2005). RF Signals Provide Additional Information on Embolic Events Recorded During TCD Monitoring. *Ultrasound in Medicine & Biology, 31*(5), 613–623. doi:10.1016/j.ultrasmedbio.2005.02.002

Cullinane, M., & Markus, H. S. (2001). Evaluation of a 1 Mhz Transducer for Transcranial Doppler Ultrasound Including Embolic Signal Detection. *Ultrasound in Medicine & Biology, 27*(6), 795–800. doi:10.1016/S0301-5629(01)00369-6

Cullinane, M., Reid, G., Dittrich, R., Kaposzta, Z., Ackerstaff, R., & Babikian, V. (2000). Evaluation of New Online Automated Embolic Signal Detection Algorithm, Including Comparison With Panel of International Experts. *Stroke, 31*(6), 1335–1341.

Daubechies, I. (1990). The Wavelet Transform, Time-Frequency Localization and Signal Analysis. *IEEE Transactions on Information Theory, 36*(5), 961–1005. doi:10.1109/18.57199

Devuyst, G., Darbellay, G. A., Vesin, J.-M., Kemeny, V., Ritter, M., & Droste, D. W. (2001). Automatic Classification of HITS Into Artifacts or Solid or Gaseous Emboli by a Wavelet Representation Combined With Dual-Gate TCD. *Stroke*, *32*(12), 2803–2809. doi:10.1161/hs1201.099714

Dongarra, J., Sterling, T., Simon, H., & Strohmaier, E. (2005). High-Performance Computing: Clusters, Constellations, MPPs, and Future Directions. *Computing in Science & Engineering*, *7*, 51–59. doi:10.1109/MCSE.2005.34

Erberich, S. G., Silverstein, J. C., Chervenak, A., Schuler, R., Nelson, M., & Kesselman, C. (2007). Globus MEDICUS - Federation of DICOM Medical Imaging Devices into Healthcare Grids. *Studies in Health Technology and Informatics*, *126*, 269–279.

Evans, D. H. (1999). Detection of Microemboli. In Babikian, V. L., & Welchser, L. R. (Eds.), *Transcranial Doppler Ultrasonography* (2nd ed., pp. 141–155). Boston: Butterworth-Heineman Medical.

Evans, D. H. (2003). Doppler Detection of Cerebral Emboli: The State-of-the-Art. *Ultrasound in Medicine & Biology*, *29*(5), S38–S39. doi:10.1016/S0301-5629(03)00200-X

Evans, D. H. (2003). Ultrasonic Detection of Cerebral Emboli. *IEEE Symposium on Ultrasonics*, *1*, 316-326. Honolulu, Hawaii.

Evans, D. H., & McDicken, W. N. (2000). *Doppler Ultrasound: Physics, Instrumentation, and Clinical Applications* (2nd ed.). New York: John Wiley & Sons.

Fan, L., & Evans, D. H. (1994). Extracting Instantaneous Mean Frequency Information from Doppler Signals Using the Wigner Distribution Function. *Ultrasound in Medicine & Biology*, *20*(5), 429–443. doi:10.1016/0301-5629(94)90098-1

Fan, L., Evans, D. H., & Naylor, R. (2001). Automated Embolus Identification Using a Rule-Based Expert System. *Ultrasound in Medicine & Biology*, *27*(8), 1065–1077. doi:10.1016/S0301-5629(01)00414-8

Foster, I. (2002, July 20). What is the Grid? A Three Point Checklist. *GRIDToday*.

Foster, I., Kesselman, C., & Tuecke, S. (2001). The anatomy of the grid: Enabling scalable virtual organizations. *International Journal of High Performance Computing Applications*, *15*(3), 200–222. doi:10.1177/109434200101500302

Frank, A., Stotzka, R., Jejkal, T., Hartmann, V., Sutter, M., & Gemmeke, H. (2007). GridIJ - A Dynamic Grid Service Architecture for Scientific Image Processing. *33rd EUROMICRO Conference on Software Engineering and Advanced Applications* (pp. 375-384).

Furui, E., Hanzawa, K., Ohzeki, H., Nakajima, T., Fukuhara, N., & Takamori, M. (1999). "Tail Sign" Associated With Microembolic Signals. *Stroke*, *30*(4), 863–866.

García-Nocetti, F., González, J. S., Acosta, E. R., & Hernández, E. M. (2001). Parallel Processing in Time-Frequency Distributions For Signal Analysis. *BioEng 2001*, (p. ID46.pdf). Faro.

Gatzoulis, L., & Iakovidis, I. (2007). Wearable and Portable eHealth Systems. Technological Issues and Opportunities for Personalized Care. *IEEE Engineering in Medicine and Biology Magazine*, *26*(5), 51–56. doi:10.1109/EMB.2007.901787

Georgiadis, D., Uhlmann, F., Lindner, A., & Zierz, S. (2000). Differentiation Between True Microembolic Signals and Artefacts Using an Arbitrary Sample Volume. *Ultrasound in Medicine & Biology*, *26*(3), 493–496. doi:10.1016/S0301-5629(99)00158-1

Girault, J.-M., Kouamé, D., Ouahabi, A., & Patat, F. (2000). Micro-Emboli Detection: An Ultrasound Doppler Signal Processing View Point. *IEEE Transactions on Bio-Medical Engineering*, *47*(11), 1431–1439. doi:10.1109/10.880094

Guetbi, C., Kouame, D., Ouahabi, A., & Remenieras, J. P. (1997). New Emboli Detection Methods. *IEEE Ultrasonics Symposium, 2*, 1119-1122. Toronto, Canada.

Güler, İ., & Übeyli, E. D. (2006). A Recurrent Neural Network Classifier for Doppler Ultrasound Blood Flow Signals. *Pattern Recognition Letters*, *27*(13), 1560–1571. doi:10.1016/j.patrec.2006.03.001

Guo, Z., Durand, L.-G., & Lee, H. C. (1994). Comparison of Time-Frequency Distribution Techniques For Analysis of Simulated Doppler Ultrasound Signals of the Femoral Artery. *IEEE Transactions on Bio-Medical Engineering*, *41*(4), 1176–1186.

Gutierrez, M. A., Lage, S. H., Lee, J., & Zhou, Z. (2007). *A Computer-Aided Diagnostic System using a Global Data Grid Repository for the Evaluation of Ultrasound Carotid Images* (pp. 840–845). CCGRID.

Hademenos, G. J. (1997). The Biophysics of Stroke. *American Scientist*, *85*(3), 226–235.

Hagen-Ansert, S. L. (2006). Society of Diagnostic Medical Sonographers: A Timeline of Historical Events in Sonography and the Development of the SDMS: In the Beginning. *Journal of Diagnostic Medical Sonography*, *22*(4), 272–278. doi:10.1177/8756479306291456

Hao, D., & Zhang, H. (2007). Detection of Doppler Embolic Signals with Hilbert-Huang Transform. *IEEE/ICME International Conference on Complex Medical Engineering* (pp. 412-415). Beijing, China.

Hoskins, P. R., Thrush, A., Martin, K., & Whittingham, T. A. (2003). *Diagnostic Ultrasound: Physics and Equipment* (Hoskins, P. R., Thrush, A., Martin, K., & Whittingham, T. A., Eds.). London, UK: Greenwich Medical Media.

Hudorović, N. (2006). Clinical significance of microembolus detection by transcranial Doppler sonography in cardiovascular clinical conditions. *International Journal of Surgery*, *4*, 232–241. doi:10.1016/j.ijsu.2005.12.001

INMOS, Limited. (n.d.). Transputer Architecture and Overview, manual of Transputer Education Kit.

Kemény, V., Droste, D. W., Hermes, S., Nabavi, D. G., Schulte-Altedorneburg, G., & Siebler, M. (1999). Automatic Embolus Detection by a Neural Network. *Stroke*, *30*(4), 807–810.

Kouamé, D., Biard, M., Girault, J.-M., & Bleuzen, A. (2006). Adaptive AR and Neurofuzzy Approaches: Access to Cerebral Particle Signatures. *IEEE Transactions on Information Technology in Biomedicine*, *10*(3), 559–566. doi:10.1109/TITB.2005.862463

Kouamé, D., Girault, J.-M., Ouahabi, A., & Patat, F. (1999). Reliability Evaluation of Emboli Detection Using a Statistical Approach. *IEEE Ultrasonics Symposium, 2*, 1601-1604. Nevada, USA.

Krishnan, A. (2004). A survey of life sciences applications on the grid. *New Gen. Comput.*, *22*(2), 111–126. doi:10.1007/BF03040950

Latt, J., & Chopard, B. (2003). An Implicitly Parallel Object-Oriented Matrix Library and its Application to Medical Physics. In *Proceedings of the International Parallel and Distributed Processing Symposium.* IEEE Computer Society.

Leiria, A. (2005). *Spectral Analysis of Embolic Signals.* PhD Thesis, University of Algarve, Faro, Portugal.

Leiria, A., Madeira, M. M., & Ruano, M. G. (1999). Aortic Valve Analyser: A Cost/Benefit Study. *International Conference on Signal Processing Applications and Technology.*

Leiria, A., Moura, M. M., Ruano, M. G., & Evans, D. H. (2005). Time, time-frequency and displacement-frequency analysis of embolic signals. *IEEE International Workshop on Intelligent Signal Processing* (pp. 49-53). Faro, Portugal.

Leiria, A., Moura, M. M., Solano, J., Ruano, M. G., & Evans, D. H. (2004). *Middle Cerebral Artery Blood Flow: Accurate Time-Frequency Evaluation* (pp. 1095–1098). João Pessoa, Brasil: Anais da Conferência Latino-Americana de Engenharia Biomédica.

Leiria, A., Ruano, M. G., & Evans, D. H. (2007). Displacement-Frequency Doppler Blood Flow Estimation. *IEEE International Symposium on Intelligent Signal Processing* (pp. 1-4). Alcalá de Henares, Spain.

Lottiaux, R., Gallard, P., Vallee, G., Morin, C., & Boissinot, B. (2005). OpenMosix, OpenSSI and Kerrighed: a comparative study. *Cluster Computing and the Grid, 2*, 1016–1023.

Mackinnon, A., Aaslid, R., & Markus, H. (2004). Long-term ambulatory monitoring for cerebral emboli using transcranial Doppler ultrasound. *Stroke, 35*(1), 73–78. doi:10.1161/01.STR.0000106915.83041.0A

Madeira, M. M., Bellis, S., Beltran, L., Solano Gonzalez, J., García-Nocceti, F., & Marnane, W. (1999). High Performance Computing for real-time Spectral Estimation. *Control Engineering Practice, 7*, 679–686. doi:10.1016/S0967-0661(98)00207-X

Madeira, M. M., Tokhi, M., & Ruano, M. G. (1997). Comparative Study of Different Doppler Spectral Estimator Implementations. *Preprints of 4th IFAC Workshop on Algorithms and Architectures for Real-Time Control*, (pp. 293-298). Vilamoura, Portugal.

Madeira, M. M., Tokhi, M., & Ruano, M. G. (2000). Real-Time Implementation of a Doppler Signal Spectral Estimator using Sequencial and Parallel Processing Techniques. *Microprocessors and Microsystems, 24*(3), 153–167. doi:10.1016/S0141-9331(00)00071-5

Markus, H. (2000). Monitoring Embolism in Real Time. *Circulation, 102*(8), 826–828.

Marvasti, S., Gillies, D., Marvasti, F., & Markus, H. (2004). Online automated detection of cerebral embolic signals using a wavelet-based system. *Ultrasound in Medicine & Biology, 30*(5), 647–653. doi:10.1016/j.ultrasmedbio.2004.03.009

Mathworks Inc. (2002). *Matlab.* MA, USA: Natick.

Matos, S., Leiria, A., & Ruano, M. G. (2000, July). Blood Flow Parameters Evaluation Using Wavelets Transforms. In *Proceedings of World Congress on Medical Physics and Biomedical Engineering* (pp. 4235-5280). Chicago, USA.

Mess, W., Willigers, J., Ledoux, L., Ackerstaff, R., & Hoeks, A. (2002). Microembolic signal description: a reappraisal based on a customized digital postprocessing system. *Ultrasound in Medicine & Biology, 28*(11-12), 1447–1455. doi:10.1016/S0301-5629(02)00618-X

Moehring, M. A., & Klepper, J. R. (1994). Pulse Doppler Ultrasound Detection, Characterisation and Size Estimation of Emboli in Flowing Blood. *IEEE Transactions on Bio-Medical Engineering, 41*(1), 35–44. doi:10.1109/10.277269

Müller, M., Pan, X., Walter, P., & Klaus, S. (1998). Variability of Velocity and Duration of Microembolic Signals Detected by Bigated Transcranial Doppler Sonography in Carotid Endarterectomy. *European Journal of Ultrasound, 41*(1), 1–6. doi:10.1016/S0929-8266(98)00044-5

Ni, Y.-J., Youn, C.-H., Kim, B.-J., Han, Y.-J., & Liu, P. (2007). A PQRM-based PACS System for Advanced Medical Services under Grid Environment. In *Proceedings of the 7th IEEE International Conference on Bioinformatics and Bioengineering* (pp. 1225-1229).

Oliveira, P., & du Buf, H. (2003). SPMD Image Processing on Beowulf Clusters: Directives and Libraries. In *IPDPS '03: Proceedings of the 17th International Symposium on Parallel and Distributed Processing* (p. 230.1). IEEE Computer Society.

Parashair, M., & Browne, J. C. (2005). Conceptual and Implementation Modules for the Grid. *Proceedings of the IEEE*, *93*(3), 653–668. doi:10.1109/JPROC.2004.842780

Ringelstein, B. E., Droste, D. W., Babikian, V. L., Evans, D. H., Grosset, D. G., & Kaps, M. (1998). Consensus on Microembolus Detection by TCD. International Consensus Group on Microembolus Detection. *Stroke*, *29*(3), 725–729.

Ringelstein, E. B., & Droste, D. W. (1999). Microembolic Signal Criteria. In Babikian, V. L., & Welchser, L. R. (Eds.), *Transcranial Doppler Ultrasonography* (2nd ed., pp. 157–166). Boston, USA: Butterworth-Heineman Medical.

Roy, E., Abraham, P., Montresor, S., & Saumet, J.-L. (2000). Comparison of Time-Frequency Estimators for Peripheral Embolus Detection. *Ultrasound in Medicine & Biology*, *26*(5), 419–423. doi:10.1016/S0301-5629(99)00142-8

Ruano, M. G. (1992). Investigation of Real Time Spectral Analysis Techniques for Use with Pulsed Ultrasound Doppler Blood Flow Detectors. PhD thesis, University College of North Wales, Bangor UK.

Sigel, B. (1998). A Brief History of Doppler Ultrasound in the Diagnosis of Peripheral Vascular Disease. *Ultrasound in Medicine & Biology*, *24*(2), 169–176. doi:10.1016/S0301-5629(97)00264-0

Sloan, J. D. (2004). *High Performance Linux Clusters with OSCAR, Rocks, OpenMosix, and MPI*. O'Reilly.

Sloan, M. A., Alexandrov, A. V., Tegeler, C. H., Spencer, M. P., Caplan, L. R., & Feldmann, E. (2004). Assessment: Transcranial Doppler ultrasonography: Report of the Therapeutics and Technology Assessment Subcommittee of the American Academy of Neurology. *Neurology*, *62*(9), 1468–1481.

Smith, J., Evans, D. H., Bell, P. R., & Naylor, A. R. (1998). Time Domain Analysis of Embolic Signals can be Used in Place of High-Resolution Wigner Analysis when Classifying Gaseous and Particulate Emboli. *Ultrasound in Medicine & Biology*, *24*(7), 989–993. doi:10.1016/S0301-5629(98)00107-0

Smith, J. L., Evans, D. H., Fan, L., Thrush, A. J., & Naylor, A. R. (1997). Processing Doppler Ultrasound Signals from Blood-Borne Emboli. *Ultrasound in Medicine & Biology*, *20*(5), 455–462. doi:10.1016/0301-5629(94)90100-7

Smith, J. L., Evans, D. H., Lingke, F., Bell, P. R., & Naylor, A. R. (1996). Differentiation Between Emboli and Artefacts Using Dual-Gated Transcranial Doppler Ultrasound. *Ultrasound in Medicine & Biology*, *22*(8), 1031–1036. doi:10.1016/S0301-5629(96)00103-2

Smith, J. L., Evans, D. H., & Naylor, A. R. (1997). Analysis of the Frequency Modulation Present in Doppler Ultrasound Signals May Allow Differentiation Between Particulate and Gaseous Cerebral Emboli. *Ultrasound in Medicine & Biology*, *26*(5), 727–734. doi:10.1016/S0301-5629(97)00003-3

Tanenbaum, A. S. (2001). *Modern Operating Systems* (2nd ed.). Prentice Hall.

Tanenbaum, A. S., & Van Steen, M. (2002). *Distributed Systems: Principles and Paradigms. Prentice Hall* (International Editions). Pearson Education.

Teixeira, C., Ruano, M., & Ruano, A. E. (2004). Emboli Classification using RBF Neural Networks. *Sixth Portuguese Conference on Automatic Control* (pp. 630-635). Faro, Portugal.

Texas Instruments. (1991). *TMS320C40 User's Guide.*

Wanous, K. (2008). *Main Page - Debian Clusters*. Obtido em 14 de 06 de 2008, de Debian Clusters for Education and Research: The Missing Manual: http://debianclusters.cs.uni.edu/index.php/Main_Page

Xilink. (1995). Xilinx - The Programmable Logic Data Book.

Xu, D., & Wang, Y. (2006). Automated Emboli Detection from Doppler Ultrasound Signals Using the GDFM and STFT. *Ultrasound in Medicine & Biology*, *32*(5Suppl 1), 100. doi:10.1016/j.ultrasmedbio.2006.02.367

Xu, D., & Wang, Y. (2007). An Automated Feature Extraction and Emboli Detection System Based on the PCA and Fuzzy Sets. *Computers in Biology and Medicine*, *37*(6). doi:10.1016/j.compbiomed.2006.09.002

Yeo, C. S., Buyya, R., Pourreza, H., Eskicioglu, R., Graham, P., & Sommers, F. (2006). Cluster Computing: High-Performance, High-Availability, and High-Throughput Processing on a Network of Computers. In Zomaya, A. Y. (Ed.), *Handbook of Nature-Inspired and Innovative Computing: Integrating Classical Models with Emerging Technologies* (pp. 521–551). doi:10.1007/0-387-27705-6_16

Zhang, Y., Zhang, H., & Zhang, N. (2005). Microembolic Signal Characterization Using Adaptive Chirplet Expansion. *IEEE Transactions on Ultrasonics, Ferroelectrics, and Frequency Control*, *52*(8), 1291–1299. doi:10.1109/TUFFC.2005.1509787

Zuilen, E. V., Gijn, J. V., & Ackerstaff, R. G. (1998). The Clinical Relevance of Cerebral Microemboli Detection by Transcranial Doppler Ultrasound. *Journal of Neuroimaging*, *8*(1), 32–36.

ADDITIONAL READING

Cowe, J., & Evans, D. H. (2006). Automatic Detection of Emboli in the TCD RF Signal Using Principal Component Analysis. *Ultrasound in Medicine & Biology*, *3*(12), 1853–1867. doi:10.1016/j.ultrasmedbio.2006.06.019

Fan, L., & Evans, D. H. (1994). Extracting Instantaneous Mean Frequency Information from Doppler Signals Using the Wigner Distribution Function. *Ultrasound in Medicine & Biology*, *20*(5), 429–443. doi:10.1016/0301-5629(94)90098-1

Furui, E., Hanzawa, K., Ohzeki, H., Nakajima, T., Fukuhara, N., & Takamori, M. (1999). "Tail Sign" Associated With Microembolic Signals. *Stroke*, *30*(4), 863–866.

García-Nocetti, F., González, J. S., Acosta, E. R., & Hernández, E. M. (2001). Parallel Processing in Time-Frequency Distributions For Signal Analysis. *BioEng 2001* (p. ID46.pdf). Faro.

Guo, Z., Durand, L.-G., & Lee, H. C. (1994). Comparison of Time-Frequency Distribution Techniques For Analysis of Simulated Doppler Ultrasound Signals of the Femoral Artery. *IEEE Transactions on Bio-Medical Engineering*, *41*(4), 1176–1186.

Matos, S., Leiria, A., & Ruano, M. G. (2000). Blood Flow Parameters Evaluation Using Wavelets Transforms. In *Proceedings of World Congress on Medical Physics and Biomedical Engineering* (pp. 4235-5280). Chicago, USA.

Ruano, M. G. (1992). Investigation of Real Time Spectral Analysis Techniques for Use with Pulsed Ultrasound Doppler Blood Flow Detectors. PhD thesis, University College of North Wales, Bangor UK.

Smith, J. L., Evans, D. H., Lingke, F., Bell, P. R., & Naylor, A. R. (1996). Differentiation Between Emboli and Artefacts Using Dual-Gated Transcranial Doppler Ultrasound. *Ultrasound in Medicine & Biology*, *22*(8), 1031–1036. doi:10.1016/S0301-5629(96)00103-2

Test of Alternative Spectral Estimators of Doppler Ultrasound Signals Cardoso, J., Ruano, M. G., & Fish, P. (1996). Non-Stationary Broadening Reduction in Pulsed Doppler Spectrum Measurements Using Time-Frequency Estimators. *IEEE Transactions on Bio-Medical Engineering*, *43*(12), 1176–1186. doi:10.1109/10.544341

Chapter 9
Massive Data Classification of Neural Responses

Pedro Tomás
INESC-ID, IST TU Lisbon, Portugal

Aleksandar Ilic
INESC-ID / IST TU Lisbon, Portugal

Leonel Sousa
INESC-ID / IST TU Lisbon, Portugal

ABSTRACT

When analyzing the neuronal code, neuroscientists usually perform extra-cellular recordings of neuronal responses (spikes). Since the size of the microelectrodes used to perform these recordings is much larger than the size of the cells, responses from multiple neurons are recorded by each micro-electrode. Thus, the obtained response must be classified and evaluated, in order to identify how many neurons were recorded, and to assess which neuron generated each spike. A platform for the mass-classification of neuronal responses is proposed in this chapter, employing data-parallelism for speeding up the classification of neuronal responses. The platform is built in a modular way, supporting multiple web-interfaces, different back-end environments for parallel computing or different algorithms for spike classification. Experimental results on the proposed platform show that even for an unbalanced data set of neuronal responses the execution time was reduced of about 45%. For balanced data sets, the platform may achieve a reduction in execution time equal to the inverse of the number of back-end computational elements.

1. INTRODUCTION

Parallel computing platforms provide researchers the means to apply computationally demanding algorithms to large sets of data. Although these algorithms can be applied in a sequential computing system, the use of parallelization techniques allows the substantial reduction of the execution time. One such case is the classification of neuronal responses for modeling neuronal systems and, at the bottom line, enabling the development of neural prostheses. With this goal, information being transmitted between neurons is recorded when the neuronal system is stimulated by a given stimulus. This information is communicated by biphasic electric pulses lasting a couple of mil-

DOI: 10.4018/978-1-60566-280-0.ch009

liseconds, usually known as action potentials or spikes[1].

In order to understand the information being transmitted or processing mechanisms of the neuronal system, large arrays of microelectrodes are employed to perform simultaneous extracellular recordings of neuronal data, i.e. of the action potentials being communicated. The problem in performing extracellular recordings is that a single electrode typically records the action potentials originated from multiple neurons (Brown, Kass, & Mitra, 2004). This makes the analysis of the neuronal data difficult, since one does not know how many cells elicited action potentials, or even which neuron is responsible for the generation of a given action potential. To overcome this difficulty, several classification algorithms have been developed to estimate the number of active neurons and to identify which neuron generated each action potential (e.g. Tomás & Sousa, 2007; Takahashi, Anzai, & Sakurai, 2003a; Shoham, Fellows & Normann, 2003; Quiroga, Nadasdy, & Ben-Shaul, 2004).

Spike classification algorithms are computationally intensive, where the classification of spikes from a single electrode can take several hours. Moreover, in typical neural recordings, several electrodes are used to capture the action potentials from multiple locations. Nowadays arrays of 100 microelectrodes are common and it is possible to record the neuronal responses using more than one microelectrode array. This makes the spike classification a time consuming task (Quiroga, Nadasdy, & Ben-Shaul, 2004). To overcome this difficulty, one can use parallel processing in order to decrease computational time and increase the availability of the data for further analysis, which is usually the intent of researchers.

Herein is proposed a platform for mass-classification of neuronal responses, using data parallelism for reducing computational time. The proposed platform is divided into three main components: *i)* a front-end part for interfacing with the user, allowing him to specify the classification parameters and to check the status of the submitted jobs; *ii)* a middleware part for supervising the classification job and ensuring that the classification algorithm is being correctly executed; and *iii)* a back-end part that supplies the platform computational power. The proposed platform design has a modular approach, which guarantees that further front-end parts can be easily added to the system, such as client applications to directly interface with the middleware part. Also, other computing systems can be explored, such as those using different job schedulers. Moreover, by adopting a data parallelization approach to reduce classification time, one can easily develop new classification algorithms and integrate them into the proposed platform.

This chapter is organized as follows. Section 2 presents the classification algorithm and file format for submitting jobs for the mass-classification platform. Section 3 describes the platform architecture, detailing each of the platform's three parts. Section 4 presents the platform implementation details, including the user interface, the mechanisms for checking the job statuses and the used back-end computing system. Experimental results are also presented, illustrating the performance of the proposed mass-classification platform. Finally, in section 5 the main conclusions are drawn.

2. THE CLASSIFICATION ALGORITHM

To perform spike classification, researchers use the knowledge that the waveform of the action potentials from a given neuron does not significantly change over the time. On the other hand, the waveforms from two different neurons are typically different enough for one to recognize which spikes are originated from each neuron. The classification of the action potential waveforms is presented in Figure 1, where the spikes from different neurons (units) are represented by dif-

Figure 1. Waveform of the action potentials

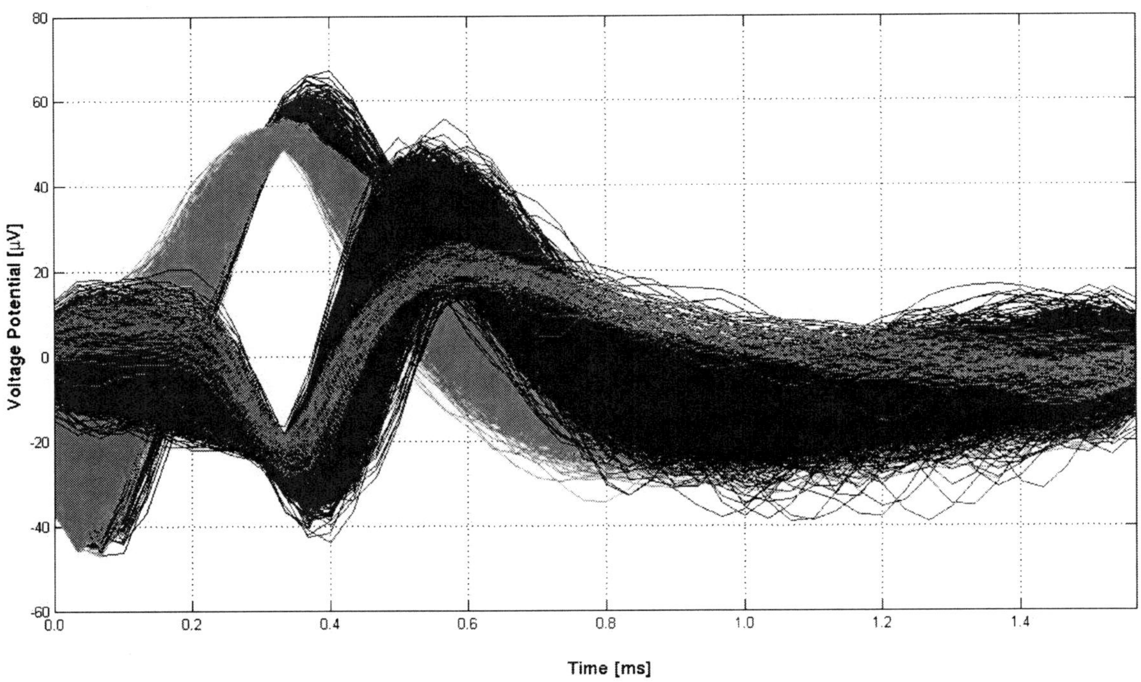

ferent grayscales. The results were obtained after applying the classification algorithm in (Tomás & Sousa, 2007), as presented in subsection 2.1.

The recording of the neuronal responses is performed by acquiring the signal corresponding to the action potentials. Since information is transmitted from neuron to neuron by action potentials, and these do not change in time, neuroscientists are mainly interested in knowing the time instants when action potentials are generated. Thus, when recording neural responses, only the time of spike generation is stored (i.e. the time stamp of occurrence) and the shape of the action potential. To detect the presence of an action potential, a usual method is to define a positive (negative) threshold and whenever the potential goes above (below) the defined threshold, the voltage potential at the microelectrode top is stored for a time period of a few milliseconds. Also, since the action potential is only recognized when it reaches near its maximum (minimum) value, the acquisition system also saves the potential trace preceding the detection of the action potential. As an example, in Figure 1 spike waveforms were detected at time t=0.32ms; and the action potential was stored during the time period ranging from -0.32ms to 1.18ms after its detection.

The actual recording of the waveforms of action potentials is however affected by several issues that must be taken into account when performing spike classification. On the one hand, the system is affected by a noise source with a significant power in comparison with action potentials' signal; in the experimental data used in this chapter, the signal to noise ratio (SNR) can be as low as 25dB on some microelectrodes. On the other hand, the threshold mechanism induces misalignment when recording the action potential signal. Furthermore, electromagnetic interference can also induce voltage peaks (burst noise), detected as spikes. Thus, in order to perform spike classification, one must first correct this misalignment and be aware that

Figure 2. Neuronal data classification algorithm

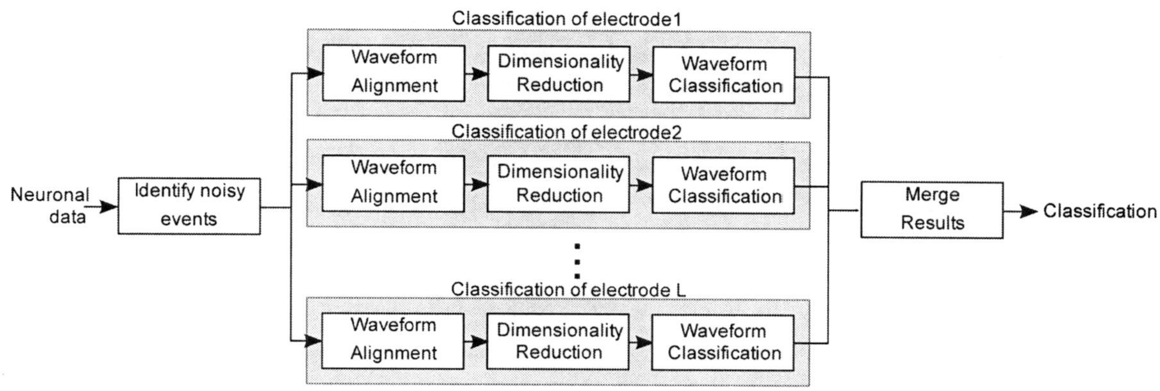

some spikes result from external noise (noisy events), as it will be discussed in the following subsection.

2.1 The Classification Algorithm

As detailed in Figure 2, the classification algorithm of neuronal data is composed by three main blocks, devoted to: *i)* identification and elimination of noisy events; *ii)* classification of spike waveforms for each available electrode; and *iii)* merging of the results into an output file. The first step, removal of noisy events, is relatively simple and attempts to simplify the overall classification of spikes. Noisy events, generated by burst noise, induce voltage peaks on the electrodes that, on occasions, become large enough to mislead the acquisition system in identifying them as action potentials. However, when this happens it simultaneously affects all electrodes, generating fake spike events on most of them. On the other hand, the probability for a large number of cells to elicit spikes in a very short amount of time (less than 1ms) is considerably small. This makes the identification of these noisy events simple: when a large number of electrodes identify a spike event in a small time window, these events are most likely noise, and can be removed.

The second step of the spike classification procedure is the most computationally demanding, but can be easily parallelized. Since a cell is so small, it cannot produce a spike event strong enough to propagate to two electrodes, thus classification of the spikes on each electrode can be made independently and in parallel. Hence, the mass-classification of spikes recorded by N electrodes can be done by exploring data parallelism: each logical or physical processor in a cluster/grid receives spike waveforms recorded in a single microelectrode and classifies it. The platform scalability is mostly limited if there are more processors in the computing environment than electrodes to classify: given a single job, there will be free computing elements. However, since the proposed platform allows multiple users to submit classification jobs, or even the same user to submit several jobs–from different neuronal datasets or with different classification parameters for the same dataset–this scalability problem is overcome.

The classification algorithm for each electrode can be decomposed in three main operations executing in series. The first operation involves the alignment of the waveforms of spike events. This step is crucial, since spikes are only saved whenever the AC electrode potential exceeds a given threshold (in modulus). This creates slight misalignments in the waveform recordings due to low noise fluctuations. In order to re-align the waveforms, two techniques can be employed.

One technique makes use of templates to estimate the spike generation times (Lewicki, M. S., 1998; Zhang, Wu, Zhou, Liang, & Yuan, 2004). The disadvantage of this technique is that, before performing actual classification, the shape of the neuron action potential (spike waveform) is not known. Therefore, either predefined templates can be used (which can lead to large classification errors) or a dual stage approach can be employed: first classification is performed using predefined templates; then the templates are extracted from the classification results and used for re-classifying the data. While this leads to small improvements in the classification results, it has a large computational penalty.

An alternative method is to align the waveforms by the time-stamp of the maximum or minimum potential of the waveform (Linderman, Santhanam, Kemere, Gilja, O'Driscoll, Yu, Afshar, Ryu, Shenoy, & Meng, 2008). Notice that one should not use the absolute AC maximum potential: in some action potentials the minimum and maximum AC voltage values have similar values. Thus, if the absolute maximum AC potential is used for spike alignment, action potentials coming from the same cell can be alternatively aligned by the (real) maximum and minimum values, causing a global miss-alignment. Therefore, alignment must be made by either the minimum or the maximum waveform potential and never by both.

After aligning the spike events, dimensionality reduction must be applied to the waveforms. In principle, the more information is given to the classification algorithm, the better it performs. However, in practice, some features can be just "noise", adding nothing to, or even degrading, the classification results. Since there is no knowledge on what cells have generated the data (spikes)–i.e. on the ground truth–or even on how many cells have generated the recorded spike events in one micro-electrode, one must apply an unsupervised classification algorithm. On the absence of the ground truth, the classification algorithm will interpret all information, including noise, as relevant information (not necessarily with the same weight). Thus, care should be taken in the choice of relevant features. Moreover, the representation of spike waveforms with features allows reducing the dimensionality of the classification problem, thus also reducing the execution time. Maximum and minimum potentials of the waveforms are the simplest features that can be extracted (Hulata, Segev, & Ben-Jacob, 2002; Lewicki, M. S., 1998). Other more complex features can be extracted by applying Principal Component Analysis (PCA) (Shoham, Fellows & Normann, 2003; Hulata, Segev, & Ben-Jacob, 2002; Lewicki, M. S., 1998), Independent Component Analysis (ICA) (Takahashi, Anzai, & Sakurai, 2003a; Quiroga, Nadasdy, & Ben-Shaul, 2004) or those extracted from wavelet-based analysis (Quiroga, Nadasdy, & Ben-Shaul, 2004; Hulata, Segev, & Ben-Jacob, 2002). Herein, ICA is used for extracting the most relevant features, by applying the FastICA algorithm proposed by (Hyvärinen, 1999).

The last step to classify spike events in a single electrode is the application of a unsupervised classification algorithm. Many algorithms have been developed to address this issue, e.g., k-means (Takahashi, Anzai, & Sakurai, 2003b; Salganicoff, Sarna, Sax, & Gerstein, 1988), fuzzy c-means (Zouridakis & Tam, 2000) and maximum likelihood procedures that typically use the Expectation-Maximization (EM) algorithm (e.g. KlustaKwik (Harris, Henze, Csicsvari, Hirase, & Buzsaki, 2000)). The assumption behind maximum likelihood approaches is that, after accounting for non-additive noise sources (e.g., spike misalignments), the real waveform is affected by a Gaussian-distributed noise source. While there has been some indications that spike statistics have wider tails than Gaussian distributions, therefore suggesting the use of other distributions (Shoham, Fellows & Normann, 2003), herein we use the Gaussian assumption. It should be noticed that the proposed platform can be easily adapted to use other algorithms and distributions. The problem regarding the EM algorithm is that it requires knowledge on the number of models generating the data. Thus, the algorithm is modified in order to incorporate the estimation on the number of cells that produced the spike events (Tomás & Sousa, 2007): see section 2.2.

When finished, the EM algorithm returns the most likely number of models (cells) that generated the spike events. Since the number of cells is blindly estimated from the spike waveforms, neuroscientists typically refer to the estimated classes as spike units. The EM algorithm also produces the probability of each spike event to have been generated by each unit. For obtaining a hard classification of the neuronal data, each spike is then assigned to the class having largest probability to have generated it.

Finally, once all electrodes are classified, results are merged together into a single output file containing *i)* the number of active units (cells) that generated spikes recorded by each electrode, and *ii)* the spike assignment to the cell that is more likely to have generated it. Moreover, the probability for the spike to belong to the assigned unit is included in the output file. This allows further analysis on the data to be aware that some spikes may have been miss-classified; in general, the lowest the probability for the spike to belong to the assigned class, the more likely it is to have been miss-classified. An example where this may be of use is in the modeling of the processing mechanisms of the neuronal system. Finally, all events identified as resulting from noise are also marked as belonging to the specific unit of noisy events.

2.2 The Expectation-Maximization Algorithm

The EM algorithm is typically used in statistics for finding maximum likelihood estimates of parameters in probabilistic models. The algorithm assumes that the observed M-dimensional dataset $\mathbf{x}_1,\mathbf{x}_2,\ldots,\mathbf{x}_N$ was generated by a mixture of K statistical models with some parameters $\mathbf{\Theta}_1, \mathbf{\Theta}_2,\ldots,\mathbf{\Theta}_K$, e.g., Gaussian distributions with means $\boldsymbol{\mu}_1,\boldsymbol{\mu}_2,\ldots,\boldsymbol{\mu}_K$ and covariance matrices $\mathbf{\Sigma}_1,\mathbf{\Sigma}_2,\ldots,\mathbf{\Sigma}_K$. The purpose of the algorithm is then to identify the unknown latent variables that state which model 1,...,K has generated each data sample $\mathbf{x}_1,\mathbf{x}_2,\ldots,\mathbf{x}_N$, and to estimate the parameters for each model. The EM algorithm operates by performing an expectation of the likelihood (E step), which includes the latent (hidden) variables as if they were observed, and a maximization (M step) of the likelihood of both the dataset and the latent variables It iterates between the two steps by using the results from one step to compute the other.

The main problem in employing the usual EM algorithm is that the total number of models (units, for the current case) is unknown. Thus, the EM algorithm must be changed in order to be able to estimate the number of active units and to assign each spike (data sample) to a unit. The method proposed in (Figueiredo & Jain, 2002) can be used for this purpose. Furthermore, since the number of samples can be limited, a weighting factor can be added to give more importance to the regions in the samples' space that are better represented (Tomás & Sousa, 2007). Thus, a smoothed data distribution function *sdd*(**x**) has to be firstly computed as:

$$sdd(x) = {}^{3}\sum_{i=1}^{N} G\left(d\left(x, x_i\right); 0; h\right), \qquad (1)$$

where d($\mathbf{x}_i$,$\mathbf{x}_j$) is the Euclidean distance between $\mathbf{x}_i$ and $\mathbf{x}_j$, γ is a constant value defined such as $\sum sdd(x) = 1$ and $G(\mathbf{x};0;h)$ is a Gaussian function with zero mean and standard deviation h, evaluated at point **x**. The parameters for each statistical model are estimated by minimizing the optimization function,

$$l(\Theta_1,\cdots,\Theta_K) = \frac{D}{2}\sum_{k=1}^{K}\log\left(\frac{N}{12}\pi_k\right) + \frac{K}{2}\log\left(\frac{N}{12}\right) + \frac{K(D+1)}{2} - \beta\sum_{i=1}^{N} sdd(x_i)\log\sum_{k=1}^{K}\pi_k p\left(x_i \mid k,\Theta_k\right) + \lambda\left(\sum_{k=1}^{K}\pi_k - 1\right) \tag{2}$$

where D is the total number of parameters required to represent each unit, i.e. the dimension of $\mathbf{\Theta}_k$, β=N is the number of samples, π_k is the probability for the statistical model k to generate a given waveform, and λ is a Lagrangian multiplier designed to guarantee that $\sum \pi_k = 1$. Also $p(\mathbf{x}_i|k,\mathbf{\Theta}_k)$ is the probability for the statistical model k to generate the sample $\mathbf{x}_i$ given the parameters $\mathbf{\Theta}_k$.

Considering that the features extracted from the spike waveforms of each neuron (class) k are distributed accordingly to a Gaussian function with mean $\boldsymbol{\mu}_k$ and covariance matrix $\boldsymbol{\Sigma}_k$, the EM algorithm works by iteratively computing the following equations (Tomás & Sousa, 2007):

$$\pi_k = \frac{\max\left\{N\sum_{i=1}^{N} sdd(x_i)p\left(x_i \mid k,\Theta_k\right) - \frac{D}{2};0\right\}}{\sum_{j=1}^{K}\max\left\{N\sum_{i=1}^{N} sdd(x_i)p\left(x_i \mid j,\Theta j\right) - \frac{D}{2};0\right\}} \tag{3}$$

$$\mu_k = \frac{\sum_{i=1}^{N} sdd(x_i)p\left(x_i \mid k,\Theta_k\right)x_i}{\sum_{i=1}^{N} sdd(x_i)p\left(x_i \mid k,\Theta_k\right)} \tag{4}$$

$$\Sigma_k = \frac{\sum_{i=1}^{N} sdd(x_i)p\left(x_i \mid k,\Theta_k\right)\left(x_i - \mu_k\right)\left(x_i - \mu_k\right)^T}{\sum_{i=1}^{N} sdd(x_i)p\left(x_i \mid k,\Theta_k\right)} \tag{5}$$

To disclose the number of active units in each electrode, an alternate merge/split method is adopted after the convergence of the EM algorithm. This method starts with a relatively high number of components, regarding the expected number of classes. Then, it applies the EM algorithm as previously described, and after convergence, the method attempts to remove/introduce units. It tries to remove a unit by merging two units together, and if it does not work it also tries to split a unit into two new ones (Tomás & Sousa, 2007). After unit merging/splitting, the EM algorithm iterates again in order to produce a new solution, which is accepted only if it decreases the optimization function. Since we start with a relatively high number of units, after the initial EM convergence, we perform unit merging and continue doing it while better solutions are reached. When no further improvement is possible, we switch to unit splitting and continue while better solutions are achieved; thus alternating between unit splitting and merging until no further improvement can be reached.

2.3 File Format

In order to submit the neuronal data to the large-scale classification platform (presented in section 3), a XML schema data file was designed, as illustrated in Figure 3. The schema file uses a hierarchical structure where the base of the structure is an Electrode, identified with a unique ID, *number*. Each electrode can have multiple *spike* elements, each defined by its time of occurrence, *time*, and by its *waveform*. To support the classification results, the XML schema also includes the information of the number of valid units found per electrode, *NumberOfUnits*, and each spike is identified with the *unit* that is most likely to have generated it. Moreover, to provide other neural data analysis tools with information regarding the classification likelihood, the sub-element *probunit* of the element *spike* includes the probability for the spike to belong to that unit.

Figure 3. Neuronal data format

```
<xs:schema xmlns:xs="http://www.w3.org/2001/XMLSchema">
    <xs:element name="electrode" type="Electrode"/>
    <xs:complexType name="Electrode">
        <xs:sequence >
            <xs:element name="number"         type="xs:decimal"/>
            <xs:element name="spike"          type="Spike"/>
            <xs:element name="NumberOfUnits"  type="xs:decimal"/>
        </xs:sequence>
    </xs:complexType>
    <xs:complexType  name="Spike">
        <xs:sequence>
            <xs:element name="time"     type="xs:decimal"/>
            <xs:element name="waveform" type="Waveform"/>
            <xs:element name="unit"     type="xs:decimal"/>
            <xs:element name="probunit" t  ype="xs:double"/>
        </xs:sequence>
    </xs:complexType>
    <xs:simpleType name="Waveform">
        <xs:list itemType="xs:integer"/>
    </xs:simpleType>
</xs:schema>
```

3. PLATFORM ARCHITECTURE FOR LARGE-SCALE CLASSIFICATION

This section presents a computational platform, which is not only an efficient implementation of the previously presented spike classification algorithm but also adopts a specific parallel environment. This increases the algorithm's computational performance, and also simplifies the process of classification management at the user level.

As shown in Figure 4, the computational platform is organized in three different parts: *i)* a Web-based user interface in the *Front-end* part, *ii)* a *Middleware* section, responsible for the classification managing mechanism, both considerably relying on a database, and *iii)* a distributed *Back-end*, comprising a grid of computers running the data classifications (*Workers*) and a scheduler to manage a queue of requested classifications through the grid (*Master*).

3.1 Front-End

A Web-based application is used as the system Front-end, which does not require the user to be familiar with the system organization and spike

Figure 4. Platform architecture

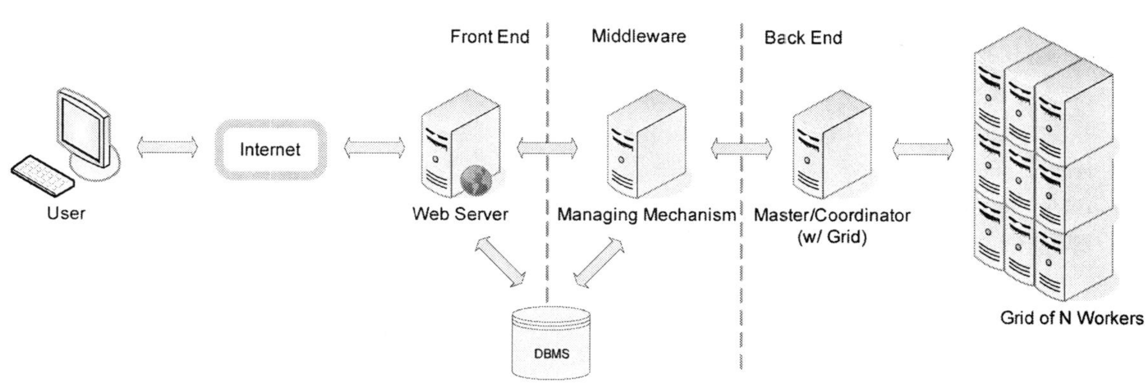

Figure 5. Simplified front-end use-case diagram

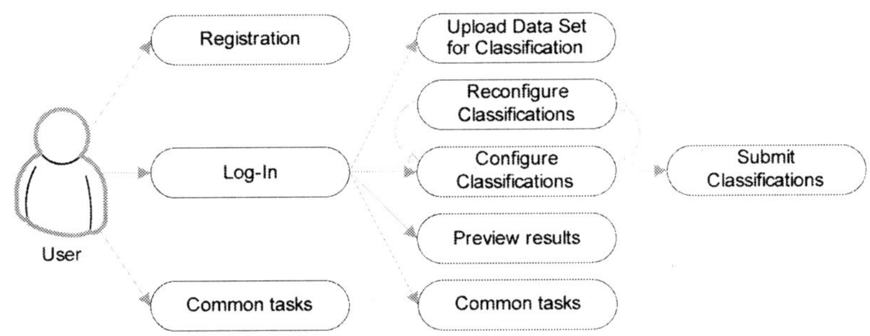

classification algorithm, but still preserves its performance and constraints. Without loss of generality, we present herein the functionality provided by the current implementation, but it can be easily adapted for different kind of applications, e.g., when the Internet connection is not required.

The platform Front-end is based on the client-server architectural model allowing interaction between the end user and the rest of the system through a standard Web interface. This part of the system is supported by a Database Management System (DBMS), in order to allow access to multiple users and store a comprehensive configuration of all aspects related with spike classification. The DBMS is also used to store all information regarding user and administrator accounts, and classification jobs. To prevent possible compromise of sensitive information, data protection should be incorporated, namely, encryption of the connection between the client and the Web server, and encryption of both user account information and user data. Furthermore, the reinforced security at the data level can significantly improve the system reliability and the related functional sections presented in the Figure 5.

The main group of user actions consists in the *Registration* process, *Log in* and a set of helper functions referred to as *Common tasks.* The first one resolves the stated security issues in order to allow access to the sequence of classification actions after a successful *Log in*. These later tasks involve the actions which are available to every platform user, whether registered or not, e.g., contact the system administrator, general platform utilization manuals, and lost password retrieval.

Registered users are allowed to upload the files containing the acquired data sets on which spike classification has to be applied, depicted as the *Upload Data Set* option. The system ensures the uploaded files are available only to the user who uploaded the file, and also provides basic manipulation on those files, including deletion.

From the user's point of view, the Web-based interface can be seen as the core of the system, since it allows the user to setup all the parameters required to perform spike classifications on previously uploaded acquired data files. The configuration process is represented in a diagram as a chain of events that includes *Configure*, *Reconfigure* and *Submit Classifications* actions. Once classifications are marked for submission, a large number of files are automatically prepared in order to support the execution in the system Back-end part and all information regarding the submitted classifications is automatically inserted in the database. This allows for the user to submit multiple jobs, as explained in Section 4. Moreover, the software application links each classification request with a user, accommodating the production of the specialized Front-end section, *Preview results*, which allows checking the job progress and status tracking, and also results retrieval upon job completion. The set of the *Common tasks* in the registered user area includes maintenance of the user account information and system log-out.

The proposed platform is capable of dealing with a large number of classification sessions at the same time, thus increasing the relevance of the management mechanism, whose generic working principle is described in the next subsection.

3.2 Middleware

To preserve the system stability and to maintain the job submissions order, the platform implements an independent *Classifications Managing Mechanism* (CMM). The CMM acts as a general job dispatcher on the top of the Back-end scheduler, which introduces a sequence of actions that are needed to be fulfilled in order to perform classification and produce the results. This management subsystem also facilitates the platform self-administration and provides secure connection between Front-end and Back-end parts. Nevertheless, the CMM is responsible for maintaining the consistency of the classifications information in the database and, at the bottom line, for notifying the user upon the classification completion.

Before describing the CMM operation, the structure of the classification process must be elaborated. In respect to the 3-steps of the algorithm presented in Figure 2, the classification is divided in three individual modules, marked as *Remove Noise*, *Classify Electrode(s)* and *Merge Results*. The mentioned modules are split on a set of jobs, each assigned to execute in the system Back-end. The number of jobs varies accordingly to the parallelized algorithm and its implementation. Nonetheless, the number of jobs in the *Classify electrode(s)* module is proportional to the number of electrodes chosen by the user during the classification configuration process.

During its life cycle, each job follows a deterministic finite-state machine in order to accomplish its correct execution. This machine has three main states, namely, *Initial, Execution* and *Terminal states,* as presented in Figure 6. A job is assigned to the *Initial states* in a period between its Front-end creation and Back-End submission; whereas *Terminal states* refer to the job while additional tasks are being performed in order to finalize its execution, i.e., after the application of the classification algorithm. To allow the Middleware to support different Back-ends, a set of *Execution states* is introduced to mark the states supplied by the Back-End environment during the actual job execution.

Figure 6. General job state transition process

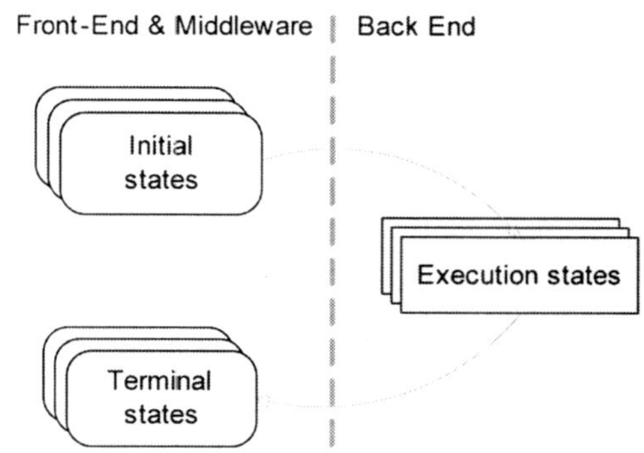

At this point, it is worth to distinguish the application of the status terms on the level of a job, module and overall classification process. Each job has its own status that marks the job's progress stage in its current execution. Status of the classification module depends on the statuses of the jobs composing it, whereas the overall classification status is evaluated by the current statuses of its modules. Moreover, the predefined transition of statuses at the job level causes a similar transitional procedure at the modules and classification levels.

Finally, the CMM comprises an autonomous procedure, which 3-steps need to be performed in sequence in order to accomplish the spike classification algorithm requirements. This procedure should efficiently incorporate all required functionalities of the platform, such as communication with the system Front-end and Back-end, job status retrieval and file transfers, database update directives, etc. Generally, the 3-step procedure is driven by the classification module presence, where the execution of a next module is preceded by the former module completion. The module is regarded as completed as soon as all included jobs have reached the completed status.

3.3 Back-End

It can be assumed, even on the level of a single classification, that the complexity of the spike classification process can achieve huge proportions. This can be perceived in multiple domains, e.g., the computational intensity, the number of automatically generated set-up files needed to sustain the process Back-end execution and the 3-step classification procedure accomplishment. In order to provide a computational environment with capacity to perform spike classification in reasonable time, we propose to use a computer grid as the Back-end platform.

As mentioned before, the sequential execution time of the classification process can be extremely high. Furthermore, the parallelization of the algorithm's tasks inside the classification modules, herein referred as *jobs*, allows the utilization of the multiple computing resources, existent in those systems, in order to reduce the overall computational time.

The core of this part of the system is made of computational elements, designated as *Workers*, which are used for direct job execution, and a *Master/Coordinator* to supervise the classification process running in the Back-end. The employed master-worker paradigm requires the existence of a job and resource management system hosted in the *Master*, mainly used for interaction with the computer grid. This manager, besides job distribution to the *Workers,* also performs execution control and tracks job progress. Moreover, the *Coordinator* may incorporate a job scheduling mechanism for efficient use of this part of the platform.

According to the nature of the spike classification process and its distributed execution in the system Back-end, special attention must be paid to the data security, data placement and the fault-tolerant job execution. Section 4 provides further discussion and the solutions to overcome these issues with implementation of the Condor system (Condor Manuals, 2008) in the Back-end part.

Due to its independent position in the presented system architecture, the Back-end part demonstrates the ability to achieve significant speedups, not only at the level of a single classification process, but also by concurrent execution of several classifications. To facilitate this achievement, full interaction with the CMM is needed. Nevertheless, the achieved speedup is restricted by the number of the *Workers* present in the system and the number of the jobs marked for execution. In addition, specific software support may be required in order to establish the required system functionality depending on the programming environment for spike classification, e.g., Octave (Octave Documentation, 2008).

4. IMPLEMENTATION AND EVALUATION

The implementation of the massive data classification platform is discussed in the next three subsections, regarding the Front-end, the Middleware and the Back-end parts, according to the architecture presented in Section 3. Description of each part is provided to underline the practical means for performing the spike classification, using the already presented general platform characteristics.

4.1 Front-End Implementation

The Front-end part is built as a Web-based application using two Open Source tools, namely, general-purpose *PHP: Hypertext Preprocessor* scripting language (PHP Documentation, 2008) and the MySQL Database System (MySQL Documentation, 2008).

As previously stated, the platform multi-user character is supported with the user accounts, which relies on the database and is fully integrated in every aspect of the system. Considering the presence of two groups of users who are admitted to access the platform, *Classification users (CUs)* and *Administrators (ADs)*, the solution assumes existence of two specifically designed interfaces. The part of the interface dedicated to the CUs is built according to the simplified use-case diagram in Figure 5.

As already mentioned, the spike classification can be performed on the multiple data sets. Albeit, this part of the system provides the tools for performing operations on the acquired data sets, such as upload, transfer and management. Once the files are successfully transferred to the local area, information regarding the uploaded files is inserted in the database to guarantee that the data set is used only by the user who submitted it. Moreover, the acquired data files are stored only in the local area, and transferred to the Back-end with classification requests, followed by its removal as soon as the execution is completed.

At this point, it is worth to emphasize the security and data placement aspects related to the Front-end part. Firstly, we strongly encourage the use of the encryption methods for storing all the provided user data accompanied by Secure Socket Layer cryptographic protocols for communication. Although this issue mainly elevates the security level of user authentication process, applying the encryption on the data sets can reinforce the security even on the data privacy and integrity levels. Secondly, separately designed interfaces for CUs and ADs reflect the different authorization levels of the two groups of platform users. Moreover, one can notice that the number of acquired data sets to upload is limited by the available disk space on the server.

The CUs are allowed to configure and submit their own classifications using several panels specially designed to cover all needed configuration aspects, i.e., acquired data sets selection and election of the electrodes per each selected data set. After the CU has marked the classifications for Back-end submission, the application automatically creates the set of the jobs. The created jobs satisfy both, the user configuration preference and 3-step classification procedure, requirements as explained in Section 2. To sustain its execution, a significant number of Condor and executable files are generated, according to the current algorithm and Back-end implementation. Finally, the insertion of appropriate job information in the database triggers the CMM to initiate the Back-end communication.

As shown in the example in Figure 7, the CU is allowed to track the progress of each submitted classification process via specifically designed interface part. Despite the current status presentation (at the job, module and classification levels), this part of the system is capable of delivering to the CU the generated Condor and executable files per each job accompanied by the job results as soon as they are produced.

According to the different authorization level of the administrators, the AD interface is designed to maintain the system correct functionality, allowing the analysis and modification of the parameters that are crucial for its correct operation. Foremost, the ADs are allowed to access important information regarding the user accounts, e.g., restricting the access of the CUs in the case of an abusive utilization that can compromise the system's performance. Moreover, the classification environment maintenance can be supervised by the ADs through a group of basic actions, namely, editing, disabling or even deleting previously submitted user classifications.

4.2 Middleware Implementation

In order to improve the overall platform stability and robustness, the Middleware is implemented as an independent part of the system. This part of the system, called *Classification Managing Mechanism* (CMM), represents a self-administrating

Figure 7. My classification option

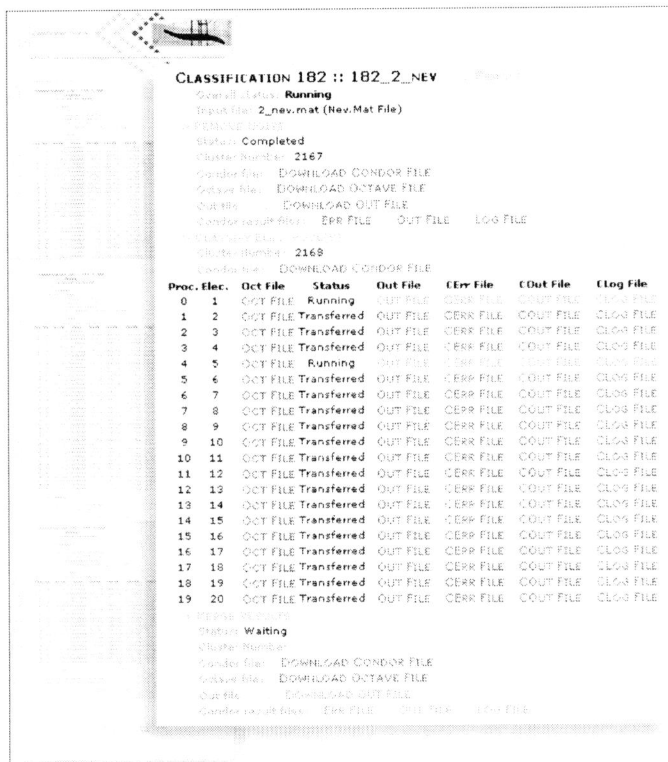

application which is built for execution of usually time-consuming tasks. Moreover, the CMM is responsible for establishing the secure connection between the Front-end and Back-end parts of the platform. All the remote computer logging in and command execution are incorporated in simple scripts which use SSH2 (OpenSSH Manual Pages, 2008) (Secure Shell) to provide secure, encrypted communication channels between two hosts over the possibly insecure network.

To reinforce its independent position and enable classification management domain, the CMM is implemented as a set of the methods which execution is performed on a regular time basis via the Unix CRON scheduling service. The methods comprise a group of actions to manage state transitions at the job, module and classification levels. The implemented classification structure is analogous to the one presented in Section 3, where the *Remove Noise* and *Merge Results* modules imply only one job, and the number of jobs inside the *Classify Electrode(s)* module depends on the number of electrodes specified by the CU.

In Figure 8, we present the implemented state machine with the transitions between states, which follow the general remarks discussed in Section 3. The *"Initial states"* group refers to the job states prior to its Back-end execution, namely, *i) Waiting* to mark the successful local storage of the set-up files and waiting for the predefined CMM action, *ii) Submitting* when the CMM transfers the set-up files to the Condor system, and *iii) Submitted* when job is submitted for its execution in the system's Back-end. In respect to the current Back-end implementation, the *"Execution states"* are provided by Condor itself, namely: *i) Idle*, when the job is waiting in the Condor queue for available resources, *ii) Running*, for the case when the job is running in the Grid system, *iii) Done*, whenever a job is finished in system's

Figure 8. Transition of states

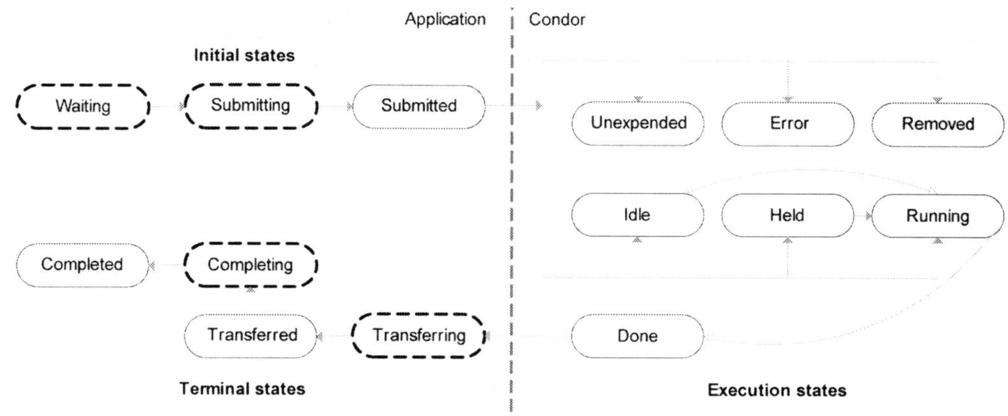

Beck-end but the results data is not yet accessible to the classification user, and *iv) Unexpanded* and *Held*, when the job encountered a problem during execution and is stopped. The states dedicated to the job in the "*Terminal state*" are: *i) Transferring*, when the CMM is transferring the result files to the local area, *ii) Transferred*, for the case when all the files were transferred and became available to the classification user, *iii) Completing* to mark execution of additional tasks needed to finalize the job, e.g., files deletion from Condor system and *iv) Completed,* when the job is completely finished.

Since different CMM methods consume different amounts of time during its execution, there is a certain probability of invoking the execution of a second CMM procedure while the previously started one is still running. This situation can produce an unpredictable outcome that affects the overall system stability and correctness. In order to prevent this violation, the transitional (*Waiting*, *Submitting*, *Transferring* and *Completing*) and terminal (*Submitted, Transferred* and *Completed*) states are used to implement the specific job's locking mechanism. A job in transitional state can spend as much time as needed to accomplish predefined actions, without being interrupted by any other method, while, at the same time, a job at the terminal state usually informs the CMM to perform assigned functions. The actions included in the lock mechanism are initiated by establishing the connection to Condor, and instantiating a set of functions to retrieve the job status, e.g. job submission, input or output files transfer, job status and execution time retrieval.

In order to fulfill the spike classification algorithm demands, the CMM performs Condor job submissions using a 3-step procedure, which is preceded by the status update for each currently running job. In the first step, the Remove Noise job is submitted to Condor. As soon as this job achieves the *Completed* status, all the jobs from the Classify Electrode(s) group are submitted in the second procedure step. The third step is performed after finishing all the Classify Electrode(s) jobs and incorporates the Merge Results job submission. Once the Merge Results job is finished, the classification is marked as *Completed.* Each of these steps is performed automatically under the CMM control. Moreover, the current implementation allows submission of the jobs from a subsequent module as soon as previous module jobs reach the "*Transferred*" status, which leads to a slight execution time speedup.

4.3 Back-End Implementation

The platform Back-end part is based on a master-worker model, as presented in Section 3. The adopted computing environment is able to support large amounts of computational parallelism over a long period of time and, thus presenting a high processing throughput environment. For efficient utilization of the computing power of the *Workers*, which communicate over a computer network, the platform is supported by the Condor software system (Condor Manuals, 2008). Moreover, the Condor provides a job and *Workers* management mechanism, scheduling policy, priority scheme, and monitoring (Thain, Tannenbaum, & Livny, 2005).

The high-level GNU Octave language (Octave Documentation, 2008), a specific programming language for numeric computation, and mostly MATLAB compatible, is used in the Back-End for spike classification. Nevertheless, the presented platform does not necessarily depend on Octave and can be adopted with any programming environment, if the classification algorithm is implemented in another programming language, e.g. C/C++.

As it has been explained, the Front-end application automatically generates a set of files needed to perform the classification process submission. Besides creating the files to ease direct job execution in Octave, the application also generates three Condor files per each classification process, in order to accomplish the necessary 3-step procedure (Remove Noise, Classify Electrode(s) and Merge Results). The Condor files contain essential information about the jobs to be used by the *Master/Coordinator* during the operation of sending the job to execution, such as the *Workers'* computer architecture and operating system, the list of input files to be transferred, path to the Octave executable and corresponding function calls as parameters. The set-up files transfer and Back-end job submissions are performed automatically by the CMM set of actions. On the Condor side, the files containing the requested jobs are parsed and the processes are scheduled according to the specified constraints and the available resources (*Workers*). Furthermore, Condor is also responsible to transfer the input files to the assigned *Worker*'s machine, start and monitor the job execution on it, and, at the bottom line, transfer back the results to the *Master* upon job completion.

During job execution, the platform Back-end provides the ability to retrieve the current job status via Condor queue and/or history file information. By periodically accessing this information the CMM updates the database with the job's current "*Execution state*" to allow the CUs to track the status of submitted jobs.

Once the job execution is completed and the CMM detects the job status as "*Done*", the CMM retrieves the respective job execution information from Condor and transfers the results to a local area where they become available to the user. It is worth to note the distinction between the two groups of output files produced by Condor, and forwarded to the user upon job completion. The first one represents the actual spike classification process result, whereas the later file group refers to the output streams and process execution details generated by Condor.

As mentioned in Section 3, the distributed execution of the spike classifications brings in focus data security, fault-tolerance and data placement issues. The proposed Back-end implementation, where Condor retains complete control over the job execution, limits the space for finding the solutions to the currently implemented Condor features. Nevertheless, Condor system is able to provide large number of techniques which help to overcome those problems. The desired security level can be achieved with the configuration of related Condor parameters. Security challenges consider many aspects, e.g., strong authentication and authorization mechanisms, encryption of the data sent across the network and data integrity check (Condor Manuals, 2008). Moreover, Condor provides flexible and secure communication, and CUs protection from errant or malicious resources (Thain, Tannenbaum, & Livny, 2005).

The fault-tolerant job execution is accommodated by Checkpoint mechanism which allows job migration from one *Worker* to another in case of any situation that violates the proper job execution, e.g., failure of the *Worker* (Condor Manuals, 2008). Nonetheless, check-pointing is not available in all Condor universes, thus the chosen programming environment for spike classification may affect the overall system's fault-tolerance.

Finally, concurrent execution of the multiple spike classification reveals the data intensive dimension of the processes, despite the computational one. The data placement issues can be resolved by the use of Stork subsystem, where data placement activities can be queued, scheduled, monitored, managed, and even check-pointed, just like computational jobs (Condor Manuals, 2008; Kosar & Livny, 2005). A further analysis of the issues related with the system reliability is addressed in (Thain & Livny, 2003).

4.4 Evaluation

For the evaluation of the proposed mass-classification platform, the complete system was implemented. The Front-end part is supported by Apache 2.2.4 and PHP 5.2.5, running on a SuSE 10.3 Linux machine. The Middleware part is also implemented on the same machine, however it runs as an independent process. Thus, the process can easily be moved to another machine if required (e.g. to face a possible overload of requests on the first machine). Both Front-end and Middleware parts use the MySQL 5.0.45 DBMS for storing users and job information. The Back-end part is implemented in a cluster composed of 14 identical computers: Pentium 4 processor, running at 3.2GHz, with 1GB of memory. These computers are connected through a dedicated 1Gbit Ethernet network. Condor 6.9.3 is used to schedule jobs for the grid, which is installed on the SuSE 10.3 Linux operating system.

The classification algorithm was implemented in Octave 2.9, an open-source numerical computing software mostly compatible with MATLAB. For performing the classification, the input XML file is firstly converted into a MATLAB 5.0 compatible file format. Once classification results are obtained, these are stored in an output XML file.

For evaluating the performance of the platform, a dataset of rabbit retina was used. This dataset consist of the responses of the retinal ganglion cells when stimulated by random stimuli. The data was obtained in the Unidad de Neuroprótesis y Rehabilitación Visual, Universidad Miguel Hernandez (Unidad de Neuroprótesis y Rehabilitacin Visual, 2008), by using a Utah array with 100 microelectrodes. The retina was repeatedly stimulated by white noise random visual stimuli. Each of the 9 trials lasted 50s. Between each period there was a 300s time where no stimulus was presented. In total, over 350.000 spikes were recorded on this experiment. However, the number of spikes per electrode is unevenly distributed: since the retina is not flat, not all electrodes captured a significant number of spikes. Thus only 16 electrodes captured over 1000 spikes, with two electrodes capturing about 75.000 and 110.000 spikes. Figure 9 presents the spikes recorded at each electrode, where valid spikes are marked with a dot and fake events (resulted from burst noise), are marked with a cross.

The graphic in Figure 10 represents the computational time for performing the classification of all electrodes in the used data set, i.e. ignoring the time for identifying noisy events and merging the results. The graphic presents three distinct times, namely the *Sequential Run Time* that corresponds to the execution time in a single grid computer (Worker), the *Grid Run Time* which is the execution time in the implemented multicomputer platform, and the *Without HW Restrictions* time that represents the predicted execution time when an unlimited number of Workers are available. All execution times are normalized are normalized by the *Sequential Run Time*. The graph illustrates that data parallelism is efficiently explored by the platform, with a reduction in the execution time of about 45%, regarding the sequential run time–corresponding to a decrease of about five hours. Notice that the achieved speed-

Figure 9. Spikes recorded at each electrode; each dot represents a valid spike and each cross represents an event identified as resultant from noise

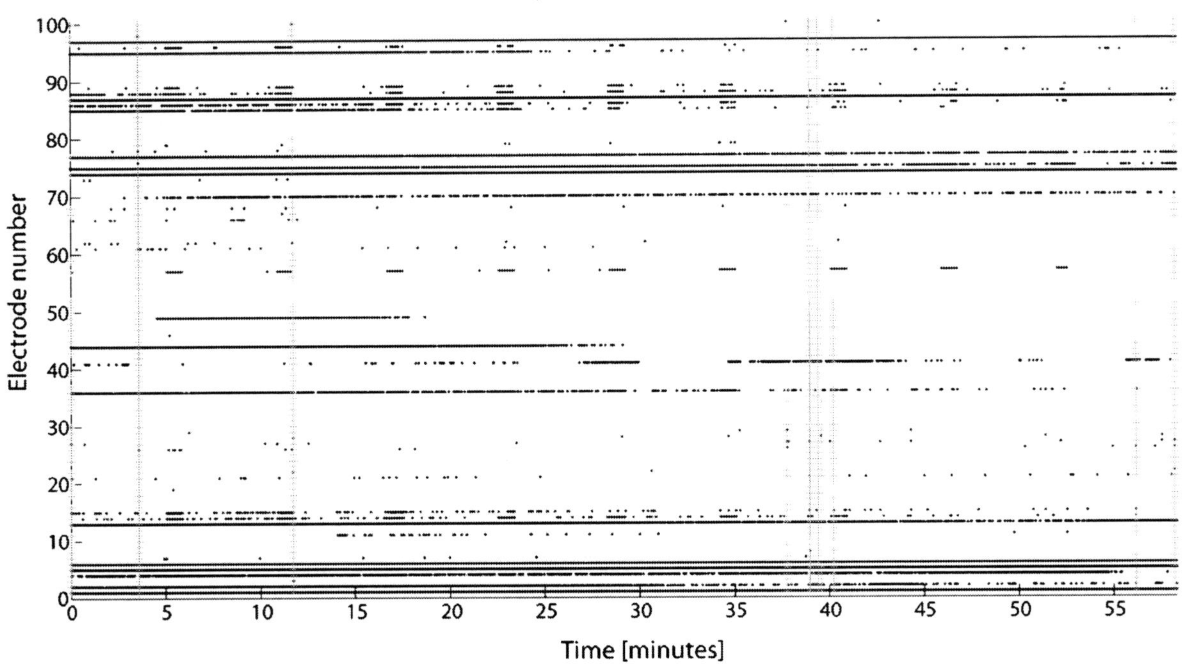

Figure 10. Reduction of the execution time in the proposed platform

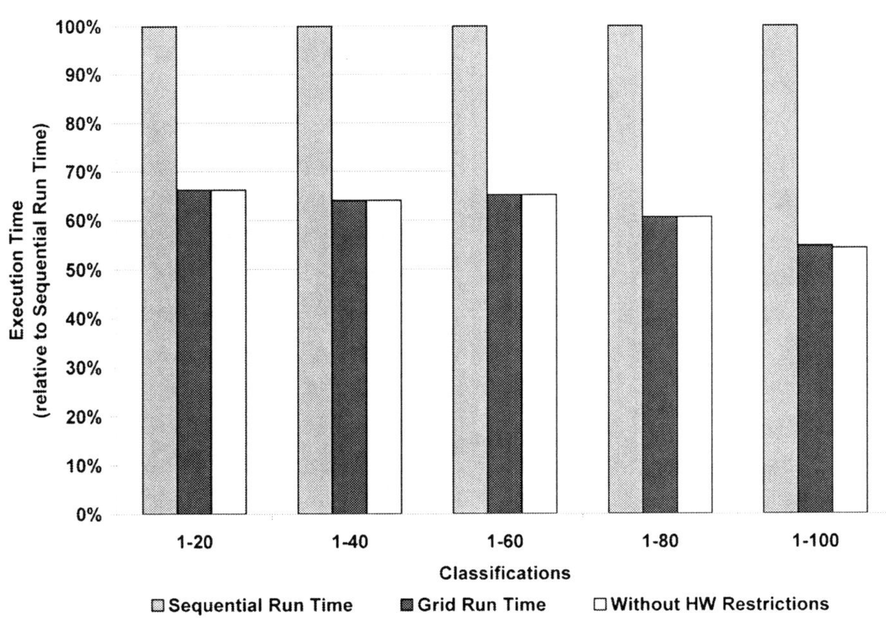

up depends on the dataset. If a completely balanced dataset is used–the number of spikes is the same for all electrodes–than one should expect that the relative execution time is equal to the inverse of the number of workers. On the other hand, if the dataset is completely unbalanced, with one electrode being responsible for the large majority of spikes, the speed-up will tend towards zero, where the speed-up is defined as:

$$\text{Speed Up} = 1 - \frac{\text{New Run Time}}{\text{Sequential Run Time}}.$$

Comparing the *Grid Run Time* and the *Without HW Restrictions* results in Figure 10 one can conclude that, even though the number of microelectrodes is larger than the number of workers, the proposed mass-classification platform is able to achieve almost the maximum speed-up possible, using the current parallelization scheme. If an unlimited number of workers were available, the execution time would decrease in less than 1%.

Considering the complete classification algorithm, i.e. including the identification of noisy events and the merging of the results, the total execution time for the used data set is, on average, 21863 seconds (around 6 hours), where 134 seconds correspond to the identification of noisy events, whereas 16 seconds are due to the merging of the results. Thus, the electrode classification part of the algorithm is the computational bottleneck, which justifies the parallelization effort.

For evaluating the electrode classification time, in Figure 11 the execution time is traced for different numbers of spikes. The dots represent real measures, while the line corresponds to a quadratic interpolation of the dots with quadratic coefficient 1.7×10^{-6} and linear coefficient 8.7×10^{-3}. This shows the quadratic behavior of the classification algorithm execution time, which is mainly due to the computation of a smoothed data distribution function in the modified EM unsupervised learning algorithm: see subsection 2.2.

Figure 11. Average execution time for the classification of one electrode

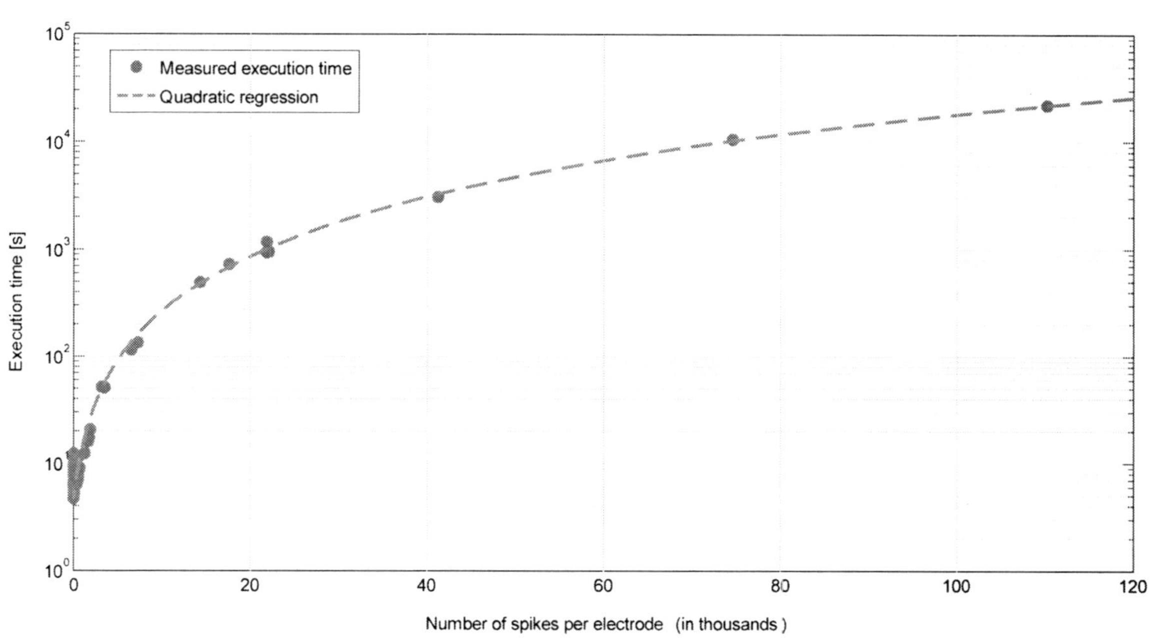

4.5. Future Work

To further decrease the execution time, other parallelization techniques could be applied, which would greatly benefit unbalanced datasets. Such techniques correspond mainly to the exploitation of data and task parallelism. Moreover other computing platforms can be explored, such as homogeneous multicore CPUs (Chapman, 2007) or heterogeneous computing of the CELL processor (Gschwind, Hofstee, Flachs, Hopkins, Watanabe, & Yamazaki, 2006). Alternatively, if the algorithm is programmed for stream computing, one can also take advantage of nowadays GPUs (Owens, Luebke, Govindaraju, Harris, Krüger, Lefohn, Purcell, 2007; Gummaraju, Coburn, Turner, & Rosenblum, 2008), which might significantly reduce execution run-time.

To improve classification results, researchers may want to explore different types of probability density functions, such as Gaussian (Tomás & Sousa, 2007) or skew t distributions (Lin, Lee, & Hsieh, 2007): see section 2. In this case, a single CU may require the classification of the same data set using different parameters. This also allows the platform to explore further parallelism since even if the data set is unbalanced, two or more classification processes can be performed in parallel using different algorithms.

6. CONCLUSION

In this chapter a platform for mass-classification of neural responses was presented. The platform is divided into 3 parts: *i)* a Front-end part that is responsible for the interaction with the user, *ii)* a Middleware part that supervises the classification of neuronal responses and *iii)* a Back-end part that corresponds to the parallel computational platform. Each part was built in a modular way, in order to facilitate its expansion and upgrade; namely to support multiple web servers or client applications for submitting jobs. Moreover, the architecture of the platform allows the integration of more computing systems to increase the computing power to the platform.

For speeding up the classification algorithm, three steps have been considered, which are sequentially executed: identification of noisy events, classification of spikes for each electrode and merging the results into an output file. By exploiting data level parallelism for the classification of the spikes in each electrode, a significant computational speed-up can be achieved. For a balanced data set, the execution time can be reduced in *(#workers–1)/#workers*, where *#workers* is the number of computational elements in the grid. Even though for unbalanced data sets the speed-up is lower. Experimental results for an unfavorable case, where most of the spikes are concentrated on few electrodes, still show a reduction of 45% in the execution time: the classification time of spikes from 100 electrodes was reduced from 11 hours to 6 hours. The experimental results also show that the non-parallelized sequential parts of the classification algorithm, namely identification of noisy events and merging of the results, account for less than 1% of the total execution time (2.5 minutes out of 6 hours). This shows that the parallelization effort has been focused on the most computationally demanding parts of the algorithm.

ACKNOWLEDGMENT

This work was partially supported by the Portuguese Foundation for Science and Technology (FCT), POSI/EEA-CPS/61779/2004. The experimental data used in this paper was acquired at Unidad de Neuroprótesis y Rehabilitación Visual, Universidad Miguel Hernandez, and gently provided by Prof. Eduardo Fernandez.

REFERENCES

Brown, E. N., Kass, R. E., & Mitra, P. P. (2004). Multiple neural spike train data analysis: state-of-the-art and future challenges. *Nature Neuroscience*, *7*, 456–461. doi:10.1038/nn1228

Chapman, B. (2007). *The Multicore Programming Challenge (LNCS)*. Springer.

Condor Manuals. (2008). Retrieved from http://www.cs.wisc.edu/condor/manual/index.html

Documentation, P. H. P. (2008). Retrieved from http://www.php.net/docs.php

Figueiredo, M., & Jain, A. (2002). Unsupervised learning of finite mixture models. *IEEE Transactions on Pattern Analysis and Machine Intelligence*, *24*(3), 381–396. doi:10.1109/34.990138

Gschwind, M., Hofstee, H. P., Flachs, B., Hopkins, M., Watanabe, Y., & Yamazaki, T. (2006). Synergistic Processing in Cell's Multicore Architecture. *IEEE Micro*, 20–24.

Gummaraju, J., Coburn, J., Turner, Y., & Rosenblum, M. (2008). Streamware: programming general-purpose multicore processors using streams. In *Proceedings of the 13th international conference on Architectural support for programming languages and operating systems* (pp. 297-307). ACM.

Harris, K. D., Henze, D. A., Csicsvari, J., Hirase, H., & Buzsaki, G. (2000). Accuracy of Tetrode Spike Separation as Determined by Simultaneous Intracellular and Extracellular Measurements. *Journal of Neurophysiology*, *84*(1), 401–414.

Hulata, E., Segev, R., & Ben-Jacob, E. (2002). A method for spike sorting and detection based on wavelet packets and Shannon's mutual information. *Journal of Neuroscience Methods*, *117*(1), 1–12. doi:10.1016/S0165-0270(02)00032-8

Hyvärinen, A. (1999). Fast and Robust Fixed-Point Algorithms for Independent Component Analysis. *IEEE Transactions on Neural Networks*, *10*(3), 626–634. doi:10.1109/72.761722

Kosar, T., & Livny, M. (2005). A framework for reliable and efficient data placement in distributed computing systems. *Journal of Parallel and Distributed Computing*.

Lewicki, M. S. (1998). A review of methods for spike sorting: the detection and classification of neural action potentials. *Network (Bristol, England)*, *9*(4), 53–78. doi:10.1088/0954-898X/9/4/001

Lin, T. I., Lee, J. C., & Hsieh, W. J. (2007). Robust mixture modeling using the skew t distribution. *Statistics and Computing*, *17*(2), 81–92. doi:10.1007/s11222-006-9005-8

Linderman, M. D., Santhanam, G., Kemere, C. T., Gilja, V., O'Driscoll, S., & Yu, B. M. (2008). Signal Processing Challenges for Neural Prostheses. *IEEE Signal Processing Magazine*, *25*(1), 18–28. doi:10.1109/MSP.2008.4408439

MySQL Documentation. (2008). Retrieved from http://dev.mysql.com/doc

Octave Documentation. (2008). Retrieved from http://www.gnu.org/software/octave/docs.html

OpenSSH Manual Pages. (2008). Retrieved from http://www.openssh.com/manual.html

Owens, J. D., Luebke, D., Govindaraju, N., Harris, M., Krüger, J., Lefohn, A. E., & Purcell, T. J. (2007). A Survey of General-Purpose Computation on Graphics Hardware. *Computer Graphics Forum*, *26*(1), 80–113. doi:10.1111/j.1467-8659.2007.01012.x

Quiroga, R. Q., Nadasdy, Z., & Ben-Shaul, Y. (2004). Unsupervised Spike Detection and Sorting with Wavelets and Superparamagnetic Clustering. *Neural Computation*, *16*(8), 1661–1687. doi:10.1162/089976604774201631

Salganicoff, M., Sarna, M., Sax, L., & Gerstein, G. L. (1988). Unsupervised waveform classification for multineuron recordings: a real-time, software-based system. I: Algorithms and implementation. *Journal of Neuroscience Methods*, *25*(3), 181–187. doi:10.1016/0165-0270(88)90132-X

Shoham, S., Fellows, M. R., & Normann, R. A. (2003). Robust, automatic spike sorting using mixtures of multivariate t-distributions. *Journal of Neuroscience Methods*, *127*(2), 111–122. doi:10.1016/S0165-0270(03)00120-1

Takahashi, S., Anzai, Y., & Sakurai, Y. (2003a). A new approach to spike sorting for multi-neuronal activities recorded with a tetrode: how ICA can be practical. *Neuroscience Research*, *46*(3), 265–272. doi:10.1016/S0168-0102(03)00103-2

Takahashi, S., Anzai, Y., & Sakurai, Y. (2003b). Automatic sorting for multi-neuronal activity recorded with tetrodes in the presence of overlapping spikes. *Journal of Neurophysiology*, *89*, 2245–2258. doi:10.1152/jn.00827.2002

Thain, D., & Livny, M. (2003). Building Reliable Clients and Servers. In Foster, I., & Kesselman, C. (Eds.), *The Grid: Blueprint for a New Computing Infrastructure* (2nd ed.). Morgan Kaufmann.

Thain, D., Tannenbaum, T., & Livny, M. (2005). Distributed Computing in Practice: The Condor Experience. *Concurrency and Computation*, *17*(2-4), 323–356. doi:10.1002/cpe.938

Tomás, P., & Sousa, L. (2007). An Efficient Expectation-Maximisation Algorithm for Spike Classification. In15th International Conference on Digital Signal Processing (DSP 2007) (pp. 203-206).

Unidad de Neuroprótesis y Rehabilitacin Visual. (2008). Universidade Miguel Hernandez. Retrieved from http://naranja.umh.es/ lab

Zhang, P. M., Wu, J. Y., Zhou, Y., Liang, P. J., & Yuan, J. Q. (2004). Spike sorting based on automatic template reconstruction with a partial solution to the overlapping problem. *Journal of Neuroscience Methods*, *135*(1-2), 55–65. doi:10.1016/j.jneumeth.2003.12.001

Zouridakis, G., & Tam, D. C. (2000). Identification of reliable spike templates in multi-unit extracellular recordings using fuzzy clustering. *Computer Methods and Programs in Biomedicine*, *61*(2), 91–98. doi:10.1016/S0169-2607(99)00032-2

ENDNOTE

1 Some neurons can also release special chemicals that interfere with the activity of other neurons; however, here we are focused on the communication being carried out in spike trains.

Selected Readings

Chapter 10
Combining Geometry and Image in Biomedical Systems:
The RT TPS Case

Thomas V. Kilindris
University of Thessaly, Greece

Kiki Theodorou
University of Thessaly, Greece

ABSTRACT

Patient anatomy, biochemical response, as well functional evaluation at organ level, are key fields that produce a significant amount of multi modal information during medical diagnosis. Visualization, processing, and storage of the acquired data sets are essential tasks in everyday medical practice. In order to perform complex processing that involves or rely on image data a robust as well versatile data structure was used as extension of the Visualization Toolkit (VTK). The proposed structure serves as a universal registration container for acquired information and post processed resulted data. The structure is a dynamic multidimensional data holder to host several modalities and/or Meta data like fused image sets, extracted features (volumetric, surfaces, edges) providing a universal coordinate system used for calculations and geometric processes. A case study of Treatment Planning System (TPS) in the stereotactic radiotherapy (RT) based on the proposed structure is discussed as an efficient medical application.

INTRODUCTION

Computer aided medical applications for diagnosis, therapy, simulation or training proliferate gradually in everyday practice heavily relying on image data (Dawson and Kaufmann, 1998; Spitzer & Whitlock, 1998). Radio therapy planning, surgery as well medical simulation requires anatomic and physical modeling of the whole or part of the human body. Further on *in silico* functional study of the human body physiology requires the interoperation of several models to approximate an as real as possible behavior (Noble, 2002; Gavaghan, Garny, Maini, & Kohl, 2006; Seemann, Hoeper, Doessel, Holden, & Zhang, 2006). Major sources of real world data related to anatomical details are tomographic image sets. Tomographic image sets of 3D solid objects are in general stacked 2D cross-sectional images of the inspected object that contain geometric information mixed with material properties of the solid in terms of radiation absorbance.

The modality used to obtain the tomographic set determines the geometric accuracy of anatomical regions, the resolution of material properties as well functional characteristics. The almost annual doubling in computer power permits today real time manipulation of simultaneous multimodal datasets representation also know as image fusion and 3D image registration. Sometimes modalities act complementary in cases of sparse acquired datasets (Shim, Pitto, Streicher, Hunter P. J. & Anderson I. A. 2007). In order to study physiological function of internal organs several models have been proposed ranging from simple calculation diagrams to complex animated 3D solid models (France et al. 2005; Noble 2002; Seemann, 2007; Selberg & Vanderploeg, 1994; Spirka & Damasa, 2007). Almost all models involve dynamics and geometry. Physiological functions rule dynamics, dynamics produce data and data become finally visualized (Freudenberg, Schiemann, Tiede, & Hoehne, 2000). Soft tissue simulation used extensively in computer assisted surgery planning or training is an example. Tissue is modeled as a deformable object while collision detection between the virtual surgery instruments or even neighbor organs is used. Deformation is modeled according to physiological data while collision detection queries the geometric models to undertake the desired action for example simulated tissue ablation, rapture (Nealen et al. 2005; Teschner et al., 2005).

The Visible Human Project is another reference project that serves educational as well research (Ackerman 1998; Robb & Hanson 2006). Using the multimodal sets of the project (CT, MRI, CRYO) volume reconstruction of the human body both female and male is possible. Especially today where computational power and special graphics hardware is widely available at the cost of regular home personal computer the realization of a virtual dissection is feasible (Spitzer et al. 2004). One successful example is the Voxel-Man navigator (Schiemann, Tiede & Hoehne, 1997). Image guided techniques can assist both surgery and diagnosis. Virtual Endoscopy is an example of simulated endoscopic examination for diagnostic purposes (Robb, 1999). Reconstruction of the anatomy is done using tomographic imagesets and a fly through visualization is adopted to provide the analogous of real endoscopy. Once again improvements in the medical scanning systems combined with progress in computer systems lead to a novel approach of diagnostic medical imaging. Finally therapy planning systems in medicine make extensive use of imageset. Either directly or indirectly used to extract volumetric – geometric characteristics and 3D models those systems become essential in calculating complex therapeutic schemes like stereotactic radiotherapy, IMRT, neurosurgery, liver surgery orthopedics surgery etc (Mock et al. 2004; Shim et al. 2007).

All these systems are relative new and are undergoing an evaluation period where knew concepts from already established knowledge areas are reused. An example mentioned above is collision detection. Collision detection concept serves gaming from the very first day when primitive bouncing ball games debuted to the virtual reality implementation of industrial standard simulators. Data structures are continuously tested in the complex field of computer visualization.

Finally the most critical part is the man machine interface. But poor human interaction with application's functional dynamics can render useless even a state of the art system. Thus a lot of new techniques, input devices, displays, and controllers exist to fulfill the principal need for as possible high reality representation of the real world.

BACKGROUND

The primary task in spatial modelling of the human body is to regain real world patient's geometry from the available image data. Since the introduction of CT and MRI image datasets in medical diagnosis this task is mentally performed by the physician. Tilling cross-sectional images across a light box can reduce the size of area in interest as well the ability of the physician to traverse in space along planar data. Computer aided reconstruction was introduced (Robb et al, 1974; Herman & Liou, 1977) known as 3D reconstruction. On the 2D interactive visual display systems (computer monitors) this is done successful using different techniques like ray tracing, volume rendering [etc.] The amount as well the nature of data are more photometric than geometric thus it is extremely difficult to perform several morphometric measurement or even distance calculation between points in those data sets. A polygonal approximation of the external surface of the ventricle can be easily used to calculate any metrics like volume or surface distance. Applying a flow approximation model that involves finite element methods on the polygonal surface modelled vena cava is more efficient and feasible than to apply the simplest flow law in a point cloud that represents spatially the amount of absorbed energy. The results of the 3D reconstruction are geometric constructs with defined spatial boundaries composed by planar polygons also called polygonal approximations. (Fig. 1)

Polygonal approximations may vary in resolution as well in the type of primitive planar polygons used. The simplest planar polygon to manipulate mathematically and handle unambiguously by graphics rendering hardware is the triangle therefore the approximation tends more to triangulation. It is shown that any polygon can be divided in triangles. As already explained for practical reasons triangles were the first and are still used as the most favoured primitive polygon type to approximate surfaces. Polygonal surface approximations can be viewed in general as a fitting problem, a point set in R^3 space has to be fitted in one ore more possible surface approximations embedded in R^3 space. In most cases the point set is derived from a tomographic image set where the sliced nature ensures that points are rather layered than arbitrarily distributed in a cloud manner like the points acquired using a 3D digitizer.

The procedure to extract an anatomical meaningful region enclosed by a planar curve, the boundary of the anatomical unit, is called contouring or contour extraction. Contour extraction plays a key role in anatomical surface reconstruction. Algorithms that directly extract a surface (also called an isosurface) from a 3D point data set are well known and are extensively optimised. The famous Marching Cubes (MC) algorithm (Lorensen & Cline, 1987) or later improvements of it (Brodlie & Wood, 2001; Lopes & Brodlie, 2003) in surface extraction speed, resolution as well accuracy are widely used to extract surface on relatively large well defined anatomical units like bones. Application of the algorithm to smaller soft tissue areas does not always supply acceptable results even if fed by MRI image datasets. Using extracted planar contours the previous mentioned problem becomes a problem to combine points of adjacent slices that are not evenly spaced along adjacent contours. Although introduced in the early day of graphical computing (Kepel 1975, Fuchs, Kedem & Uselton, 1977) it is still an active research topic (Jones & Chen, 1994; Berzin 2002). Contouring algorithms often produce high detail contours. In order to reduce the level of detail, unnecessary or redundant vertices have to be removed using Vertex reduction filters applied to each contour line. These filters operate at each point that forms the polygonal contour line. A very simple one is the n-th point where the every n-th point is part of the output contour line but has the disadvantage that it is sensitive to the start point as well essential characteristics of the contour line might be lost arbitrarily. More complex algo-

Figure 1. Demonstrating part of the external surface of the head triangulated and embedded into a CT slice

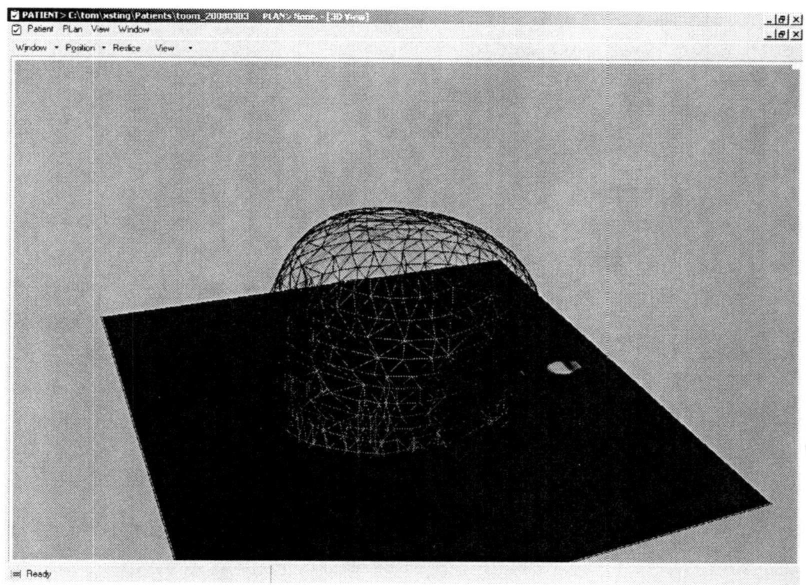

rithms preserve local geometrical characteristics (ie curvature) according to predefined tolerance metrics (distance, energy functions etc) without sacrificing global geometry of the processed line (Douglas and Peuckert 1973; Reuman and Witkam 1974). The reduction can be also done at a later stage on higher dimension by merging/eliminating triangular elements based on spatial smoothing criteria or other restrictions or requirements. Sometimes regeneration of the triangular mesh is needed. A collection of some classical algorithms to achieve polygonal mesh manipulation can be found in several survey and reviews (Heckbert & Garland 1997; Luebke, 2001).

Unlike geometric surfaces that can be described using equation sets in general point reconstructed surfaces do not have straight forward analytical expressions that can participate in transformations, actual processing is performed on their corresponding surface points. A set of powerful and well explored surface categories are the implicit surfaces. These surfaces can be expressed as the zero level set of a function $f(x,y,z)$. Implicit surfaces have some useful properties that are exploited in computer graphics as implicit surface modelling, especially in solids modelling, animation and simulation. One of their property extensively used is the intrinsic space division they provide. Consider the equation of a sphere of radius r in 3D space placed at the origin

$$x^2 + y^2 + z^2 = r^2 \qquad (1)$$

Rewriting the equation as the zero level set we can classify every point in $\Re^3$ according to the spheres surface as "inside"/ "outside" or at surface by checking the sign of $f(x,y,z)$. Thus an implicit surface divides the 3D space in a known way. It is also easy to combine implicit surfaces and form more complex surfaces or solid shapes by setting a tree like structure where the leaves are surfaces and the branches are operators in this case the root will represent the resulted final stage of construction. This method is know as Construc-

Figure 2. Visualizing the «inside/outside» property of the universal matrix voxels. Grey voxels are inside black voxels are outside. The implicit surface (patch) used to classify the voxels is also visible. Voxels have been intentionally shrinked for better visual perception

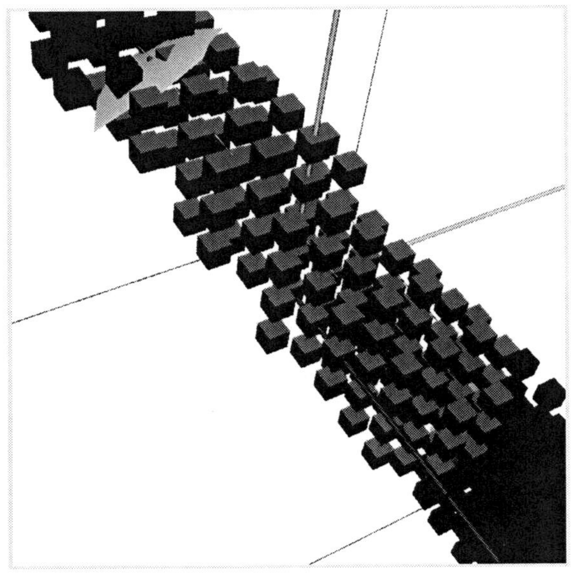

tive Solid Geometry (CSG). The resulted construct has the same property regarding classification of points in space therefore it is easy to built complex constructs approximating real world constructs and interact , manipulate or perform collision detection. We have successfully expanded this property to polygonal reconstructed shapes by imitating the classification behavior of implicit surfaces permitting the participation of these functions to CSG driven simulation applications. Fig. 2 and Fig. 3

REGISTRATION AND FUSION OF MODALITIES AND GRAPHICS IN STEREOTACTIC RADIOTHERAPY

Stereotactic Radiotherapy as well Radiosurgery make intensive use of image extracted features. Main concerns in therapy planning and irradiation procedure are proper localisation of the lesion in terms of diagnosis and definition in real world coordinate system as well calculation of the spatial distribution of deposited energy, called dose, on the lesion and healthy tissue. Further on possible successive sessions required need also follow up evaluation and verification based on new datasets and physical examinations acquired. Special systems are developed to assist this procedure called Treatment Planning Systems (TPS). Those systems simulate the irradiation room world by modelling precisely all devices involved in the plan like the linear accelerator (LINAC) the patient table and the patient itself to perform geometric verification in 3D space of patient placement, lesion targeting, functional feasibility and finally accepted volume dose distribution. The data input to the system are single or multimodal tomographic image sets representing the desired body anatomy where the lesion is located. Stereotactic radiotherapy is widely known for successful treatment of malignances into the head. Its almost spherical geometry that

Figure 3. A closer look at the implicit surface patch

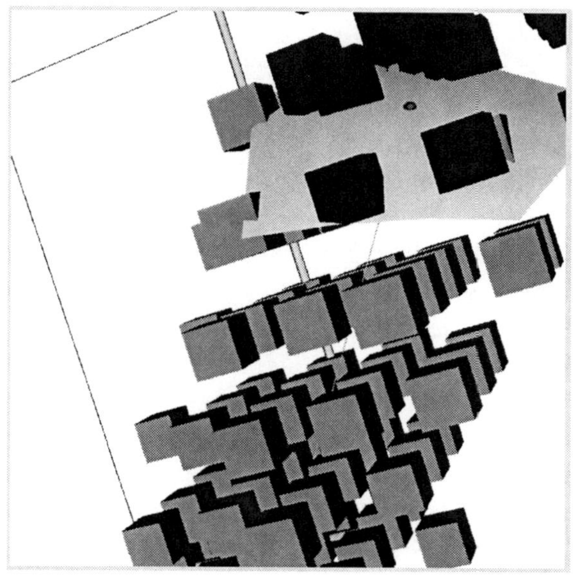

is easily accessed by the rotational LINAC as well the homogeneity of the brain tissue that allows fast dose calculation made it an excellent field of therapeutic application. Stereotactic radiotherapy can be also applied to treat almost any part the human body (Stereotactic Body Radiotherapy). Specific areas with high spatial density of different anatomical structures (spinal cord, blood vessels, trachea, lymphatic network etc) like the neck require sophisticated calculating power demanding TPS to achieve feasibility of irradiation within the required therapeutic, safety and geometrical constraints. A novel mounting approach of the LINAC on a robotic arm combined with a six freedom degree patient table and a patient movement synchronisation system is the state of the art in radiotherapy. The CyberKnife as it is called has been applied to lung (Brown et al. 2007; Cessaretti et al. 2008), pancreas, prostate (Fuller et al. 2008), neck, and spinal cord (Sahgal, Larson, & Chang, 2008) cancer treatment promising higher dose accuracy and almost total body access.

The patient images used for the simulated reconstruction presented were axial scans of the head. The image size was 256 x 256 or 512 x 512 pixels. Two types of slices are used fine and normal slices with 1.0 and 5.0 mm thickness respectively. The total size of the stack is 40 to 80 slices. Normal slices are used to define the exterior of the head and provide also landmarks for proper localisation of the imageset regarding the real world coordinate system. Fine slices include the lesion which is usual soft tissue. After successful localisation contour extraction (also know as delineation) of all organs or anatomic areas has to be performed in order to reconstruct their models in 3D space. Contour extraction can be done manually, semi automatically and automatically. In case of manual contour extraction the physician marks every point that belongs to the contour trying to follow it based on visual distinction of the boundaries. Proper contrast level is applied using window and slope settings in order to locate anatomic areas. All the points are linearly connected and form a closed contour.

The semi automatic way works also in planar mode but for every contour on a particular slice a physician indicates the point that is part of the external surface of desired organ or anatomical area. The selected Hounsfield Unit (HU) selected is used by a contour extraction algorithm as the isoline value and the points that belong to the corresponding isoline are generated. It is possible that more than one closed isoline exist, in this case manual intervention determines the correct one although automatic detection and correction can be implemented by advising already delineated contours or anatomic atlas retrieved prototypes. (Falcao & Udupa 2000; Faerber, Ehrhardt, & Handels 2007). The last method can be also used for automatic contour extraction. Pateint slices are registered with an anatomic atlas and necessary seed points are automatically transferred to initiate contouring algorithms. (Faerber, Ehrhardt, & Handels 2005) Physicians have to review the generated contours and accept or modify them to the anatomical detail desired.

Intermediate slice imaging data can be artificially generated using several classical interpolation methods (Lehmann, Goenner, & Spitzer 1999) or image registration techniques (Penney et al. 2004; Frakes et al 2008). Once delineation process is complete the image stack contains overlaid planar curves or to be more accurate a point set that is line connected to form a linear approximation of a set of contour curves. There are no interslice connections yet established. All these contour curves will be used to form a closed, watertight hull that encloses the area of interest in 3D space. The hull surface is composed by triangular elements that interconnect points of adjacent slices. A lot of hull generation algorithms exist. Some of them can directly operate on point clouds (points distributed in 3D space) were other require a planar layout of points. The connection element between points is still a linear segment and the representation is a connectivity list that indicates a traversal direction from one point to the next. While constructing contours and hulls the problem of direction is important because a lot of other issues like normals direction on planar elements are directly related. In order to ensure that the reconstructed hulls normals direction is consistent all contour lines extracted are filtered to maintain clockwise or counter clockwise connection. Once the global direction is set the connection of the points of the individual triangles has to be the same to ensure that each normal vector on every triangle will point outside the hull. This convention is stressed because the characterization algorithm used to determine and construct the models inside/outside map requires consistent normals direction. Also the light and transform algorithm of the render engine will produce a messy image (obscured and darkened areas) making 3D image perception difficult (Borodin, Zachmann & Klein, 2004).

The user saved structures that model organs and anatomic units are automatically saved as implicit surface constructs. These constructs consist of the polygonal data that is needed to represent the surface; the point set an octtree and normals cache. The octtree is a treelike data structure for space subdivision like the quad trees in planar subdivision. The use of octtrees speeds up point, elementary triangle retrieval of the polygonal surface. The normals cache is actually an array holding the normal vectors for every individual triangular element. Generation of the normals cache and the octtree is done upon creation of the implicit surface. Both of them are needed to speedup the point classification algorithm. As already mentioned any given point in 3D space can be characterized relative to an implicit surface. The implicit surface construct using its own classification algorithm replies to the call surfA->InOut() returning only three values 1, -1 and 0 representing outside, inside and "at surface" respectively.

All structures are embedded into a particular 3D data structure that acts as the universal container for the modeling environment. The structure has rectilinear grid for space subdivision. The cells composing this grid are called voxels. Depending on the implemented simulation, the size of the hexahedral voxels may be non equal for every side of the cell allowing a more dense resolution in areas required. Once an implicit surface construct is embedded into the universal container a new attribute is generated and added to the voxels that is used to label all voxels of the container as inside/outside the embedded surface or to be more concrete if the implicit surface represents the patient left eye "belongs to LE". Subsequent embedding of implicit surface structures causes a universal voxel to be multiple labeled. Specific volume data can be easily queried out of the universal data structure by counting the voxel labeled to the organ of interest. The particular developed TPS for radiotherapy uses a complex hexahedral grid based on the acquired patient image spatial resolution. The hexahedral cells have quadratic section matched to image resolution while the height of each cell depends whether the cells have normal or fine slice embedded into them. It is also possible to work entirely on the fine resolution by interpolating missing slices between normal slices but the result does not justify the computation overhead. In stereotactic radiotherapy the therapeutic dose is delivered partially to the patient using more irradiation beams that form fans rather than single beams. The benefit of this concept is that all irradiation beams are positioned to converge to a common area accumulating maximum energy as close as possible at the lesion. The placement of the beams as well the arcs traversed by individual beams is a problem that does not have a single solution. Restrictions apply to the path of every beam regarding sensitive or even forbidden anatomic units. These have to be either totally omitted or the dose should be kept below an upper limit. As already mentioned irradiation beams are generated by LINACs that are machines with a rotating gantry around a center called the isocenter. The gantry can rotate either clockwise or counterclockwise up to 180 degrees. The patient table rotates as well around the same the isocenter but the semi circle drawn is always on a plane perpendicular to the rotation plane of the gantry. It is obvious that while the gantry rotates to irradiate it should not in any way collide with the patient. Thus operational restrictions and machine limitations have to be taken in account during therapy planning. Using a simulated view of the beam also called "beams eye view" (BEV) the physician can see how the beam will interact with anatomic structures. Visual guidance ensures that the beams avoid them and a proper set of starting and ending angle are chosen for the rotating gantry position.

Isocenter placement is also a critical planning stage. Sometimes more than one isocenter are needed to cover adequately the whole volume of the lesion. Every isocenter has its own set of beams and has to be verified as already mentioned.

Once all preconditions are set the simulation starts firing beams passing through the isocenter across our geometric constructs registering energy deposition on the respectively cells contained into the beam's path. The calculation of the dose *D (v)* on a given voxel *v* is given by the following simplified formula:

$$D(v) = TPR(d(v)) \cdot OAR(d(v), offset(v)) \cdot C \qquad (2)$$

Function *d(v)* is the depth of voxel(cell) *v* referred to the beams entry point in patients external surface (skin). The function *offset(v)* is the distance of voxel *v* to the beams centerline. *TPR(d)* is the Tissue Phantom Ratio at phantom depth *d* while *OAR(d, off)* is the off-axis ratio at depth *d* and distance *off* from the beam's centerline entering the phantom. *C* is a collimator specific precalculated correction constant that justifies the circular field of the beams to a predefined square sectioned radiation field at a standard source detector distance.

The dose contents of the the voxels involved are added up and stored as new attribute to the voxel representing the total dose. Quality evaluation of the treatment plan requires visualization of the total dose as well computation some metrics. The total dose data is a volumetric dataset like the initial imageset. Visualization of dose data can be done either in 2D or 3D after normalization against a special user selected point (max. dose, dose at isocenter, specific point in patients body) Both of them require overlay with acquired patient images as well any delineated organs to percept the actual effect. In 2D visualization the dose is usually color coded in contrast to the gray scaled CT/MRI images. Radiotherapists prefer to view isodose curves instead of colored areas overlaid on grey scaled images. At this point automatic multiple contour extraction algorithms give a set of isodose lines. Every isodose line is carefully examined traversing through CT/MRI slices for the anatomic structures enclosed.

In 3D the only meaningful visualization of the total dose data is the extracted isosurfaces (Fig. 4). These isosurfaces show the volume of lesion enclosed that receives the specific dose. Only one surface at a time is meaningful to be displayed. Control on the isosurface opacity can highly contribute to spatial perception of the relative volume covered. Usually more than one treatment plans are generated as a result of optimization. Dose profiles are compared and the best plan is set for implementation.

Stereotactic Radiotherapy is in its nature an extended registration and fusion process. (Pellizari 1998). Multimodality coordinates (CT, MRI, PET, MR-Spectroscopy etc), machine – room coordinates (LINAC, table), patient body coordinates (lesion) as well the therapeutic plan (expected dose) have to be co-registered on the physical patient. Therefore spatial precision is essential in stereotactic radiotherapy. Proper positioning of the patient has to be ensured by any means. Any movement of the patient during dose delivery should be avoided. Specially designed frames have been developed and applied to patients to achieve this goal as well to provide a physical reference coordinates frame that is also used for fast registration of patient multimodal images. It is known that CT scans provide accurate anatomical information with high spatial resolution while MRI, has excellent soft tissue contrast and PET, MR-Spectroscopy etc reveal functional disorders sometimes down to metabolic level. This mutual information derived from the multimodality can be combined to precisely locate the lesion using the delineation process described above. (Maintz and Viergever 1998;. Pluim, Maintz, & Viergever, 2003);

Advanced image registration techniques promise frameless treatment (Eggers, Muehling, & Marmulla, 2006) while real time registration might compensate respiration movement that elastically deforms the torso geometry affecting internal organs boundaries. (Rietzel, Chen, Choi, & Willet, 2005; Lu et al 2006; McClelland et al. 2006).

The whole simulation environment of the TPS was coded in C++. Imageset and dataset processing, environment modeling and graphics realization was done using kitware's Visualization Toolkit (VTK). (Schroeder, Martin, & Lorensen, 1998). The proposed structures were designed according to VTK's interface model ensuring seamless integration and easy usage to already experienced developers.

FUTURE TRENDS

Geometric concepts in biomedical systems are intrinsically related to biomedical images. In most cases images are the starting point to lead to representation of world's real models. In prototyping the order is reversed but the common point is still high fidelity representation. Following the chain from the acquired image sets to 3D representation and user interaction almost all points need constant improvement. Multi slice medical scanners may increase spatial resolution and scanning speed producing more data to be processed at later processing stage. Consider

Figure 4. Demonstrating 3D dose representation. The object in red is the target volume while the olive colored surface embedded in it is the isosurface of a specific user selected dose level. The arcs are the 4 beam used to deliver dose to the target. The external surface of the head is colored orange.

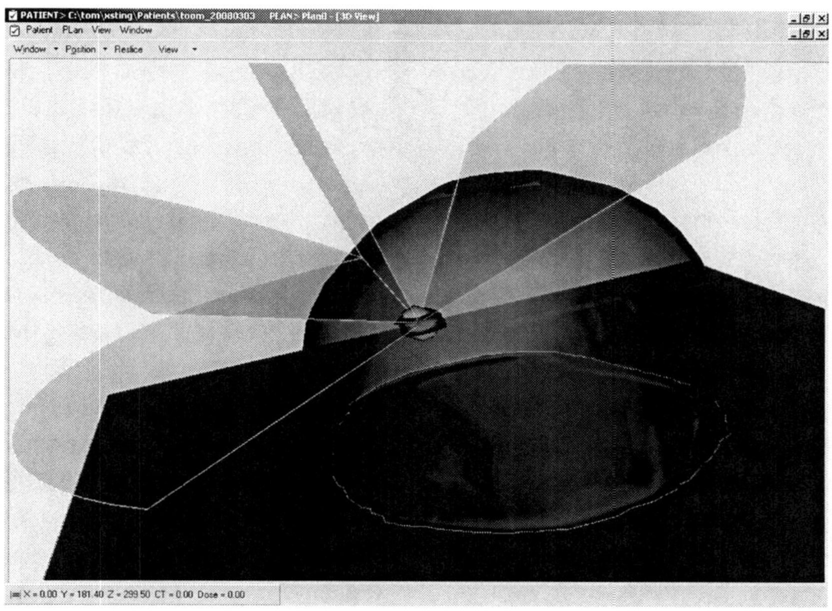

dynamic, real time processing of the imageset generated and existing graphic hardware reaches its limits. This data flooding overwhelms today's multicore general purpose CPU as well volatile memory bandwidth and size. Also processing software should encourage the development and use of well defined, high quality libraries, toolkits, classes even total development platforms stressing constant optimization and reusability of code. Dynamics in models might be handled by specialized hardware. Recall in early 90's the term GPU was more fiction than fact while the first SuperVGA adapters proudly displayed true color images to CRT monitors. Today's dedicated graphics processors pose units that perform higher than general purpose CPU raising the interest for general purpose GPU.

Constructional limits posed by solid state physics have been always the nightmare of microelectronics to disturb/cancel Moore's law. Core redesign of CPUs entering parallelism using multiple identical cores and promising novel nanomaterials might keep the Moore's law valid for the near future. Specialized processors might strongly support some highly repeatable tasks. Today PhysX, a dedicated physics processor unit (PPU) starts offering physics calculation offering universal collision detection, rigid-body dynamics, soft-body dynamics and deformation, fluid dynamics, and smart particle systems in gaming industry. But hardware is not a sole contributor, software needs also redesign and refactoring to exploit as more as possible the available or future GPU hardware platform. Thus the co-evolution algorithms-architecture leads to a Chicken/Egg problem.

Although fundamental limits of image registration are continuously studied (Robinson & Milanfar, 2004; Yetik & Nehorai 2006) the topic is still an open research and application field

(Orchard 2008). New and old hardware platforms (GPU, VLSI) are investigated promising high performance for sophisticated registration algorithms (Gupta & Gupta 2007; Samant, Xia, Muyan-Oezcelik & Owens, 2008). New optimization techniques and parallel implementation of the registration process (Wachowiak & Peters, 2006) show significant speed up maintaining robustness and accuracy.

The final part of the chain is human visual perception and interaction. Beside tremendous improvement in imaging and processing hardware the terminal visualization display remains 2-dimensional. The demand for real 3D display system is an old but still active research field for wide area of applications. There exist some implementations with acceptable spatial perception of the objects displayed. A commercially available system using dome shaped display unit offers color 3D projection for RT planning (Napoli et al., 2008). Some recent research has announced the development of an updatable flat monochrome holographic display (Tay et al. 2008).

Finally virtual reality environments offer a new perception in medical training and treatment planning. In some surgical operations instead of looking to an image guiding display system information is directly projected in front of the surgeons view field (Lorensen et al. 1993). Wearing a special head mounted display (HMD) visual system graphical information is overlayed to the surgeons view field (Grimson et al 1996). The information may be a CT/MRI image or synthetic graphical simulated information. This is a typical application of augmented reality. In general augmented reality is actually an image registration problem in real time. A visual system (camera) is used to provide the real world image while a computer is synthesizing the composed – overlaid image to be projected. The problems to be solved in real time are real scene light matching, real world – object coordinate systems transformation and matching (Uenohora & Kanade, 1995). The benefits of augmented reality eliminate the use of stereotactic frames because solving the coordinate transformation a virtual universal real time coordinate system accompanies the patient thus any externally attached positioning devices can be omitted (Grimson et al, 1996). Total immersion virtual reality is also promising a new dimension in medical training and education. Simulating a complete environment (i.e. operation room) by synthesizing the scene with graphically modeled 3D objects enhances spatial reality perception. A radiotherapy room has been simulated (Philips, Ward & Beavis, 2005) using this type of virtual reality for training. The linac movement was controlled by a real handheld device. Although VR systems progress in the visual part of reality the lack of proper human interaction. User interaction is mainly done using keyboard and pointing device. In some cases joysticks are used to move or traveling through 3D scenes. In surgical and laparoscopy simulators the sense of touch is essential. Special controls that imitate force feedback using haptics technology are explored (Westerbring-van der Putten, Goossens, Jakimowicz, & Dankelman, 2008).

CONCLUSION

Visualization of geometric features embedded in biomedical images is essential for medical spatial perception. We have presented an application framework for image and geometry coregistration by extending functionality of an already existing, reliable and widely used visualization toolkit. High speed computing at medium cost permits to switch from the classic 2 dimensional patient images to 3 dimensional patient anatomy reconstruction. Establishing a universal matrix where all geometrical structures and image reside, interact and register topological and functional data might serve as basic framework to build simulation application. A real application in stereotactic radiotherapy treatment planning that is based on the particular framework was presented in detail. There are functional topics in the application that can be optimized to increase performance in repeated treatment planning. To enhance the framework the parameter of time to support motion could be a possible extension serving real time dynamics where needed. On the other hand evolving hardware like virtual reality supporting devices could give another perspective of design and simulation in biomedical systems.

REFERENCES

Ackerman, M. (1998). The visible human project. *Proceedings of the IEEE, 86*(3), 504–511.

Berzin, D., & Hagiwara, I. (2002). Minimal area for surface reconstruction from crosssections, *The Visual Computer, 18*, 437–444.

Borodin, P., Zachmann, G., & Klein, R. (2004). Consistent Normal Orientation for Polygonal Meshes. *Computer Graphics International 2004* (CGI), June 16–19, Crete, Greece. IEEE Computer Society Press.

Brodlie, K., & Wood, J. (2001). Recent Advantages in Volume Visualization. *Computer Graphics Forum, 20*(2), 125-148.

Brown, W. T., Wu, X., Amendola, B., Perman, M., Han, H., Fayad, F., Garcia, S., Lewin, A., Abitbol, A., de la Zerda, A., & Schwade, J. G. (2007). Treatment of early non-small cell lung cancer, stage IA, by image-guided robotic stereotactic radioablation--CyberKnife. *The Cancer Journal, 13*(2), 75-7.

Cesaretti, J., Pennathur, A., Rosenstein, B. S., Swanson, S. J., & Fernando, H. (2008). Stereotactic Radiosurgery for Thoracic Malignancies. *The Annals of Thoracic Surgery, 85*(2), 785–791.

Dawson, S. L., & Kaufman, J. A. (1998). The imperative for medical simulation. *Proceedings of the IEEE 8*(3), 479–483.

Douglas, D. H., & Peucker, T. K. (1973). Algorithms for the Reduction of the Number of Points Required to Represent a Line or its Character. *The American Cartographer, 10*(2), 112-123.

Eggers, G., Mühling, J., & Marmulla, R. (2006). Image-to-patient registration techniques in head surgery. *International Journal of Oral and Maxillofacial Surgery, 35*(12), 1081-95.

Faerber, M., Ehrhardt, J., & Handels, H. (2005). Automatic atlas-based contour extraction of anatomical structures in medical images. *International Congress Series, 1281*, 272–277.

Faerber, M., Ehrhardt, J., & Handels, H. (2007). Live-wire-based segmentation using similarities between corresponding image structures. *Computerized Medical Imaging and Graphics, 31*, 549–560.

Falcao, A., & Udupa, J. (2000). A 3D generalization of user-steered live-wire segmentation. *Medical. Image Analysis, 4*(4) 89–402.

Frakes, D. H., Dasi, L. P., Pekkan, K., Kitajima, H. D., Sundareswaran, K., Yoganathan, A. P., & Smith, M. J. T. (2008). A New Method for Registration-Based Medical Image Interpolation. *IEEE Transactions on Medical Imaging, 27*(3), 370-377.

France, L., Lenoir, J., Angelidis, A., Meseure, P., Cani, M.-P., Faure, F., & Chaillou, C. (2005). A layered model of a virtual human intestine for surgery simulation. *Medical Image Analysis,* (9).

Freudenberg, J., Schiemann, T., Tiede, U., & Hoehne, K. H. (2000). Simulation of cardiac excitation patterns in a three-dimensional anatomical heart atlas. *Computers in Biology and Medicine, 30*, 191-205.

Fuchs, H., Kedem, Z. M., & Uselton, S. P. (1977). Optimal surface reconstruction from planar contours. *Commun ACM, 20*, 693–702.

Fuller, D. B., Naitoh, J., Lee, Ch., Hardy, S., & Jin, H. (2008). Virtual HDR CyberKnife Treatment for Localized Prostatic Carcinoma: Dosimetry Comparison With HDR Brachytherapy and Preliminary Clinical Observations. *International Journal of Radiation Oncology, Biology, Physics, 70*(5), 1588-1597.

Gavaghan, D., Garny, A., Maini, P. K., & Kohl, P. (2006). Mathematical models in physiology. *Phil. Trans. R. Soc. A 364*, 1099–1106.

Grimson, W. E. L., Ettinger, G. J., White, S. J., Lozano-Perez, T., Wells, W. M., III., & Kikinis, R. (1996, April). An Automated Registration Methods for Frameless Stereotaxy, Image Guided Surgery, and Enhanced Reality Visulatization. *Medical Imaging, IEEE Transactions, 15*(2), 129-140.

Gupta, N., & Gupta, N. (2007). A VLSI Architecture for Image Registration in Real Time. *IEEE Transactions on VLSI, 15*(9), 981-989.

Heckbert, P., & Garland, M. (1997). Survey of Polygonal Surface Simplification Algorithms. *Siggraph 97 Course Notes, 25*. ACM Press.

Herman, G. T., & Liu, H. K. (1977). Display of three dimensional information in computed tomography. *J Comput Assist Tomogr, 1*, 155–160.

Jones, M. W., & Chen, M. (1994). A new approach to the construction of surfaces from contour data. *Comput Graph Forum, 13*, 75–84.

Keppel, E. (1975). Approximating complex surfaces by triangulation of contour lines. *IBM J Res Dev 19*(1), 2–11.

Lu, W., Olivera, G. H., Chen, Q., Chen M-L., & Ruchala, K. J. (2006). Automatic re-contouring in 4D radiotherapy. *Physics in Medicine and Biology, 51*, 1077–1099.

Lehmann, T. Goenner, C., & Spitzer K. (1999). Survey: Interpolation Methods in Medical Image Processing. *IEEE Transactions on Medical Imaging,18*(11), 1049-1075.

Lopes, A., & Brodlie, K.(2003). Improving the robustness and accuracy of the marching cubes algorithm for isosurfacing. *IEEE Transactions on Visualization and ComputerGraphics, 9*, 16–29.

Lorensen, W. E., & Cline, H. E. (1987). Marching cubes: A high resolution 3D surface construction algorithm. *In Proceedings of the 14th annual conference on Computer graphics and interactive techniques*. (pp. 163–169). ACM Press.

Lorensen, W., Cline, H., Nafis, C., Kikinis, R., Altobelli, D., & Gleason, L. (1993). Enhancing Reality in the Operating Room. *Proceedings of the 1993 IEEE Visualization Conference* (pp. 410-415).

Luebke, D. (2001). A Developer's Survey of Polygonal Simplification Algorithms. *IEEE Computer Graphics &Applications,* (pp. 24-35).

McClelland, J. R., Blackall, J. M., Tarte, S., Chandler, A. C., Hughes, S., Ahmad, S., Landau, D. B., &Hawkes, D. J. (2006). A continuous 4D motion model from multiple respiratory cycles for use in lung radiotherapy. *Medical Physics, 33*, 3348–3358.

Mock, U., Georg, D., Bogner, J., Auberger, T., & Potter, R. (2004). Treatment planning comparison of conventional, 3D conformal, and intensity-modulated photon (IMRT) and proton therapy for paranasal sinuscarcinoma. *Int J Radiat Oncol Biol Phys, 58*(1), 147–154. [3D reduces dose delivered].

Maintz, J. B. A., & Viergever, M. A. (1998). *A Survey of Medical Image Registration Medical Image Analysis, 2*(1), 1–37.

Napoli, J., Stutsman, S., Chu, J. C. H., Gong, X., Rivard, M. J., Cardarelli, G., Ryan, T. P., & Favalora, G. E. (2008). Radiation therapy planning using a volumetric 3-D display: PerspectaRAD. *Proceedings of SPIE-IS&T Electronic Imaging, SPIE, 6803.*

Nealen, A., Muller, M., Keiser, R., Boxerman, E., & Carlson, M. (2005). Physically based deformable models in computer graphics. In *Eurographics 2005, State of the Art Report* 2005.

Noble, D. (2002). Modeling the Heart from Genes to Cells to the Whole Organ. Science, *295*(5560), 1678-1682.

Pelizzari, C. A. (1998). Image Processing in Stereotactic Planning: Volume Visualization and Image Registration. *Medical Dosimetry*, *23*(3), 137–145.

Penney, G. P., Schnabel, J. A., Rueckert, D., Viergever, M. A., & Niessen, W. J. (2004). Registration-Based Interpolation. *IEEE Transactions on Medical Imaging, 23*(7), 922-926.

Phillips, R., Ward, R., & Beavis, A. (2005). Immersive visualization training of radiotherapy treatment. In *Medicine Meets Virtual Reality Conference (MMVR 13)* (pp. 390–396) (Long-Beach, California), IOS Press.

Pluim, J. P. W., Maintz, J. B. A., & Viergever, M. A. (2003). Mutual-Information-Based Registration of Medical Images: A Survey. *IEEE Transactions on Medical Imaging, 22*(8), 986-1004.

Reumann, K., & Witkam, A. P. M. (1974). Optimizing Curve Segmentation in Computer Graphics. I*nternational Computing Symposium. Amsterdam, North Holland*, (pp. 467- 472).

Rietzel, E., Chen, G. T., Choi, N. C., & Willet, C. G. (2005). Four-dimensional image-based treatment planning: Target volume segmentation and dose calculation in the presence of respiratory motion. *International Journal of Radiation Oncology Biology and Physics, 61*, 1535–1550.

Robb, R. A., Greenleaf, J. F., Ritman, E. L., Johnson, S. A., Sjostrand, J. D., Herman, G. T., & Wood, E. H. (1974). Three-dimensional visualization of the intact thorax and contents: a technique for cross-sectional reconstruction from multiplanar x-ray views. *Comput Biomed Res, 7*, 395–419.

Robb, R. A. (1999). Virtual endoscopy: development and evaluation using the Visible Human Datasets, *Computerized Medical Imaging and Graphics,* (24), 133–151.

Robb, R. A., & Hanson, D. P. (2006). Biomedical Image Visualization Research Using the Visible Human Datasets. *Clinical Anatomy, 19*, 240–253.

Robinson, D., & Milanfar, P. (2004). Fundamental Performance Limits in Image Registration. *IEEE Transactions on Image Processing,13*(9), 1185-1199.

Sahgal, A., Larson, D. A., & Chang, E. L. (2008). Stereotactic body radiosurgery for spinal metastases: a critical review. *International Journal of Radiation Oncology, Biology, Physics., 71*(3), 652-65.

Samant, S. S., Xia, J., Muyan-Özçelik, P., & Owens, J. D. (2008). High performance computing for deformable image registration: Towards a new paradigm in adaptive radiotherapy. *Medical. Physics., 35*(8), 3546-3553.

Seemann, G., Hoeper, Ch., Doessel, O., Holden, A. V., & Zhang, H. (2006). Heterogeneous three-dimensional anatomical and electrophysiological model of human atria. *Phil. Trans. R. Soc., A 364*, 1465–1481.

Sellberg, M. S., & Vanderploeg, M. J. (1994). Virtual human: A computer graphics model for biomechanical simulations and computer-aided instruction. *Proceedings of the 16th Annual International Conference of the IEEE Engineering in Medicine and Biology Society, Engineering Advances: New Opportunities for Biomedical Engineers, IEEE*, New York, NY, (pp. 329–330).

Schroeder, W., Martin, K., & Lorensen, W. (1998). *The Visualization Toolkit: An Object-Oriented Approach to 3D Graphics*. Prentice Hall.

Schiemann, T., Tiede, U., & Höhne, K. H. (1997). Segmentation of the visible human for high-quality volume-based visualization. *Medical Image Analysis, 1*(4), 263-70.

Shim, V. B., Pitto, R. P., Streicher, R. M., Hunter, P. J., & Anderson, I. A. (2007). The use of sparse CT datasets for auto-generating accurate FE models of the femur and pelvis. *Journal of Biomechanics, 40*, 26–35.

Spirka, T. A., & Damaser, M. S. (2007). Modeling physiology of the urinary tract. *Journal of Endourology, 21*(3), 294-299.

Spitzer, V. M., & Whitlock, D. G. (1998). The visible human data set: the anatomical platform for human simulation. *Anat. Rec. (New Anat.,) 253*, 49–57.

Spitzer, V., Spitzer, G., Lee, C., Reinig, K., Granas, L., Graus, K., & Smyth, P. (2004). VH Dissector: A platform for curriculum development and presentation for the anatomical arts and sciences. In *Medicine Meets Vitual Reality 12* (Newport Beach, California), IOS Press, (pp. 127–129).

Tay, S., Blanche, P.-A., Voorakaranam, R. A., Tunc, V., Lin, W., Rokutanda, S., Gu, T., Flores, D., Wang, P., Li, G., St Hilaire, P., Thomas, J., Norwood, R. A., Yamamoto, M., & Peyghambarian, N. (2008). An updatable holographic three-dimensional display. *Nature Letters, 451*, 694-698.

Teschner, M., Kimmerle, S., Heidelberger, B., Zachmann, G., Raghupathi, L., Fuhrmann, A., Cani, P. M., Faure, F., Magenat-Thalmann, N., Strasser, W., & Volino, P. (2005). Collision detection for deformable objects. *Computer Graphics Forum, 24*(1), 61–81.

Uenohara, M., & Kanade, T. (1995). Vision-Based Object Registration for Real-Time Image Overlay. In N. Ayache (Ed.), *Computer Vision, Virtual Reality and Robotics in Medicine: CVRMed '95* (pp. 14-22). Berlin: Springer-Verlag.

Wachowiak, M. P., & Peters, T. M. (2006). High-Performance Medical Image Registration Using New Optimization Techniques. *IEEE Transactions on Information Technology in Biomedicine, 10*(2), 344-353.

Westerbring-van der Putten, E. P., Goossens, R. H. M., Jakimowicz, J. J., & Dankelman, J. (2008). Haptics in minimally invasive surgery – a review. *Minimally Invasive Therapy, 17*(1), 3–16.

Yetik, I. S., & Nehorai, A. (2006). Performance Bounds on Image Registration. *IEEE Transactions on Signal Processing, 54*(5), 1737-1749.

KEY TERMS AND DEFINITIONS

Contouring: A subdivision process where a set of points logically connected forms a construct that represents a common characteristic feature in general. On a 2D space contouring generates lines while on a 3D space beside lines and surfaces.

Dose Calculation/Optimization: The procedure to determine the body absorbed energy in both the lesion and healthy tissue. The optimization of the process is inherent due to steep dose delivery around the target.

Image Fusion: Simultaneous presentation of multimodal registered images on a visual media.

Image Registration: Registration of images in a common known reference coordinate system.

Implicit Surface Modeling: Specific modeling process that approximates every geometrical model using implicit mathematical functions as analytical surface representation constructing complex geometric representations maintaining mathematical functionality of the final model.

Multimodal Imaging (Multispectral): Images of the same object using different physical acquisition technology the term is widely used for medical imaging while multispectral refers to satellite imaging and survey.

Octtrees: 3D space divison data structures analogous to 2D quad trees. Used for storage, compression, collision detection, point search etc.of 3D models.

Stereotactic Radiotherapy: A Radiation therapy procedure that requires precise localization of the target area to deliver fractioned prescribed dose by means of convergent or not beams.

Surface Reconstruction: The reconstrunction of geometrical surface The surface might by a point cloud, know contours of the recoctructed surface, known gradients.

Treatment Planning System (TPS): A computer based system used to simulate, calculate and optimize the radiotherapy treatment of patients. The main tasks are lesion localization, radiation plan generation according to safety and health constaints and geometric feasibility plan optimization.

Visualization Toolkit (VTK): An open source graphical toolkit widely used as a common extendable customizable platform for scientific visualization.

This work was previously published in Handbook of Research on Advanced Techniques in Diagnostic Imaging and Biomedical Applications, edited by T. Exarchos and D. Fotiadis, pp. 197-212, copyright 2009 by Medical Information Science Reference (an imprint of IGI Global).

Chapter 11
Image Registration for Biomedical Information Integration

Xiu Ying Wang
The University of Sydney, Australia

Dagan Feng
The University of Sydney, Australia;
Hong Kong Polytechnic University, Hong Kong

ABSTRACT

The rapid advance and innovation in medical imaging techniques offer significant improvement in healthcare services, as well as provide new challenges in medical knowledge discovery from multi-imaging modalities and management. In this chapter, biomedical image registration and fusion, which is an effective mechanism to assist medical knowledge discovery by integrating and simultaneously representing relevant information from diverse imaging resources, is introduced. This chapter covers fundamental knowledge and major methodologies of biomedical image registration, and major applications of image registration in biomedicine. Further, discussions on research perspectives are presented to inspire novel registration ideas for general clinical practice to improve the quality and efficiency of healthcare.

INTRODUCTION

With the reduction of cost in imaging data acquisition, biomedical images captured from anatomical imaging modalities, such as Magnetic Resonance (MR) imaging, Computed Tomography (CT) and X-ray, or from functional imaging modalities, such as Positron Emission Tomography (PET) and Single Photon Emission Computed Tomography (SPECT), are widely used in modern clinical practice. However, these ever-increasing huge amounts of datasets unavoidably cause information repositories to overload and pose substantial challenges in effective and efficient medical knowledge management, imaging data retrieval, and patient management.

Biomedical image registration is an effective mechanism for integrating the complementary and valuable information from diverse image datasets. By searching the optimal correspondence among the multiple datasets, biomedical image registration enables a more complete insight and full utilization of heterogeneous imaging resources (Wang and Feng, 2005) to facilitate knowledge discovery and management of patients with a variety of diseases.

Biomedical image registration has important applications in medical database management, for instance, patient record management, medical image retrieval and compression. Image registration is essential in constructing statistical atlases and templates to extract common patterns of morphological or functional changes across a large specific population (Wang and Feng, 2005). Therefore, registration and fusion of diverse imaging resources is important component for clinical image data warehouse and clinical data mining.

Due to its research significance and crucial role in clinical applications, biomedical image registration has been extensively studied during last three decades (Brown, 1992; Maintz et al., 1998; Fitzpatrick et al. 2000). The existing registration methodologies can be catalogued into different categories according to criteria such as image dimensionality, registration feature space, image modality, and subjects involved (Brown, 1992). Different Region-of-Interests (ROIs) and various application requirements and scenarios are key reasons for continuously introducing new registration algorithms. In addition to a large number of software-based registration algorithms, more advanced imaging devices such as combined PET/CT and SPECT/CT scanners provide hardware-based solutions for the registration and fusion by performing the functional and anatomical imaging in the one imaging session with the one device. However, it remains challenging to generate clinically applicable registration with improved performance and accelerated computation for biomedical datasets with larger imaging ranges, higher resolutions, and more dimensionalities.

CONCEPTS AND FUNDAMENTALS OF BIOMEDICAL IMAGE REGISTRATION

Definition

Image registration is to compare or combine multiple imaging datasets captured from different devices, imaging sessions, or viewpoints for the purpose of change detection or information integration. The major task of registration is to search for an appropriate transformation to spatially relate and simultaneously represent the images in a common coordinate system for further analysis and visualization. Image registration can be mathematically expressed as (Brown, 1992):

$$I_R(X_R) = g(I_S(T(X_S))) \qquad (1)$$

where I_R and I_S are the reference (fixed) image and study (moving) image respectively; $T:(X_S) \rightarrow (X_R)$is the transformation which sets up spatial correspondence between the images so that the study image X_S can be mapped to and represented in the coordinate system of reference image X_R ; $g:(I_s) \rightarrow (I_R)$ is one-dimensional intensity calibration transformation.

Framework

As illustrated in Figure 1, in registration framework, the study dataset is firstly compared to the reference dataset according to a pre-defined similarity measure. If the convergence has not been achieved yet, the optimization algorithm estimates a new set of transformation parameters to calculate a better spatial match between the images. The study image is interpolated and transformed with the updated transformation parameters, and then compared with the reference image again. This procedure is iterated until the optimum transformation parameters are found, which are then used to register and fuse the study image to the reference image.

Major Components of Registration

Input Datasets

The characteristics of input datasets, including modality, quality and dimensionality, determine the choice of similarity measure, transformation, interpolation and optimization strategy, and eventually affect the performance, accuracy, and application of the registration.

The input images for registration may originate from identical or different imaging modality, and accordingly, registration can be classified as monomodal registration (such as CT-CT registration, PET-PET registration, MRI-MRI registration) or multimodal registration (such as CT-MRI registration, CT-PET registration, and MRI-PET registration). Monomodal registration is required to detect changes over time due to disease progression or treatment. Multimodal registration is used to correlate and integrate the complementary information to provide a more complete insight into the available data. Comparatively, multimodal registration proves to be more challenging than monomodal, due to the heterogeneity of data sources, differing qualities (including spatial resolution and gray-level resolution) of the images, and insufficient correspondence.

Registration algorithms for the input datasets with different dimensionalities are used for other applications and requirements. For instance, two-dimensional image registration is applied to construct image mosaics to provide a whole view of a sequence of partially overlapped images, and is used to generate atlases or templates for a specific group of subjects. Although three-dimensional image registration is required for most clinical applications, it is challenging to produce an automatic technique with high computational efficiency for routine clinical usages. Multidimensional registration is demanded to align a series of three-dimensional images acquired from different sessions for applications such as tumor growth monitoring, cancer staging and treatment assessment (Fitzpatrick et al, 2000).

Figure 1. Framework of image registration

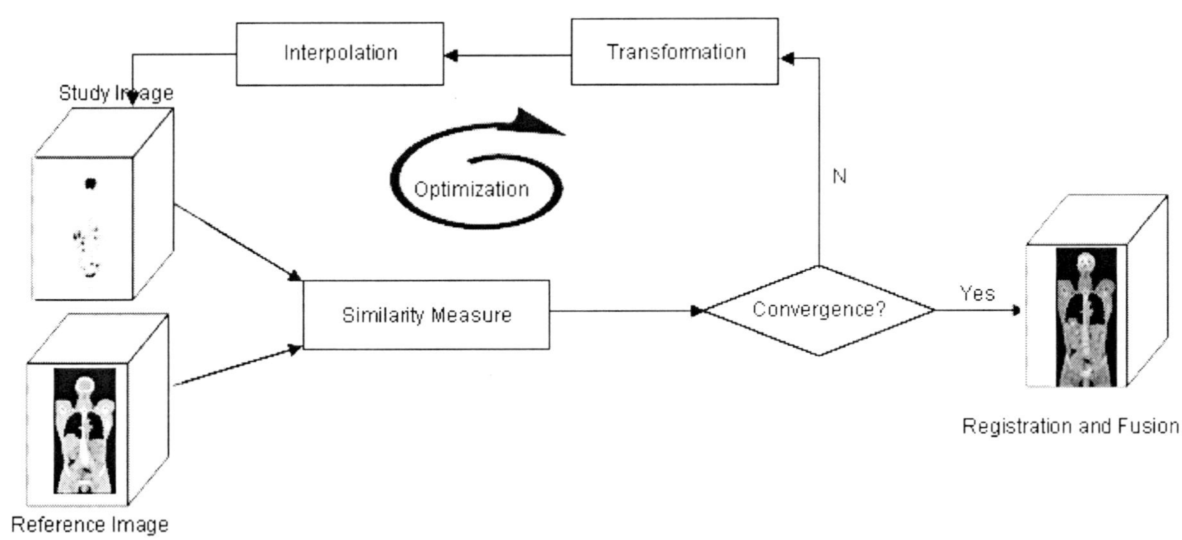

Registration Transformations

The major task of registration is to find a transformation to align and correlate the input datasets with differences and deformations, introduced during imaging procedures. These discrepancies occur in the form of variations in the quality, content, and information within the images, therefore posing a significant obstacle and challenge in the area of image registration. In addition, motions, either voluntary or involuntary, require special attention and effort during the registration procedure (Wang et al., 2007; Fitzpatrick et al., 2000).

- **Rigid-body Transformations** include rigid and affine transformations, and are mainly used to correct simple differences or to provide initial estimates for more complex registration procedures. Rigid transformation is used to cope with differences due to positional changes (such as translations and rotations) in the imaging procedure and is often adopted for the registration of brain images, due to the rigid nature of the skull structure. In addition, affine transformation can be used to deal with scaling deformations. However, these transformations are usually limited outside of the brain.
- **Deformable Transformations** are used to align the images with more complex deformations and changes. For instance, motions and changes of organs such as lung, heart, liver, bowel, need to be corrected by more comprehensive non-linear transformations. The significant variance between subjects and changes due to disease progression and treatment intervention require nonlinear transformations with more degrees of freedom. In deformable registration, a deformation field which is composed of deformation vectors, needs to be computed. One displacement vector is decided for each individual image element (pixel for 2D or voxel for 3D). Compared to rigid-body transformations, the complexity of deformable transformations will slow down the registration speed, and efficient deformable registration remains a challenging research area.

Interpolation Algorithms

Interpolation is an essential component in registration, and is required whenever the image needs to be transformed or there are resolution differences between the datasets to be registered. After the transformation, if the points are mapped to non-grid positions, interpolation is performed to approximate the values for these transformed points. For the multimodal image registration, the sample space of the lower-resolution image is often interpolated (up-sampled) to the sample space of the higher-resolution image. In the interpolation procedure, the more neighbouring points are used for the calculation, the better accuracy can be achieved, and the slower the computation. To balance interpolation accuracy and computational complexity, bilinear interpolation technique which calculates the interpolated value based on four points, and trilinear interpolation, are often used in registration (Lehmann et al., 1999).

Optimization Algorithms

Registration can be defined as an iterative optimization procedure (Equation 2) for searching the optimal transformation to minimize a cost function for two given datasets:

$$T_{optimal} = \underset{(T)}{\arg\min}\, f(T(X_S), X_R) \qquad (2)$$

where T is the registration transformation; f is the cost function to be minimized.

- **Gradient-based optimization methods** are often used in registration, in which the gradient vector at each point is calculated to determine the search direction so that the value of the cost function can be decreased locally. For instance, Quasi-Newton methods such as Broyden-Fletcher-Goldfarb-Shanno (BFGS), has been investigated and applied in medical image registration (Unser, Aldroubi, 1993; Mattes et al., 2003).

- **Powell optimization** (Powell, 1964) is another frequently adopted searching strategy in registration. Powell method performs a succession of one-dimensional searches to find the best solution for each transformation parameter, and then the single-variable optimizations are used to determine the new search direction. This procedure is iterative until no better solution or further improvement over the current solution can be found. Because of no derivatives required for choosing the searching directions, computational cost is reduced in this algorithm.
- **Downhill Simplex optimization** (Press et al., 1992) does not require derivatives either. However, compared with Powell algorithm, Downhill Simplex is not so efficient due to more evaluations involved. For a given n-dimensional problem domain, the Simplex method searches the optimum solution downhill through a complex n-dimensional topology through operations of reflection, expansion, contraction, and multiple contractions. Because it is more robust in finding the optimal solution, Simplex optimization has been widely used in medical registration.
- **Multi-resolution optimization schemes** have been utilized to avoid being trapped into a local optimum and to reduce computational times of the registration (Thévenaz ,Unser, 2000; Borgefors, 1988; Bajcsy, Kovacic, 1989; Unser, Aldroubi, 1993). In multi-resolution registration, the datasets to be registered are firstly composed into multiple resolution levels, and then the registration procedure is carried out from low resolution scales to high resolution scales. The initial registration on the global information in the low resolution provides a good estimation for registration in higher resolution scales and contributes to improved registration performance and more efficient computation (Wang et al, 2007).

Spline based multi-resolution registration has been systematically investigated by Thévenaz (Thévenaz, Unser, 2000) , and Unser (Unser, Aldroubi, 1993). In these Spline-based registration, the images are filtered by B-spline or cubic spline first and then down-sampled to construct multi-resolution pyramids. Multi-resolution B-spline method provides a faster and more accurate registration result for multimodal images when using mutual information as a similarity measure.

BIOMEDICAL IMAGE REGISTRATION METHODOLOGIES AND TECHNIQUES

Registration methods seek to optimize values of a cost function or similarity measure which define how well two image sets are registered. The similarity measures can be based on the distances between certain homogeneous features and differences of gray values in the two image sets to be registered (Wang et al, 2007). Accordingly, biomedical image registration can be classified as feature-based or intensity-based methods (Brown, 1992).

Feature-Based Registration

In feature-based registration, the transformation required to spatially match the features such as landmark points (Maintz, et al, 1996), lines (Subsol, et al, 1998) or surfaces (Borgefors, 1988), can be determined efficiently. However, in this category of registration, a preprocessing step is usually necessary to extract the features manually or semi-automatically, which makes the registration, operator- intensive and dependent (Wang et al, 2007).

Landmark-Based Registration

Landmark-based registration includes identifying homologous points which should represent the same features in different images as the first step, and then the transformation can be estimated based on these corresponding landmarks to register the images. The landmark points can be artificial markers attached to the subject which can be detected easily or anatomical feature points.

- **Extrinsic landmarks (fiducial markers)**, such as skin markers, can be noninvasive. However, skin markers cannot provide reliable landmarks for registration due to elasticity of human skin. The invasive landmarks such as stereotactic frames are able to provide robust basis for registration, and can be used in Image Guided Surgery (IGS) where registration efficiency and accuracy are the most important factors. Since they are easily and automatically detectable in multiple images to be registered, extrinsic landmarks can be used in both monomodal and multimodal image registration.
- **Intrinsic landmarks** can be anatomically or geometrically (such as corner points, intersection points or local extrema) salient points in the images. Since landmarks are required to be unique and evenly distributed over the image, and to carry substantial information, automatic landmark selection is challenging task. Intensive user interaction is often required to manually identify the feature points for registration (Wang et al, 2007). Iterative closest point (ICP) algorithm (Besl, MaKey 1992) is one of most successful landmark-based registration methods. Because no prior knowledge on correspondence between the features is required, ICP eases the registration procedure greatly.

Line-Based Registration and Surface-Based Registration

- **Line-based registration** utilizes line features such as edges and boundaries extracted from images to determine the transformation. "Snakes" or active contours (Kass et al, 1988) provide effective contour extraction techniques and have been widely applied in image segmentation and shape modelling, boundary detection and extraction, motion tracking and analysis, and deformable registration (Wang and Feng 2005). Active contours are energy-minimizing splines, which can detect the closest contour of an object. The shape deformation of an active contour is driven by both internal forces, image forces and external forces. To handle the difficulties of concavity and sensitivity during initialization, classic snakes, balloon model (Cohen and Cohen 1993) and gradient vector flow (GVF) (Xu and Prince 1998) were proposed.
- **Surface-based registration** uses the distinct surfaces as a registration basis to search the transformation. The "Head-and-Hat" algorithm (Chen, et al, 1987) is a well-known surface fitting technique for registration. In this method, two equivalent surfaces are identified in the images to be registered. The surface extracted from the higher-resolution images, is represented as a stack of discs, and is referred to as "head", and the surface extracted from the lower-resolution image volume, is referred to as "hat", which is represented as a list of unconnected 3D points. The registration is determined by iteratively transforming the hat surface with respect to the head surface, until the closest fit of the hat onto the head is found. Because the segmentation task is comparatively easy, and the computational cost is relatively low, this method remains popular. More details

of surface-based registration algorithms can be found in the review by Audette et al, 2000.

Intensity-Based Registration

Intensity-based registration can directly utilize the image intensity information without segmentation or intensive user interaction required, and thereby can achieve fully automatic registration. In intensity-based registration, a similarity measure is defined on the basis of raw image content and is used as a criterion for optimal registration. Several well-established intensity-based similarity measures have been used in the biomedical image registration domain.

Similarity measures based on intensity differences including sum of squared differences (SSD) (Equ. 3) and sum of absolute differences (SAD) (Equ.4) (Brown, 1992), are the simplest similarity criteria which exhibit minimum value for perfect registration. As these methods are too sensitive to the intensity changes and significant intensity differences may lead to false registration, SAD and SSD are limited in application and as such, are mainly used to register monomodal images (Wang et al, 2007):

$$SSD = \sum_{i}^{N} (I_R(i) - T(I_S(i)))^2 \quad (3)$$

$$SAD = \frac{1}{N} \sum_{i}^{N} \left| I_R(i) - T(I_S(i)) \right| \quad (4)$$

where $I_R(i)$ is the intensity value at position i of reference image R and $I_S(i)$ is the corresponding intensity value in study image S; T is geometric transformation.

Correlation techniques were proposed for multimodal image registration (Van den Elsen, et al, 1995) on the basis of assumption of linear dependence between the image intensities. However, as this assumption is easily violated by the complexity of images from multiple imaging devices, correlation measures are not always able to find optimal solution for multimodal image registration.

Mutual information (MI) was simultaneously and independently introduced by two research groups of Collignon et al (1995) and Viola and Wells (1995) to measure the statistical dependence of two images. Because of no assumption on the feature of this dependence and no limitation on the image content, MI is widely accepted as multimodal registration criterion (Pluim et al., 2003).

For two intensity sets $R = \{r\}$ and $S = \{s\}$, mutual information is defined as:

$$I(R,S) = \sum_{r,s} p_{RS}(r,s) \log \frac{p_{RS}(r,s)}{p_R(r) \cdot p_S(s)} \quad (5)$$

where $p_R(r,s)$ is the joint distribution of the intensity pair (r,s); $p_R(r)$ and $p_S(s)$ are the marginal distributions of r and s.

Mutual information can be calculated by entropy:

$$\begin{aligned} I(R,S) &= H(R) + H(S) - H(R,S) \\ &= H(R) - H(R \mid S) \\ &= H(S) - H(S \mid R) \end{aligned} \quad (6)$$

$H(S|R)$ is the conditional entropy which is the amount of uncertainty left in S when R is known, and is defined as:

$$H(S \mid R) = \sum_{r \in R} \sum_{s \in S} p_{RS}(r,s) \log p_{S|R}(s \mid r) \quad (7)$$

If R and S are completely independent, $p_{RS}(r,s) = p_R(r) \cdot p_S(s)$ and $I(R,S) = 0$ reaches its minimum; if R and S are identical, $I(R,S) = H(R) = H(S)$ arrives at its maximum. Registration can be achieved by searching the transformation parameters which maximize the mutual information. In implementation, the joint entropy and marginal entropies can be estimated by normalizing the joint and marginal histograms of the overlapped sections of the images. Although maximization of MI is a powerful registration measure, it cannot always generate accurate result. For instance, the changing overlap between the images may lead to false registration with maximum MI (Studholme, et al., 1999).

Case Study: Inter-Subject Registration of Thorax CT Image Volumes Based on Image Intensity

The increase in diagnostic information is critical for early detection and treatment of disease and provides better patient management. In the context of a patient with non-small cell lung cancer (NSCLC), registered data may mean the difference between surgery aimed at cure and a palliative approach by the ability to better stage the patient. Further, registration of studies from healthy lung and the lung with tumor or lesion is critical to better tumor detection.

In the example (Figure 2), the registration between healthy lung and the lung with tumor is performed based on image intensity, and normalized MI is used as similarity measure. Figure 2 shows that affine registration is not able to align the common structures from different subjects correctly and therefore deformable registration by using spline (Mattes, et al 2003) is carried out to further improve the registration accuracy.

Hardware Registration

Although continued progress in image registration algorithms (software-based registration) has been achieved, the software-based registration might be labor intensive, computationally expensive, and with limited accuracy, and thus is impractical to be applied routinely (Townsend, et al, 2003). Hardware registration, in which the functional imaging device, such as PET is combined with an anatomical imaging device such as CT in the one instrument, largely overcomes the current limitations of software-based techniques. The functional and anatomical imaging are performed in the one imaging session on the same imaging table, which minimizes the differences in patient positioning and locations of internal organs between the scans. The mechanical design and calibration procedures ensure that the CT and PET data are inherently accurately registered if the patient does not move. However, patient motion can be encountered between the CT and PET. This not only results in incorrect anatomical localization, but also artifacts from the attenuation correction based on the misaligned CT data (Wang et al, 2007). Misalignment between the PET and CT data can also be due to involuntary motion, such as respiratory or cardiac motion. Therefore, although the combined PET/CT scanners are becoming more and more popular, there is a clear requirement for software-registration to remove the motions and displacements from the images captured by the combined imaging scanners.

APPLICATIONS OF BIOMEDICAL IMAGE REGISTRATION

Biomedical image registration is able to integrate relevant and heterogeneous information contained in multiple and multimodal image sets, and is important for clinical database management. For instance, registration is essential to mining the large medical imaging databases for constructing statistical atlas of specific disease to reveal the functional and morphological characteristics and changes of the disease, and to facilitate a more suitable patient care. The dynamic atlas in turn is used as a pattern template for automated segmentation and classification of the disease. Image registration is also critical for medical image retrieval of a specific type of disease in a large clinical image database, and in such a scenario, the functional or anatomical atlas provides prior knowledge and is used as a template for early-stage disease detection and identification (Toga, Thompson, 2001).

Registration has a broad range of clinical applications to improve the quality and safety of healthcare. Early detection of tumors or disease

Figure 2. Registration for thoracic CT volumes from different subjects

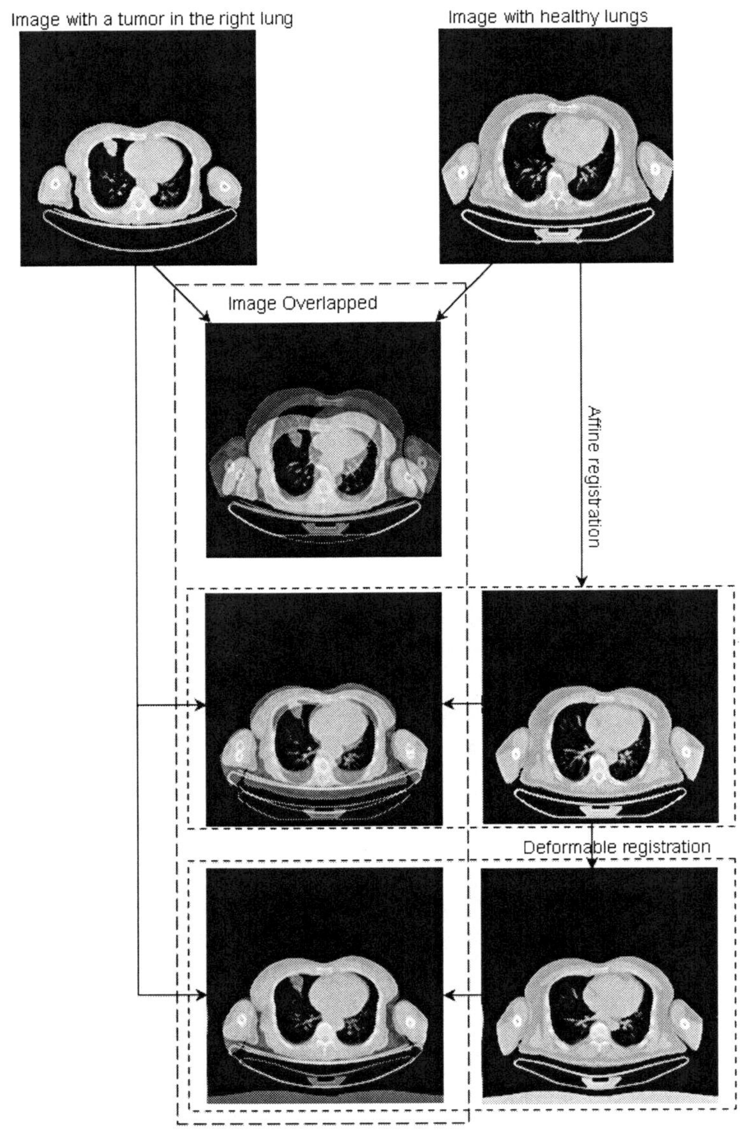

offers the valuable opportunity for early intervention to delay or halt the progression of the disease, and eventually to reduce its morbidity and mortality. Biomedical image registration plays an important role in detection of a variety of diseases at an early stage, by combining and fully utilizing complementary information from multimodal images. For instance, dementias are the major causes of disability in the elderly population, while Alzheimer's disease (AD) is the most common cause of dementia (Nestor, et al, 2004).. Registration of longitudinal anatomical MR studies (Scahill, et al, 2003) allows the identification of probable AD (Nestor, et al, 2004) at an early stage to assist an early, effective treatment. Breast cancer is one of major cause of cancer-related death. Registration of pre- and post-contrast of a MR sequence can effectively distinguish different types of malignant and normal tissues (Rueckert, et al, 1998) to offer a better opportunity to cure the patient with the disease (Wang et al, 2007).

Biomedical image registration plays an indispensable role in the management of different diseases. For instance, heart disease is the main cause of death in developed counties (American Heart Association 2006) and cardiac image registration provides a non-invasive method to assist in the diagnosis of heart diseases. For instance, registration of MR and X-ray images is a crucial step in the image guided cardiovascular intervention, as well as in therapy and treatment planning (Rhode, et al, 2005). Multimodal image registration such as CT-MR, CT-PET allows a more accurate definition of the tumor volume during the treatment planning phase (Scarfone et al 2004). These datasets can also be used later to assess responses to therapy and in the evaluation of a suspected tumor recurrence (Wang et al, 2007).

FUTURE TRENDS

Image registration is an enabling technique for fully utilizing heterogeneous image information. However, the medical arena remains a challenging area due to differences in image acquisition, anatomical and functional changes caused by disease progression and treatment, variances and differences across subjects, and complex deformations and motions of internal organs. It is particularly challenging to seamlessly integrate diverse and complementary image information in an efficient, acceptable and applicable manner for clinical routine. Future research in biomedical image registration would need to continuously focus on improving accuracy, efficiency, and usability of registration.

Deformable techniques are in high demand for registering images of internal organs such as liver, lung, and cardiac. However, due to complexity of the registration transformation, this category of registration will continuously hold research attention.

Insufficient registration efficiency is a major barrier to clinical applications, and is especially prevalent in the case of whole-body images from advanced imaging devices such as the combined PET/CT scanners. For instance, whole-body volume data may consist of more than 400 slices for each modality from the combined PET/CT machine. It is a computationally expensive task for registering these large data volumes. With rapid advance in medical imaging techniques, greater innovation will be achieved, for instance, it is expected that a combined MRI/PET will be made available in near future, which will help to improve the quality of healthcare significantly, but also pose a new set of challenges for efficiently registering the datasets with higher resolution, higher dimensionality, and wider range of scanning areas. Multi-scale registration has the potential to find a more accurate solution with greater efficiency.

Graphics Processing Units (GPUs) may provide a high performance hardware platform for real-time and accurate registration and fusion for clinical use. With its superior memory bandwidth, massive parallelism, improvement in the programmability, and stream architecture, GPUs are becoming the most powerful computation hardware and are attracting more and more research attention. The improvement in floating point format provides sufficient computational accuracy for applications in medical areas. However, effective use of GPUs in image registration is not a simple issue (Strzodka, et al 2004). Knowledge about its underlying hardware, design, limitations, evolution, as well as its special programming model is required to map the proposed medical image registration to the GPU pipeline and fully utilize its attractive features. Medical image registration, particularly for high-dimensional data, which fully utilizes the outstanding features of graphics hardware to facilitate fast and cost-saving real-time clinical applications, is new and yet to be fully explored.

CONCLUSION

Registration of medical images from multiple imaging devices and at multiple imaging times is able to integrate and to facilitate a full utilization of the useful image information, and is essential to clinical diagnosis, treatment planning, monitoring and assessment. Image registration is also important in making the medical images more ready and more useful to improve the quality of healthcare service, and is applicable in a wide array of areas including medical database management, medical image retrieval, telemedicine and e-health.

Biomedical image registration has been extensively investigated, and a large number of software-based algorithms have been proposed alongside the developed hardware-based solutions (for instance, the combined PET/CT scanners). Among the comprehensive software-based registration, the feature-based techniques are more computationally efficient, but require a preprocessing step to extract the features to be used in registration, which make this category of registration user-intensive and user-dependent. The intensity-based scheme provides an automatic solution to registration. However, this type of registration is computationally costly. Particularly, image registration is a data-driven and case-orientated research area. It is challenging to select the most suitable and usable technique for specific requirement and datasets from various imaging scanners. For instance, although maximization of MI has been recognized as one of the most powerful registration methods, it cannot always generate accurate solution. A more general registration is more desirable. The combined imaging devices such as PET/CT provide an expensive hardware-based solution. However, even this expensive registration method is not able to always provide the accurate registration, and software-based solution is required to fix the mis-registration caused by patient motions between the imaging sessions. The rapid advance in imaging techniques raises more challenges in registration area to generate more accurate and efficient algorithms in a clinically acceptable time frame.

ACKNOWLEDGMENT

This work is supported by the ARC and UGC grants.

REFERENCES

American Heart Association (2006). *Heart and stroke statistical update.* Http://www.americanheart.org

Audette, M., Ferrie, F., & Peters, T. (2000). An algorithm overview of surface registration techniques for medical imaging. *Medical Image Analysis*, 4(4), 201-217.

Bajcsy, R., & Kovacic, S. (1989). Multiresolution elastic matching. *Comp Vision Graphics Image Processing*, *46*, 1–21, April 1989

Besl, P. J., & MaKey, N. D. (1992). A method for registration of 3-D shapes. *IEEE Trans. PAMI*, 14(2), 239-256.

Borgefors, G. (1988). Hierarchical Chamfer Matching: A Parametric Edge Matching Algorithm. *IEEE Transactions on Pattern Analysis and Machine Intelligence, 10*, 849-865.

Brown, L. G. (1992). A survey of image registration techniques. *ACM Computing Surveys, 24*(4), 325-376.

Chen, C., Pellizari, C. A., Chen, G. T. Y., Cooper, M. D., & Levin, D. N. (1987). Image analysis of PET data with the aid of CT and MR images. *Information processing in medical imaging*, 601-611.

Cohen, I., & Cohen, I. (1993, November). Finite-element methods for active contour models and balloons for 2-D and 3-D images. *IEEE Pattern Anal. Machine Intelligence*, 15, 1131-1147.

Collignon, A., Maes, F., Delaere, D., Vandermeulen, D., Suetens, P., & Marchal, G. (1995). Automated multimodality image registration based on information theory. In *Proc. 14th International Conference of Information Processing in Medical Imaging 1995,* vol.3, (Bizais, Y., Barillot, C. and Di Paola, R. eds.), Ile Berder, France, pp. 263–274, June 1995.

Fitzpatrick, J.M., Hill, D.L.G. & Maurer, C.R. (2000). *Handbook of medical imaging*, (pp. 375-435). Bellingham, WA: SPIE Press.

Kass, M., Witkin, A., & Terzopoulos, D. (1988). Snakes: active contour models. *International Journal of Computer Vision*, pp.321-331.

Lehmann, T. M., Gönner, C., & Spitzer, K. (1999). Survey: Interpolation methods in medical image processing. *IEEE Transactions on Medical Imaging, 18*(11), 1049-1075.

Maintz, J. B. A., van den Elsen, P. A. & Viergever, M. A. (1996). Evaluation of ridge seeking operators for multimodality medical image registration. *IEEE Trans. PAMI, 18*(4), 353-365.

Maintz, J. B. A. & Viergever, M. A. (1998). A Survey of Medical Image Registration. *Medical Image Analysis, 2*(1), 1-36.

Mattes, D., Haynor, D. R., Vesselle, H., Lewellen, T. K., & Eubank, W. (2003) PET-CT image registration in the chest using free-form deformations. *IEEE Transactions on Medical Imaging*, 23(1), 120-128.

Nestor, P. J., Scheltens, P., & Hodges, J. R. (2004, July). Advances in the early detection of Alzheimer's disease. *Nature Reviews Neuroscience, 5*(Supplement), S34-S41.

Pluim, J. P., Maintz, J. B. A., & Viergever, M. A. (2003, August) Mutual-information-based registration of medical images: a survey. *IEEE Transactions on Medical Imaging*, 22(8), 986-1004.

Powell, M. J. D. (1964). An efficient method for finding the minimum of a function of several variables without calculating derivatives. *Comput. J., 7,* 155-163.

Press, W. H., Teukolsky, S. A., Vetterling, W. T., & Flannery, B. P. (1992). *Numerical Recipes in C.* Cambridge Univ. Press, Cambridge, U.K.

Rhode, K. S., Sermesant, M., Brogan, D., Hegde, S., Hipwell, J., Lambiase, P., Rosenthsal, E., bucknall, C., Qureshi, S. A., Gill, J.S., Razavi, R., & Hill, D. L.G. (2005, November). A system for real-time XMR guided cardiovascular intervention. *IEEE Transactions on Medical Imaging,* 24(11), 1428-1440.

Rueckert, D., Hayes, C., Studholme, C., Summers, P., Leach, M., & Hawkes, D. J. (1998). Non-rigid registration of breast MR images using mutual information. *MICCAI'98 lecture notes in computer science*, Cambridge, pp.1144-1152.

Scahill, R. I. Frost, C., Jenkins, R., Whitwell, J. L., Rossor, M. N., & Fox, N.C. (2003, July). A longitudinal study of brain volume changes in normal aging using serial registered magnetic resonance imaging. *Archives of Neurology*, 60(7), 989-994.

Scarfone, C., Lavely, W. C., Cmelak, A. J., Delbeke, D., Martin, W. H., Billheimer, D., & Hallahan, D. E. (2004). Prospective feasibility trial of radiotherapy target definition for head and neck cancer using 3-dimensional PET and CT imaging. *Journal of Nuclear Medicine*, 45(4), 543-552, Apr 2004.

Subsol, G., Thirion, J. P., & Ayache, N. (1998). A scheme for automatically building three dimensional morphometric anatomical atlases: application to a skull atlas. *Medical Image Analysis*, 2(1), 37-60.

Strzodka, R., Droske, M., & Rumpf, M. (2004) Image registration by a regularized gradient flow - a streaming implementation in DX9 graphics hardware. *Computing, 73*(4), 373–389.

Studholme, C., Hill, D. L. G., & Hawkes, D. J. (1999) An overlap invariant entropy measure of 3D medical image alignment. *Pattern Recognition, 32*, 71–86.

Thévenaz, P., & Unser, M. (2000). Optimization of mutual information for multiresolution registration. *IEEE Transaction on Image Processing*, 9(12), 2083-2099.

Toga, A. W., & Thompson P. M. (2001, september) The role of image registration in brain mapping. *Image and Vision Computing Journal*, 19, 3–24.

Townsend, D. W., Beyer, T., & Blodgett, T. M. (2003). PET/CT Scanners: A Hardware Approach to Image Fusion. *Semin Nucl Med* XXXIII(3), 193-204.

Unser, M., & Aldroubi, A. (1993, November). A multiresolution image registration procedure using spline pyramids. Proc. of SPIE 2034, 160-170, Wavelet Applications in Signal and Image Processing, ed. Laine, A. F.

Van den Elsen, P. A., Maintz, J. B. A., Pol, E. -J. D., & Viergever, M. A. (1995, June). Automatic registration of CT and MR brain images using correlation of geometrical features. *IEEE Transactions on Medical Imaging, 14*(2), 384 – 396.

Viola, P. A., & Wells, W. M. (1995, June) Alignment by maximization of mutual information. In *Proc. 5th International Conference of Computer Vision*, Cambridge, MA, 16-23.

Wang, X., S. Eberl, Fulham, M., Som, S., & Feng, D. (2007) Data Registration and Fusion, Chapter 8 in D. Feng (Ed.) *Biomedical Information Technology*, pp.187-210, Elsevier Publishing

Wang, X., & Feng, D. (2005). Active Contour Based Efficient Registration for Biomedical Brain Images. *Journal of Cerebral Blood Flow & Metabolism*, *25*(Suppl), S623.

Wang, X., & Feng, D. (2005). Biomedical Image Registration for Diagnostic Decision Making and Treatment Monitoring. Chapter 9 in R. K. Bali (Ed.) *Clinical Knowledge Management: Opportunities and Challenges*, pp.159-181, Idea Group Publishing

Xu, C., & Prince, J. L. (1998, March). Snakes, shapes, and gradient vector flow. *IEEE Trans. Image Processing*, *7*, 359-369.

KEY TERMS AND DEFINITIONS

Image Registration: The process to search for an appropriate transformation to spatially align the images in a common coordinate system.

Intra-Subject Registration: Registration for the images from same subject/person.

Inter-Subject Registration: Registration for the images from different subjects/persons.

Monomodal Images: Refers to images acquired from same imaging techniques.

Multimodal Images: Refers to images acquired from different imaging.

This work was previously published in Data Mining and Medical Knowledge Management: Cases and Applications, edited by P. Berka, J. Rauch and D. Zighed, pp. 122-136, copyright 2009 by Medical Information Science Reference (an imprint of IGI Global).

Compilation of References

Acha, B., Serrano, C., Acha, J. I., & Roa, L. M. (2003). CAD tool for burn diagnosis. In Taylor, C., & Noble, A. (Eds.), *Proceedings of information processing in medical imaging* (pp. 282–293). Ambleside, UK.

Ackerstaff, R. G., Babikian, V. L., Georgiadis, D., Russell, D., Siebler, M., & Spencer, M. P. (1995). Basic identification criteria of Doppler microembolic signals. Consensus Committee of the Ninth International Cerebral Hemodynamic Symposium. *Stroke*, *26*(6), 1123.

Afsharpour, S. (1985). Light microscopic analysis of Golgi-impregnated rat subthalamic neurons. *The Journal of Comparative Neurology*, *236*, 1–13. doi:10.1002/cne.902360102

Alan, P. M., & Ross, T. W. (1999). Partitioning 3D Surface Meshes Using Watershed Segmentation. *IEEE Transactions on Visualization and Computer Graphics*, *5*(4), 308–321. doi:10.1109/2945.817348

Alberto, M. (1976). An application of heuristic search methods to edge and contour detection. *Communications of the ACM*, *19*(2), 73–83. doi:10.1145/359997.360004

Albin, R. L., Young, A. B., & Penney, J. B. (1989). The functional anatomy of basal ganglia disorders. *Trends in Neurosciences*, *12*, 366–375. doi:10.1016/0166-2236(89)90074-X

Aldridge, J. W., Berridge, K. C., & Rosen, A. R. (2004). Basal ganglia neural mechanisms of natural movement sequences. *Canadian Journal of Physiology and Pharmacology*, *82*, 732–739. doi:10.1139/y04-061

Alex Parallel Computers, Inc. (1996). *Sharc1000 user's manual.*

Alexander, G., & Crutcher, M. (1991). Reply: letter to the editor. *Trends in Neurosciences*, *14*, 2.

Alexander, G. E., DeLong, & M. R., Strick, P. L. (1986). Parallel organization of functionally segregated circuits linking basal ganglia and cortex. *Annual Review of Neuroscience*, *9*, 357–381. doi:10.1146/annurev.ne.09.030186.002041

Alexander, G. E., & Crutcher, M. D. (1990). Functional architecture of basal ganglia circuits: neural substrates of parallel processing. *Trends in Neurosciences*, *13*, 266–271. doi:10.1016/0166-2236(90)90107-L

Alliez, P., & Gotsman, C. (2003). Recent advances in compression of 3D meshes. In *Symposium on Multiresolution in Geometric Modeling*.

Alparonte, L., Argenti, F., & Benelli, G. (1990). Fast calculation of co-occurrence matrix parameters for image segmentation. *Electronics Letters*, *26*(1), 23–24. doi:10.1049/el:19900015

Alvarez, R. E., & Macovski, A. (1976). Energy-Selective Reconstructions in X-Ray CT. *Physics in Medicine and Biology*, *21*(5), 733–744. doi:10.1088/0031-9155/21/5/002

Amendolia, S., Bisogni, M., Bottigli, U., Ceccopieri, A., Delogu, P., & Fantacci, M. (2001). The CALMA project: a CAD tool in breast radiography. *Nuclear Instruments and Methods*, *A460*, 107–112.

Amini, A. A., Tehrani, S., & Weymouth, T. E. (1988). *Using Dynamic Programming For Minimizing The Energy Of Active Contours In The Presence Of Hard Constraints.* Paper presented at the Second International Conference onComputer Vision.

Andr, Gu, ziec, & Nicholas, A. (1994). Smoothing and matching of 3-D space curves. *International Journal of Computer Vision, 12*(1), 79–104. doi:10.1007/BF01420985

Andraka, R. (2006). Hybrid Floating Point Technique Yields 1.2 Gigasample Per Second 32 to 2048 point Floating Point FFT in a single FPGA (37K). *Proceedings of the 10th Annual High Performance Embedded Computing Workshop.*

Angelini, E., Song, T., Mensh, B., & Laine, A. F. (2007). Brain MRI Segmentation with multiphase minimal partitioning: a comparative study. *Int.l Journal of Biomedical Imaging.*

Ansia, F. M., Lopez, J., Penedo, M. G., & Mosquera, A. (2000). *Automatic 3D shape reconstruction of bones using active nets based segmentation.* Paper presented at the 15th International Conference on Pattern Recognition, 2000.

Ardon, R., & Cohen, L. (2006). Fast Constrained Surface Extraction by Minimal Paths. *International Journal of Computer Vision, 69*(1), 127–136. doi:10.1007/s11263-006-6850-z

Ardon, R., Cohen, L. D., & Yezzi, A. (2007). A New Implicit Method for Surface Segmentation by Minimal Paths in 3D Images. *Applied Mathematics & Optimization, 55*(2), 127–144. doi:10.1007/s00245-006-0885-y

Ardon, R., Cohen, L., & Yezzi, A. (2005). A New Implicit Method for Surface Segmentation by Minimal Paths: Applications in 3D Medical Images. In *Energy Minimization Methods in Computer Vision and Pattern Recognition* (pp. 520-535).

Arneodo, A., Bacry, E., & Muzy, J. (1995). The thermodynamics of fractals revisited with wavelets. *Physica A, 213*, 232–275. doi:10.1016/0378-4371(94)00163-N

Ashby, P., Kim, Y. J., Kumar, R., Lang, A. E., & Lozano, A. M. (1999). Neurophysiological effects of stimulation through electrodes in the human subthalamic nucleus. *Brain, 122*(Pt 10), 1919–1931. doi:10.1093/brain/122.10.1919

Aspert, N., Santa-Cruz, D., & Ebrahimi, T. (2002). Mesh: Measuring errors between surfaces using the Hausdorff distance. In *International Conference on Multimedia & Expo*, (Vol. 1, pp. 705-708).

Aubert, G., Barlaud, M., Faugeras, O., & Jehan-Besson, S. (2003). Image segmentation using active contours: Calculus of variations or shape gradients? *SIAM Applied Mathematics, 63*(6), 2128–2154. doi:10.1137/S0036139902408928

Audit, B. (1999). *Analyse statistique des séquences d'ADN par l'intermédiaire de la transformée en ondelettes.* PhD dissertation, Université de Paris VI Pierre et Marie Curie.

Aujol, J.-F., Aubert, G., & Blanc-Féraud, L. (2003). Wavelet-based level set evolution for classification of textured images. *IEEE Transactions on Image Processing, 12*(12), 1634–1641. doi:10.1109/TIP.2003.819309

Aydin, N., & Markus, H. S. (2000). Optimization of processing parameters for the analysis and detection of embolic signals. *European Journal of Ultrasound, 12*(1), 69–79. doi:10.1016/S0929-8266(00)00104-X

Aydin, N., Padayachee, S., & Markus, H. S. (1999). The use of the wavelet transform to describe embolic signals. *Ultrasound in Medicine & Biology, 25*(6), 953–958. doi:10.1016/S0301-5629(99)00052-6

Azarpazhooh, M. R., & Chambers, B. R. (2006). Clinical Application of Transcranial Doppler Monitoring for Embolic Signals. *Journal of Clinical Neuroscience, 6*(8), 799–810. doi:10.1016/j.jocn.2005.12.026

Banerjee, A., Dhillon, I., Ghosh, J., & Merugu, S. (2004). An information theoretic analysis of maximum likelihood mixture estimation for exponential families. In *International Conference on Machine Learning,* 57–64.

Bar-Gad, I., Morris, G., & Bergman, H. (2003). Information processing, dimensionality reduction and reinforcement learning in the basal ganglia. *Progress in Neurobiology, 71*, 439–473. doi:10.1016/j.pneurobio.2003.12.001

Barral, J., & Seuret, S. (2007). *The singularity spectrum of levy processes in multifractal time.* Advances in Mathematics.

Barreira, N., Penedo, M. G., Mariño, C., & Ansia, F. M. (2003). Topological Active Volumes. In *Computer Analysis of Images and Patterns* (pp. 337-344).

Basu, S., & Bresler, Y. (2000). An O(N^2/log N) Filtered Backprojection Reconstruction Algorithm for Tomography. *IEEE Transactions on Medical Imaging*, *9*, 1760–1773.

Bay, B. K. (1995). Texture correlation. A method for the measurement of detailed strain distributions within trabecular bone. *Journal of Orthopaedic Research*, *13*(2), 258–267. doi:10.1002/jor.1100130214

Bay, B. K., Smith, T. S., Fyhrie, D. P., Martin, R. B., Reimann, D. A., & Saad, M. (1998). Three-dimensional texture correlation measurement of strain in trabecular bone. In *Orthopaedic research society, transactions of the 44th annual meeting* (p. 109). New Orleans, Louisiana.

Beare, R. (2006). A Locally Constrained Watershed Transform. *IEEE Transactions on Pattern Analysis and Machine Intelligence*, *28*(7), 1063–1074. doi:10.1109/TPAMI.2006.132

Beekman, F. J., & Kamphuis, C. (2001). Ordered Subset Reconstruction for X-Ray CT. *Physics in Medicine and Biology*, *46*, 1835–1844. doi:10.1088/0031-9155/46/7/307

Beil, M., Irinopoulou, T., Vassy, J., & Rigaut, J. P. (1995). Chromatin texture analysis in three-dimensional images from confocal scanning laser microscopy. *Analytical and Quantitative Cytology and Histology*, *17*(5), 323–331.

Benabid, A., Benazzous, A., & Pollak, P. (2002). Mechanisms of Deep Brain Stimulation. *Movement Disorders*, *17*, S73–S74. doi:10.1002/mds.10145

Benabid, A. L., Krack, P., Benazzouz, A., Limousin, P., Koudsie, A., & Pollak, P. (2000). Deep brain stimulation of the subthalamic nucleus for Parkinson's disease: Methodologic aspects and clinical criteria. *Neurology*, *55*, S40–S44.

Benabid, A. L., Pollak, P., Gervason, C., Hoffman, D., Gao, D. M., & Hommel, M. (1991). Long-term suppression of tremor by chronic stimulation of the ventral intermediate thalamic nucleus. *Lancet*, *337*, 403–406. doi:10.1016/0140-6736(91)91175-T

Benazzouz, A., Breit, S., Koudsie, A., Pollak, P., Krack, P., & Benabid, A. (2002). Intraoperative Microrecordings of the Subthalamic Nucleus in Parkinson's Disease. *Movement Disorders*, *17*, S145–S149. doi:10.1002/mds.10156

Benazzouz, A., Gao, D. M., Ni, Z. G., Piallat, B., Bouali-Benazzouz, R., & Benabid, A. L. (2000). Effect of high-frequency stimulation of the subthalamic nucleus on the neuronal activities of the substantia nigra pars reticulate and ventroalteral nucleus of the thalamus in the rat. *Neuroscience*, *99*, 289–295. doi:10.1016/S0306-4522(00)00199-8

Bennett, B., & Wilson, C. (1999). Spontaneous Activity of Neostriatal Cholinergic Interneurons In Vitro. *The Journal of Neuroscience*, *19*, 5586–5596.

Beran, J. (1992). Statistical Methods for Data with Long-Range Dependence. *Statistical Science*, 7.

Beran, J. (1994). *Statistics for Long-Memory Processes*. New York: Chapman & Hal.

Beran, J., Sherman, R., Taqqu, M. S., & Willinger, W. (1992). *Variable-Bit-Rate Video Traffic and Long-Range Dependence*. IEEE Transactions on Networking.

Beran, J., & Terrin, N. (1992). *A Multivariate Central limit Theorem for Long-Memory Processes with Statistical Applications* [White paper].

Bergman, H., Feingold, A., Nini, A., Raz, A., Slovin, H., Abeles, M., & Vaadia, E. (1998). Physiological aspects of information processing in the basal ganglia of normal and parkinsonian primates. *Trends in Neurosciences*, *21*, 32–38. doi:10.1016/S0166-2236(97)01151-X

Bergman, H., Wichmann, T., Karmon, B., & De Long, M. R. (1994). The Primate Subthalamic Nucleus II. Neuronal Activity in the MPTP Model of Parkinsonism. *Journal of Neurophysiology*, *72*, 507–520.

Bernasconi, A., Antel, S. B., Collins, D. L., Bernasconi, N., Olivier, A., & Dubeau, F. (2001). Texture analysis and morphological processing of MRI assist detection of focal cortical dysplasia in extra-temporal partial epilepsy. *Annals of Neurology*, *49*(6), 770–775. doi:10.1002/ana.1013

Berns, G. S., & Sejnowski, T. J. (1998). A Computational Model of How the Basal Ganglia Produce Sequences. *Journal of Cognitive Neuroscience*, *10*(1), 108–121. doi:10.1162/089892998563815

Bertram, M. (2004). Biorthogonal loop-subdivision wavelets. *Computing*, *72*(1-2), 29–39. doi:10.1007/s00607-003-0044-0

Beurrier, C., Congar, P., Bioulac, B., & Hammond, C. (1999). Subthalamic nucleus neurons switch from single spike activity to burst-firing mode. *The Journal of Neuroscience*, *19*, 599–609.

Bevan, M. D., & Wilson, C. J. (1999). Mechanisms underlying spontaneous oscillation and rhythmic firing in rat subthalamic neurons. *The Journal of Neuroscience*, *19*, 7617–7628.

Bezard, E., Gross, C. E., & Brotchie, J. M. (2003). Presymptomatic compensation in Parkinson's disease is not dopamine-mediated. *Trends in Neurosciences*, *26*, 215–221. doi:10.1016/S0166-2236(03)00038-9

Bickel, P. J., & Docksum, K. A. (2001). *Mathematical statistics: basic ideas and selected topics* (2nd ed., *Vol. I*). London: Prentice Hall.

Bigun, J. (1991). Multidimensional orientation estimation with applications to texture analysis and optical flow. *IEEE Transactions on Pattern Analysis and Machine Intelligence*, *13*(8), 775–790. doi:10.1109/34.85668

Bigun, J., & du-Buf, J. M. H. (1994). N-folded symmetries by complex moments in Gabor space and their application to unsupervised texture segmentation. *IEEE Transactions on Pattern Analysis and Machine Intelligence*, *16*(1), 80–87. doi:10.1109/34.273714

Blandini, F., Nappi, G., Tassorelli, C., & Martignoni, E. (2000). Functional changes of the basal ganglia circuitry in Parkinson's disease. *Progress in Neurobiology*, *62*, 63–88. doi:10.1016/S0301-0082(99)00067-2

Blanks, R., Wallis, M., & Moss, S. (1998). A Comparison of Cancer Detection Rates Achieved by Breast Cancer Screening Programmes by Number of Readers, for One and Two-View Mammography: Results from the UK National Health Breast Screening Programme. *J Med S*, *5*, 195–201.

Blanquer, I., Hernández, V., Mas, F., & Segrelles, D. (2004). A Middleware Grid for Storing, Retrieving and Processing DICOM Medical Images. *Working Notes of the Workshop on Distributed Databases and Processing in Medical Image Computing (DIDAMIC)*. Rennes, France.

Blot, L., & Zwiggelaar, R. (2002). Synthesis and analysis of solid texture: Application in medical imaging. In *Texture 2002: The 2nd international workshop on texture analysis and synthesis* (pp. 9-14). Copenhagen.

Boashash, B. (1992). Estimating and interpreting the instantaneous frequency of a signal; part i: Fundamentals, part ii: Algorithms. *Proceedings of the IEEE*, *80*(4), 519–569.

Bockenbach, O., Knaup, M., & Kachelriess, M. (2007). Real Time Adaptive Filtering for Computed Tomography Applications. *IEEE Medical Imaging Conference Proceedings 2007.*

Boggis, C., & Astley, S. (2000). Computer-assisted mammographic imaging. *Breast Cancer Research*, *2*, 392–395. doi:10.1186/bcr84

Boskovitz, V., & Guterman, H. (2002). An adaptive neuro-fuzzy system for automatic image segmentation and edge detection. *Fuzzy Systems. IEEE Transactions on*, *10*(2), 247–262.

Bouman, C. A., & Shapiro, M. (1994). A multiscale random field model for Bayesian image segmentation. *IEEE Transactions on Image Processing*, *3*(2), 162–177. doi:10.1109/83.277898

Bouman, C., & Liu, B. (1991). Multiple resolution segmentation of textured images. *IEEE Transactions on Pattern Analysis and Machine Intelligence*, *13*(2), 99–113. doi:10.1109/34.67641

Bovik, A. C., Clark, M., & Geisler, W. S. (1990). Multichannel texture analysis using localized spatial filters. *IEEE Transactions on Pattern Analysis and Machine Intelligence*, *12*(1), 55–73. doi:10.1109/34.41384

Braak, H., Ghebremedhin, E., Rub, U., Bratzke, H., & Del Ttredici, K. (2004). Stages in the development of Parkinson's disease-related pathology. *Cell and Tissue Research*, *318*, 124–134. doi:10.1007/s00441-004-0956-9

Brain Lord, & Walton, J.N. (1969). *Brain's Diseases of the nervous system*. London: Oxford University Press.

Breit, S., Lessmann, L., Benazzouz, A., & Schulz, J. B. (2005). Unilateral lesion of the pedunculopontine nucleus induces hyperactivity in the subthalamic nucleus and substantia nigra in the rat. *The European Journal of Neuroscience*, *22*, 2283–2294. doi:10.1111/j.1460-9568.2005.04402.x

Breit, S., Schulz, J. B., & Benabid, A. (2004). Deep brain stimulation. *Cell and Tissue Research*, *318*, 275–288. doi:10.1007/s00441-004-0936-0

Brown, J., Bullock, D., & Grossberg, S. (1999). How the Basal Ganglia Use Parallel Excitatory and Inhibitory Learning Pathways to Selectively Respond to Unexpected Rewarding Cues. *The Journal of Neuroscience*, *19*(23), 10502–10511.

Brown, P. (2003). Oscillatory nature of human basal ganglia activity: relationship to the pathophysiology of Parkinson's disease. *Movement Disorders*, *18*, 357–363. doi:10.1002/mds.10358

Brown, E. N., Kass, R. E., & Mitra, P. P. (2004). Multiple neural spike train data analysis: state-of-the-art and future challenges. *Nature Neuroscience*, *7*, 456–461. doi:10.1038/nn1228

Budaev, V., Takamura, S., Ohno, N., & Masuzaki, S. (2006). Superdiffusion and multifractal statistics of edge plasma turbulence in fusion devices. *Nuclear Fusion*, *46*, 181. doi:10.1088/0029-5515/46/4/S10

Buecher, S., & Lantuéjoul, C. (1979, September 1979). *Use of watershed in contour detection*. Paper presented at the Int. Workshop Image Processing, Real-Time Edge and Motion Detection/Estimation, Rennes, France.

Bullock, D., & Grossberg, S. (1988). Neural Dynamics of Planned Arm Movements: Emergent Invariants and Speed-Accuracy Properties During Trajectory Formation. *Psychological Review*, *95*, 49–90. doi:10.1037/0033-295X.95.1.49

Burt, P. J., & Adelson, E. H. (1983). The Laplacian pyramid as a compact image code. *IEEE Transactions on Communications*, *31*(4), 532–540. doi:10.1109/TCOM.1983.1095851

Cagnan, H., Meijer, H. E., van Gils, S. A., Krupa, M., Heida, T., Rudolph, M., Wadman, W. J., & Martens, H. C. F. (2009). Frequency-selectivity of a thalamocortical relay neuron during Parkinson's disease and Deep Brain Stimulation: a computational study. *European Journal of Neuroscience*, 30,1306-1317 (DOI:10.1111/j.1460-9568.2009.06922.x)Calabresi, P., Centonze, D., & Bernardi, G. (2000). Electrophysiology of dopamine in normal and denervated striatal neurons. *Trends in Neurosciences, 23*, S57-S63.

Cardoso, J., Ruano, M. G., & Fish, P. (1996). Non-Stationary Broadening Reduction in Pulsed Doppler Spectrum Measurements Using Time-Frequency Estimators. *IEEE Transactions on Bio-Medical Engineering*, *43*(12), 1176–1186. doi:10.1109/10.544341

Carlson, J., & Ortendahl, D. (1987). *Segmentation of Magnetic Resonance Images Using Fuzzy Clustering*. Paper presented at the Proc. Information Processing in Medical Imaging.

Carrillat, A., Randen, T., Sönneland, L., & Elvebakk, G. (2002). Seismic stratigraphic mapping of carbonate mounds using 3D texture attributes. In *Extended abstracts, annual meeting, European association of geoscientists and engineers*. Florence, Italy.

Caselles, V., Catte, F., Coll, T., & Dibos, F. (1993). A geometric model for active contours. *Numerische Mathematik*, *66*, 1–31. doi:10.1007/BF01385685

Caselles, V., Kimmel, R., & Sapiro, G. (1997). Geodesic active contours. *International Journal of Computer Vision*, *22*(1), 61–79. doi:10.1023/A:1007979827043

Caselles, V., Kimmel, R., & Sapiro, G. (1995). *Geodesic active contours*. Paper presented at the Proceedings of the Fifth International Conference on Computer Vision.

Chakraborty, A., Staib, L. H., & Duncan, J. S. (1996). Deformable boundary finding in medical images by integrating gradient and region information. *IEEE Transactions on Medical Imaging*, *15*(6), 859–870. doi:10.1109/42.544503

Chakraborty, A., Staib, L., & Duncan, J. (1996). Deformable boundary finding in medical images by integrating gradient and region information. *IEEE Transactions on Medical Imaging*, *15*, 859–870. doi:10.1109/42.544503

Chalana, V., & Kim, Y. (1997). A methodology for evaluation of boundary detection algorithms on medical images. *IEEE Transactions on Medical Imaging*, *16*(5), 642–652. doi:10.1109/42.640755

Chan, T. F., & Vese, L. A. (2001). Active contours without edges. *IEEE Transactions on Image Processing*, *10*(2), 266–277. doi:10.1109/83.902291

Chan, T., & Vese, L. (2001). Active contours without edges. *IEEE Transactions on Image Processing*, *10*(2), 266–277. doi:10.1109/83.902291

Chang, T., & Kuo, C. C. J. (1993). Texture analysis and classification with tree-structured wavelet transform. *IEEE Transactions on Image Processing*, *2*(4), 429–441. doi:10.1109/83.242353

Chantler, M. J. (1995). Why illuminant direction is fundamental to texture analysis. *IEEE Proceedings in Vision. Image and Signal Processing*, *142*(4), 199–206. doi:10.1049/ip-vis:19952065

Chapman, B. (2007). *The Multicore Programming Challenge (LNCS)*. Springer.

Chen, T., & Metaxas, D. (2000). Image Segmentation Based on the Integration of Markov Random Fields and Deformable Models. In *Medical Image Computing and Computer-Assisted Intervention* (pp. 256–265). MICCAI.

Chen, T., & Metaxas, D. (2003). A Hybrid Framework for 3D Medical Image Segmentation. In *Medical Image Computing and Computer-Assisted Intervention - MICCAI 2003* (pp. 703–710). Gibbs Prior Models, Marching Cubes, and Deformable Models. doi:10.1007/978-3-540-39903-2_86

Chen, Y., & Wang, Y. (2008). Doppler Embolic Signal Detection Using the Adaptive Wavelet Packet Basis and Neurofuzzy Classification. *Pattern Recognition Letters*, *29*(10), 1589–1595. doi:10.1016/j.patrec.2008.03.015

Chen, G. H. (2003). From Tuy's Inversion Scheme to Katsevich's Inversion Scheme: Pulling a Rabbit out of the Hat. *Proceedings of the 7th Int. Meeting on Fully 3D Image Reconstruction, Saint Malo, France.*

Cheng, L., Yang, J., & Fan, X. (2005). A new region-based active contour for object extraction using level set method. *Pattern Recognition and Image Analysis*, *3522*, 285–291.

Chenyang, X., & Jerry, L. P. (1997). *Gradient Vector Flow: A New External Force for Snakes*. Paper presented at the Proceedings of the 1997 Conference on Computer Vision and Pattern Recognition (CVPR '97).

Choi, H.-I., & Williams, W. J. (1989). Improved Time-Frequency of Multicomponent Signals using Exponential Kernels. *IEEE Transactions on Acoustics, Speech, and Signal Processing*, *37*(6), 862–871. doi:10.1109/ASSP.1989.28057

Chui, C. K. (1992). *An introduction to wavelets*. Boston: Academic Press Inc.

Chung, A. C. S., Noble, J. A., & Summers, P. (2002). Fusing magnitude and phase information for vascular segmentation in phase contrast MR angiography. *Medical Image Analysis Journal*, *6*(2), 109–128. doi:10.1016/S1361-8415(02)00057-9

Chung, E., L., F., Degg, C., & Evans, D. H. (2005). Detection of Doppler embolic signals: Psychoacoustic considerations. *Ultrasound in Medicine & Biology*, *31*(9), 1177–1184. doi:10.1016/j.ultrasmedbio.2005.05.001

Clausi, D. A., & Jernigan, M. E. (1998). A fast method to determine co-occurrence texture features. *IEEE Transactions on Geoscience and Remote Sensing*, *36*(1), 298–300. doi:10.1109/36.655338

Cohen, L. D. (1991). On active contour models and balloons. *Computer Vision, Graphics, and Image Processing. Image Understanding*, *53*(2), 211–218. doi:10.1016/1049-9660(91)90028-N

Cohen, L. (1989). Time-Frequency Distributions – A Review. *Proceedings of the IEEE*, *77*(7), 941–981. doi:10.1109/5.30749

Cohen, L. D., & Kimmel, R. (1996). *Global Minimum for Active Contour Models: A Minimal Path Approach*. Paper presented at the Proceedings of the 1996 Conference on Computer Vision and Pattern Recognition (CVPR '96).

Cohen, L., Bardinet, E., & Ayache, N. (1993). Surface reconstruction using active contour models. *SPIE Conference on Geometric Methods in Computer Vision*.

Coleman, G. B., & Andrews, H. C. (1979). Image segmentation by clustering. *Proceedings of the IEEE*, *67*(5), 773–785. doi:10.1109/PROC.1979.11327

Coleman, G. B., & Andrews, H. C. (1979). Image segmentation by clustering. *Proceedings of the IEEE*, *67*(5), 773–785. doi:10.1109/PROC.1979.11327

Collins, D. L., Zijdenbos, A. P., Kollokian, V., Sled, J. G. A. S. J. G., Kabani, N. J. A. K. N. J., & Holmes, C. J. A. H. C. J. (1998). Design and construction of a realistic digital brain phantom. *IEEE Transactions on Medical Imaging*, *17*(3), 463–468. doi:10.1109/42.712135

Collins, D. L., Terence, M. P., Weiqian, D., & Alan, C. E. (1992). *Model-based segmentation of individual brain structures from MRI data*.

Condor Manuals. (2008). Retrieved from http://www.cs.wisc.edu/condor/manual/index.html

Contreras-Vidal, J. L., & Stelmach, G. E. (1995). A neural model of basal ganglia-thalamocortical relations in normal and Parkinsonian movement. *Biological Cybernetics*, *73*, 467–476. doi:10.1007/BF00201481

Cootes, T. F., Beeston, C., Edwards, G. J., & Taylor, C. J. (1999). *A Unified Framework for Atlas Matching Using Active Appearance Models*. Paper presented at the Proceedings of the 16th International Conference on Information Processing in Medical Imaging.

Coulouris, G., Dollimore, J., & Kindberg, T. (2001). *Distributed Systems: Concepts and Design* (3rd ed.). Addison Wesley, Pearson Education.

Cowe, J., & Evans, D. H. (2006). Automatic Detection of Emboli in the TCD RF Signal Using Principal Component Analysis. *Ultrasound in Medicine & Biology*, *3*(12), 1853–1867. doi:10.1016/j.ultrasmedbio.2006.06.019

Cowe, J., Gittins, J., Naylor, A., & Evans, D. (2005). RF Signals Provide Additional Information on Embolic Events Recorded During TCD Monitoring. *Ultrasound in Medicine & Biology*, *31*(5), 613–623. doi:10.1016/j.ultrasmedbio.2005.02.002

Cox, D. (1984). Long-range dependence: A review. *Statistics: An Appraisa*.

Cremers, D., Rousson, M., & Deriche, R. (2007). A review of statistical approaches to level set segmentation: Integrating color, texture, motion and shape. *International Journal of Computer Vision*, *72*(2), 195–215. doi:10.1007/s11263-006-8711-1

Cremers, D., Tischhäuser, F., Weickert, J., & Schnörr, C. (2002). Diffusion snakes: Introducing statistical shape knowledge into the Mumford-Shah functional. *IJCV*, *50*, 295–313. doi:10.1023/A:1020826424915

Cross, G. R., & Jain, A. K. (1983). Markov random field texture models. *IEEE Transactions on Pattern Analysis and Machine Intelligence*, *5*(1), 25–39. doi:10.1109/TPAMI.1983.4767341

Cuisenaire, O., J.-P., T., Macq, B. M., Michel, C., de Volder, A., & Marques, F. (1996). Automatic registration of 3D MR images with a computerized brain atlas. *Medical Imaging 1996. Image Processing*, *2710*, 438–448.

Cula, O. G., & Dana, K. J. (2004). 3D texture recognition using bidirectional feature histograms. *International Journal of Computer Vision*, *59*(1), 33–60. doi:10.1023/B:VISI.0000020670.05764.55

Cullinane, M., & Markus, H. S. (2001). Evaluation of a 1 Mhz Transducer for Transcranial Doppler Ultrasound Including Embolic Signal Detection. *Ultrasound in Medicine & Biology*, *27*(6), 795–800. doi:10.1016/S0301-5629(01)00369-6

Cullinane, M., Reid, G., Dittrich, R., Kaposzta, Z., Ackerstaff, R., & Babikian, V. (2000). Evaluation of New Online Automated Embolic Signal Detection Algorithm, Including Comparison With Panel of International Experts. *Stroke*, *31*(6), 1335–1341.

Dana, K. J., van-Ginneken, B., Nayar, S. K., & Koenderink, J. J. (1999). Reflectance and texture of real-world surfaces. *ACM Transactions on Graphics*, *18*(1), 1–34. doi:10.1145/300776.300778

Danielsson, P. E., & Ingerhed, M. (1998). Backprojection in O(N^2/log N) Time. *IEEE Nuclear Science Symposium Record, 2,* 1279-1283.

Daras, P., Zarpalas, D., Axenopoulos, A., Tzovaras, D., & Strintzis, M. G. (2006). Three-dimensional shape-structure comparison method for protein classification. *IEEE/ACM Transactions on Computational Biology and Bioinformatics*, *3*(3), 193–207. doi:10.1109/TCBB.2006.43

Dathe, A., Tarquis, A., & Perrier, E. (2006). Multifractal analysis of the pore and solid phases in binary twodimensional images of natural porous structures.

Daubechies, I. (1990). The Wavelet Transform, Time-Frequency Localization and Signal Analysis. *IEEE Transactions on Information Theory*, *36*(5), 961–1005. doi:10.1109/18.57199

Davis, G. C., Williams, A. C., & Markey, S. P. (1979). Chronic parkinsonism secondary to intravenous injection of meperidine analogues. *Psychiatry Research*, *1*, 249–254. doi:10.1016/0165-1781(79)90006-4

Dawant, B. M., Hartmann, S. L., Thirion, J. P., Maes, F., Vandermeulen, D., & Demaerel, P. (1999). Automatic 3-D segmentation of internal structures of the head in MR images using a combination of similarity and free-form transformations. I. Methodology and validation on normal subjects. *IEEE Transactions on Medical Imaging*, *18*(10), 909–916. doi:10.1109/42.811271

Debreuve, E., Gastaud, M., Barlaud, M., & Aubert, G. (2007). Using the shape gradient for active contour segmentation: from the continuous to the discrete formulation. *Journal of Mathematical Imaging and Vision*, *28*(1), 47–66. doi:10.1007/s10851-007-0012-y

Delfour, M. C., & Zolésio, J. P. (2001). *Shape and geometries. Advances in Design and Control.* SIAM.

DeLong, M. R. (1990). Primate models of movement disorders of basal ganglia origin. *Trends in Neurosciences*, *13*, 281–285. doi:10.1016/0166-2236(90)90110-V

Demetri, T. (1999). Artificial life for computer graphics. *Communications of the ACM*, *42*(8), 32–42. doi:10.1145/310930.310966

Demetri, T., Xiaoyuan, T., & Radek, G. (1994). Artificial fishes: autonomous locomotion, perception, behavior, and learning in a simulated physical world. *Artificial Life*, *1*(4), 327–351. doi:10.1162/artl.1994.1.4.327

Denny-Brown, D. (1962). *The Basal Ganglia and their relation to disorders of movement.* Oxford: Oxford University Press.

Destexhe, A., Neubig, M., Ulrich, D., & Huguenard, J. (1998). Dendritic low-threshold calcium currents in thalamic relay cells. *The Journal of Neuroscience*, *18*, 3574–3588.

Devuyst, G., Darbellay, G. A., Vesin, J.-M., Kemeny, V., Ritter, M., & Droste, D. W. (2001). Automatic Classification of HITS Into Artifacts or Solid or Gaseous Emboli by a Wavelet Representation Combined With Dual-Gate TCD. *Stroke*, *32*(12), 2803–2809. doi:10.1161/hs1201.099714

Ding, F., Leow, W., & Wang, S.-C. (2005). 3D CT Volume Images Using a Single 2D Atlas. In *Computer Vision for Biomedical Image Applications* (pp. 459–468). Segmentation of. doi:10.1007/11569541_46

Do, M. T. H., & Bean, B. P. (2003). Subthreshold sodium currents and pacemaking of subthalamic neurons: modulation by slow inactivation. *Neuron, 39*, 109–120. doi:10.1016/S0896-6273(03)00360-X

Documentation, P. H. P. (2008). Retrieved from http://www.php.net/docs.php

Dongarra, J., Sterling, T., Simon, H., & Strohmaier, E. (2005). High-Performance Computing: Clusters, Constellations, MPPs, and Future Directions. *Computing in Science & Engineering, 7*, 51–59. doi:10.1109/MCSE.2005.34

Dostrovsky, J., & Lozano, A. (2002). Mechanisms of Deep Brain Stimulation. *Movement Disorders, 17*(3), S63–S68. doi:10.1002/mds.10143

Dryden, L. (2005). *Statistical analysis on high-dimensional spheres and shape spaces*. Annals of Statistics.

Dryden, L., & Zempleni, A. (2004). Extreme shape analysis - Technical report. *Journal of the Royal Statistical Society, Series C, Applied Statistics*.

Duda, R., & Hart, P. (1973). *Pattern Classification and Scene Analysis*. John Wiley & Sons.

Dunn, J. C. (1973). A fuzzy relative of the ISODATA process and its use in detecting compact well-sparated clusters. *Journal of Cybernetics, 3*, 32–57. doi:10.1080/01969727308546046

Dunn, D., & Higgins, W. E. (1995). Optimal Gabor filters for texture segmentation. *IEEE Transactions on Image Processing, 4*(7), 947–964. doi:10.1109/83.392336

Dunn, D., Higgins, W. E., & Wakeley, J. (1994). Texture segmentation using 2-D Gabor elementary functions. *IEEE Transactions on Pattern Analysis and Machine Intelligence, 16*(2), 130–149. doi:10.1109/34.273736

Dydenko, I., Jamal, F., Bernard, O., D'Hooge, J., Magnin, I. E., & Friboulet, D. (2006). A level set framework with a shape and motion prior for segmentation and region tracking in echocardiography. [Bas du formulaire]. *Medical Image Analysis, 10*(2), 162–177. doi:10.1016/j.media.2005.06.004

Erberich, S. G., Silverstein, J. C., Chervenak, A., Schuler, R., Nelson, M., & Kesselman, C. (2007). Globus MEDICUS - Federation of DICOM Medical Imaging Devices into Healthcare Grids. *Studies in Health Technology and Informatics, 126*, 269–279.

Ercoli, A., Battaglia, A., Raspaglio, G., Fattorossi, A., Alimonti, A., & Petrucci, F. (2000). Activity of cisplatin and ici 182,780 on estrogen receptor negative ovarian cancer cells: Cell cycle and cell replication rate perturbation, chromatin texture alteration and apoptosis induction. *International Journal of Cancer, 85*(1), 98–103. doi:10.1002/(SICI)1097-0215(20000101)85:1<98::AID-IJC18>3.0.CO;2-A

Evans, D. H. (2003). Doppler Detection of Cerebral Emboli: The State-of-the-Art. *Ultrasound in Medicine & Biology, 29*(5), S38–S39. doi:10.1016/S0301-5629(03)00200-X

Evans, D. H., & McDicken, W. N. (2000). *Doppler Ultrasound: Physics, Instrumentation, and Clinical Applications* (2nd ed.). New York: John Wiley & Sons.

Evans, D. H. (1999). Detection of Microemboli. In Babikian, V. L., & Welchser, L. R. (Eds.), *Transcranial Doppler Ultrasonography* (2nd ed., pp. 141–155). Boston: Butterworth-Heineman Medical.

Fan, Y., Jiang, T., & David, E. (2002). Volumetric segmentation of brain images using parallel genetic algorithms. *IEEE Transactions on Medical Imaging, 21*(8), 904–909. doi:10.1109/TMI.2002.803126

Fan, L., & Evans, D. H. (1994). Extracting Instantaneous Mean Frequency Information from Doppler Signals Using the Wigner Distribution Function. *Ultrasound in Medicine & Biology, 20*(5), 429–443. doi:10.1016/0301-5629(94)90098-1

Fan, L., Evans, D. H., & Naylor, R. (2001). Automated Embolus Identification Using a Rule-Based Expert System. *Ultrasound in Medicine & Biology*, *27*(8), 1065–1077. doi:10.1016/S0301-5629(01)00414-8

Fatemi-Ghomi, N. (1997). *Performance measures for wavelet-based segmentation algorithms*. Centre for Vision, Speech and Signal Processing, University of Surrey.

Feldkamp, L. A., Davis, L. C., & Kress, J. W. (1984). Practical Cone-Beam Algorithm. *Journal of the Optical Society of America*, *1*, 612–619. doi:10.1364/JOSAA.1.000612

Fernández, M., Mavilio, A., & Tejera, M. (2000). Texture segmentation of a 3D seismic section with wavelet transform and Gabor filters. In *International conference on pattern recognition, ICPR 00* (Vol. 3, pp. 358-361). Barcelona.

Figueiredo, M., & Jain, A. (2002). Unsupervised learning of finite mixture models. *IEEE Transactions on Pattern Analysis and Machine Intelligence*, *24*(3), 381–396. doi:10.1109/34.990138

Filion, M., & Tremblay, L. (1991). Abnormal spontaneous activity of globus pallidus neurons in monkeys with MPTP-induced parkinsonism. *Brain Research*, *547*, 142–151.

Filion, M., Tremblay, L., & Bedard, P. J. (1988). Abnormal influences of passive limb movement on the activity of globus pallidus neurons in parkinsonian monkeys. *Brain Research*, *444*, 165–176. doi:10.1016/0006-8993(88)90924-9

Flachs, B., Asano, S., Dhong, S. H., Hofstee, H. P., Gervais, G., Kim, R., et al. (2005). A Streaming Processing Unit for a Cell Processor. *IEEE International Solid-State Circuits Conference 2005.*

Florio, T., Scarnati, E., Confalone, G., Minchella, D., Galati, S., & Stanzione, P. (2007). High frequency stimulation of the subthalamic nucleus modulates theactivity of pedunculopontine neurons through direct activation of excitatory fibers as well as through indirect activation of inhibitory pallidal fibers in the rat. *The European Journal of Neuroscience*, *25*, 1174–1186. doi:10.1111/j.1460-9568.2007.05360.x

Foster, I., Kesselman, C., & Tuecke, S. (2001). The anatomy of the grid: Enabling scalable virtual organizations. *International Journal of High Performance Computing Applications*, *15*(3), 200–222. doi:10.1177/109434200101500302

Foster, I. (2002, July 20). What is the Grid? A Three Point Checklist. *GRIDToday*.

Foulonneau, A., Charbonnier, P., & Heitz, F. (2003). Geometric shape priors for region-based active contours. *In International Conference on Image Processing.*

Frank, J., Verschoor, A., & Boublik, M. (1981). Computer averaging of electron micrographs of 40S ribosomal subunits. *Science*, *214*, 1353–1355. doi:10.1126/science.7313694

Frank, M. J. (2005). Dynamic dopamine modulation in the basal ganglia: a neurocomputational account of cognitive deficits in medicated and nonmedicated Parkinsonism. *Journal of Cognitive Neuroscience*, *17*, 51–72. doi:10.1162/0898929052880093

Frank, A., Stotzka, R., Jejkal, T., Hartmann, V., Sutter, M., & Gemmeke, H. (2007). GridIJ - A Dynamic Grid Service Architecture for Scientific Image Processing. *33rd EUROMICRO Conference on Software Engineering and Advanced Applications* (pp. 375-384).

Fritscher, K., & Schubert, R. (2006). 3D image segmentation by using statistical deformation models and level sets. *International Journal of Computer Assisted Radiology and Surgery*, *1*(3), 123–135. doi:10.1007/s11548-006-0048-2

Furui, E., Hanzawa, K., Ohzeki, H., Nakajima, T., Fukuhara, N., & Takamori, M. (1999). "Tail Sign" Associated With Microembolic Signals. *Stroke*, *30*(4), 863–866.

Gabor, D. (1946). Theory of communication. *Journal of the IEE*, *93*(26), 429–457.

Galland, F., Bertaux, N., & Réfrégier, P. (2005). Multicomponent image segmentation in homogeneous regions based on description length minimization: Application to speckle, Poisson and Bernoulli noise. *Pattern Recognition*, *38*, 1926–1936. doi:10.1016/j.patcog.2004.10.002

Garcia, L., D'Alessandro, G., Bioulac, B., & Hammond, C. (2005b). High-frequency stimulation in Parkinson's disease: more or less? *Trends in Neurosciences*, *28*, 4. doi:10.1016/j.tins.2005.02.005

Garcia, L., D'Alessandro, G., Fernagut, P., Bioulac, B., & Hammond, C. (2005a). Impact of High-Frequency Stimulation Parameters on the Pattern of Discharge of Subthalamic Neurons. *Journal of Neurophysiology*, *94*, 3662–3669. doi:10.1152/jn.00496.2005

García-Nocetti, F., González, J. S., Acosta, E. R., & Hernández, E. M. (2001). Parallel Processing in Time-Frequency Distributions For Signal Analysis. *BioEng 2001*, (p. ID46.pdf). Faro.

Garcia-Rill, E. (1991). The pedunculopontine nucleus. *Progress in Neurobiology*, *36*, 363–389. doi:10.1016/0301-0082(91)90016-T

Gastaud, M., Barlaud, M., & Aubert, G. (2003). Tracking video objects using active contours and geometric priors, In *IEEE Workshop on Image Analysis and Multimedia Interactive Services*, 170-175.

Gatzoulis, L., & Iakovidis, I. (2007). Wearable and Portable eHealth Systems. Technological Issues and Opportunities for Personalized Care. *IEEE Engineering in Medicine and Biology Magazine*, *26*(5), 51–56. doi:10.1109/EMB.2007.901787

Georgiadis, D., Uhlmann, F., Lindner, A., & Zierz, S. (2000). Differentiation Between True Microembolic Signals and Artefacts Using an Arbitrary Sample Volume. *Ultrasound in Medicine & Biology*, *26*(3), 493–496. doi:10.1016/S0301-5629(99)00158-1

Gerfen, C. R., & Wilson, C. J. (1996). The basal ganglia. In L. W. Swanson (Ed.) *Handbook of Chemical Neuroanatomy vol 12: Integrated systems of the CNS, Part III* (pp. 371-468).

Gibson, S., & Mirtich, B. (1997). *A Survey of Deformable Modeling in Computer Graphics*. Cambridge: Mitsubishi Electric Research Lab.

Giger, M. (1999). Computer-aided diagnosis. *RSNA Categorial Course in Breast Imaging*, 249-72.

Gilchrist, C. L., Xia, J. Q., Setton, L. A., & Hsu, E. W. (2004). High-resolution determination of soft tissue deformations using MRI and first-order texture correlation. *IEEE Transactions on Medical Imaging*, *23*(5), 546–553. doi:10.1109/TMI.2004.825616

Gilles, A., & Laure Blanc, F., & raud. (1999). Some Remarks on the Equivalence between 2D and 3D Classical Snakes and Geodesic Active Contours. *International Journal of Computer Vision*, *34*(1), 19–28. doi:10.1023/A:1008168219878

Gillies, A., & Willshaw, D. (2006). Membrane channel interactions underlying rat subthalamic projection neuron rhythmic and bursting activity. *Journal of Neurophysiology*, *95*, 2352–2365. doi:10.1152/jn.00525.2005

Giordano, S., Pagano, M., Russo, F., & Sparano, D. (1996). *A Novel Multiscale Fractal Image Coding Algorithm based on SIMD Parallel Hardware*. Paper presented at Picture Coding Symposium PCS '96, Australia.

Girault, J.-M., Kouamé, D., Ouahabi, A., & Patat, F. (2000). Micro-Emboli Detection: An Ultrasound Doppler Signal Processing View Point. *IEEE Transactions on Bio-Medical Engineering*, *47*(11), 1431–1439. doi:10.1109/10.880094

Goddard, I., & Trepanier, M. (2002). High-Speed Cone-Beam Reconstruction: An Embedded Systems Approach. *SPIE Medical Imaging Proceedings*, *4681*, 483–491.

Goldberg, D. (1989). *Genetic Algorithms in Search, Optimization, and Machine Learning*. Addison-Wesley Professional.

Goldberger, A., Amaral, L., Hausdorff, J., Ivanov, P., Peng, C., & Stanley, H. (2002). Fractal dynamics in physiology: Alterations with disease and aging. In *Proceedings of the National Academy of Sciences*.

Gomes, J., & Faugeras, O. (2000). Reconciling distance functions and level sets. *Journal of Visual Communication and Image Representation*, *11*, 209–223. doi:10.1006/jvci.1999.0439

Gomez-Gallego, M., Fernandez-Villalba, E., Fernandez-Barreiro, A., & Herrero, M. T. (2007). Changes in the neuronal activity in the pedunculopontine nucleus in chronic MPTP-treated primates: an in situ hybridization study of cytochrome oxidase subunit I, choline acetyl transferase and substance P mRNA expression. *Journal of Neural Transmission*, *114*, 319–326. doi:10.1007/s00702-006-0547-x

Gonzalez, R. C., & Woods, R. E. (1992). *Digital image processing*. Reading, MA: Addison Wesley.

Goodman, J. W. (1976). Some fundamental properties of speckle. *Journal of the Optical Society of America*, *66*, 1145–1150. doi:10.1364/JOSA.66.001145

Gordon, R. A. (1974). Tutorial on ART (Algebraic Reconstruction Techniques). *IEEE Transactions on Nuclear Science*, *NS-21*, 78–93.

Grady, L., & Funka-Lea, G. (2004). Multi-label Image Segmentation for Medical Applications Based on Graph-Theoretic Electrical Potentials. In *Computer Vision and Mathematical Methods in Medical and Biomedical Image Analysis* (pp. 230-245).

Grangeat, P. (1987). *Analyse d'un système d'imagerie 3D par reconstruction à partir de radiographies X en géométrie conique.* Doctoral dissertation, Ecole Nationale Supérieure des Télécommunications, France.

Graps, A. (1995). An introduction to wavelets. *IEEE Computational Science & Engineering*, *2*(2), 50–61. doi:10.1109/99.388960

Grau, V., Mewes, A. U. J., Alcaniz, M., Kikinis, R., & Warfield, S. K. (2004). Improved watershed transform for medical image segmentation using prior information. *Medical Imaging. IEEE Transactions on*, *23*(4), 447–458.

Grill, M. W., & McIntyre, C. C. (2001). Extracellular excitation of central neurons: implications for the mechanisms of deep brain stimulation. *Thalamus & Related Systems*, *1*, 269–277.

Groenewegen, H. J., & Van Dongen, Y. C. (2008). Role of the Basal Ganglia. In Wolters, E. C., van Laar, T., & Berendse, H. W. (Eds.), *Parkinsonism and related disorders*. Amsterdam: VU University Press.

Gschwendtner, A., Hoffmann-Weltin, Y., Mikuz, G., & Mairinger, T. (1999). Quantitative assessment of bladder cancer by nuclear texture analysis using automated high resolution image cytometry. *Modern Pathology*, *12*(8), 806–813.

Gschwind, M., Hofstee, H. P., Flachs, B., Hopkins, M., Watanabe, Y., & Yamazaki, T. (2006). Synergistic Processing in Cell's Multicore Architecture. *IEEE Micro*, 20–24.

Gubjartsson, H., & Patz, S. (1995). *The Rician distribution of noisy MRI data*. Magnetic Resonance Medecine.

Guetbi, C., Kouame, D., Ouahabi, A., & Remenieras, J. P. (1997). New Emboli Detection Methods. *IEEE Ultrasonics Symposium*, *2*, 1119-1122. Toronto, Canada.

Güler, İ., & Übeyli, E. D. (2006). A Recurrent Neural Network Classifier for Doppler Ultrasound Blood Flow Signals. *Pattern Recognition Letters*, *27*(13), 1560–1571. doi:10.1016/j.patrec.2006.03.001

Gummaraju, J., Coburn, J., Turner, Y., & Rosenblum, M. (2008). Streamware: programming general-purpose multicore processors using streams. In *Proceedings of the 13th international conference on Architectural support for programming languages and operating systems* (pp. 297-307). ACM.

Guo, Y., Rubin, J., McIntyre, C., Vitek, J., & Terman, D. (2008). Thalamocortical relay fidelity varies across subthalamic nucleus deep brain stimulation protocols in a data driven computational model. *Journal of Neurophysiology*, *99*, 1477–1492. doi:10.1152/jn.01080.2007

Guo, Z., Durand, L.-G., & Lee, H. C. (1994). Comparison of Time-Frequency Distribution Techniques For Analysis of Simulated Doppler Ultrasound Signals of the Femoral Artery. *IEEE Transactions on Bio-Medical Engineering*, *41*(4), 1176–1186.

Gurney, K., Prescott, T. J., & Redgrave, P. (2001a). A computational model of action selection in the basal ganglia. I. A new functional anatomy. *Biological Cybernetics*, *84*, 401–410. doi:10.1007/PL00007984

Gurney, K., Prescott, T. J., & Redgrave, P. (2001b). A computational model of action selection in the basal ganglia. II. Analysis and simulation of behaviour. *Biological Cybernetics*, *84*, 411–423. doi:10.1007/PL00007985

Gurney, K., Redgrave, P., & Prescott, A. (1998). *Analysis and simulation of a model of intrinsic processing in the basal ganglia (Technical Report AIVRU 131)*. Dept. Psychology, Sheffield University.

Guskov, I. (2007). Manifold-based approach to semi-regular remeshing. *Graphical Models*, *69*(1), 1–18. doi:10.1016/j.gmod.2006.05.001

Guskov, I., Vidimce, K., Sweldens, W., & Schröder, P. (2000). Normal Meshes. In *Computer Graphics Proceedings* (pp. 95-102).

Gutierrez, M. A., Lage, S. H., Lee, J., & Zhou, Z. (2007). *A Computer-Aided Diagnostic System using a Global Data Grid Repository for the Evaluation of Ultrasound Carotid Images* (pp. 840–845). CCGRID.

Hademenos, G. J. (1997). The Biophysics of Stroke. *American Scientist*, *85*(3), 226–235.

Haeri, M., Sarbaz, Y., & Gharibzadeh, S. (2005). Modeling the Parkinson's tremor and its treatments. *Journal of Theoretical Biology*, *236*, 311–322. doi:10.1016/j.jtbi.2005.03.014

Hagen-Ansert, S. L. (2006). Society of Diagnostic Medical Sonographers: A Timeline of Historical Events in Sonography and the Development of the SDMS: In the Beginning. *Journal of Diagnostic Medical Sonography*, *22*(4), 272–278. doi:10.1177/8756479306291456

Hamarneh, G., McInerney, T., & Terzopoulos, D. (2001). *Deformable Organisms for Automatic Medical Image Analysis*. Paper presented at the Proceedings of the 4th International Conference on Medical Image Computing and Computer-Assisted Intervention.

Hampel, F. R. (1987). Data Analysis and Self-Similar Processes. In *Proceedings of 46th Session ISI*.

Hand, D. J. (1981). *Discrimination and classification*. Chichester: Wiley.

Hao, D., & Zhang, H. (2007). Detection of Doppler Embolic Signals with Hilbert-Huang Transform. *IEEE/ICME International Conference on Complex Medical Engineering* (pp. 412-415). Beijing, China.

Haralick, R. M. (1979). Statistical and structural approaches to texture. *Proceedings of the IEEE*, *67*(5), 786–804. doi:10.1109/PROC.1979.11328

Haralick, R. M., Shanmugam, K., & Dinstein, I. h. (1973). Textural features for image classification. *IEEE Transactions on Systems, Man, and Cybernetics*, *3*(6), 610–621. doi:10.1109/TSMC.1973.4309314

Harris, K. D., Henze, D. A., Csicsvari, J., Hirase, H., & Buzsaki, G. (2000). Accuracy of Tetrode Spike Separation as Determined by Simultaneous Intracellular and Extracellular Measurements. *Journal of Neurophysiology*, *84*(1), 401–414.

Harwood, D., Ojala, T., Petrou, P., Kelman, S., & Davis, S. (1993). *Texture classification by center-symmetric auto-correlation, using kullback discrimination of distributions*. College Park, Maryland: Computer Vision Laboratory, Center for Automation Research, University of Maryland.

Hashimoto, T., Elder, C. M., Okun, M. S., Patrick, S. K., & Vitek, J. L. (2003). Stimulation of the subthalamic nucleus changes firing pattern of pallidal neurons. *The Journal of Neuroscience*, *23*, 1916–1923.

Hashimoto, A., & Kudo, H. (2000). Ordered-subsets EM algorithm for image segmentation with application to brain MRI. In *IEEE Nuclear Symposium and Medical Imaging Conference*.

Hassler, R. (1937). Zur Normalanatomie der Substantia nigra. *Journal für Psychologie und Neurologie*, *48*, 1–55.

Hassler, R. (1938). Zur Pathologie der Paralysis agitans und des postencephalitischen Parkinsonismus. *Journal für Psychologie und Neurologie*, *48*, 387–476.

Hassler, R. (1939). Zur pathologischen Anatomie des senilen und des parkinsonistischen Tremor. *Journal für Psychologie und Neurologie*, *49*, 193–230.

Hawkins, J. K. (1970). Textural properties for pattern recognition. In Lipkin, B., & Rosenfeld, A. (Eds.), *Picture processing and psychopictorics* (pp. 347–370). New York.

Haykin, S. (2002). *Adaptive Filter Theory.* Prentice Hall Information and System Science Series, ISBN 0-130-90126-1, 4th Edition.

He, D. C., & Wang, L. (1991). Textural filters based on the texture spectrum. *Pattern Recognition*, *24*(12), 1187–1195. doi:10.1016/0031-3203(91)90144-T

Heida, T., Marani, E., & Usunoff, K. G. (2008). The subthalamic nucleus: Part II, Modeling and simulation of activity. *Advances in Anatomy, Embryology, and Cell Biology*, 199.

Heimer, L., Switzer, R. D., & Van Hoesen, G. W. (1982). Ventral striatum and ventral pallidum. Components of the motor system? *Trends in Neurosciences*, *5*, 83–87. doi:10.1016/0166-2236(82)90037-6

Henkelman, R. M. (1985). Measurement of signal intensities in the presence of noise in MR images. *Medical Physics*, 232–233. doi:10.1118/1.595711

Herlidou, S., Grebve, R., Grados, F., Leuyer, N., Fardellone, P., & Meyer, M. E. (2004). Influence of age and osteoporosis on calcaneus trabecular bone structure: A preliminary in vivo MRI study by quantitative texture analysis. *Magnetic Resonance Imaging*, *22*(2), 237–243. doi:10.1016/j.mri.2003.07.007

Herlidou, S., Rolland, Y., Bansard, J. Y., Le-Rumeur, E., & Certaines, J. D. (1999). Comparison of automated and visual texture analysis in MRI: Characterization of normal and diseased skeletal muscle. *Magnetic Resonance Imaging*, *17*(9), 1393–1397. doi:10.1016/S0730-725X(99)00066-1

Herlidou-Même, S., Constans, J. M., Carsin, B., Olivie, D., Eliat, P. A., & Nadal Desbarats, L. (2001). MRI texture analysis on texture text objects, normal brain and intracranial tumors. *Magnetic Resonance Imaging*, *21*(9), 989–993. doi:10.1016/S0730-725X(03)00212-1

Herman, G. T. (1980). *Image Reconstruction from Projections: The Fundamentals of Computerized Tomography.* Computer Science and Applied Mathematics, Academic Press, New York, ISBN 0-123-42050-4.

Hertz, L., & Schafer, R. W. (1988). Multilevel thresholding using edge matching. *Computer Vision Graphics and Image Processing*, *44*, 279–295. doi:10.1016/0734-189X(88)90125-9

Hodgkin, A., & Huxley, A. F. (1952). A quantative description of membrane current and its application to conduction and excitation in nerve. *The Journal of Physiology*, *117*, 500–544.

Hoffman, E. A., Reinhardt, J. M., Sonka, M., Simon, B. A., Guo, J., & Saba, O. (2003). Characterization of the interstitial lung diseases via density-based and texture-based analysis of computed tomography images of lung structure and function. *Academic Radiology*, *10*(10), 1104–1118. doi:10.1016/S1076-6332(03)00330-1

Hofstee, H. P. (2005). Power Efficient Processor Architecture and the Cell Processor. *Proceedings of the 11th International Symposium on High-Performance Computer Architecture.*

Hojjatoleslami, S. A., & Kittler, J. (1998). Region growing: a new approach. *Image Processing. IEEE Transactions on*, *7*(7), 1079–1084.

Holsheimer, J., Demeulemeester, H., Nuttin, B., & De Sutter, P. (2000). Identification of the target neuronal elements in electrical deep brain stimulation. *The European Journal of Neuroscience*, *12*, 4573–4577.

Hoppe, H. (1996). Progressive Meshes. In *ACM SIGGRAPH Conference* (pp. 99-108).

Hornykiewicz, O. (1989). The Neurochemical Basis of the Pharmacology of Parkinson's Disease. Handbook of Experimental Pharmacology 88. *Drugs for the Treatment of Parkinson's Disease* (pp. 185-204). Calne, D.B.: Springer-Verlag.

Hoskins, P. R., Thrush, A., Martin, K., & Whittingham, T. A. (2003). *Diagnostic Ultrasound: Physics and Equipment* (Hoskins, P. R., Thrush, A., Martin, K., & Whittingham, T. A., Eds.). London, UK: Greenwich Medical Media.

Hounsfield, G. N. (1972). *A Method of and Apparatus for Examination of a Body by Radiation such as X or Gamma Radiation. Patent Specification 1283915*. London: The Patent Office.

Hsu, T. I., Calway, A., & Wilson, R. (1992). *Analysis of structured texture using the multiresolution Fourier transform*. Department of Computer Science, University of Warwick.

Hua, L., & Yezzi, A. (2005). *A hybrid medical image segmentation approach based on dual-front evolution model*. Paper presented at the IEEE International Conference on Image Processing, 2005. ICIP 2005.

Hudorović, N. (2006). Clinical significance of microembolus detection by transcranial Doppler sonography in cardiovascular clinical conditions. *International Journal of Surgery*, *4*, 232–241. doi:10.1016/j.ijsu.2005.12.001

Huguenard, J. R., & McCormick, D. A. (1992). Simulation of the currents involved in rhythmic oscillations in thalamic relay neurons. *Journal of Neurophysiology*, *68*, 1373–1383.

Huguenard, J. R., & Prince, D. A. (1992). A novel T-type current underlies prolonged calcium-dependent burst firing in GABAergic neurons of rat thalamic reticular nucleus. *The Journal of Neuroscience*, *12*, 3804–3817.

Hulata, E., Segev, R., & Ben-Jacob, E. (2002). A method for spike sorting and detection based on wavelet packets and Shannon's mutual information. *Journal of Neuroscience Methods*, *117*(1), 1–12. doi:10.1016/S0165-0270(02)00032-8

Hyunjin, P., Bland, P. H., & Meyer, C. R. (2003). Construction of an abdominal probabilistic atlas and its application in segmentation. *IEEE Transactions on Medical Imaging*, *22*(4), 483–492. doi:10.1109/TMI.2003.809139

Hyvärinen, A. (1999). Fast and Robust Fixed-Point Algorithms for Independent Component Analysis. *IEEE Transactions on Neural Networks*, *10*(3), 626–634. doi:10.1109/72.761722

Iakovidis, D. K., Maroulis, D. E., & Karkanis, S. A. (2006). An intelligent system for automatic detection of gastrointestinal adenomas in video endoscopy. *Computers in Biology and Medicine*, *36*(10), 1084–1103. doi:10.1016/j.compbiomed.2005.09.008

Ibáñez, O., Barreira, N., Santos, J., & Penedo, M. (2006). Topological Active Nets Optimization Using Genetic Algorithms. In *Image Analysis and Recognition* (pp. 272-282).

INMOS, Limited. (n.d.). Transputer Architecture and Overview, manual of Transputer Education Kit.

Ip, H. H. S., & Lam, S. W. C. (1994). Using an octree-based rag in hyper-irregular pyramid segmentation of texture volume. In *Proceedings of the IAPR workshop on machine vision applications* (pp. 259-262). Kawasaki, Japan.

Jafari-Khouzani, K., Soltanian-Zadeh, H., Elisevich, K., & Patel, S. (2004). Comparison of 2D and 3D wavelet features for TLE lateralization. In A. A. Amir & M. Armando (Eds.), *Proceedings of SPIE vol. 5369, medical imaging 2004: Physiology, function, and structure from medical images* (pp. 593-601). San Diego, CA, USA.

Jain, A. K., Duin, R. P. W., & Jianchang, M. (2000). Statistical pattern recognition: a review. *IEEE Transactions on Pattern Analysis and Machine Intelligence*, *22*(1), 4–37. doi:10.1109/34.824819

Jain, A. K., & Farrokhnia, F. (1991). Unsupervised texture segmentation using Gabor filters. *Pattern Recognition*, *24*(12), 1167–1186. doi:10.1016/0031-3203(91)90143-S

Jain, A. K., & Farrokhnia, F. (1990). *Unsupervised texture segmentation using Gabor filters.* Paper presented at the IEEE International Conference on Systems, Man and Cybernetics, 1990.

James, S. D., & Nicholas, A. (2000). Medical Image Analysis: Progress over Two Decades and the Challenges Ahead. *IEEE Transactions on Pattern Analysis and Machine Intelligence*, *22*(1), 85–106. doi:10.1109/34.824822

James, D., Clymer, B. D., & Schmalbrock, P. (2002). Texture detection of simulated microcalcification susceptibility effects in magnetic resonance imaging of the breasts. *Journal of Magnetic Resonance Imaging*, *13*(6), 876–881. doi:10.1002/jmri.1125

Jean-Francois, R., Serge, B., & Delhomme, J. (1992). Marker-controlled segmentation: an application to electrical borehole imaging. *Journal of Electronic Imaging*, *1*(2), 136–142. doi:10.1117/12.55184

Jehan-Besson, S., Barlaud, M., & Aubert, G. (2003). DREAM^{2}S: Deformable regions driven by an Eulerian accurate minimization method for image and video segmentation. *International Journal of Computer Vision*, *53*, 45–70. doi:10.1023/A:1023031708305

Jehan-Besson, S., Barlaud, M., & Aubert, G. (2001). Video object segmentation using eulerian region-based active contours. In *International Conference on Computer Vision*.

Jehan-Besson, S., Barlaud, M., & Aubert, G. (2003). Shape gradients for histogram segmentation using active contours. In *International Conference on Computer Vision*.

Jenkins, N., Nandi, D., Oram, R., Stein, J. F., & Aziz, T. Z. (2006). Pedunculopontine nucleus electric stimulation alleviates akinesia independently of dopaminergic mechanisms. *Neuroreport*, *17*, 639–641. doi:10.1097/00001756-200604240-00016

Jenkinson, N., Nandi, D., Miall, R. C., Stein, J. F., & Aziz, T. Z. (2004). Pedunculopontine nucleus stimulation improves akinesia in a Parkinsonian monkey. *Neuroreport*, *15*, 2621–2624. doi:10.1097/00001756-200412030-00012

Joel, D., & Weiner, I. (2000). The connections of the dopaminergic system with the striatum in rats and primates: an analysis with respect to the functional and compartmental organization of the striatum. *Neuroscience*, *96*, 451–474. doi:10.1016/S0306-4522(99)00575-8

Jones, O. (2004). Analyzing self-similarity in network traffic via the crossing tree. In *Proceedings of Mathematics of Networks*. Ipswich, UK: BT Martlesham.

Jorgensen, T., Yogesan, K., Tveter, K. J., Skjorten, F., & Danielsen, H. E. (1996). Nuclear texture analysis: A new prognostic tool in metastatic prostate cancer. *Cytometry*, *24*(3), 277–283. doi:10.1002/(SICI)1097-0320(19960701)24:3<277::AID-CYTO11>3.0.CO;2-N

Joseph, P. M. (1982). An Improved Algorithm for Reprojecting Rays through Pixel Images. *IEEE Transactions on Medical Imaging*, *2*(3), 192–196. doi:10.1109/TMI.1982.4307572

Jouck, P. (2004). *Application of the Wavelet Transform Modulus Maxima method to T-wave detection in cardiac*. Maastricht University.

Julesz, B. (1981). A theory of preattentive texture discrimination based on first-order statistics of textons. *Biological Cybernetics*, *41*, 131–138. doi:10.1007/BF00335367

Kachelrieß, M., Knaup, M., & Bockenbach, O. (2007). Hyperfast Parallel-Beam and Cone-Beam Backprojection using the Cell General Purpose Hardware. *Medical Physics*, *34*, 1474–1486. doi:10.1118/1.2710328

Kachelrieß, M., Knaup, M., & Kalender, W. A. (2004). Extended parallel backprojection for standard 3D and phase-correlated 4D axial and spiral cone-beam CT with arbitrary pitch and 100% dose usage. *Medical Physics*, *31*(6), 1623–1641. doi:10.1118/1.1755569

Kachelrieß, M., Watzke, O., & Kalender, W. A. (2001). Generalized multi-dimensional adaptive filtering (MAF) for conventional and spiral single-slice, multi-slice and cone-beam CT. *Medical Physics*, *28*(4), 475–490. doi:10.1118/1.1358303

Kaczmarz, S. (1937). Angenäherte Auflösung von Systemen Linearer Gleichungen. *Bull. Acad. Polon. Sci. Lett. A*, *35*, 335–357.

Kadyrov, A., & Petrou, M. (2001). The trace transform and its applications. *IEEE Transactions on Pattern Analysis and Machine Intelligence*, *23*(8), 811–828. doi:10.1109/34.946986

Kadyrov, A., Talepbour, A., & Petrou, M. (2002). Texture classification with thousand of features. In *British machine vision conference* (pp. 656–665). Cardiff, UK: BMVC.

Kak, A. C., & Slaney, M. (1988). *Principles of Computerized Tomographic Imaging.* Society of Industial and Applied Mathematics, Philadelphia, ISBN 0-898-71494-X.

Kalender, W. A. (2005). *Computed Tomography.* Wiley & Sons, ISBN 3-89578-216-5, 2nd Edition.

Kaplan, L. M. (1999). Extended Fractal Analysis for Texture Classification and Segmentation. *IEEE Transactions on Image Processing*, *8*, 1572–1585. doi:10.1109/83.799885

Kaplan, L., & Murenzi, R. (1997). Texture segmentation using multiscale Hurst features. *International Conference on Image Processing, 1997.* Santa Barbara, CA, USA.

Kapur, J. N., Sahoo, P. K., & Wong, A. K. C. (1985). A new method for gray-level picture thresholding using the entropy of the histogram. *Graph. Models Image Process.*, *29*, 273–285. doi:10.1016/0734-189X(85)90125-2

Kapur, T. (1999). *Model-based three dimensional medical image segmentation.* AI Lab, Massachusetts Institute of Technology.

Karkanis, S. A., Iakovidis, D. K., Maroulis, D. E., Karras, D. A., & Tzivras, M. (2003). Computer-aided tumor detection in endoscopic video using color wavelet features. *IEEE Transactions on Information Technology in Biomedicine*, *7*(3), 141–152. doi:10.1109/TITB.2003.813794

Karoui, I., Fablet, R., Boucher, J. M., & Augustin, J. M. (2006). *Region-based image segmentation using texture statistics and level-set methods In.* ICASSP.

Kasner, J., Marcellin, M., & Hunt, B. (1999). Universal trellis coded quantization. *IEEE Transactions on Image Processing*, *8*(12), 1677–1687. doi:10.1109/83.806615

Kass, M., Witkin, A., & Terzopoulos, D. (1988). Snakes: Active contour models. *International Journal of Computer Vision*, *1*(4), 321–331. doi:10.1007/BF00133570

Katsevich, A. (2002). Analysis of an Exact Inversion Algorithm for Spiral Cone-Beam CT. *Physics in Medicine and Biology*, *47*, 2583–2597. doi:10.1088/0031-9155/47/15/302

Katsevich, A. (2003). A General Scheme for Constructing Inversion Algorithms for Cone Beam CT. *International Journal of Mathematics and Mathematical Sciences*, *21*, 1305–1321. doi:10.1155/S0161171203209315

Kelly, A. E., Domesick, V. B., & Nauta, W. J. H. (1982). The amygdalostriatal projection in the rat – an anatomical study by anterograde and retrograde tracing methods. *Neuroscience*, *7*, 615–630. doi:10.1016/0306-4522(82)90067-7

Kemény, V., Droste, D. W., Hermes, S., Nabavi, D. G., Schulte-Altedorneburg, G., & Siebler, M. (1999). Automatic Embolus Detection by a Neural Network. *Stroke*, *30*(4), 807–810.

Kenney, C., Fernandez, H. H., & Okum, M. S. (2007). *Role of deep brain stimulation targeted to the pedunculopontine nucleus in Parkinson's disease* (pp. 585-589). Editorial in: Future Drugs Ltd.

Kervrann, C., & Heitz, F. (1995). A Markov random field model-based approach to unsupervised texture segmentation using local and global spatial statistics. *IEEE Transactions on Image Processing*, *4*(6), 856–862. doi:10.1109/83.388090

Kestener, P., Lina, J., Saint-Jean, P., & Arneodo, A. (2001). Wavelet-based multifractal formalism to assist in diagnosis in digitized mammograms.

Khodakovsky, A., & Guskov, I. (2002). Normal mesh compression. In *Geometric Modeling for Scientific Visualization.* Springer-Verlag.

Khodakovsky, A., Schröder, P., & Sweldens, W. (2000). Progressive Geometry Compression. In *Computer Graphics Proceedings, SIGGRAPH 2000* (pp. 271-278).

Kippenhan, J. S., Barker, W. W., Pascal, S., Nagel, J., & Duara, R. (1992). Evaluation of a Neural-Network Classifier for PET Scans of Normal and Alzheimer's Disease Subjects. *Journal of Nuclear Medicine*, *33*(8), 1459–1467.

Kirby, R. L., & Rosenfeld, A. (1979). A note on the use of ~gray level, local average gray level! space as an aid in threshold selection. *IEEE Transactions on Systems, Man, and Cybernetics*, *SMC-9*, 860–864.

Kita, H., Chang, H. T., & Kitai, S. T. (1983). The morphology of intracellularly labeled rat subthalamic neurons: a light microscopic analysis. *The Journal of Comparative Neurology*, *215*, 245–257. doi:10.1002/cne.902150302

Kita, H., Nambu, A., Kaneda, K., Tachibana, Y., & Takada, M. (2004). Role of Ionotropic Glutamatergic and GABAergic Inputs on the Firing Activity of Neurons in the External Pallidum in Awake Monkeys. *Journal of Neurophysiology*, *92*, 3069–3084. doi:10.1152/jn.00346.2004

Kittler, J. (1986). Feature selection and extraction. In Fu, Y. (Ed.), *Handbook of pattern recognition and image processing* (pp. 59–83). New York: Academic Press.

Klauschen, F., Goldman, A., Barra, V., Meyer-Lindenberg, A., & Lundervold, A. (2008). Evaluation of Automated Brain MR Image Segmentation and Volumetry methods. *Human Brain Mapping*, *30*, 1310–1327. doi:10.1002/hbm.20599

Knaup, M., & Kachelriess, M. (2007). Acceleration techniques for 2D Parallel and 3D perspective Forward- and Backprojections. *Proceedings of the HPIR Workshop at the 9th Int. Meeting on Fully 3D Image Reconstruction, Lindau, Germany.*

Knaup, M., Kalender, W. A., & Kachelrieß, M. (2006). Statistical cone-beam CT image reconstruction using the Cell broadband engine. *IEEE Medical Imaging Conference Program, M11-422,* 2837-2840.

Knutsson, H., & Granlund, G. H. (1983). Texture analysis using two-dimensional quadrature filters. In *IEEE computer society workshop on computer architecture for pattern analysis and image database management - capaidm* (pp. 206-213). Pasadena.

Knutsson, H., Westin, C. F., & Granlund, G. H. (1994). Local multiscale frequency and bandwidth estimation. In *Proceedings of the IEEE international conference on image processing* (pp. 36-40). Austin, Texas: IEEE.

Kole, J. S., & Beekman, F. J. (2006). Evaluation of Accelerated Iterative X-Ray CT Image Reconstruction Using Floating Point Graphics Hardware. *Physics in Medicine and Biology*, *51*, 875–889. doi:10.1088/0031-9155/51/4/008

Koopman, P. O. (1936). On distributions admitting a sufficient statistic. *Transactions of the American Mathematical Society*, *39*, 399–409.

Kosar, T., & Livny, M. (2005). A framework for reliable and efficient data placement in distributed computing systems. *Journal of Parallel and Distributed Computing*.

Kouamé, D., Biard, M., Girault, J.-M., & Bleuzen, A. (2006). Adaptive AR and Neurofuzzy Approaches: Access to Cerebral Particle Signatures. *IEEE Transactions on Information Technology in Biomedicine*, *10*(3), 559–566. doi:10.1109/TITB.2005.862463

Kouamé, D., Girault, J.-M., Ouahabi, A., & Patat, F. (1999). Reliability Evaluation of Emboli Detection Using a Statistical Approach. *IEEE Ultrasonics Symposium, 2*, 1601-1604. Nevada, USA.

Kovalev, V. A., Kruggel, F., Gertz, H.-J., & von Cramon, D. Y. (2001). Three-dimensional texture analysis of MRI brain datasets. *IEEE Transactions on Medical Imaging*, *20*(5), 424–433. doi:10.1109/42.925295

Kovalev, V. A., Kruggel, F., & von Cramon, D. Y. (2003a). Gender and age effects in structural brain asymmetry as measured by MRI texture analysis. *NeuroImage*, *19*(3), 895–905. doi:10.1016/S1053-8119(03)00140-X

Kovalev, V. A., & Petrou, M. (1996). Multidimensional co-occurrence matrices for object recognition and matching. *Graphical Models and Image Processing*, *58*(3), 187–197. doi:10.1006/gmip.1996.0016

Kovalev, V. A., Petrou, M., & Bondar, Y. S. (1999). Texture anisotropy in 3D images. *IEEE Transactions on Image Processing*, *8*(3), 346–360. doi:10.1109/83.748890

Kovalev, V. A., Petrou, M., & Suckling, J. (2003b). Detection of structural differences between the brains of schizophrenic patients and controls. *Psychiatry Research: Neuroimaging*, *124*(3), 177–189. doi:10.1016/S0925-4927(03)00070-2

Krishnan, A. (2004). A survey of life sciences applications on the grid. *New Gen. Comput.*, *22*(2), 111–126. doi:10.1007/BF03040950

Kropinsky, E. (2003). The Future of Image Perception in Radiology. *Academic Radiology*, *10*(1).

Krupinskia, E., & Nodine, C. (1994). Gaze Duration Predicts the Locations of Missed Lesions in Mammography. In Gale, A. G., Astley, S. M., Dance, D. R., & Cairns, A. Y. (Eds.), *Digital Mammography* (pp. 399–405). Elsevier.

Kullback, S. (1959). *Information Theory and Statistics*. New York: Wiley.

Kumar, P. K., Yegnanarayana, B., & Das, S. (2000). 1-d Gabor for edge detection in texture images. In *International conference on communications, computers and devices (ICCCD 2000)* (pp. 425-428). IIT Kharagpur, INDIA.

Laine, A., & Fan, J. (1993). Texture classification by wavelet packet signatures. *IEEE Transactions on Pattern Analysis and Machine Intelligence*, *15*(11), 1186–1191. doi:10.1109/34.244679

Lang, Z., Scarberry, R. E., Zhang, Z., Shao, W., & Sun, X. (1991). A texture-based direct 3D segmentation system for confocal scanning fluorescence microscopic images. In *Twenty-third southeastern symposium on system theory* (pp. 472-476). Columbia, SC.

Langston, J. W., Ballard, P., Tetrud, J., & Irwin, I. (1983). Chronic parkinsonism in humans due to a product of meperidine-analog synthesis. *Science*, *219*, 979–980. doi:10.1126/science.6823561

Langston, J. W., Forno, L. S., Tetrud, J., Reeves, A. G., Kaplan, J. A., & Karluk, D. (1999). Evidence of active nerve cell degeneration in the substantia nigra of humans years after 1-Methyl-4-phenyl- 1,2,3,6- tertahydropyridine exposure. *Annals of Neurology*, *46*, 598–605. doi:10.1002/1531-8249(199910)46:4<598::AID-ANA7>3.0.CO;2-F

Latt, J., & Chopard, B. (2003). An Implicitly Parallel Object-Oriented Matrix Library and its Application to Medical Physics. In *Proceedings of the International Parallel and Distributed Processing Symposium*. IEEE Computer Society.

Lau, P. Y., & Ozawa, S. (2004). A region-based approach combining marker-controlled active contour model and morphological operator for image segmentation. *In IEEE engineering in Medicine and Biology Society, 165–170.*

Laws, K. (1980). *Textured image segmentation*. University of Southern California.

Le, H. (2003). Unrolling shape curves. *Journal of the London Mathematical Society*, *2*, 511–526. doi:10.1112/S0024610703004393

Lecellier, F., Fadili, J., Jehan-Besson, S., Aubert, G., & Revenu, M. (2010). Region-based active contours with exponential family observations. *International Journal on Mathematical Imaging and Vision*, *36*, 28–45. doi:10.1007/s10851-009-0168-8

Lecellier, F., Jehan-Besson, S., Fadili, J., Aubert, G., & Revenu, M. (2006). *Statistical region-based active contours with exponential family observations*. ICASSP.

Lecellier, F., Jehan-Besson, S., Fadili, J., Aubert, G., Revenu, M., & Saloux, E. (2006). *Region-based active contours with noise and shape priors*. ICIP.

Lee, A., Sweldens, W., Schröder, P., Cowsar, P., & Dobkin, D. (1998). Multiresolution adaptive parameterization of surfaces. In *SIGGRAPH '98*. MAPS.

Leeser, M., Coric, S., Miller, E., Yu, H., & Trepanier, M. (2002). Parallel-Beam Backprojection: An FPGA Implementation Optimized for Medical Imaging. *Proceedings of the 10th Int. Symposium on FPGA, Monterey, CA.*

Lefèvre, S. (2007). Knowledge from Markers in Watershed Segmentation. In *Computer Analysis of Images and Patterns* (pp. 579-586).

Leiria, A., Moura, M. M., Solano, J., Ruano, M. G., & Evans, D. H. (2004). *Middle Cerebral Artery Blood Flow: Accurate Time-Frequency Evaluation* (pp. 1095–1098). João Pessoa, Brasil: Anais da Conferência Latino-Americana de Engenharia Biomédica.

Leiria, A. (2005). *Spectral Analysis of Embolic Signals.* PhD Thesis, University of Algarve, Faro, Portugal.

Leiria, A., Madeira, M. M., & Ruano, M. G. (1999). Aortic Valve Analyser: A Cost/Benefit Study. *International Conference on Signal Processing Applications and Technology.*

Leiria, A., Moura, M. M., Ruano, M. G., & Evans, D. H. (2005). Time, time-frequency and displacement-frequency analysis of embolic signals. *IEEE International Workshop on Intelligent Signal Processing* (pp. 49-53). Faro, Portugal.

Leiria, A., Ruano, M. G., & Evans, D. H. (2007). Displacement-Frequency Doppler Blood Flow Estimation. *IEEE International Symposium on Intelligent Signal Processing* (pp. 1-4). Alcalá de Henares, Spain.

Lerski, R. A., Straughan, K., Schad, L. R., Boyce, D., Bluml, S., & Zuna, I. (1993). MR image texture analysis - an approach to tissue characterization. *Magnetic Resonance Imaging, 11*(6), 873–887. doi:10.1016/0730-725X(93)90205-R

Létal, J., Jirák, D., Šuderlová, L., & Hájek, M. (2003). MRI 'texture' analysis of MR images of apples during ripening and storage. *Lebensmittel-Wissenschaft und-Technologie, 36*(7), 719-727.

Leung, T. K., & Malik, J. (1999). Recognizing surfaces using three-dimensional textons. In *ICCV (2)* (pp. 1010-1017). Corfu, Greece.

Leventon, M. (2000). *Statistical Models for Medical Image Analysis*. Ph.D. thesis, MIT.

Leventon, M. E., Grimson, W. E. L., & Faugeras, O. (2000). *Statistical shape influence in geodesic active contours.* Paper presented at the IEEE Conference on Computer Vision and Pattern Recognition, 2000.

Lewicki, M. S. (1998). A review of methods for spike sorting: the detection and classification of neural action potentials. *Network (Bristol, England), 9*(4), 53–78. doi:10.1088/0954-898X/9/4/001

Lewy, F. H. (1913). Zur pathologischen Anatomie der Paralysis agitans. *Deutsch Zeitschr Nervenheilk, 50*, 50–55.

Lewy, F. H. (1912). Paralysis agitans. I Pathalogische Anatomie. In Lewandowsky, M. H. (Ed.), *Handbuch der Neurologie* (*Vol. 3*, pp. 920–933). Berlin: Springer.

Li, C. H., & Lee, C. K. (1993). Minimum cross-entropy thresholding. *Pattern Recognition, 26*, 617–625. doi:10.1016/0031-3203(93)90115-D

Li, H., Liu, K., Lo, S., Inc, O., & Jessup, M. (1997). Fractal Modeling and Segmentation for the Enhancement of Microcalcifications in Digital Mammograms. *IEEE Transactions on Medical Imaging, 16*, 785–798. doi:10.1109/42.650875

Li, C.-T. (1998). *Unsupervised texture segmentation using multiresolution Markov random fields*. Coventry: Department of Computer Science, University of Warwick.

Li, D., Qin, K., & Sun, H. (2004). Unlifted loop subdivision wavelets. In *Pacific Graphics Conference on Computer Graphics and Applications* (pp. 25-33).

Li, H., Yezzi, A., & Cohen, L.D. (2006). 3D Brain cortex segmentation using dual-front active contours with optional user-interaction. *International Journal of Biomedical Imaging.*

Lin, T. I., Lee, J. C., & Hsieh, W. J. (2007). Robust mixture modeling using the skew t distribution. *Statistics and Computing, 17*(2), 81–92. doi:10.1007/s11222-006-9005-8

Linderman, M. D., Santhanam, G., Kemere, C. T., Gilja, V., O'Driscoll, S., & Yu, B. M. (2008). Signal Processing Challenges for Neural Prostheses. *IEEE Signal Processing Magazine*, *25*(1), 18–28. doi:10.1109/MSP.2008.4408439

Lingrand, D., & Montagnat, J. (2005). A Pragmatic Comparative Study. In *Image Analysis* (pp. 25–34). Levelset and B-Spline Deformable Model Techniques for Image Segmentation. doi:10.1007/11499145_4

Lladó, X., Oliver, A., Petrou, M., Freixenet, J., & Mart, J. (2003). Simultaneous surface texture classification and illumination tilt angle prediction. In *British machine vision conference* (pp. 789–798). Norwich, UK: BMVC.

Lo, A. W. (1991). Long-Term Memory in Stock Market Prices. *Econometrica*, *59*, 1279–1313. doi:10.2307/2938368

Lorigo, L. M., Faugeras, O. D., Grimson, W. E. L., Keriven, R., & Kikinis, R. (1998). Segmentation of bone in clinical knee MRI using texture-based geodesic active contours. In *Medical image computing and computer-assisted interventions* (pp. 1195–1204). Cambridge, USA: MICCAI.

Lottiaux, R., Gallard, P., Vallee, G., Morin, C., & Boissinot, B. (2005). OpenMosix, OpenSSI and Kerrighed: a comparative study. *Cluster Computing and the Grid*, *2*, 1016–1023.

Lozano, A., Dostrovsky, J., Chen, R., & Ashby, P. (2002). Deep brain stimulation for Parkinson's disease: disrupting the disruption. *The Lancet Neurology*, *1*, 225–231. doi:10.1016/S1474-4422(02)00101-1

Lutz, R., Pun, T., & Pellegrini, C. (1991). Colour displays and look-up tables: real time modification of digital images. *Computerized Medical Imaging and Graphics*, *15*(2), 73–84. doi:10.1016/0895-6111(91)90029-U

Mackinnon, A., Aaslid, R., & Markus, H. (2004). Long-term ambulatory monitoring for cerebral emboli using transcranial Doppler ultrasound. *Stroke*, *35*(1), 73–78. doi:10.1161/01.STR.0000106915.83041.0A

Madeira, M. M., Bellis, S., Beltran, L., Solano Gonzalez, J., García-Nocceti, F., & Marnane, W. (1999). High Performance Computing for real-time Spectral Estimation. *Control Engineering Practice*, *7*, 679–686. doi:10.1016/S0967-0661(98)00207-X

Madeira, M. M., Tokhi, M., & Ruano, M. G. (2000). Real-Time Implementation of a Doppler Signal Spectral Estimator using Sequencial and Parallel Processing Techniques. *Microprocessors and Microsystems*, *24*(3), 153–167. doi:10.1016/S0141-9331(00)00071-5

Madeira, M. M., Tokhi, M., & Ruano, M. G. (1997). Comparative Study of Different Doppler Spectral Estimator Implementations. *Preprints of 4th IFAC Workshop on Algorithms and Architectures for Real-Time Control*, (pp. 293-298). Vilamoura, Portugal.

Magnin, M., Morel, A., & Jeanmonod, D. (2000). Single-unit analysis of the pallidum, thalamus and subthalamic nucleus in parkinsonian patients. *Neuroscience*, *96*(3), 549–564. doi:10.1016/S0306-4522(99)00583-7

Mahmoud-Ghoneim, D., Grégoire, T., Constans, J. M., & Certaines, J. D. d. (2003). Three dimensional texture analysis in MRI: A preliminary evaluation in gliomas. *Magnetic Resonance Imaging*, *21*(9), 983–987. doi:10.1016/S0730-725X(03)00201-7

Mairinger, T., Mikuz, G., & Gschwendtner, A. (1999). Are nuclear texture features a suitable tool for predicting non-organ-confined prostate cancer? *The Journal of Urology*, *162*(1), 258–262. doi:10.1097/00005392-199907000-00078

Malik, J., & Perona, P. (1990). Preattentive texture discrimination with early vision mechanisms. *Journal of the Optical Society of America. A, Optics and Image Science*, *7*(5), 923–932. doi:10.1364/JOSAA.7.000923

Malladi, R., Sethian, J. A., & Vemuri, B. C. (1995). Shape modeling with front propagation: a level set approach. *IEEE Transactions on Pattern Analysis and Machine Intelligence*, *17*(2), 158–175. doi:10.1109/34.368173

Mallat, S. G. (1989). A Theory for Multiresolution Signal Decomposition: The Wavelet Representation. *IEEE Transactions on Pattern Analysis and Machine Intelligence*, *11*(7), 674–693. doi:10.1109/34.192463

Mallat, S. (1999). *A Wavelet Tour of Signal Processing* (2nd ed.). Academic Press.

Mandelbrot, B. (1982). *The fractal geometry of nature*. WH Freeman.

Marani, E., Heida, T., Lakke, E. A. J. F., & Usunoff, K. G. (2008). The subthalamic nucleus: Part I, Development, cytology, topography and connections. *Advances in Anatomy, Embryology, and Cell Biology*, 198.

Marc, D., Bernhard, M., Martin, R., & Carlo, S. (2001). *An Adaptive Level Set Method for Medical Image Segmentation*. Paper presented at the Proceedings of the 17th International Conference on Information Processing in Medical Imaging.

Margaret, M. F. (1992). Some Defects in Finite-Difference Edge Finders. *IEEE Transactions on Pattern Analysis and Machine Intelligence*, *14*(3), 337–345. doi:10.1109/34.120328

Markus, H. (2000). Monitoring Embolism in Real Time. *Circulation*, *102*(8), 826–828.

Marroquin, J. L., Vemuri, B. C., Botello, S., Calderon, F., & Fernandez-Bouzas, A. (2002). An accurate and efficient Bayesian method for automatic segmentation of brain MRI. *IEEE Transactions on Medical Imaging*, *21*(8), 934–945. doi:10.1109/TMI.2002.803119

Martin, P., Réfrégier, P., Goudail, F., & Guérault, F. (2004). Influence of the noise model on level set active contour segmentation. *IEEE PAMI*, *26*, 799–803.

Marvasti, S., Gillies, D., Marvasti, F., & Markus, H. (2004). Online automated detection of cerebral embolic signals using a wavelet-based system. *Ultrasound in Medicine & Biology*, *30*(5), 647–653. doi:10.1016/j.ultrasmedbio.2004.03.009

Masters, B. R., & So, P. T. C. (2004). Antecedents of two-photon excitation laser scanning microscopy, microscopy research and technique. *Microscopy Research and Technique*, *63*, 3–11. doi:10.1002/jemt.10418

Mathias, J. M., Tofts, P. S., & Losseff, N. A. (1999). Texture analysis of spinal cord pathology in multiple sclerosis. *Magnetic Resonance in Medicine*, *42*(5), 929–935. doi:10.1002/(SICI)1522-2594(199911)42:5<929::AID-MRM13>3.0.CO;2-2

Mathworks Inc. (2002). *Matlab*. MA, USA: Natick.

Matos, S., Leiria, A., & Ruano, M. G. (2000, July). Blood Flow Parameters Evaluation Using Wavelets Transforms. In *Proceedings of World Congress on Medical Physics and Biomedical Engineering* (pp. 4235-5280). Chicago, USA.

Mattfeldt, T., Vogel, U., & Gottfried, H. W. (1993). Three-dimensional spatial texture of adenocarcinoma of the prostate by a combination of stereology and digital image analysis. *Verhandlungen der Deutschen Gesellschaft fur Pathologie*, *77*, 73–77.

Mazzone, P., Lozano, A., Stanzione, P., Galati, S., Scarnati, E., Peppe, A., & Stefani, A. (2005). Implantation of human pedunculopontine nucleus: a safe and clinically relevant target in Parkinson's disease. *Neuroreport*, *16*, 1877–1881. doi:10.1097/01.wnr.0000187629.38010.12

McCormick, D. A., & Huguenard, J. R. (1992). A model of the electrophysiological properties of thalamocortical relay neurons. *Journal of Neurophysiology*, *68*, 1384–1400.

Mcinerney, T., & Terzopoulos, D. (1995). A dynamic finite element surface model for segmentation and tracking in multidimensional medical images with application to cardiac 4D image analysis. *Computerized Medical Imaging and Graphics*, *19*, 69–83. doi:10.1016/0895-6111(94)00040-9

McInerney, T., & Terzopoulos, D. (1996). Deformable models in medical image analysis: a survey. *Medical Image Analysis*, *1*(2), 91–108. doi:10.1016/S1361-8415(96)80007-7

McIntosh, C., & Hamarneh, G. (2006). *Spinal Crawlers: Deformable Organisms for Spinal Cord Segmentation and Analysis.* Paper presented at the MICCAI (1).

McIntosh, C., & Hamarneh, G. (2006). *Vessel Crawlers: 3D Physically-based Deformable Organisms for Vasculature Segmentation and Analysis.* Paper presented at the Computer Vision and Pattern Recognition, 2006 IEEE Computer Society Conference on.

McIntyre, C. (2001). Extracellular excitation of central neurons: implications for the mechanisms of deep brain stimulation. *Thalamus & Related Systems, 1,* 269–277.

McIntyre, C. C., Grill, W. M., Sherman, D. L., & Thakor, N. V. (2004b). Cellular effects of Deep Brain Stimulation: Model-Based Analysis of Activation and Inhibition. *Journal of Neurophysiology, 91,* 1457–1469. doi:10.1152/jn.00989.2003

McIntyre, C. C., Savasta, M., Kerkerian-Le Goff, L., & Vitek, J. L. (2004a). Uncovering the mechanism(s) of action of deep brain stimulation: activation, inhibition, or both. *Clinical Neurophysiology, 115,* 1239–1248. doi:10.1016/j.clinph.2003.12.024

Mehmet, S., & Bulent, S. (2004). Survey over image thresholding techniques and quantitative performance evaluation. *Journal of Electronic Imaging, 13*(1), 146–168. doi:10.1117/1.1631315

Meier, U., Lopez, O., Monserrat, C., Juan, M. C., & Alcaniz, M. (2005). Real-time deformable models for surgery simulation: a survey. *Computer Methods and Programs in Biomedicine, 77*(3), 183–197. doi:10.1016/j.cmpb.2004.11.002

Meijer, H. G. E., Krupa, M., Cagnan, H., Heida, T., Martens, H., & Van Gils, S. A. (in prep.). Mathematical studies on the frequency response of a model for a thalamic neuron. *Journal of Computational Neuroscience.*

Mena-Segovia, J., Bolam, J. P., & Magill, P. J. (2004). Pedunculopontine nucleus and basal ganglia: distant relatives or part of the same family? *Trends in Neurosciences, 27,* 585–588. doi:10.1016/j.tins.2004.07.009

Merceron, G., Taylor, S., Scott, R., Chaimanee, Y., & Jaeger, J. J. (2006). Dietary characterization of the hominoid khoratpithecus (Miocene of Thailand): Evidence from dental topographic and microwear texture analyses. *Naturwissenschaften, 93*(7), 329–333. doi:10.1007/s00114-006-0107-0

Mess, W., Willigers, J., Ledoux, L., Ackerstaff, R., & Hoeks, A. (2002). Microembolic signal description: a reappraisal based on a customized digital postprocessing system. *Ultrasound in Medicine & Biology, 28*(11-12), 1447–1455. doi:10.1016/S0301-5629(02)00618-X

Metaxas, D., & Ting, C. (2004). *A hybrid 3D segmentation framework.* Paper presented at the Biomedical Imaging: Nano to Macro, 2004. IEEE International Symposium on.

Mettler, F. A. (1944). Physiologic consequences and anatomic degeneration following lesions of primate brain stem. *The Journal of Comparative Neurology, 80,* 69–148. doi:10.1002/cne.900800107

Mettler, F. A. (1946). Experimental production of static tremor. *Proceedings of the National Academy of Sciences of the United States of America, 89,* 3859–3863.

Mettler, F. A. (1968). Anatomy of the basal ganglia. In Vinken, P. J., & Bruyn, G. W. (Eds.), *Handbook of Clinical Neurology* (*Vol. 6*, pp. 1–55). Amsterdam: North Holland Publ. Co.

Meyers, R. (1968). Ballismus. In Vinken, P. J., & Bruyn, G. W. (Eds.), *Handbook of Clinical Neurology* (pp. 476–490). Amsterdam: North Holland Publ. Co.

Michailovich, O., Rathi, Y., & Tannenbaum, A. (2007). Image segmentation using active contours driven by the Bhattacharyya gradient flow. *IEEE Trans.s on Image Processing, 16,* 2787-2801.

Mink, J. W. (1996). The basal ganglia: focused selection and inhibition of competing motor programs. *Progress in Neurobiology, 50,* 381–425. doi:10.1016/S0301-0082(96)00042-1

Moehring, M. A., & Klepper, J. R. (1994). Pulse Doppler Ultrasound Detection, Characterisation and Size Estimation of Emboli in Flowing Blood. *IEEE Transactions on Bio-Medical Engineering*, *41*(1), 35–44. doi:10.1109/10.277269

Montagnat, J., & Delingette, H. (2000). *Space and Time Shape Constrained Deformable Surfaces for 4D Medical Image Segmentation*. Paper presented at the Proceedings of the Third International Conference on Medical Image Computing and Computer-Assisted Intervention.

Montgomery, E., & Gale, J. (2005). *Mechanisms of Deep Brain Stimulation: Implications for Physiology, Pathophysiology and Future Therapies*. 10th Annual Conference of the International FES Society.

Moroney, R., Heida, T., & Geelen, J. A. G. (2008). Modeling of bradykinesia in Parkinson's disease during simple and complex movements. *Journal of Computational Neuroscience*, *25*, 501–519. doi:10.1007/s10827-008-0091-9

Mudigonda, N., Rangayyan, R., & Desautels, J. (2000). Gradient and texture analysis for the classification of mammographic masses. *IEEE Transactions on Medical Imaging*, 1032–1043.

Mühlenbein, H., Schomisch, M., & Born, J. (1991). The parallel genetic alghorithm as function optimizer. *Parallel Computing*, *17*(6-7), 619–632. doi:10.1016/S0167-8191(05)80052-3

Müller, K., Yagel, R., & Wheller, J. J. (1999). Fast Implementation of Algebraic Methods for Three-Dimensional Reconstruction from Cone-Beam Data. *IEEE Transactions on Medical Imaging*, *18*, 538–548. doi:10.1109/42.781018

Müller, M., Pan, X., Walter, P., & Klaus, S. (1998). Variability of Velocity and Duration of Microembolic Signals Detected by Bigated Transcranial Doppler Sonography in Carotid Endarterectomy. *European Journal of Ultrasound*, *41*(1), 1–6. doi:10.1016/S0929-8266(98)00044-5

Müller, K., & Xu, F. (2006). Practical Considerations for GPU-Accelerated CT. *IEEE International Symposium on Biomedical Imaging 2006*.

Muzy, J., Bacry, E., & Arneodo, A. (1991). Wavelets and multifractal formalism for singular signals: application to turbulence data. *Physical Review Letters*, *67*, 3515–3518. doi:10.1103/PhysRevLett.67.3515

MySQL Documentation. (2008). Retrieved from http://dev.mysql.com/doc

Nakagawa, Y., & Rosenfeld, A. (1979). Some experiments on variable thresholding. *Pattern Recognition*, *11*(11), 191–204. doi:10.1016/0031-3203(79)90006-2

Nakanishi, H., Kita, H., & Kitai, S. T. (1987). Electrical membrane properties of rat subthalamic neurons in an in vitro slice preparation. *Brain Research*, *437*, 35–44. doi:10.1016/0006-8993(87)91524-1

Nambu, A., Tokuno, H., Hamada, I., Kita, H., Imanishi, M., & Akazawa, T. (2000). Excitatory cortical inputs to pallidal neurons via the subthalamic nucleus in the monkey. *Journal of Neurophysiology*, *84*, 289–300.

Nambu, A., Tokuno, H., & Takada, M. (2002). Functional significance of the cortico-subthalamo-pallidal 'hyperdirect' pathway. *Neuroscience Research*, *43*, 111–117. doi:10.1016/S0168-0102(02)00027-5

Nambu, A. (2005). A new approach to understand the pathophysiology of Parkinson's disease. *Journal of Neurology 252*, IV/1-IV/4.

Nandi, D., Aziz, T. Z., Giladi, N., Winter, J., & Stein, F. (2002a). Reversal of akinesia in experimental parkinsonism by GABA antagonist microinjections in the pedunculopontine nucleus. *Brain*, *123*, 2418–2430. doi:10.1093/brain/awf259

Nandi, D., Liu, X., Winter, J. L., Aziz, T. Z., & Stein, J. F. (2002b). Deep brain stimulation of the pedunculopontine region in the normal non-human primate. *Journal of Clinical Neuroscience*, *9*, 170–174. doi:10.1054/jocn.2001.0943

Natterer, F. (1989). *The Mathematics of Computerized Tomography*. B.G. Teubner, Stuttgart, ISBN 0-898-71493-1.

Neyret, F. (1995). *A general and multiscale model for volumetric textures.* Paper presented at the Graphics Interface, Canadian Human-Computer Communications Society, Québec, Canada.

Ni, Y.-J., Youn, C.-H., Kim, B.-J., Han, Y.-J., & Liu, P. (2007). A PQRM-based PACS System for Advanced Medical Services under Grid Environment. In *Proceedings of the 7th IEEE International Conference on Bioinformatics and Bioengineering* (pp. 1225-1229).

Nieuwenhuys, R., Voogd, J., & van Huijzen, C. (2008). *The human central nervous system.* Berlin: Springer.

O'Reilly, R. C., & Frank, M. J. (2006). Making working memory work: a computational model of learning in the prefrontal cortex and basal ganglia. *Neural Computation, 18*, 283–328. doi:10.1162/089976606775093909

Octave Documentation. (2008). Retrieved from http://www.gnu.org/software/octave/docs.html

O'Donnell, T., Dubuisson-Jolly, M. P., & Gupta, A. (1998). *A cooperative framework for segmentation using 2D active contours and 3D hybrid models as applied to branching cylindrical structures.* Paper presented at the Sixth International Conference on Computer Vision, 1998.

Ohanian, P. P., & Dubes, R. C. (1992). Performance evaluation for four classes of tectural features. *Pattern Recognition, 25*, 819–833. doi:10.1016/0031-3203(92)90036-I

Ojala, T., Pietikinen, M., & Harwood, D. (1996). A comparative study of texture measures with classification based on feature distributions. *Pattern Recognition, 29*(1), 51–59. doi:10.1016/0031-3203(95)00067-4

Ojala, T., Valkealahti, K., Oja, R., & Pietikinen, M. (2001). Texture discrimination with multidimensional distributions of signed gray level differences. *Pattern Recognition, 34*(3), 727–739. doi:10.1016/S0031-3203(00)00010-8

Olabarriaga, S. D., & Smeulders, A. W. M. (2001). Interaction in the segmentation of medical images: A survey. *Medical Image Analysis, 5*(2), 127–142. doi:10.1016/S1361-8415(00)00041-4

Oldershaw, R. L. (2002). *Nature adores Self-Similarity.* Retrieved December 2008 from http://www3.amherst.edu/~rloldershaw/nature.html

Oliveira, P., & du Buf, H. (2003). SPMD Image Processing on Beowulf Clusters: Directives and Libraries. In *IPDPS '03: Proceedings of the 17th International Symposium on Parallel and Distributed Processing* (p. 230.1). IEEE Computer Society.

OpenSSH Manual Pages. (2008). Retrieved from http://www.openssh.com/manual.html

Orieux, G., Francois, C., Féger, J., Yelnik, J., Vila, M., & Ruberg, M. (2000). Metabolic activity of excitatory parafascicular and pedunculopontine inputs to the subthalamic nucleus in a rat model of Parkinson's disease. *Neuroscience, 97*, 79–88. doi:10.1016/S0306-4522(00)00011-7

Osher, S., & Sethian, J. A. (1988). Fronts propagating with curvature-dependent speed: Algorithms based on Hamilton-jacobi formulation. *Journal of Computational Physics, 79*, 12–49. doi:10.1016/0021-9991(88)90002-2

Otsu, N. (1979). A Threshold Selection Method from Gray-Level Histograms. *IEEE Transactions on Systems, Man, and Cybernetics, 9*(1), 62–66. doi:10.1109/TSMC.1979.4310076

Otsuka, T., Abe, T., Tsukagawa, T., & Song, W. J. (2000). Single compartment model of the voltage-dependent generation of a plateau potential in subthalamic neurons. *Neuroscience Research. Supplement, 24*, 581.

Otsuka, T., Abe, T., Tsukagawa, T., & Song, W.-J. (2004). Conductance-based model of the voltage-dependent generation of a plateau potential in subthalamic neurons. *Journal of Neurophysiology, 92*, 255–264. doi:10.1152/jn.00508.2003

Otsuka, T., Murakami, F., & Song, W. J. (2001). Excitatory postsynaptic potentials trigger a plateau potential in rat subthalamic neurons at hyperpolarized states. *Journal of Neurophysiology, 86*, 1816–1825.

Owens, J. D., Luebke, D., Govindaraju, N., Harris, M., Krüger, J., Lefohn, A. E., & Purcell, T. J. (2007). A Survey of General-Purpose Computation on Graphics Hardware. *Computer Graphics Forum*, *26*(1), 80–113. doi:10.1111/j.1467-8659.2007.01012.x

Paelinck, B. P., & Kasprzak, J. D. (1999). Contrast-enhanced echocardiography: review and current role. *Acta Cardiologica*, *54*(4), 195–201.

Pagano, M., Giordano, S., Russo, F., & Sparano, D. (1996). Parallel Implementation of a Progressive Fractal Image Compression System. *IEEE International Workshop on Intelligent Signal Processing & Communication Systems ISPACS '96*.

Pahapill, P. A., & Lozano, A. M. (2000). The pedunculopontine nucleus and Parkinson's disease. *Brain*, *123*, 1767–1783. doi:10.1093/brain/123.9.1767

Paragios, N. (2002). A Variational Approach for the Segmentation of the Left Ventricle. *International Journal of Computer Vision*, 345–362. doi:10.1023/A:1020882509893

Paragios, N., & Deriche, R. (2002). Geodesic active regions and level set methods for supervised texture segmentation. *International Journal of Computer Vision*, *46*(3), 223. doi:10.1023/A:1014080923068

Paragios, N., & Deriche, R. (2002). Geodesic active regions: A new paradigm to deal with frame partition problems in computer vision. *Journal of Visual Communication and Image Representation*, *13*, 249–268. doi:10.1006/jvci.2001.0475

Paragios, N., & Deriche, R. (2000). Coupled geodesic active regions for image segmentation: A level set approach. In *European Conference in Computer Vision*.

Parashair, M., & Browne, J. C. (2005). Conceptual and Implementation Modules for the Grid. *Proceedings of the IEEE*, *93*(3), 653–668. doi:10.1109/JPROC.2004.842780

Parisot, C., Antonini, M., & Barlaud, M. (2003). *3D scan based wavelet transform and quality control for video coding*. EURASIP Journal on Applied Signal Processing.

Payan, F., & Antonini, M. (2005). An efficient bit allocation for compressing normal meshes with an error-driven quantization. *Elsevier Computer Aided Geometric Design*, *22*, 466–486. doi:10.1016/j.cagd.2005.04.001

Payan, F., & Antonini, M. (2006). Mean Square Error Approximation for Wavelet-based Semi-regular Mesh Compression. [TVCG]. *IEEE Transactions on Visualization and Computer Graphics*, *12*(4). doi:10.1109/TVCG.2006.73

Payan, F., & Antonini, M. (2003). 3D multiresolution context-based coding for geometry compression. In *IEEE International Conference in Image Processing (ICIP)*, Barcelona, Spain (pp. 785-788).

Pellerin, D., & Taylor, D. (1997). *VHDL Made Easy.* Prentice Hall, ISBN 0-13-650763-8.

Peng, C. K., Havlin, S., Simons, M., Stanley, H. E., & Goldberger, A. L. (1994). Mosaic organizatino of DNA nucleotides. *Physical Review E: Statistical Physics, Plasmas, Fluids, and Related Interdisciplinary Topics*, *49*, 49–54. doi:10.1103/PhysRevE.49.1685

Percheron, G., & Filion, M. (1991). Parallel processing in the basal ganglia: up to a point (letter to the editor). *Trends in Neurosciences*, *14*, 55–56. doi:10.1016/0166-2236(91)90020-U

Pesquet-Popescu, B., & Vehel, J. (2002). Stochastic fractal models for image processing.

Pessiglione, M., Guehl, D., Rollard, A., Francois, C., Hirsch, E., Feger, J., & Tremblay, L. (2005). Thalamic neuronal activity in dopamine-depleted primates: evidence for a loss of functional segregation within basal ganglia circuits. *The Journal of Neuroscience*, *25*, 1523–1531. doi:10.1523/JNEUROSCI.4056-04.2005

Peters, G. (2007). Computer-aided detection for digital breast tomosynthesis.

Petrou, M., & Kadyrov, A. (2004). Affine invariant features from the trace transform. *IEEE Transactions on Pattern Analysis and Machine Intelligence*, *26*(1), 30–44. doi:10.1109/TPAMI.2004.1261077

Pham, D., Asano, S., Bolliger, M., Day, M. N., Hofstee, H. P., Johns, C., et al. (2005). The Design and Implementation of a First-Generation Cell Processor. *Proceedings of the IEEE International Solid-State Circuits Conference 2005.*

Pichler, O., Teuner, A., & Hosticka, B. J. (1996). A comparison of texture feature extraction using adaptive Gabor filtering, pyramidal and tree structured wavelet transforms. *Pattern Recognition, 29*(5), 733–742. doi:10.1016/0031-3203(95)00127-1

Pickard, J. E., Hossack, J. A., & Acton, S. T. (2006). Shape model segmentation of long-axis contrast enhanced echocardiography. *IEEE Int. Symp. on Biomedical Imaging Nano to Macro.*

Pieranzotti, M., Palmieri, M. G., Galati, S., Stanzione, P., Peppe, A., & Tropepi, D. (2008). Pedunculopontine nucleus deep brain stimulation changes spinal cord excitability in Parkinson's disease patients. *Journal of Neural Transmission, 115*, 731–735. doi:10.1007/s00702-007-0001-8

Pisano, E. (2000). Current status of full-field digital mammography. *Academic Radiology, 7*, 266–280. doi:10.1016/S1076-6332(00)80478-X

Pisano, E., Hendrick, R., Yaffe, M., Baum, J., Acharyya, S., & Cormack, J. (2008). Diagnostic accuracy of digital versus film mammography: exploratory analysis of selected population subgroups in DMIST. *Radiology, 246*(2), 376. doi:10.1148/radiol.2461070200

Plaha, P., & Gill, S. S. (2005). Bilateral deep brain stimulation of the pedunculopontine nucleus for Parkinson's disease. *Neuroreport, 16*, 1883–1887. doi:10.1097/01.wnr.0000187637.20771.a0

Plenz, D., & Kitai, S. T. (1999). A basal ganglia pacemaker formed by the subthalamic nucleus and external globus pallidus. *Nature, 400*, 677–682. doi:10.1038/23281

Porteneuve, C., Korb, J.-P., Petit, D., & Zanni, H. (2000). Structure-texture correlation in ultra high performance concrete: A nuclear magnetic resonance study. In *Franco-Italian conference on magnetic resonance.* France: La Londe Les Maures.

Potlapalli, H., & Luo, R. (1998). Fractal-based classification of natural textures. *IEEE Transactions on Industrial Electronics, 45*, 142–150. doi:10.1109/41.661315

Precioso, F., & Barlaud, M. (2002). B-spline active contour with handling of topology changes for fast video segmentation. *EURASIP Journal on Applied Signal Processing*, (1): 555–560. doi:10.1155/S1110865702203121

Prescott, T. J., Gurney, K., Montes-Gonzalez, F., Humphries, M., & Redgrave, P. (2002). The robot basal ganglia: action selection by an embedded model of the basal ganglia. In Nicholson, L., & Faull, R. (Eds.), *Basal Ganglia VII.* Plenum Press.

Prêteux, F., Rougon, N., & Discher, A. (2006). Region-based statistical segmentation using informational active contours. In *Proceedings SPIE Conference on Mathematics of Data/Image Pattern Recognition, Compression, and Encryption with Applications IX.*

Priest, E., & Forbes, T. (2007). The Bursty Nature Of Solar Flare X-Ray Emission. *The Astrophysical Journal*, 662-691Y700.

Pujol, O., & Radeva, P. (2005). On the assessment of texture feature descriptors in intravascular ultrasound images: A boosting approach to a feasible plaque classification. *Studies in Health Technology and Informatics, 113*, 276–299.

Pun, T., Hochstrasser, D. F., Appel, R. D., Funk, M., & Villars-Augsburger, V. (1988). Computerized classification of two-dimensional gel electrophoretograms by correspondence analysis and ascendant hierarchical clustering. *Applied and Theoretical Electrophoresis, 1*(1), 3–9.

Pun, T., Gerig, G., & Ratib, O. (1994). Image analysis and computer vision in medicine.

Quiroga, R. Q., Nadasdy, Z., & Ben-Shaul, Y. (2004). Unsupervised Spike Detection and Sorting with Wavelets and Superparamagnetic Clustering. *Neural Computation, 16*(8), 1661–1687. doi:10.1162/089976604774201631

Radon, J. (1986). On the Determination of Functions From Their Integral Values Along Certain Manifolds. *IEEE Transactions on Medical Imaging*, *MI-5*, 170–176. doi:10.1109/TMI.1986.4307775

Rajpoot, N. M. (2002). Texture classification using discriminant wavelet packet subbands. In *Proceedings 45th IEEE Midwest symposium on circuits and systems (MWSCAS 2002)*. Tulsa, OK, USA.

Ramachandran, G. N., & Lakshminarayanan, A. V. (1971). Three-Dimensional Reconstruction from Radiographs and Electron Micrographs: Application of Convolution instead of Fourier Transforms. *Proceedings of the National Academy of Sciences of the United States of America*, *68*, 2236–2240. doi:10.1073/pnas.68.9.2236

Ranck, J. B. (1975). Which elements are excited in electrical stimulation of mammalian central nervous system? *Annual Review Brain Research*, *98*, 417–440.

Randen, T., & Husøy, J. H. (1994). Texture segmentation with optimal linear prediction error filters. *Piksel'n*, *11*(3), 25–28.

Randen, T., & Husøy, J. H. (1999). Filtering for texture classification: A comparative study. *IEEE Transactions on Pattern Analysis and Machine Intelligence*, *21*(4), 291–310. doi:10.1109/34.761261

Randen, T., Monsen, E., Abrahamsen, A., Hansen, J. O., Shlaf, J., & Sønneland, L. (2000). Three-dimensional texture attributes for seismic data analysis. In *Ann. Int. Mtg., soc. Expl. Geophys., exp. Abstr.* Calgary, Canada.

Randen, T., Sønneland, L., Carrillat, A., Valen, S., Skov, T., Pedersen, S. I., et al. (2003). Preconditioning for optimal 3D stratigraphical and structural inversion. In *65th EAGE conference & exhibition*. Stavanger.

Rathi, Y., Michailovich, O., Malcolm, J., & Tannenbaum, A. (2006). Seeing the unseen: Segmenting with distributions. In *International Conference on Signal and Image Processing*.

Ravishankar-Rao, A., & Lohse, G. L. (1993). Towards a texture naming system: Identifying relevant dimensions of texture. In *Proceedings of the 4th conference on visualization* (pp. 220-227). San Jose, California.

Reljin, I., & Reljin, B. (2002). Fractal geometry and multifractals in analyzing and processing medical data and images.

Reyes Aldasoro, C. C. (2004). *Multiresolution volumetric texture segmentation*. Coventry: The University of Warwick.

Reyes Aldasoro, C. C., & Bhalerao, A. (2006). The Bhattacharyya space for feature selection and its application to texture segmentation. *Pattern Recognition*, *39*(5), 812–826. doi:10.1016/j.patcog.2005.12.003

Reyes Aldasoro, C. C., & Bhalerao, A. (2007). Volumetric texture segmentation by discriminant feature selection and multiresolution classification. *IEEE Transactions on Medical Imaging*, *26*(1), 1–14. doi:10.1109/TMI.2006.884637

Riddell, C., & Trousset, Y. (2006). Rectification for Cone-Beam Projection and Backprojection. *IEEE Transactions on Medical Imaging*, *25*, 950–962. doi:10.1109/TMI.2006.876169

Ringelstein, B. E., Droste, D. W., Babikian, V. L., Evans, D. H., Grosset, D. G., & Kaps, M. (1998). Consensus on Microembolus Detection by TCD. International Consensus Group on Microembolus Detection. *Stroke*, *29*(3), 725–729.

Ringelstein, E. B., & Droste, D. W. (1999). Microembolic Signal Criteria. In Babikian, V. L., & Welchser, L. R. (Eds.), *Transcranial Doppler Ultrasonography* (2nd ed., pp. 157–166). Boston, USA: Butterworth-Heineman Medical.

Romanelli, P., Esposito, V., Schaal, D. W., & Heit, G. (2005). Somatotopy in the basal ganglia: experimental and clinical evidence for segrated sensorimotor channels. *Brain Research. Brain Research Reviews*, *48*, 112–128. doi:10.1016/j.brainresrev.2004.09.008

Romo, R., & Schultz, W. (1992). Role of primate basal ganglia and frontal cortex in the internal generation of movements. III. Neuronal activity in the supplementary motor area. *Experimental Brain Research*, *91*, 396–407. doi:10.1007/BF00227836

Ronfard, R. (1994). Region-based strategies for active contour models. *International Journal of Computer Vision*, *13*(2), 229–251. doi:10.1007/BF01427153

Rosito, M. A., Moreira, L. F., da Silva, V. D., Damin, D. C., & Prolla, J. C. (2003). Nuclear chromatin texture in rectal cancer. Relationship to tumor stage. *Analytical and Quantitative Cytology and Histology*, *25*(1), 25–30.

Rougon, N., Petitjean, C., Preteux, F., Cluzel, P., & Grenier, P. (2005). A non-rigid registration approach for quantifying myocardial contraction in tagged MRI using generalized information measures. *Medical Image Analysis*, *9*(4), 353–375. doi:10.1016/j.media.2005.01.005

Rousson, M., Lenglet, C., & Deriche, R. (2004). Level set and region based surface propagation for diffusion tensor MRI segmentation, In *Computer Vision Approaches to Medical Image Analysis nd Mathematical Methods in Biomedical Image Analysis Workshop*.

Roy, E., Abraham, P., Montresor, S., & Saumet, J.-L. (2000). Comparison of Time-Frequency Estimators for Peripheral Embolus Detection. *Ultrasound in Medicine & Biology*, *26*(5), 419–423. doi:10.1016/S0301-5629(99)00142-8

Ruan, S., Jaggi, C., Xue, J., Fadili, J., & Bloyet, D. (2000). Brain Tissue classification of magnetic resonance images using partial volume modeling. *IEEE Transactions on Medical Imaging*, *19*(12), 1179–1187. doi:10.1109/42.897810

Ruano, M. G. (1992). Investigation of Real Time Spectral Analysis Techniques for Use with Pulsed Ultrasound Doppler Blood Flow Detectors. PhD thesis, University College of North Wales, Bangor UK.

Rubin, J., & Terman, D. (2004). High frequency stimulation of the subthalamic nucleus eliminates pathological rhythmicity in a computational model. *Journal of Computational Neuroscience*, *16*, 211–235. doi:10.1023/B:JCNS.0000025686.47117.67

Rudy, B., & McBain, C. J. (2001). Kv3 channels: voltage-gated K^+ channels designed for high-frequency repetitive firing. *Trends in Neurosciences*, *24*, 517–526. doi:10.1016/S0166-2236(00)01892-0

Rueckert, D., Lorenzo-Valdes, M., Chandrashekara, R., Sanchez-Ortiz, G. L., & Mohiaddin, R. (2002). *Non-rigid registration of cardiac MR: application to motion modelling and atlas-based segmentation.* Paper presented at the 2002 IEEE International Symposium on Biomedical Imaging.

Rui, H., Pavlovic, V., & Metaxas, D. (2006). *A tightly coupled region-shape framework for 3D medical image segmentation.* Paper presented at the 3rd IEEE International Symposium on Biomedical Imaging: Nano to Macro.

Saeed, N., & Puri, B. K. (2002). Cerebellum segmentation employing texture properties and knowledge based image processing: Applied to normal adult controls and patients. *Magnetic Resonance Imaging*, *20*(5), 425–429. doi:10.1016/S0730-725X(02)00508-8

Salfity, M., Kaufmann, G., Granitto, P., & Ceccatto, H. (2001). *Automated detection and classification of clustered microcalcifications using morphological filtering and statistical techniques. IWDM2000*. Medical Physics Publishing.

Salganicoff, M., Sarna, M., Sax, L., & Gerstein, G. L. (1988). Unsupervised waveform classification for multineuron recordings: a real-time, software-based system. I: Algorithms and implementation. *Journal of Neuroscience Methods*, *25*(3), 181–187. doi:10.1016/0165-0270(88)90132-X

Samet, H. (1984). The quadtree and related hierarchical data structures. *Computing Surveys*, *16*(2), 187–260. doi:10.1145/356924.356930

Sayeed, A., Petrou, M., Spyrou, N., Kadyrov, A., & Spinks, T. (2002). Diagnostic features of Alzheimer's disease extracted from PET sinograms. *Physics in Medicine and Biology*, *47*(1), 137–148. doi:10.1088/0031-9155/47/1/310

Schad, L. R., Bluml, S., & Zuna, I. (1993). MR tissue characterization of intracranial tumors by means of texture analysis. *Magnetic Resonance Imaging*, *11*(6), 889–896. doi:10.1016/0730-725X(93)90206-S

Schaller, S., Flohr, T., & Steffen, P. (1998). An Efficient Fourier method in 3D reconstruction from cone-beam data. *IEEE Transactions on Medical Imaging*, *17*, 244–250. doi:10.1109/42.700736

Schiller, N. B., Shah, P. M., Crawford, M., DeMaria, A., Devereux, R., & Feigenbaum, H. (1989). Recommendations for quantitation of the left ventricle by two-dimensional echocardiography. American Society of Echocardiography Committee on Standards, Subcommittee on Quantitation of Two-Dimensional Echocardiograms. *Journal of the American Society of Echocardiography*, *2*(5), 358–367.

Schröder, P., & Sweldens, W. (1995). Efficiently Representing Functions on the Sphere. In *SIGGRAPH'95* (pp. 161–172). Spherical Wavelets.

Schroeter, P., & Bigun, J. (1995). Hierarchical image segmentation by multi-dimensional clustering and orientation-adaptive boundary refinement. *Pattern Recognition*, *28*(5), 695–709. doi:10.1016/0031-3203(94)00133-7

Schuurman, P. R., Bosch, A. D., Bossuyt, P. M. M., Bonsel, G. J., van Someren, E. J. W., & de Bie, R. M. A. (2000). A comparison of continuous thalamic stimulation and thalatomy for suppression of severe tremor. *The New England Journal of Medicine*, *342*, 461–468. doi:10.1056/NEJM200002173420703

Scott, R. S., Ungar, P. S., Bergstrom, T. S., Brown, C. A., Childs, B. E., & Teaford, M. F. (2006). Dental microwear texture analysis: Technical considerations. *Journal of Human Evolution*, *51*(4), 339–349. doi:10.1016/j.jhevol.2006.04.006

Segovia-Martínez, M., Petrou, M., Kovalev, V. A., & Perner, P. (1999). Quantifying level of brain atrophy using texture anisotropy in ct data. In *Medical imaging understanding and analysis* (pp. 173-176). Oxford, UK.

Sezan, M. I. (1985). A peak detection algorithm and its application to histogram-based image data reduction. *Graph. Models Image Process.*, *29*, 47–59.

Shattuck, D. W., & Leahy, R. M. (2002). BrainSuite: an automated cortical surface identification tool. *Medical Image Analysis*, *6*(2), 129–142. doi:10.1016/S1361-8415(02)00054-3

Shen, H., Shi, Y., & Peng, Z. (2005). 3D Complex Anatomic Structures. In *Computer Vision for Biomedical Image Applications* (pp. 189–199). Applying Prior Knowledge in the Segmentation of. doi:10.1007/11569541_20

Shepp, L. A., & Logan, B. F. (1974). The Fourier Reconstruction of a Head Section. *IEEE Transactions on Nuclear Science*, *NS-21*, 21–43.

Sheppard, C. J., & Wilson, T. (1981). The theory of the direct-view confocal microscope. *Journal of Microscopy*, *124*(Pt 2), 107–117.

Shink, E., Bevan, M. D., Bolam, J. P., & Smith, Y. (1996). The subthalamic nucleus and the external pallidum: two tightly interconnected structures that control the output of the basal ganglia in the monkey. *Neuroscience*, *73*, 335–357. doi:10.1016/0306-4522(96)00022-X

Shoham, S., Fellows, M. R., & Normann, R. A. (2003). Robust, automatic spike sorting using mixtures of multivariate t-distributions. *Journal of Neuroscience Methods*, *127*(2), 111–122. doi:10.1016/S0165-0270(03)00120-1

Siddon, R. (1985). Fast calculation of the exact radiological path length for a three-dimensional CT array. *Medical Physics*, *12*, 252–255. doi:10.1118/1.595715

Sigel, B. (1998). A Brief History of Doppler Ultrasound in the Diagnosis of Peripheral Vascular Disease. *Ultrasound in Medicine & Biology*, *24*(2), 169–176. doi:10.1016/S0301-5629(97)00264-0

Sivaramakrishna, R., Powell, K. A., Lieber, M. L., Chilcote, W. A., & Shekhar, R. (2002). Texture analysis of lesions in breast ultrasound images. *Computerized Medical Imaging and Graphics*, *26*(5), 303–307. doi:10.1016/S0895-6111(02)00027-7

Sloan, J. D. (2004). *High Performance Linux Clusters with OSCAR, Rocks, OpenMosix, and MPI*. O'Reilly.

Sloan, M. A., Alexandrov, A. V., Tegeler, C. H., Spencer, M. P., Caplan, L. R., & Feldmann, E. (2004). Assessment: Transcranial Doppler ultrasonography: Report of the Therapeutics and Technology Assessment Subcommittee of the American Academy of Neurology. *Neurology*, *62*(9), 1468–1481.

Smith, S. M. (2002). Fast robust automated brain extraction. *Human Brain Mapping*, *17*(3), 143–155. doi:10.1002/hbm.10062

Smith, Y., Bevan, M. D., Shink, E., & Bolam, J. P. (1998). Microcircuitry of the direct and indirect pathways of the basal ganglia. *Neuroscience*, *86*, 353–387.

Smith, Y., Wichmann, T., & DeLong, M. R. (1994). Synaptic innervation of neurons in the internal pallidal segment by the subthalamic nucleusand the external pallidum in monkeys. *The Journal of Comparative Neurology*, *343*, 297–318. doi:10.1002/cne.903430209

Smith, J., Evans, D. H., Bell, P. R., & Naylor, A. R. (1998). Time Domain Analysis of Embolic Signals can be Used in Place of High-Resolution Wigner Analysis when Classifying Gaseous and Particulate Emboli. *Ultrasound in Medicine & Biology*, *24*(7), 989–993. doi:10.1016/S0301-5629(98)00107-0

Smith, J. L., Evans, D. H., Fan, L., Thrush, A. J., & Naylor, A. R. (1997). Processing Doppler Ultrasound Signals from Blood-Borne Emboli. *Ultrasound in Medicine & Biology*, *20*(5), 455–462. doi:10.1016/0301-5629(94)90100-7

Smith, J. L., Evans, D. H., Lingke, F., Bell, P. R., & Naylor, A. R. (1996). Differentiation Between Emboli and Artefacts Using Dual-Gated Transcranial Doppler Ultrasound. *Ultrasound in Medicine & Biology*, *22*(8), 1031–1036. doi:10.1016/S0301-5629(96)00103-2

Smith, J. L., Evans, D. H., & Naylor, A. R. (1997). Analysis of the Frequency Modulation Present in Doppler Ultrasound Signals May Allow Differentiation Between Particulate and Gaseous Cerebral Emboli. *Ultrasound in Medicine & Biology*, *26*(5), 727–734. doi:10.1016/S0301-5629(97)00003-3

Soares, F., & Andruszkiewicz, P. M., F., P, C., & Pereira, M. (2007). Self-Similarity Analysis Applied to 2D Breast Cancer Imaging. *The First International Workshop on High Performance Computing Applied to Medical Data and Bioinformatics (HPC-Bio 2007)*. IEEE.

Sokolowski, J., & Zolésio, J. P. (1992). *Introduction to shape optimization* (Vol. 16 of Springer series in computational mathematics). Springer-Verlag.

Song, W.-J., Baba, Y., Otsuka, T., & Murakami, F. (2000). Characterization of Ca^{2+} channels in rat subthalamic nucleus neurons. *Journal of Neurophysiology*, *84*, 2630–2637.

Sonka, M., Hlavac, V., & Boyle, R. (1998). *Image processing, analysis and machine vision*. Pacific Grove, USA: PWS.

Spruston, N., Stuart, G., & Häusser, M. (2008). Dendritic integration. In Stuart, G. (Ed.), *Dendrites* (pp. 351–399). Oxford University Press.

Squire, L. R., Bloom, F. E., McConnell, S. K., Roberts, J. L., Spitzer, N. C., & Zigmond, M. J. (2003). The Basal Ganglia. In *Fundamental Neuroscience* (2nd ed., pp. 815–839). Academic Press.

Srisuk, S., Ratanarangsank, K., Kurutach, W., & Waraklang, S. (2003). Face recognition using a new texture representation of face images. In *Proceedings of electrical engineering conference* (pp. 1097-1102). Cha-am, Thailand.

Staib, L. H., & Duncan, J. S. (1992). Boundary finding with parametrically deformable models. *IEEE Transactions on Pattern Analysis and Machine Intelligence*, *14*(11), 1061–1075. doi:10.1109/34.166621

Staib, L. H., & Duncan, J. S. (1996). Model-based deformable surface finding for medical images. *IEEE Transactions on Medical Imaging*, *15*(5), 720–731. doi:10.1109/42.538949

Stefani, A., Lozano, A. M., Peppe, A., Stanzione, P., Galati, S., & Tropepi, D. (2007). Bilateral deep brain stimulation of the pedunculopontine and subthalamic nuclei in severe Parkinson's disease. *Brain*, *130*, 1596–1607. doi:10.1093/brain/awl346

Stegmann, M. B., Olafsdottir, H., & Larsson, H. B. W. (2005). Unsupervised motion-compensation of multi-slice cardiac perfusion MRI. *Medical Image Analysis*, *9*(4), 394–410. doi:10.1016/j.media.2004.10.002

Strafella, A., Ko, J. H., Grant, J., Fraraccio, M., & Monchi, O. (2005). Corticostriatal functional interactions in Parkinson's disease: a rTMS/[11C]raclopride PET study. *The European Journal of Neuroscience*, *22*, 2946–2952. doi:10.1111/j.1460-9568.2005.04476.x

Subramanian, K. R., Brockway, J. P., & Carruthers, W. B. (2004). Interactive detection and visualization of breast lesions from dynamic contrast enhanced MRI volumes. *Computerized Medical Imaging and Graphics*, *28*(8), 435–444. doi:10.1016/j.compmedimag.2004.07.004

Suri, R. E., Albani, C., & Glattfelder, A. H. (1997). A dynamic model of motor basal ganglia functions. *Biological Cybernetics*, *76*, 451–458. doi:10.1007/s004220050358

Suri, R. E., & Schultz, W. (1998). Learning of sequential movements by neural network model with dopamine-like reinforcement signal. *Experimental Brain Research*, *121*, 350–354. doi:10.1007/s002210050467

Sweldens, W. (1998). The lifting scheme: A construction of second generation wavelets. *SIAM Journal on Mathematical Analysis*, *29*(2), 511–546. doi:10.1137/S0036141095289051

Székely, G., Kelemen, A., Brechbühler, C., & Gerig, G. (1995). 3D objects from MRI volume data using constrained elastic deformations of flexible Fourier surface models. In *Computer Vision, Virtual Reality and Robotics in Medicine* (pp. 493–505). Segmentation of. doi:10.1007/BFb0034992

Tai, C. W., & Baba-Kishi, K. Z. (2002). Microtexture studies of pst and pzt ceramics and pzt thin film by electron backscatter diffraction patterns. *Textures and Microstructures*, *35*(2), 71–86. doi:10.1080/07303300210000001 91

Takahashi, S., Anzai, Y., & Sakurai, Y. (2003a). A new approach to spike sorting for multi-neuronal activities recorded with a tetrode: how ICA can be practical. *Neuroscience Research*, *46*(3), 265–272. doi:10.1016/S0168-0102(03)00103-2

Takahashi, S., Anzai, Y., & Sakurai, Y. (2003b). Automatic sorting for multi-neuronal activity recorded with tetrodes in the presence of overlapping spikes. *Journal of Neurophysiology*, *89*, 2245–2258. doi:10.1152/jn.00827.2002

Takakusaki, K., Saitoh, K., Harada, H., & Kashiwayanagi, M. (2004). Role of the basal ganglia-brainstem pathways in the control of motor behaviours. *Neuroscience Research*, *50*, 137–151. doi:10.1016/j.neures.2004.06.015

Tamura, H., Mori, S., & Yamawaki, T. (1978). Texture features corresponding to visual perception. *IEEE Transactions on Systems, Man, and Cybernetics*, *8*(6), 460–473. doi:10.1109/TSMC.1978.4309999

Tanenbaum, A. S. (2001). *Modern Operating Systems* (2nd ed.). Prentice Hall.

Tanenbaum, A. S., & Van Steen, M. (2002). *Distributed Systems: Principles and Paradigms. Prentice Hall* (International Editions). Pearson Education.

Tang, J., Moro, E., Lozano, A., Lang, A., Hutchison, W., Mahant, N., & Dostrovsky, J. (2005). Firing rates of pallidal neurons are similar in Huntington's and Parkinson's disease patients. *Experimental Brain Research*, *166*, 230–236. doi:10.1007/s00221-005-2359-x

Taqqu, M. S. (1985). A Bibliographical Guide to Self-Similar Processes and Long-Range Dependence. *Dependence in Probability and Statistic*, 137-165.

Tarquis, A., McInnes, K., Key, J., Saa, A., Garcia, M., & Diaz, M. (2006). Multiscaling analysis in a structured clay soil using 2D images.

Teixeira, C., Ruano, M., & Ruano, A. E. (2004). Emboli Classification using RBF Neural Networks. *Sixth Portuguese Conference on Automatic Control* (pp. 630-635). Faro, Portugal.

Temel, Y., Blokland, A., Steinbusch, H. W., & Visser-Vandewalle, V. (2005). The functional role of the subthalamic nucleus in cognitive and limbic circuits. *Progress in Neurobiology*, *76*, 393–413. doi:10.1016/j.pneurobio.2005.09.005

ter Haar Romeny, B., Florack, L., Koenderink, J., & Viergever, M. (1991). Scale space: Its natural operators and differential invariants. In *Information Processing in Medical Imaging* (pp. 239-255).

Terman, D., Rubin, J. E., Yew, A. C., & Wilson, C. J. (2002). Activity patterns in a model for subthalamopallidal network of the basal ganglia. *The Journal of Neuroscience*, *22*, 2963–2976.

Terzopoulos, D., Witkin, A., & Kass, M. (1988). Constraints on deformable models: Recovering 3d shape and nonrigid motion. *Artificial Intelligence*, 35.

Texas Instruments. (1991). *TMS320C40 User's Guide.*

Thain, D., Tannenbaum, T., & Livny, M. (2005). Distributed Computing in Practice: The Condor Experience. *Concurrency and Computation*, *17*(2-4), 323–356. doi:10.1002/cpe.938

Thain, D., & Livny, M. (2003). Building Reliable Clients and Servers. In Foster, I., & Kesselman, C. (Eds.), *The Grid: Blueprint for a New Computing Infrastructure* (2nd ed.). Morgan Kaufmann.

The, C. H., & Chin, R. T. (1988). On image analysis by the methods of moments. *IEEE Pattern Analysis and Machine Intelligence*, *10*, 496–513. doi:10.1109/34.3913

Thenien, C. (1983). An estimation-theoretic approach to terrain image segmentation. *Computer Vision Graphics and Image Processing*, *22*, 313–326. doi:10.1016/0734-189X(83)90079-8

Thybo, A. K., Szczypiński, P. M., Karlsson, A. H., Dønstrup, S., Stødkilde-Jorgensen, H. S., & Andersen, H. J. (2004). Prediction of sensory texture quality attributes of cooked potatoes by NMR-imaging (MRI) of raw potatoes in combination with different image analysis methods. *Journal of Food Engineering*, *61*, 91–100. doi:10.1016/S0260-8774(03)00190-0

Thybo, A. K., Andersen, H. J., Karlsson, A. H., Dønstrup, S., & Stødkilde-Jorgensen, H. S. (2003). Low-field NMR relaxation and NMR-imaging as tools in different determination of dry matter content in potatoes. *Lebensmittel-Wissenschaft und-Technologie, 36*(3), 315-322.

Timothy, F. C., Gareth, J. E., & Christopher, J. T. (2001). Active Appearance Models. *IEEE Transactions on Pattern Analysis and Machine Intelligence*, *23*(6), 681–685. doi:10.1109/34.927467

Timothy, F. C., Hill, A., Christopher, J. T., & Haslam, J. (1993). *The Use of Active Shape Models for Locating Structures in Medical Images*. Paper presented at the Proceedings of the 13th International Conference on Information Processing in Medical Imaging.

Tomás, P., & Sousa, L. (2007). An Efficient Expectation-Maximisation Algorithm for Spike Classification. In15th International Conference on Digital Signal Processing (DSP 2007) (pp. 203-206).

Touma, C., & Gotsman, C. (1998). Triangle mesh compression. In *Graphics Interface'98* (pp. 26-34).

Trepanier, M., & Goddard, I. (2002). Adjunct Processors in Embedded Medical Imaging Systems. *SPIE Medical Imaging Proceedings*, *4681*, 416–424.

Tretriakoff, C. (1919). *Contribution a l'étude de l'anatomie pathologique du locus niger de Soemmering avec quelques déductions relatives a la pathogenie des troubles du tonus musculaire et de la maladie du Parkinson.* Thesis No 293, Jouve et Cie, Paris.

Tronstad, L. (1973). Scanning electron microscopy of attrited dentinal surfaces and subjacent dentin in human teeth. *Scandinavian Journal of Dental Research*, *81*(2), 112–122.

Trovero, M. (2003). Long Range Dependence: a Light Tale for the Practitioner. In *Proceedings of Statistics students' seminar at UNC.*

Tsai, A., Yezzi, A., & Wells, W. (2003). A shape-based approach to the segmentation of medical imagery using level sets. *IEEE Transactions on Medical Imaging, 22*, 137–154. doi:10.1109/TMI.2002.808355

Tsechpenakis, G., Wang, J., Mayer, B., & Metaxas, D. A. M. D. (2007). *Coupling CRFs and Deformable Models for 3D Medical Image Segmentation.* Paper presented at the 11th International Conference on Computer Vision, 2007. ICCV 2007.

Tsumiyama, Y., Sakaue, K., & Yamamoto, K. (1989). Active Net: Active Net Model for Region Extraction. *Information Processing Society of Japan, 39*(1), 491–492.

Tuceryan, M., & Jain, A. K. (1998). Texture analysis. In Chen, C. H., Pau, L. F., & Wang, P. S. P. (Eds.), *Handbook of pattern recognition and computer vision* (pp. 207–248). World Scientific Publishing.

Tunstall, M. J., Oorschot, D. E., Kean, A., & Wickens, J. R. (2002). Inhibitory interactions between spiny projection neurons in the rat striatum. *Journal of Neurophysiology, 88*, 1263–1269.

Turbell, H. (2001). *Cone Beam Reconstruction using filtered Backprojection.* Doctoral dissertation, University of Linköping, Sweden.

Tuy, H. K. (1983). An Inversion Formula for Cone-Beam Reconstruction. *SIAM Journal on Applied Mathematics, 43*, 546–552. doi:10.1137/0143035

Udupa, J. K., & Saha, P. K. (2003). Fuzzy connectedness and image segmentation. *Proceedings of the IEEE, 91*(10), 1649–1669. doi:10.1109/JPROC.2003.817883

Uma, K., Ramakrishnan, K., & Ananthakrishna, G. (1996). Image analysis using multifractals. *ICASSP, 4*, 2188–2190.

Unidad de Neuroprótesis y Rehabilitacin Visual. (2008). Universidade Miguel Hernandez. Retrieved from http:// naranja.umh.es/ lab

Unser, M. (1995). Texture classification and segmentation using wavelet frames. *IEEE Transactions on Image Processing, 4*(11), 1549–1560. doi:10.1109/83.469936

Usevitch, B. (1996). Optimal Bit Allocation for Biorthogonal Wavelet Coding. In *IEEE Data Compression Conference.*

Ushizima Sabino, D. M., Da Fontoura Costa, L., Gil Rizzati, E., & Zago, M. A. (2004). A texture approach to leukocyte recognition. *Real-time imaging, 10*, 205-216.

Usunoff, K. G., Itzev, D. E., Ovtscharoff, W. A., & Marani, E. (2002). Neuromelanin in the Human Brain: A review and atlas of pigmented cells in the substantia nigra. *Archives of Physiology and Biochemistry, 110*, 257–369. doi:10.1076/apab.110.4.257.11827

Vannier, M. W., Butterfield, R. L., Jordan, S., Murphy, W. A., Levitt, R. G., & Gado, M. (1988). Multispectral analysis of magnetic resonance images. *Radiology, 154*, 221–224.

Véhel, J. L. (1997). *Introduction to the multifractal analysis of images.* Fractal Image Encoding and Analysis.

Vese, L. A., & Chan, T. (2002). A multiphase level set framework for image segmentation using the Mumford and Shah model. *International Journal of Computer Vision, 50*, 271–293. doi:10.1023/A:1020874308076

Vincent, L., & Soille, P. (1991a). Watersheds in digital spaces: an efficient algorithm based on immersion simulations. *IEEE Transactions on Pattern Analysis and Machine Intelligence, 13*(6), 583–598. doi:10.1109/34.87344

Vincent, L., & Soille, P. (1991b). Watersheds in digital spaces: An efficient algorithm based on immersion simulations. *IEEE Transactions on Pattern Analysis and Machine Intelligence, 13*(6), 583–598. doi:10.1109/34.87344

Vitek, J. (2002). Mechanisms of Deep Brain Stimulation: Excitation or Inhibition. *Movement Disorders, 17*, S69–S72. doi:10.1002/mds.10144

Von Economo, C. J. (1917). Neue Beitrage zur Encephalitis lethargica. *Neurologisches Zentralblatt, 36*(21), 866–878.

Von Economo, C. J. (1918). Wilsons Krankheit und das "Syndrome du corpse strie". *Zentralblatt für die gesamte. Neurologie et Psychiatrie*, *44*, 173–209.

Wang, Z., Zheng, W., Wang, Y., Ford, J., Makedon, F., & Pearlman, J. D. (2006). Neighboring Feature Clustering. In *Advances in Artificial Intelligence* (*Vol. 3955*, pp. 605–608). Springer Berlin / Heidelberg. doi:10.1007/11752912_79

Wang, L., & He, D. C. (1990). Texture classification using texture spectrum. *Pattern Recognition*, *23*(8), 905–910. doi:10.1016/0031-3203(90)90135-8

Wanous, K. (2008). *Main Page - Debian Clusters*. Obtido em 14 de 06 de 2008, de Debian Clusters for Education and Research: The Missing Manual: http://debianclusters.cs.uni.edu/index.php/Main_Page

Warren Burhenne, L., Wood, S., D'Orsi, C., Feig, S., Kopans, D., & O'Shaugnessy, K. (2000). The Potential Contribution of Computer Aided Detection to the Sensitivity of Screening Mammography. *Radiology*, *215*, 554–562.

Webster, M. (2004). *Merriam-Webster's collegiate dictionary*. USA: NY.

Weldon, T. P., Higgins, W. E., & Dunn, D. F. (1996). Efficient Gabor filter design for texture segmentation. *Pattern Recognition*, *29*(12), 2005–2015. doi:10.1016/S0031-3203(96)00047-7

Wen, C., & Acharya, R. (1996). Fractal Analysis of Self-Similar Textures Using a Fourier-Domain Maximum Likelihood Estimation Method. *International Conference on Image Processing*. Lausanne, Switzerland.

Wen, C., & Acharya, R. (1996). Self-Similar Texture Charcaterization Using Wigner-Ville Distribution. *International Conference on Image Processing*. Lausanne, Switzerland.

Westin, C. F., Abhir, B., Knutsson, H., & Kikinis, R. (1997). Using local 3D structure for segmentation of bone from computer tomography images. In *Proceedings of IEEE computer society conference on computer vision and pattern recognition*. San Juan, Puerto Rico: IEEE.

Weszka, J. S., & Rosenfeld, A. (1978). Threshold evaluation techniques. *IEEE Transactions on Systems, Man, and Cybernetics*, *SMC-8*, 627–629.

Weszka, J. S., Dyer, C. R., & Rosenfeld, A. (1976). A comparative study of texture measures for terrain classification. *IEEE Transactions on Systems, Man, and Cybernetics*, *6*(4), 269–285.

Wichmann, T., & DeLong, M. R. (1996). Functional and pathophysiological models of the basal ganglia. *Current Opinion in Neurobiology*, *6*, 751–758. doi:10.1016/S0959-4388(96)80024-9

Wigmore, M. A., & Lacey, M. G. (2000). A Kv3-like persistent, outwardly rectifying, Cs^+-permeable, K^+ current in rat subthalamic nucleus neurones. *The Journal of Physiology*, *527*, 493–506. doi:10.1111/j.1469-7793.2000.t01-1-00493.x

Williams, D., & Shah, M. (1992). A Fast algorithm for active contours and curvature estimation. *CVGIP: Image Understanding*, *55*(1), 14–26. doi:10.1016/1049-9660(92)90003-L

Wilson, R. G., & Spann, M. (1988). Finite prolate spheroidal sequences and their applications: Image feature description and segmentation. *IEEE Transactions on Pattern Analysis and Machine Intelligence*, *10*(2), 193–203. doi:10.1109/34.3882

Wilson, T. (1989). Three-dimensional imaging in confocal systems. *Journal of Microscopy*, *153*(Pt 2), 161–169.

Winkler, G. (1995). *Image analysis, random fields and dynamic Monte Carlo methods*. Berlin, Germany: Springer.

Withey, D. J., & Koles, Z. J. (2007). *Medical Image Segmentation: Methods and Software*. Paper presented at the Joint Meeting of the 6th International Symposium on Noninvasive Functional Source Imaging of the Brain and Heart and the International Conference on Functional Biomedical Imaging, 2007. NFSI-ICFBI 2007.

Wu, K.-L., & Yang, M.-S. (2002). Alternative c-means clustering algorithms. *Pattern Recognition*, *35*(10), 2267–2278. doi:10.1016/S0031-3203(01)00197-2

Wu, Y., Levy, R., Ashby, P., Tasker, R., & Dostrovsky, J. (2001). Does Stimulation of the GPi Control Dyskinesia by Activating Inhibitory Axons? *Movement Disorders*, *16*, 208–216. doi:10.1002/mds.1046

Xilink. (1995). Xilinx - The Programmable Logic Data Book.

Xu, K., Bastia, E., & Schwarzschild, M. (2005). Therapeutic potential of adenosine A2A receptor antagonists in Parkinson's disease. *Pharmacology & Therapeutics*, *105*(3), 267–310. doi:10.1016/j.pharmthera.2004.10.007

Xu, F., & Mueller, K. (2005). Accelerating Popular Tomographic Reconstruction Algorithms on Commodity PC Graphics Hardware. *IEEE Transactions on Nuclear Science*, *52*(3), 654–663. doi:10.1109/TNS.2005.851398

Xu, D., & Wang, Y. (2006). Automated Emboli Detection from Doppler Ultrasound Signals Using the GDFM and STFT. *Ultrasound in Medicine & Biology*, *32*(5Suppl 1), 100. doi:10.1016/j.ultrasmedbio.2006.02.367

Xu, D., & Wang, Y. (2007). An Automated Feature Extraction and Emboli Detection System Based on the PCA and Fuzzy Sets. *Computers in Biology and Medicine*, *37*(6). doi:10.1016/j.compbiomed.2006.09.002

Xue, X., Cheryauka, A., & Tubbs, D. (2006). Acceleration of Fluoro-CT Reconstruction for a Mobile C-Arm on GPU and FPGA Hardware: A Simulation Study. *SPIE Medical Imaging Proceedings*, *6142*, 494–1501.

Yachida, M., Ikeda, M., & Tsuji, S. (1980). Plan-Guided Analysis of Cineangiograms for Measurement of Dynamic Behavior of Heart Wall. *Ieee Trans. Pattern Analy. And Mach. Intellig*, *2*(6), 537–542.

Yalamanchili, S. (1998). *VHDL Starter's Guide.* Prentice Hall, ISBN 0-13-519802-X.

Yang, J., & Duncan, J. (2003). 3D Image Segmentation of Deformable Objects with Shape-Appearance Joint Prior Models. In *Medical Image Computing and Computer-Assisted Intervention* (pp. 573–580). MICCAI. doi:10.1007/978-3-540-39899-8_71

Yeo, C. S., Buyya, R., Pourreza, H., Eskicioglu, R., Graham, P., & Sommers, F. (2006). Cluster Computing: High-Performance, High-Availability, and High-Throughput Processing on a Network of Computers. In Zomaya, A. Y. (Ed.), *Handbook of Nature-Inspired and Innovative Computing: Integrating Classical Models with Emerging Technologies* (pp. 521–551). doi:10.1007/0-387-27705-6_16

Yifei, Z., Shuang, W., Ge, Y., & Daling, W. (2007). *A Hybrid Image Segmentation Approach Using Watershed Transform and FCM.* Paper presented at the Fuzzy Systems and Knowledge Discovery, 2007. FSKD 2007. Fourth International Conference on.

Ying, L. (1995). *Document image binarization based on texture analysis*. State University of New York at Buffalo.

Yu, R., Ning, R., & Chen, B. (2001). High-Speed Cone-Beam Reconstruction on PC. *SPIE Medical Imaging Proceedings*, *4322*, 964–973.

Yu, O., Mauss, Y., Namer, I. J., & Chambron, J. (2001). Existence of contralateral abnormalities revealed by texture analysis in unilateral intractable hippocampal epilepsy. *Magnetic Resonance Imaging*, *19*(10), 1305–1310. doi:10.1016/S0730-725X(01)00464-7

Yu, O., Roch, C., Namer, I. J., Chambron, J., & Mauss, Y. (2002). Detection of late epilepsy by the texture analysis of MR brain images in the lithium-pilocarpine rat model. *Magnetic Resonance Imaging*, *20*(10), 771–775. doi:10.1016/S0730-725X(02)00621-5

Zavaljevski, A., Dhawan, A. P., Gaskil, M., Ball, W., & Johnson, J. D. (2000). Multi-level adaptative segmentation of multi-parameter MR brain images. *Computerized Medical Imaging and Graphics*, *24*(2), 87–98. doi:10.1016/S0895-6111(99)00042-7

Zeng, X., Staib, L. H., Schultz, R. T., & Duncan, J. S. (1999). Segmentation and measurement of the cortex from 3D MR images using coupled-surfaces propagation. *IEEE Transactions on Medical Imaging*, *18*(10), 927–937. doi:10.1109/42.811276

Zhan, Y., & Shen, D. (2003). Automated segmentation of 3D US prostate images using statistical texture-based matching method. In *Medical image computing and computer-assisted intervention* (pp. 688–696). Canada: MICCAI. doi:10.1007/978-3-540-39899-8_84

Zhang, Y., Brady, M., & Smith, S. (2001). Segmentation of brain MR images through a hidden Markov random field model and the expectation-maximisation algorithm. *IEEE Transactions on Medical Imaging*, *20*(1), 45–57. doi:10.1109/42.906424

Zhang, Y., Zhang, H., & Zhang, N. (2005). Microembolic Signal Characterization Using Adaptive Chirplet Expansion. *IEEE Transactions on Ultrasonics, Ferroelectrics, and Frequency Control*, *52*(8), 1291–1299. doi:10.1109/TUFFC.2005.1509787

Zhang, P. M., Wu, J. Y., Zhou, Y., Liang, P. J., & Yuan, J. Q. (2004). Spike sorting based on automatic template reconstruction with a partial solution to the overlapping problem. *Journal of Neuroscience Methods*, *135*(1-2), 55–65. doi:10.1016/j.jneumeth.2003.12.001

Zhong, S., & Mallat, S. (1992). Characterization of signals from multiscale edges. *IEEE Transactions on Pattern Analysis and Machine Intelligence*, *14*(7), 710–732. doi:10.1109/34.142909

Zhu, S., & Yuille, A. (1996). Region competition: unifying snakes, region growing, and bayes/MDL for multiband image segmentation. *IEEE Transactions on Pattern Analysis and Machine Intelligence*, *18*, 884–900. doi:10.1109/34.537343

Zhu, Z., Bartol, M., Shen, K., & Johnson, S. W. (2002). Excitatory effects of dopamine on subthalamic nucleus neurons: in vitro study of rats pretreated with 6-hydroxydopamine and levodopa. *Brain Research*, *945*, 31–40. doi:10.1016/S0006-8993(02)02543-X

Zorin, D., Schröder, P., & Sweldens, W. (1997). Interactive multiresolution mesh editing. In [Annual Conference Series]. *Computer Graphics*, *31*, 259–268.

Zouridakis, G., & Tam, D. C. (2000). Identification of reliable spike templates in multi-unit extracellular recordings using fuzzy clustering. *Computer Methods and Programs in Biomedicine*, *61*(2), 91–98. doi:10.1016/S0169-2607(99)00032-2

Zrinzo, L., Zrinzo, L. V., & Hariz, M. (2007). The pedunculopontine and peripeduncular nuclei: a tale of two structures. *Brain*, *130*, E73. doi:10.1093/brain/awm079

Zucker, S. W., & Hummel, R. A. (1981). A three-dimensional edge operator. *IEEE Transactions on Pattern Analysis and Machine Intelligence*, *3*(3), 324–331. doi:10.1109/TPAMI.1981.4767105

Zuilen, E. V., Gijn, J. V., & Ackerstaff, R. G. (1998). The Clinical Relevance of Cerebral Microemboli Detection by Transcranial Doppler Ultrasound. *Journal of Neuroimaging*, *8*(1), 32–36.

About the Contributors

Manuela Pereira received the 5-year B.S. degree in Mathetmatics and Computer Science in 1994 and the M. Sc. degree in Computational Mathematics in 1999, both from the University of Minho, Portugal. She received the Ph. D. degree in Signal and Image Processing in 2004 from the University of Nice Sophia Antipolis, France. She is an Assistant Professor at the Department of Computer Science of the University of Beira Interior, Portugal. Her main research interests include: multiple description coding, joint source/channel coding, image and video coding, wavelet analysis, information theory, image segmentation and real-time video streaming.

Mário M. Freire received the 5-year B.S. degree in Electrical Engineering and the M. Sc. degree in Systems and Automation in 1992 and 1994, respectively, from the University of Coimbra, Portugal. He received the Ph. D. degree in electrical engineering and the aggregated title in computer science in 2000 and 2007, respectively, both from the University of Beira Interior, Portugal. He is an Associate Professor of Computer Science at the University of Beira Interior. Presently, he is head of the Department of Computer Science of University of Beira Interior. He was the co-editor of 3 books in the LNCS book series of Springer, co-editor of 3 proceedings in IEEE Computer Society Press, and has authored or co-authored 4 interatinonal patents and around 100 papers in international refereed journals and conferences. His main research interests include: medical image processing, telemedicine, high-performance networking, network security, and peer-to-peer networks.

* * *

José Fernandes received his B.Sc. and Ph.D. degrees from the University of Aveiro, Portugal, both in Electrical Engineering, in 1990 and 1997, respectively. He joined the Department of Electrical Engineering of the same University, where he became an assistant professor in 1997. Since September 2000 to August 2003 he was with the European Commission, DG Information Society, in Belgium, where he worked in the field of Mobile and Personal Communications. From September 2003 until March 2005 he served UMIC (Innovation and Knowledge Society Unit) as an adviser to the Director. From September 2003 until January 2007 he was also with FCCN (Foundation for National Scientific Computing) as member of board of Directors, both in Lisbon, Portugal. He joined Microsoft Portugal on February 1st, 2007, as Director of Dept of development support and relations with academia.

Przemyslaw Lenkiewicz has received his BSc degree in Computer Science from the Technical University of Bialystok in Poland, where he has lived and studied for a bigger part of his life. After that he has taken an opportunity to study at the University of Beira Interior in Portugal, where he was later offered a chance to participate in several research projects and finally to pursue his PhD. During 2005/2006 he has worked with optical networks at Siemens Research and Development in Amadora, Portugal and since February 2007 he carries out his PhD work at Microsoft Portugal. His main research interests include medical image processing and high performance computing. He is an author of several documents at international conferences and journals as well as a co-author of an international patent.

S. Jehan-Besson received the engineering degree from École Centrale de Nantes in 1996 and the M.Sc. and PhD degrees in computer vision and image processing from the University of Nice-Sophia Antipolis. She was an associate professor of image processing from 2003 until 2008 at ENSICAEN, France. She is currently a CNRS research scientist working in the Laboratory LIMOS, University of Clermont-Ferrand, France. Her research interests include shape optimization tools for segmentation, statistical region descriptors and significance tests, region-based active contours and medical image analysis.

F. Lecellier received the Engineering degree in computer science from ENSICAEN, France in 2005 and the Master's degree in computer science from the University of Caen, France, in 2005. He is currently Ph.D. student in computer science and image processing at University of Caen, France, since 2005. His research interests include region-based active contours, segmentation of texture, segmentation with shape prior and segmentation of echocardiographic images.

Jalal M. Fadili graduated from the Ecole Nationale Supérieure d'Ingénieurs (ENSI) de Caen, Caen, France, and received the M.Sc. and Ph.D. degrees in signal and image processing from the University of Caen. He was a Research Associate with the University of Cambridge (MacDonnel-Pew Fellow), Cambridge, UK, from 1999 to 2000. He has been an Associate Professor of signal and image processing since September 2001 at ENSI. He was a Visitor at the Queensland University of Technology, Brisbane, Australia, and Stanford University, Stanford, CA, in 2006. His research interests include statistical approaches in signal and image processing, inverse problems in image processing, multiscale methods, and sparse representations in signal and image processing. Areas of application include medical and astronomical imaging.

Guillaume Née received the Master's degree in computer science from the University of Caen, France, in 2006. He is currently Ph.D. student in computer science and image processing at University of Caen, France, since 2006. His research interests include region-based active contour models, significance tests, and analysis of p-MRI sequences.

Gilles Aubert received his These d'Etat es-Sciences Mathematiques from the University of Paris 6, France, in 1986. He is currently professor of mathematics at the University of Nice Sophia Antipolis and member of the J.A. Dieudonné Laboratory at Nice, France. His research interests are nonlinear partial differential equations, calculus of variations. Fields of application include image processing and, in particular, restoration, segmentation, decomposition models, and optical flow.

Ciska Heida (1972), assistant professor at the Faculty of Electrical Engineering, Mathematics & Computer Science and the Institute for BioMedical Technology (BMTI) of the University of Twente, the Netherlands. She received the MSc. and PhD. degrees in electrical engineering in 1997 and 2002, respectively, both at the BSS-group (Biomedical Signals & Systems) on 'Dielectrophoretic trapping of neuronal cells'. Currently, her primary research interests focus on the theoretical, experimental and clinical aspects of deep brain stimulation (DBS) in Parkinson's disease patients. Research activities include modeling basal ganglia functioning in motor control, developing volume conduction model and neuron models in order to estimate the volume of activation resulting from electrical stimulation, and movement registrations of Parkinson's patients to observe the effectiveness of stimulation and/or medication.

Enrico Marani (1946) was trained as a neuroanatomist at Leiden University where he received his PhD in 1982 on the structure and function of the cerebellum. In 1986 he became head of the Neuroregulation group at the Leiden University Medical Center. From 1990 onwards he studied regeneration of the central nervous system. Applications from 1996 onwards are: the artificial biodegradable nerve for implantation in destructed peripheral nerves and the study of neuronal networks on a chip (in co-operation with the University of Twente). He has published more than 130 international papers and is editor of Archives of Physiology and Biochemistry, Advances in Anatomy, Embryology and Cell Biology, co-editor of Bio Medical Reviews and was or is board member of several international journals. His current research interests focus on the application of Neurotechnology in Medicine.

Rachel Moroney (1974) began her undergraduate studies in the University of Limerick, Ireland. Graduating with first class honours in Computer Engineering, she received a medal for best overall results in the faculty of Informatics & Electronics. After having worked for 6 years as a software engineer in the telecommunications and consumer electronics industries in Ireland, Belgium and the USA, and a sabbatical during which she travelled through Latin America and Africa, she moved to the Netherlands to pursue a Masters in Electrical Engineering with biomedical specialisation at the University of Twente, Enschede. Her research interests include the modelling of Parkinson's disease and Deep Brain Stimulation. Rachel is currently based in Rotterdam, the Netherlands where she works as a software engineer.

Olivier Bockenbach received his Engineer degree in computer science from the Institut National des Sciences Appliquées (Lyon, France) in 1985. He specialized in real time operating systems as well as multi processor architectures. In 1996, he joined the Marben company. As a consultant, he designed dedicated multi processor architectures for major defense programs such as the Radar for the Rafale aircraft. In 1997, he joined Mercury Computer Systems to design complex real time systems destined at Digital Radiography and Computed Tomography. He became an expert in implementing high performance algorithms on FPGAs, Multi Core architectures and GPUs.

Michael Knaup was born in 1969 in Nürnberg, Germany. In 1990 he began to study physics at the Friedrich-Alexander University Erlangen-Nürnberg with a focus on theoretical plasma physics. He received his Ph.D. in 2002 at the Institute of Theoretical Physics II under the guidance of Prof. Dr. Christian Toepffer. In 2003 he joined the Institute of Medical Physics (IMP) of the Friedrich-Alexander University Erlangen-Nürnberg. The main focus of his work is cardiac imaging, image reconstruction of cone-beam CT data and iterative image reconstruction. In particular, he developed high-performance implementations of various CT image reconstruction algorithms on dedicated hardware like the Cell Broadband Engine (CBE) and Graphics Processing Units (GPUs).

Sven Steckmann received his diploma in Electrical Engineering at the Georg-Simon Ohm University of Applied Sciences (Nuremberg, Germany) in 2006. The title of his diploma thesis was "Cone-beam CT image reconstruction using distributed computing." In 2006 Sven Steckmann joined the Ph.D. program at the Institute of Medical Physics, University of Erlangen-Nürnberg where works on "High performance reconstruction in spiral Computed Tomography using manycore architectures."

Marc Kachelrieß was born in 1969 in Nürnberg, Germany. In 1989 he began to study physics with a focus on theoretical particle physics. He received his Ph.D. in 1998 at the Institute of Medical Physics (IMP) under the guidance of Prof. Willi A. Kalender. Since then, he focuses on cardiac imaging, image reconstruction of cone-beam CT data, iterative image reconstruction, methods to reduce CT artifacts, patient dose reduction techniques and automatic exposure control (AEC) for CT. His work also includes the design and development of micro-CT scanner hard- and software, micro-CT pre- and postprocessing software and image quality optimization techniques. Since 2005 Marc Kachelrieß is appointed W2-Professor of Medical Imaging at the Friedrich-Alexander University Erlangen-Nürnberg. On the basis of his university teaching position he lectures in medical imaging technology, physics and algorithms.

Frédéric Payan received his PhD degree in 2004 from the University of Nice-Sophia Antipolis. His topic was "Rate Distortion Optimization for Geometry Compression of Triangular Meshes." Then, he did a postdoctoral stage at LMC-IMAG (Laboratoire de Modélisation et de Calcul, Institut des Mathématiques Appliquées de Grenoble). During this year, his work concerned the spatiotemporal analysis of dynamic meshes. He is currently Associate Professor at the Technical Institue of Nice-Côte d'Azur (University of Nice-Sophia Antipolis). Member of the project CReATIVe (IMAGES, I3S Laboratory), his current interests include multiresolution analysis, processing and compression of static meshes and 3D animations. He is author of 1 book chapter, 3 international journals (Elsevier Computer Aided Geometric Design 2005, IEEE Transactions on Visualization and Computer Graphics 2006, and Elsevier Computer & Graphics 2007), and 15 international conferences.

Marc Antonini received the Ph. D degree in electrical engineering from the University of Nice-Sophia Antipolis (France) in 1991. He joined the CNRS in 1993 at the I3S laboratory (University of Nice-Sophia Antipolis). He is Research Director (CNRS) since 2004. Since January 2008, he is also scientific director of the CReATIVe project, head of the IMAGES research group and co-director of the <<Signal, Images, Systems>> (SIS) department of the I3S laboratory. His main research interest is compression for image, video, mesh and 3D animation. Member IEEE, he is the author of 170 publications between 1998 and 2008 including 6 book chapters, 1 paper in the CNRS journal, 22 publications in refereed journals, 124 conference papers, 10 invited conference papers. He is co-inventor of 7 international patents.

Filipe Soares received the 5-year B.S. degree in Computer Science and Engineering in 2006 from University of Beira Interior, Portugal. He was awarded with a merit scholarship for having the best final classification for this degree. Currently, he is working as a researcher at Top+ Innovation & Excellence department of Siemens S.A. Healthcare Sector, Portugal. His main research interests include: breast cancer, medical imaging processing, multifractal and wavelet analysis, computer-aided diagnoses, pattern recognition, artificial intelligence, computer security, computer networks, and bioinformatics.

Filepe Janela received the 5-year B.S. degree in Chemical Engineering in 2004 from the Instituto Superior Técnico, Portugal. He worked in the Oil & Energy Sector at Norsk Hydro Company (Norway), as process engineer with special focus in dynamic process simulation. Currently, he is the Manager for Innovation & Excellence in Siemens S.A. Healthcare Sector, Portugal, being responsible for the development of R&D activities, Innovation projects, and the establishment of relations with scientific and technological institutions (Universities and R&D centers).

João Seabra received the 5-year B.S. in Electronics and Computer Science Engineering in 1997 at Faculty of Engineering of University of Porto, Specialization in Instrumentation, Control and Computer Science. He is the General Manager of Siemens S.A. Healthcare Sector, Portugal.

Constantino Carlos Reyes-Aldasoro (BS Mechanical and Electrical Engineering UNAM, MSc Communications and Signal Processing Imperial College of Science Technology and Medicine, PhD Computer Science Warwick University) is a Research Fellow at the University of Sheffield. Between 1995 and 2000 he worked as a Lecturer in Mexico at ITESM and ITAM. From 2001 until 2004 he was as a Graduate Teaching Assistant at Warwick and in 2005 he joined the Tumour Microcirculation Group at School of Medicine, Sheffield University. His main interest is the application of image analysis in biomedical areas, in particular tumor vasculature microcirculation: tissue texture characterization, tracking and modeling of cells, vascular segmentation and permeability estimation. He was co-chair of the Angiogenesis Network Conference Angionet 2007. He has published 35 publications, of which 15 are refereed journal articles, and 3 have received best publication awards.

Abhir Bhalerao is an Associate Professor in Computer Science, University of Warwick. He joined as staff in 1998 having completed 5 years as a post-doctoral research scientist with the NHS and Kings Medical School, London including two years as a Research Fellow at Harvard Medical School Boston. His research was focused on applications of image analysis and computer vision techniques to computer aided radiology, data visualization for surgical planning. At Warwick, Dr Bhalerao has been principal and co-investigator on two EPSRC sponsored projects related to multi-resolution segmentation and modeling of vasculature from MR and use of stochastic methods for statistical image modeling. His current interests are in modeling flow in 3D X-ray imagery, characterization of the morphology of folding structures in MRI, real-time visualization of tensor data and light-estimation methods from multi-camera scenes. He has published over 50 refereed articles in image analysis, medical imaging, graphics and computer vision. He was the general co-chair and local organizer of the British Machine Vision Conference, 2007.

Ana Leiria received the Lic. Eng. Degree in Decision Systems from COCITE, Portugal, in 1993, and the PhD in Electronic Eng. & Computer Science, Signal Processing, from the University of Algarve, Portugal, in 2005. From 1991 to 1993 she worked in data analysis in TLP, SA. She worked as Assistant Lecturer from 1993-1998 and as a Lecturer from 1998 to Jan 2005, and presently as assistant professor in the Electronic Engineering and Computing Department of the University of Algarve. Her research interests are biomedical digital signal processing, particularly on modelling and characterization of blood flow signals, and telemedicine.

Maria Margarida Madeira e Moura received the Lic. Eng. Degree in Computer Science from COCITE, Lisbon, Portugal, in 1993 and the PhD in Electronic Eng. & Computer Science from the University of Algarve, Faro, Portugal, in 2004. Since 1989, before joining the University of Algarve, she worked in industrial automation and in software development and consultancy. Since 1993 she works in the Electronic Engineering and Computing Department of the University of Algarve, Portugal, teaching and researching. She is currently assistant professor, her main research interests being high-performance applications and digital signal processing of biomedical signals.

Pedro Tomás received his five-year degree and MSc in electrical and computer engineering from the Instituto Superior Técnico (IST), Technical University of Lisbon, Portugal, in 2003 and 2006, respectively. Currently, he is pursuing his Ph.D. degree in electrical engineering at IST and is developing his work with the Signal Processing Systems Group (SIPS) at Instituto de Engenhario de Sistemas e Computadores—R&D (INESC-ID). His research activities include statistical signal processing, modeling of physiological systems and algorithms for estimation and classification. He is also interested in general signal processing and in computer architectures, parallel and distributed computing.

Aleksandar Ilic received his five-year degree and M.Sc. in Electrical and Computer Engineering from Faculty of Electrical Engineering, University of Nis, Serbia, in 2007. He is currently pursuing his Ph.D. studies at Instituto Superior Técnico, Technical University of Lisbon, and doing research at the Signal Processing Systems Group (SiPS) of Instituto de Engenhario he Sistemas e Computadores R&D (INESC-ID), Portugal. His research interests include parallel and distributed computing, task scheduling and heterogeneous computer architectures.

Leonel Augusto Sousa received the PhD degree in Electrical and Computer Engineering from the Instituto Superior Técnico (IST), Technical University of Lisbon (Portugal), in 1996. He is currently an associate professor of the Electrical and Computer Engineering Department at IST, and a Senior Researcher at INESC-ID. His research interests include computer architectures, parallel and distributed computing, and multimedia and biomedical systems. He has contributed more than 150 papers to international journals and conferences and he is a member of HiPEAC European Network of Excellence. He is a senior member of IEEE and a member of ACM.

Thomas Kilindris received his Electrical Engineering Diploma in 1991 from the Aristotelian University of Thessaloniki. He is occupied at the Laboratory of Medical Phyhsics and Informatics at the Medical School of the University of Thessaly, Hellas. His research interests include biomedical image and signal processing, parallel processing methods for dose calculation and design and optimization of treatment planning systems for stereotactic radiotherapy. He is the co-author of "PARALLEL EIKONA: a parallel digital image processing package" (John Wiley & Sons, Inc., 1993).

Kiki Theodorou received her Bachelor degree in Physics in 1994, a Masters degree in Medical Physics in 1996 and her PhD in Medical Physics in 1999. She is an Assistant Professor in the Medical School at the University of Thessaly, in Medical Physics and Medical Informatics. Her main research interests are focused on Medical Imaging, Medical Image Processing, High Field Magnetic Resonance Imaging, Stereotactic Radiotherapy and Monte Carlo Simulations in Radiation Dosimetry.

Xiu Ying Wang received her Ph.D in Computer Science from The University, of Sydney in 2005. Currently she is working in the School of Information Technologies, The University of Sydney. She is a member of IFAC and executive secretary of IFAC TC on BioMed. Her research interests include image registration for applications in biomedicine and multimedia, and computer graphics.

Dagan Feng received his ME in Electrical Engineering & Computing Science (EECS) from Shanghai Jiao Tong University in 1982, MSc and Ph.D in Computer Science / Biocybernetics from the University of California, Los Angeles (UCLA) in 1985 and 1988 respectively. He joined the University of Sydney at the end of 1988, as Lecturer, Senior Lecturer, Reader, Professor and Head of Department of Computer Science / School of Information Technologies. He is currently Associate Dean of Faculty of Science at the University of Sydney, Chair-Professor of Information Technology, Hong Kong Polytechnic University and Advisory or Guest Professor at several universities in China. His research area is Biomedical & Multimedia Information Technology (BMIT). He is the Founder and Director the BMIT Research Group. He has published over 500 scholarly research papers, pioneered several new research directions, and received the Crump Prize for Excellence in Medical Engineering from UCLA. He is a Fellow of Australian Academy of Technological Sciences and Engineering, ACS, HKIE, IET, and IEEE, Special Area Editor of IEEE Transactions on Information Technology in Biomedicine, and is the current Chairman of International Federation of Automatic Control (IFAC) Technical Committee on Biological and Medical Systems.

Index

D

E

F

G

H

I

K

L

M

N

O

P

Q

R

S

T

V

W

X

Breinigsville, PA USA
28 October 2010
248290BV00005B/6/P